CLINICAL CHEMISTRY & METABOLIC MEDICINE

Seventh edition

Martin A. Crook BSc MB BS PhD FRCPath FRCPI FRCP

Consultant Chemical Pathologist and Lipidologist
Guy's Hospital, St Thomas Hospital and University Hospital Lewisham, London, UK

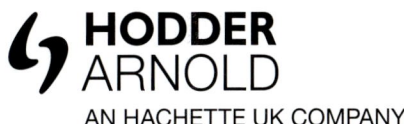

First published in Great Britain in 1971 by Lloyd-Luke (Medical Books) Ltd; reprinted in 1971, 1973.
Second edition 1975; reprinted 1978.
Third edition 1979; reprinted 1981, 1982, 1983.
Fourth edition 1984; reprinted 1985, 1987.
Fifth edition published in 1988 by Edward Arnold (Publishers) Ltd; reprinted 1989, 1990, 1991, 1992.
Sixth edition 1994; reprinted 1996, 1998, 2000, 2001, 2002, 2005.
This seventh edition published in 2006 by Hodder Arnold, an imprint of Hodder Education, an Hachette UK Company,
338 Euston Road, London, NW1 3BH.

http://www.hoddereducation.com

© 2006 Edward Arnold (Publishers) Ltd

All rights reserved. Apart from any use permitted under UK copyright law, this publication may only be reproduced, stored or transmitted, in any form, or by any means with prior permission in writing of the publishers or in the case of reprographic production in accordance with the terms of licences issued by the Copyright Licensing Agency. In the United Kingdom such licences are issued by the Copyright Licensing Agency: Saffron House, 6-10 Kirby Street, London EC1N 8TS.

Whilst the advice and information in this book are believed to be true and accurate at the date of going to press, neither the author nor the publisher can accept any legal responsibility or liability for any errors or omissions that may be made. In particular (but without limiting the generality of the preceding disclaimer) every effort has been made to check drug dosages; however, it is still possible that errors have been missed. Furthermore, dosage schedules are constantly being revised and new side-effects recognized. For these reasons the reader is strongly urged to consult the drug companiesí printed instructions before administering any of the drugs recommended in this book and to check protocols of dynamic function testing and medical treatment with their hospital guidelines.

British Library Cataloguing in Publication Data
A catalogue record for this book is available from the British Library

Library of Congress Cataloging-in-Publication Data
A catalog record for this book is available from the Library of Congress

ISBN-10 [normal]   0 340 90616 2
ISBN-13 [normal]   978 0 340 90616 3
ISBN-10 [ISE]   0 340 90617 0 (International Students, Edition, restricted territorial availability)
ISBN-13 [ISE]   978 0 340 90617 0

4 5 6 7 8 9 10

Commissioning Editors: Georgina Bentliff
Project Editors: Heather Smith and Clare Weber
Production Controller: Lindsay Smith
Cover Designer: Nichola Smith
Indexer: Laurence Errington

Cover: © Clouds Hill Imaging Ltd./ CORBIS

Typeset in 11/13 pt AGaramond by Charon Tec Ltd, Chennai, India
www.charontec.com
Printed and bound in India.

What do you think about this book? Or any other Hodder Arnold title?
Please send your comments to www.hoddereducation.com

CONTENTS

Preface   v

1. Requesting laboratory tests and interpreting the results   1
2. Water and sodium   7
3. The kidneys   36
4. Acid–base disturbances   58
5. Potassium   82
6. Calcium, phosphate and magnesium   94
7. The hypothalamus and pituitary gland   115
8. The adrenal cortex   127
9. The reproductive system   144
10. Pregnancy and infertility   155
11. Thyroid function   162
12. Carbohydrate metabolism   174
13. Plasma lipids and lipoproteins   198
14. Nutrition   214
15. Vitamins, trace elements and metals   222
16. The gastrointestinal tract   233
17. Liver disorders and gallstones   250
18. Plasma enzymes in diagnosis (clinical enzymology)   268
19. Proteins in plasma and urine   280
20. Purine and urate metabolism   301
21. Disorders of haem metabolism: iron and the porphyrias   308
22. Cardiovascular disease   323
23. Cerebrospinal and pleural fluid   329
24. Metabolic effects of tumours   335
25. Therapeutic drug monitoring and poisoning   344
26. Clinical biochemistry at the extremes of age   355
27. Inborn errors of metabolism   368
28. Genetics and DNA-based technology in clinical biochemistry   380
29. Patient sample collection and use of the laboratory   387
30. Point of care testing   393

Appendix 1   Units in clinical chemistry   397
Appendix 2   Abbreviations used in the text   399

Index   403

PREFACE

Were it not for the textbook *Clinical Chemistry in Diagnosis and Treatment* by Joan Zilva and Peter Pannall, I would not be a chemical pathologist. As a medical student, I was so struck by its clarity, depth and clinical relevance that I decided that theirs was the medical field I wished to work in.

Over the years, the field of clinical chemistry has changed radically. Confusingly, there is no consensus agreement as to the name for this field of medicine, which is known variously as clinical chemistry, chemical pathology or clinical biochemistry, to name but a few. Additionally, the field now overlaps with that of metabolic medicine, a clinical specialty involved with the management and treatment of patients with disorders of metabolism. Clinical chemistry laboratories have become further automated, molecular biology technologies have entered the diagnostic arena, and chemical pathologists have become more clinically orientated towards running out-patient clinics for a variety of biochemical disturbances. This book aims to address these new changes. Indeed, it is difficult to imagine a branch of medicine that does not at some time require clinical chemistry tests, which may not be too surprising, given the fact that every body cell is composed of chemicals!

Unfortunately, there have been some difficulties in recent times, with a relative shortage of graduates entering the specialty, which has not been helped by some people's attitude that clinical chemistry is merely a laboratory factory churning out results that anyone can interpret. There are also concerns that medical student clinical chemistry teaching may become 'diluted' as part of an expanding curriculum. It is hoped that this book will excite a new generation to enter this fascinating and essential field as well as benefit patients as their doctors learn more about their biochemical and metabolic problems.

I am particularly grateful to Dr Wijeratne, Dr Garrib (particularly for molecular biology expertise) and Dr Eldridge for constructive criticism of the text. I am also grateful to Dr Mayne for his earlier contributions and the anonymous medical student reviewer(s) who commented on the text. Although every effort has been made to avoid inaccuracies and errors, it is inevitable that some may still be present, and feedback from readers is therefore welcome.

Martin Crook
London, May 2006

Disclaimer. The publishers and author accept no responsibility for errors in the text or misuse of the material presented. Drugs and their doses should be checked with a pharmacy and the investigation protocols with an appropriate clinical laboratory. Dynamic test protocols should be checked with an accredited clinical investigation unit and may require different instructions in the elderly, children and the obese.

1 REQUESTING LABORATORY TESTS AND INTERPRETING THE RESULTS

Requesting laboratory tests	1	Is the abnormality of diagnostic value?	4
How often should I investigate the patient?	1	Has there been a clinically significant change in the laboratory test?	4
When is a laboratory investigation 'urgent'?	2		
Interpreting results	2		

REQUESTING LABORATORY TESTS

There are many laboratory tests available to the clinician. Correctly used, these may provide useful information, but if used inappropriately, they are at best useless and at worst misleading and dangerous.

In general, laboratory investigations are used:

- to help diagnosis or, when indicated, to screen for metabolic disease,
- to monitor treatment or detect complications,
- occasionally for medico-legal reasons or, with due permission from the patient, for research.

Patient over-investigation may be harmful, causing the patient unnecessary discomfort or inconvenience, delaying treatment or using resources that might be more usefully spent on other aspects of patient care. Before requesting an investigation, clinicians should consider whether its result would influence their clinical management of the patient.

Close liaison with laboratory staff is essential; they may be able to help determine the best and quickest procedure for investigation, interpret results and discover reasons for anomalous findings.

HOW OFTEN SHOULD I INVESTIGATE THE PATIENT?

This depends on the following.

- How quickly numerically significant changes are likely to occur. For example, concentrations of the main plasma protein fractions are unlikely to change significantly in less than a week (see Chapter 19), and the plasma urea concentration will not change significantly during the first 12 hours of oliguria (see Chapter 3).
- Whether a change, even if numerically significant, will alter treatment. For example, plasma transaminase activities may alter within 24 hours in the course of acute hepatitis, but once the diagnosis has been made, this is unlikely to affect treatment (see Chapter 17). By contrast, plasma potassium concentrations may alter rapidly in patients given large doses of diuretics and these alterations *may* indicate the need to instigate or change treatment (see Chapter 5).

Laboratory investigations are very rarely needed more than once daily, except for some patients receiving intensive therapy. If they are, only those that are essential should be repeated.

WHEN IS A LABORATORY INVESTIGATION 'URGENT'?

The main reason for asking for an investigation to be performed 'urgently' is that an early answer will alter the patient's clinical management. This is rarely the case. Laboratory staff should be consulted when an urgent test is required. Point-of-care testing can shorten result turnaround time and is discussed in Chapter 30.

Laboratories usually have 'panic limits', when highly abnormal test results indicate a potentially life-threatening condition that necessitates contacting of the relevant medical staff immediately. To do so, laboratory staff must have accurate information about the location of the patient and the person to notify.

INTERPRETING RESULTS

When interpreting laboratory results, the clinician should ask the following questions.

- Is the result the correct one for the patient?
- Does the result fit with the clinical findings? Remember to treat the patient and not the 'laboratory numbers'.
- If it is the first time the test has been performed on this patient, is the result normal when the appropriate reference range is taken into account?
- If the result is abnormal, is the abnormality of diagnostic significance or is it a non-specific finding?
- If it is one of a series of results, has there been a change and, if so, is this change clinically significant?

Abnormal results, particularly if unexpected and indicating the need for clinical intervention, are best repeated.

Test reference ranges

By convention, a reference ('normal') range (or interval) usually includes 95 per cent of the test results obtained from a healthy and sometimes age-defined and sex-defined population. For the majority of tests, the individual's results for any constituent are distributed around this mean in a 'normal' (Gaussian) distribution, the 95 per cent limits being about two standard deviations from the mean. For other tests, the reference distribution may be skewed, either to the right or to the left, around the population median.

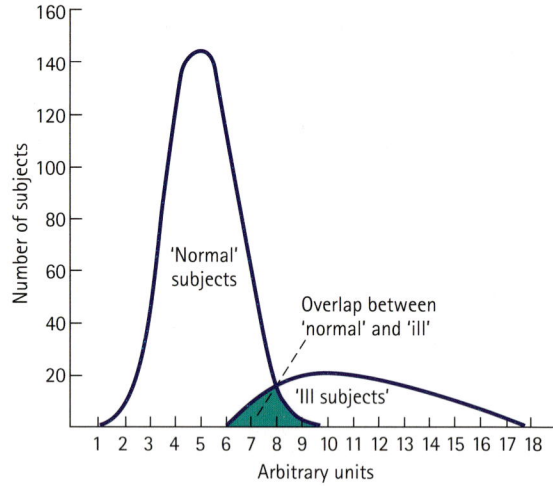

Fig. 1.1 Theoretical distribution of values for 'normal' and 'abnormal' subjects, showing overlap at the upper end of the reference range.

Remember that 2.5 per cent of the results at either end will be outside the reference range; such results are not necessarily abnormal for that individual. All that can be said with certainty is that the *probability* that a result is abnormal increases the further it is from the mean or median until, eventually, this probability approaches 100 per cent. Furthermore, a normal result does not necessarily exclude the disease that is being sought; a test result within the population reference range may be abnormal for that individual.

Very few biochemical tests clearly separate a 'normal' population from an 'abnormal' population. For most there is a range of values in which 'normal' and 'abnormal' overlap (Fig. 1.1), the extent of the overlap differing for individual tests. There is a 5 per cent chance that one result will fall outside the reference range and with 20 tests a 64 per cent chance, i.e. the more tests done, the more likely one will be statistically abnormal.

No result of any investigation should be interpreted without consulting the reference range issued by the laboratory carrying out the assay. Some analytes have risk limits for treatment, such as plasma glucose (see Chapter 12), or target or therapeutic limits, such as plasma cholesterol (see Chapter 13).

Various non-pathological factors may affect the results of investigations, the following being some of the more important ones.

Between-individual differences

Physiological factors such as the following affect the interpretation of results.

Age-related differences

These include, for example, plasma urea concentration (see Chapter 3), which tends to rise with age, especially in men, and plasma alkaline phosphatase, which is higher in children and the elderly (see Chapter 18).

Sex differences

Examples of sex differences include plasma urate, which is higher in males, and high-density lipoprotein cholesterol, which is higher in pre-menopausal women than in men (see Chapters 13 and 20). Obviously, sex-hormone concentrations also differ between the sexes (see Chapter 9).

Ethnic differences

These may occur because of either racial or environmental factors, for example plasma creatine kinase may be higher in Africans than in Caucasians (see Chapter 18).

Within-individual variations

There are biological variations of both plasma concentrations and urinary excretion rates of many constituents, and test results may be incorrectly interpreted if this is not taken into consideration. Biological variations may be regular or random.

Regular

Such changes occur throughout the 24-hour period (circadian or diurnal rhythms, like those of body temperature) or throughout the month.

The time of meals affects plasma glucose concentrations, and therefore correct interpretation is often only possible if the blood is taken when the patient is fasting or at a set time after a standard dose of glucose (see Chapter 12).

The daily (circadian) variation of plasma cortisol is of diagnostic value, but superimposed on this regular variation, 'stress' will cause an acute rise (see Chapter 8). Plasma iron concentrations may fall by 50 per cent between morning and evening (see Chapter 21). To eliminate the unwanted effect of circadian variations, blood should ideally always be taken at the same time of day, preferably in the early morning and, if indicated, with the patient fasting. This is not usually possible, and these variations should be taken into account when serial results are interpreted.

Some constituents vary monthly, especially in women. These variations can be very marked, as in the results of sex-hormone assays, for example plasma oestradiol, which can only be interpreted if the stage of the menstrual cycle is known; plasma iron may fall to very low concentrations just before the onset of menstruation. Other constituents may also vary seasonally. For example vitamin D concentrations may be highest in summer months. Some of these changes, such as the relation between plasma glucose and meals, have obvious causes, but some appear to be regulated by the so-called 'biological clock', which is often predominantly affected by the alternation of light and dark.

Random

Day-to-day variations, for example in plasma iron concentrations, can be very large and may swamp regular cycles. The causes of these are not clear, but they should be allowed for when serial results are interpreted – for example the effect of 'stress' on plasma cortisol concentrations.

Methodological differences between laboratories

It has been pointed out that, even if the same method is used throughout a particular laboratory, it is difficult to

---

CASE 1

A blood sample from a 4-year-old boy with abdominal pain was sent to the laboratory from an accident and emergency department. Some of the results were as follows.

Plasma
Bilirubin 14 μmol/L (<20)
Alanine transaminase 14 U/L (<42)
Alkaline phosphatase 326 U/L (<250)
Albumin 40 g/L (35–45)
Gamma-glutamyl transferase 14 U/L (<55)
'Corrected' calcium 2.34 mmol/L (2.15–2.55)

DISCUSSION
The patient's age was not given on the request form and the laboratory computer system 'automatically' used the reference ranges for adults. The plasma alkaline phosphatase concentration is raised if compared with the adult reference range, but in fact is within 'normal limits' for a child of 4 years (see also Chapters 6 and 18).

define normality clearly. Interpretation may sometimes be even more difficult if the results obtained in different laboratories, using different analytical methods, are compared. Agreement between laboratories is close for many constituents. However, for others, such as plasma enzymes, different methods may give different results. For various technical reasons, different laboratories may use different assay temperatures, and the results of tests on the same specimen at different temperatures will differ significantly, although apparently being expressed in the same units. Even if temperatures were standardized, the results would still vary unless the substrate, pH and all the other variables were the same.

IS THE ABNORMALITY OF DIAGNOSTIC VALUE?

Relation between plasma and cellular concentrations

Intracellular constituents are not easily sampled, and plasma concentrations do not always reflect the situation in the cells; this is particularly true for those constituents, such as potassium and phosphate, which are at much higher concentrations intracellularly than extracellularly. A normal, or even high, plasma potassium concentration may be associated with cellular depletion if equilibrium across cell membranes is abnormal, such as in diabetic ketoacidosis. Analyte concentrations may differ between plasma (the aqueous phase of anticoagulated blood produced when erythrocytes have been removed) and serum (the aqueous phase of clotted blood). The concentration of potassium, for example, is higher in serum than in plasma samples because of leakage from cells during clotting.

Non-specific abnormalities

The concentrations of all protein fractions, including immunoglobulins, and of protein-bound substances may fall by as much as 15 per cent after as little as 30 minutes' recumbency, possibly due to fluid redistribution in the body. This may account, at least in part, for the low plasma albumin concentrations found in even quite minor illnesses. In-patients often have blood taken early in the morning, while recumbent, and plasma concentrations of protein and protein-bound substances tend to be lower than in out-patients (see Chapter 19).

HAS THERE BEEN A CLINICALLY SIGNIFICANT CHANGE IN THE LABORATORY TEST?

Before one can interpret day-to-day changes in results and decide whether the patient's biochemical state has altered, one must know the degree of variation to be expected in the results derived from a normal population. We have already discussed intra-individual (same person) analyte variation. However, there is also unavoidable analytical variation.

CASE 2

A 54-year-old Nigerian male was seen in an accident and emergency department because of chest pain. His electrocardiogram (ECG) was normal. The following results were returned from the laboratory, 6 hours after his chest pain started.

Plasma
Creatine kinase 498 U/L (<250)
Troponin T 0.01 ng/L (<0.02)

DISCUSSION

The raised plasma creatine kinase concentration suggested an acute myocardial infarction (see also Chapters 18 and 22). The patient was, however, subsequently found not to have had a myocardial infarction (confirmed by a normal troponin T result) and the raised plasma creatine kinase concentration was thought to be due to his racial origin. (The reference range of <250 U/L was based on that of the predominantly Caucasian UK population; normal plasma creatine kinase concentrations may be two to three times higher in Africans than in Caucasians.)

Reproducibility of laboratory estimations

Most laboratory estimations should give results that are reproducible to well within 5 per cent; some, such as those for sodium and calcium, should be even more precise, but the variability of some hormone assays, for example, may be greater. Changes of less than the precision of the method are not likely to be clinically significant.

Precision or random changes describe the agreement between replicate assay measurements. This can be considered in terms of the within-assay precision, which is the assay variability when the same material is assayed repeatedly within the same assay batch, or day-to-day precision, which is the variability when the same material is assayed on different days.

The assay coefficient of variation (CV) is used to express precision and can be calculated by the following equation:

$$\text{CV\%} = \frac{\text{standard deviation of the assay}}{\text{mean of the assay results}} \times 100\% \quad (1.1)$$

This should be as small as possible for each assay and can be expressed as intra-assay CV%.

Test sensitivity and specificity

Diagnostic sensitivity is a measure of the frequency of a test being positive when a particular disease is present, i.e. the percentage of true-positive (TP) results. Diagnostic specificity is a measure of the frequency of a test being negative when a certain disease is absent, i.e. percentage of true-negative (TN) results. Ideally, a test would have 100 per cent specificity and 100 per cent sensitivity.

The usefulness of tests can be expressed visually as receiver operator curves (ROCs) (Fig. 1.2).

Unfortunately, in population screening, some subjects with a disorder may have negative tests (false negatives, FN); conversely, some subjects without the condition in question will show an abnormal or positive result (false positive, FP).

The predictive value of a negative result is the percentage of all negative results that are true negatives, i.e. the frequency of subjects without the disorder in all subjects with negative test results. A high negative predictive value is important in screening programmes if affected individuals are not to be missed. This can be expressed as:

$$\frac{\text{TN}}{\text{TN} + \text{FN}} \times 100\% \quad (1.2)$$

The predictive value of a positive result is the percentage of all positive results that are true positives: in other words, the proportion of screening tests that are correct. A high positive predictive value is important to minimize the number of false-positive individuals being treated unnecessarily. This can be expressed as:

$$\frac{\text{TP}}{\text{TP} + \text{FP}} \times 100\% \quad (1.3)$$

The overall efficiency of a test is the percentage of patients correctly classified by the test. This should be as high as possible and can be expressed as:

$$\frac{\text{TP} + \text{TN}}{\text{TP} + \text{FP} + \text{TN} + \text{FN}} \times 100\% \quad (1.4)$$

If the cut-off, or action, limit of a diagnostic test is set too low, more falsely positive individuals will be included and its sensitivity will increase and its specificity decline. Conversely, if a diagnostic test has its cut-off or action limit set too high, fewer falsely positive individuals will be encompassed but more individuals will be falsely defined as negative, i.e. its sensitivity will decrease and its specificity will increase.

Likelihood ratios of laboratory tests

Some may find predictive values confusing, and the likelihood ratio (LR) may be preferable. This can be defined

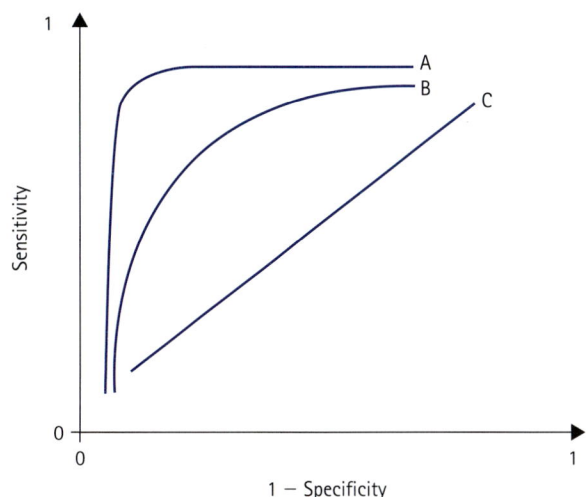

Fig. 1.2 Receiver operator curve (ROC). The greater the area under the curve, the more useful the diagnostic test. Test B is less useful than test A, which has greater sensitivity and specificity. C depicts chance performance (0.5).

as the statistical odds of a factor occurring in one individual with a disorder compared with it occurring in an individual without that disorder.

The LR for a negative test is expressed as:

$$\frac{1 - \text{sensitivity}}{\text{specificity}} \quad (1.5)$$

The LR for a positive test is expressed as:

$$\frac{\text{sensitivity}}{1 - \text{specificity}} \quad (1.6)$$

The greater the LR, the more clinically useful is the test in question.

CASE 3

100 patients with chest pain were screened with a new biochemical test which showed 80 to be positive for chest pain. What is the test's sensitivity?

$$\text{Answer} \quad \frac{80}{100}\% = 80\%$$

The same test was used on 100 patients without chest pain and 95 had a negative screening result. What is the test's specificity?

$$\text{Answer} \quad \frac{95}{100}\% = 95\%$$

DISCUSSION

Sensitivity is true positive rate per total affected.
Specificity is true negative rate per total unaffected.

CONCLUSIONS

- Careful thought is required when it comes to requesting and interpreting clinical biochemistry tests.
- Communication with the laboratory is essential to ensure optimal result interpretation and patient management.
- The laboratory reference range should be consulted when interpreting biochemical results, and results should be interpreted in the light of the clinical findings.
- Just because a result is 'abnormal' does not mean the patient has an illness; conversely, a 'normal' result does not exclude a disease process.

2 WATER AND SODIUM

Total sodium and water balance	7	Urinary sodium estimation	16
Control of water and sodium balance	8	Disturbances of water and sodium metabolism	16
Distribution of water and sodium in the body	10		

It is essential to understand the linked homeostatic mechanisms controlling water and sodium balance when interpreting the plasma sodium concentration and managing the clinically common disturbances of water and sodium balance. This is of major importance in deciding on the composition and amount, if any, of intravenous fluid to give. It must also be remembered that plasma results may be affected by such intravenous therapy, and can be dangerously misunderstood.

Water is an essential body constituent, and homeostatic processes are important to ensure that the total water balance is maintained within narrow limits and the distribution of water between the vascular, interstitial and intracellular compartments is maintained. This depends on hydrostatic and osmotic forces acting across cell membranes.

Sodium is the most abundant extracellular cation and, with its associated anions, accounts for most of the osmotic activity of the extracellular fluid (ECF); it is important in determining water distribution across cell membranes.

Osmotic activity depends on concentration, and therefore on the relative amounts of sodium and water in the ECF compartment, rather than on the absolute quantity of either constituent. An imbalance may cause hyponatraemia (low plasma sodium concentration) or hypernatraemia (high plasma sodium concentration), and therefore changes in osmolality. If water and sodium are lost or gained in equivalent amounts, the plasma sodium, and therefore the osmolal concentration, is unchanged; symptoms are then due to extracellular volume depletion or overloading (Table 2.1).

As the metabolism of sodium is so inextricably related to that of water, the two are discussed together in this chapter.

Table 2.1 Approximate contributions of solutes to plasma osmolality

	Osmolality (mmol/kg)	Total (%)
Sodium and anions	270	92
Potassium and anions	7	
Calcium (ionized) and anions	3	
Magnesium and anions	1	8
Urea	5	
Glucose	5	
Protein	1 (approx.)	
Total	292 (approx.)	

TOTAL SODIUM AND WATER BALANCE

In a 70-kg man, the total body water (TBW) is about 42 L and contributes about 60 per cent of the total body weight; there are approximately 3000 mmol of sodium, mainly in the ECF (Table 2.2). Water and electrolyte intake usually balance output in urine, faeces, sweat and expired air.

Water and sodium intake

The daily water and sodium intakes are variable, but in an adult amount to about 1.5–2 L and 60–150 mmol, respectively.

Table 2.2 The approximate volumes in different body compartments through which water is distributed in a 70-kg adult

	Volume (L)
Intracellular fluid compartment	24
Extracellular fluid compartment	18
Interstitial	(13)
Intravascular (blood volume)	(5)
Total body water	42

Water and sodium output

Kidneys and gastrointestinal tract

The kidneys and intestine deal with water and electrolytes in a similar way. Net loss through both organs depends on the balance between the volume filtered proximally and that reabsorbed more distally. Any factor affecting either passive filtration or epithelial cellular function may disturb this balance.

Approximately 200 L of water and 30 000 mmol of sodium are filtered by the kidneys each day; a further 10 L of water and 1500 mmol of sodium enter the intestinal lumen. The whole of the extracellular water and sodium could be lost by passive filtration in little more than an hour, but under normal circumstances about 99 per cent is reabsorbed. Consequently, the net daily losses amount to about 1.5–2 L of water and 100 mmol of sodium in the urine, and 100 mL and 15 mmol, respectively, in the faeces.

Fine adjustment of the relative amounts of water and sodium excretion occurs in the distal nephron and the large intestine, often under hormonal control. The effects of antidiuretic hormone (ADH) or vasopressin and the mineralocorticoid hormone aldosterone on the kidney are the most important physiologically, although atrial natriuretic peptides are also important.

Sweat and expired air

About 1 L of water is lost daily in sweat and in expired air, and less than 30 mmol of sodium a day is lost in sweat. The volume of sweat is primarily controlled by skin temperature, although ADH and aldosterone have some effect on its composition. Water loss in expired air depends on the respiratory rate. Normally, losses in sweat and expired air are rapidly corrected by changes in renal and intestinal loss. However, neither of these losses can be controlled to meet sodium and water requirements and thus they may contribute considerably to abnormal balance when homeostatic mechanisms fail.

CONTROL OF WATER AND SODIUM BALANCE

Control of water balance

Both the intake and loss of water are controlled by osmotic gradients across cell membranes in the brain's hypothalamic osmoreceptor centres. These centres, which are closely related anatomically, control thirst and the secretion of ADH.

Antidiuretic hormone (arginine vasopressin)

Antidiuretic hormone is a polypeptide with a half-life of about 20 minutes that is synthesized in the supraoptic and paraventricular nuclei of the hypothalamus and, after transport down the pituitary stalk, is secreted from the posterior pituitary gland (see Chapter 7).

Control of ADH secretion

The secretion of ADH is stimulated by flow of water out of cerebral cells caused by a relatively high extracellular osmolality. If intracellular osmolality is unchanged, an extracellular increase of only 2 per cent quadruples ADH output; an equivalent fall almost completely inhibits it. This represents a change in plasma sodium concentration of only about 3 mmol/L. In more chronic changes, when the osmotic gradient has been minimized by solute redistribution, there may be little or no effect. In addition, stretch receptors in the left atrium and baroreceptors in the aortic arch and carotid sinus influence ADH secretion in response to the low intravascular pressure of severe hypovolaemia, stimulating ADH release. The stress due to, for example, nausea, vomiting and pain may also increase ADH secretion. Inhibition of ADH secretion occurs if the extracellular osmolality falls, for whatever reason.

Actions of ADH

Antidiuretic hormone enhances water reabsorption in excess of solute from the collecting ducts of the kidney and so dilutes the extracellular osmolality. When ADH secretion is a response to a high extracellular osmolality with the danger of cell dehydration, this is an appropriate response. However, if its secretion is in response to a low circulating volume alone, it is inappropriate to the osmolality. The retained water is then distributed throughout the TBW space, entering cells along the osmotic gradient; the correction of extracellular depletion with water alone is thus relatively inefficient in correcting hypovolaemia. Plasma osmolality normally varies by less than 1–2 per cent, despite great variation in water intake, which is largely due to the action of ADH.

In some circumstances, the action of ADH is opposed by other factors. For example, during an osmotic diuresis the urine, although not hypo-osmolal, contains more water than sodium. Patients being fed intravenously, or who are breaking down more tissue protein than usual, and are therefore producing more urea from the released amino acids, may become water depleted even if there is adequate ADH; urinary osmolality will be high in these cases.

Control of sodium balance

The major factors controlling sodium balance are renal blood flow and aldosterone. This hormone controls loss of sodium from the distal tubule and colon.

Aldosterone

Aldosterone, a mineralocorticoid hormone, is secreted by the zona glomerulosa of the adrenal cortex (see Chapter 8). It affects sodium–potassium and sodium–hydrogen ion exchange across *all* cell membranes. Its main effect is on renal tubular cells, but it also affects loss in faeces, sweat and saliva. Aldosterone stimulates sodium reabsorption from the lumen of the distal renal tubule in exchange for either potassium or hydrogen ions (Fig. 2.1). The net result is the retention of more sodium than water, and the loss of potassium and hydrogen ions. If the circulating aldosterone concentration is high and tubular function is normal, the urinary sodium concentration is low.

Many factors are involved in the feedback control of aldosterone secretion. These include local electrolyte concentrations, such as that of potassium in the adrenal gland, but they are probably of less physiological and clinical importance than the effect of the renin–angiotensin system.

The renin–angiotensin system

Renin is an aspartyl protease secreted by the juxtaglomerular apparatus, a cellular complex, adjacent to the renal glomeruli, lying between the afferent arteriole and the distal convoluted tubule. Secretion increases in response to a reduction in renal artery blood flow, possibly mediated by changes in the mean pressure in the afferent arterioles, and beta-adrenergic stimulation. Renin splits* a decapeptide (angiotensin I) from a circulating α_2-globulin known as renin substrate. Another proteolytic enzyme,

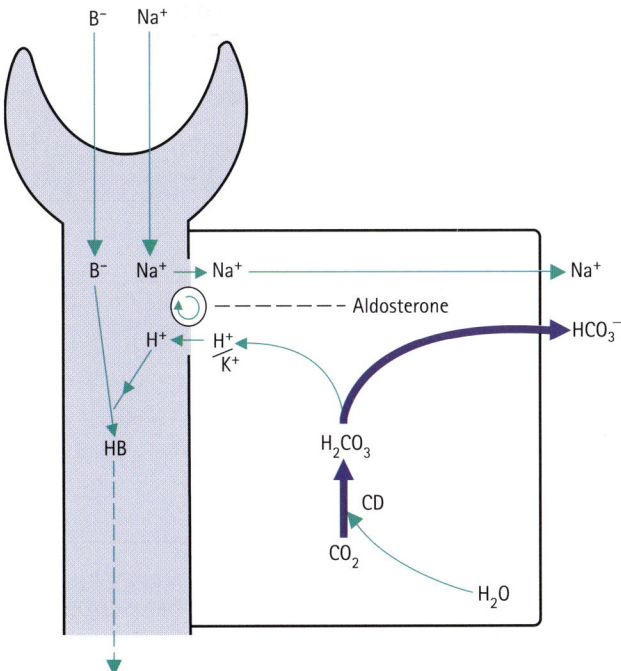

Fig. 2.1 The action of aldosterone on the reabsorption of Na^+ in exchange for either K^+ or H^+ from the distal renal tubules. See text for details. (CD = carbonate dehydratase.)

angiotensin-converting enzyme (ACE), which is located predominantly in the lungs but is also present in other tissues such as the kidneys, splits off a further two amino acid residues. This is the enzyme that ACE inhibitors (used to treat hypertension and congestive cardiac failure) act on. The remaining octapeptide, angiotensin II, has a number of important actions.

- It acts directly on capillary walls, causing vasoconstriction, and so probably helps to maintain blood pressure and alter the glomerular filtration rate (GFR). Vasoconstriction may raise the blood pressure before the circulating volume can be restored.
- It stimulates the cells of the zona glomerulosa to synthesize and secrete aldosterone.
- It stimulates the thirst centre and so promotes oral fluid intake.

Poor renal blood flow is often associated with an inadequate systemic blood pressure. The release of renin (derived from prorenin by proteolytic action) results in the production of angiotensin II, which tends to correct this by causing aldosterone release, which stimulates sodium and subsequently water retention and hence restores the circulating volume.

Table 2.3 Hypothetical cumulative fluid balance chart assuming an insensible daily loss of 500 mL

	Measured intake (mL)	Measured output (mL)	Total output (minimum mL)	Daily balance (mL)	Cumulative balance (mL)
Day 1	2000	1900	2400	−400	−400
Day 2	2000	2000	2500	−500	−900
Day 3	2100	1900	2400	−300	−1200
Day 4	2200	2000	2500	−300	−1500

Thus aldosterone secretion responds, via renin, to a reduction in renal blood flow. Sodium excretion is not directly related to total body sodium content or to plasma sodium concentration.

Atrial natriuretic peptides

A peptide hormone (or hormones) secreted from the right atrial wall in response to the stimulation of stretch receptors may cause high sodium excretion (natriuresis) by increasing the GFR and by inhibiting renin and aldosterone secretion. However, the importance of this hormone (or hormones) in the physiological control of sodium excretion and in pathological states has not yet been fully elucidated (see Chapter 22).

Monitoring fluid balance

The most important factor in assessing changes in day-to-day fluid balance is accurate records of fluid intake and output; this is particularly pertinent for unconscious patients. 'Insensible loss' is usually assumed to be about 1 L/day, but there is endogenous water production of about 500 mL/day as a result of metabolic processes. Therefore the net daily 'insensible loss' is about 500 mL. The required daily intake may be calculated from the output during the previous day plus 500 mL to allow for 'insensible loss'; this method is satisfactory if the patient is normally hydrated before day-to-day monitoring is started. Serial patient body weight determination can also be useful in the assessment of changes in fluid balance.

A pyrexial patient may lose 1 L or more of fluid in sweat and, if he or she is also hyperventilating, respiratory water loss may be considerable. In such cases an allowance of about 500 mL for 'insensible loss' may be totally inadequate. In addition, very ill patients are often incontinent of urine, which makes the accurate assessment of fluid losses very difficult.

Inaccurate measurement and charting are useless and may be dangerous.

Keeping a cumulative fluid balance record is a useful way of detecting a trend, which may then be corrected before serious abnormalities develop.

In the example shown in Table 2.3, 500 mL has been allowed for as net 'insensible daily loss'; calculated losses are therefore more likely to be under-estimated than over-estimated. This shows how insidiously a serious deficit can develop over a few days.

The volume of fluid infused should be based on the calculated cumulative balance and on clinical evidence of the state of hydration, and its composition adjusted to maintain normal plasma electrolyte concentrations.

Assessment of the state of hydration of a patient relies on clinical examination and on laboratory evidence of haemodilution or haemoconcentration.

- *Haemodilution*: increasing plasma volume with protein-free fluid leads to a fall in the concentrations of proteins and haemoglobin. However, these findings may be affected by pre-existing abnormalities of protein or red cell concentrations.
- *Haemoconcentration*: ECF is usually lost from the vascular compartment first and, unless the fluid is whole blood, depletion of water and small molecules results in a rise in the concentration of large molecules, such as proteins and blood cells, with a rise in blood haemoglobin concentration and haematocrit.

Table 2.4 shows various intravenous fluid regimens that can be used clinically.

DISTRIBUTION OF WATER AND SODIUM IN THE BODY

In mild disturbances of the balance of water and electrolytes, their total amounts in the body may be of less importance than their distribution between body compartments (see Table 2.2).

Table 2.4 Some electrolyte-containing fluids for intravenous infusion

	Na⁺ (mmol/L)	K⁺ (mmol/L)	Cl⁻ (mmol/L)	HCO₃⁻ (mmol/L)	Glucose (g/dL)	Ca²⁺ (mmol/L)	Approximate osmolarity × plasma
Saline							
'Normal' (physiological 0.9%)	154	–	154	–	–	–	×1
Twice 'normal' (1.8%)	308	–	308	–	–	–	×2
Half 'normal' (0.45%)	77	–	77	–	–	–	×0.5
'Dextrose' saline							
5%, 0.45%	77	–	77	–	278	–	×1.5
Sodium bicarbonate							
1.4%	167	–	–	167	–	–	×1
8.4%[a]	1000	–	–	1000	–	–	×6
Complex solutions							
Ringer's	147	4.2	156	–	–	2.2	×1
Hartmann's	131	5.4	112	29[b]	–	1.8	×1

[a] Most commonly used bicarbonate solution. Note marked hyperosmolarity. Only used if strongly indicated.
[b] As lactate.

Water is distributed between the main body fluid compartments, in which different electrolytes contribute to the osmolality. These compartments are:

- *intracellular*, in which potassium is the predominant cation, and
- *extracellular*, in which sodium is the predominant cation and which can be subdivided into:
  - interstitial space, with very low protein concentration, and
  - intravascular (plasma) space, with a relatively high protein concentration.

Electrolyte distribution between cells and interstitial fluid

Sodium is the predominant extracellular cation, its intracellular concentration being less than one-tenth of that within the ECF. The intracellular potassium concentration is about 30 times that of the ECF. About 95 per cent of the osmotically active sodium is outside cells, and about the same proportion of potassium is intracellular. Cell-surface energy-dependent sodium/potassium adenosine triphosphatase pumps maintain these differential concentrations.

Other ions tend to move across cell membranes in association with sodium and potassium. (The movement of hydrogen ions is discussed in Chapter 4.) Magnesium and phosphate ions are predominantly intracellular and chloride ions extracellular.

Distribution of electrolytes between plasma and interstitial fluid

The cell membranes of the capillary endothelium are more permeable to small ions than those of tissue cells. The plasma protein concentration is relatively high, but that of interstitial fluid is very low. The osmotic effect of the intravascular proteins is balanced by very slightly higher interstitial electrolyte concentrations (Gibbs–Donnan effect); this difference is small and, for practical purposes, plasma electrolyte concentrations can be assumed to be representative of those in the ECF as a whole.

Distribution of water

Over half the body water is intracellular (see Table 2.2). About 15–20 per cent of the extracellular water is intravascular; the remainder constitutes the interstitial fluid. The distribution of water across biological membranes depends on the balance between the hydrostatic pressure and the in-vivo effective osmotic pressure differences on each side of the membrane.

Osmotic pressure

The net movement of water across a membrane that is permeable only to water depends on the concentration gradient of particles – either ions or molecules – across that membrane and is known as the osmotic gradient. For any weight-to-volume ratio, the larger the particles, the fewer there are per unit volume, and therefore the lower the osmotic effect they exert. If the membranes were freely permeable to ions and smaller particles as well as to water, these diffusible particles would exert no osmotic effect across membranes and therefore the larger ones would become more important in effecting water movement. This action gives rise to the effective colloid osmotic (oncotic) gradient. Water distribution in the body is thus dependent largely on three factors, namely:

- the number of particles per unit volume,
- particle size relative to membrane permeability,
- concentration gradient across the membrane.

Units of measurement of osmotic pressure

Osmolar concentration can be expressed as:

- the *osmolarity* (in mmol/L) of solution,
- the *osmolality* (in mmol/kg) of solvent.

If solute is dissolved in pure water at concentrations such as those in body fluids, osmolarity and osmolality will hardly differ. However, as plasma is a complex solution containing large molecules such as proteins, the total volume of solution (water + protein) is greater than the volume of solvent only (water) in which the small molecules are dissolved. At a protein concentration of 70 g/L, the volume of water is about 6 per cent less than the total volume of the solution (that is, the molarity should theoretically be about 6 per cent less than the molality). Most methods for measuring individual ions assess them in molarity (mmol/L). If the concentration of proteins in plasma is markedly increased, the volume of solvent is significantly reduced but the volume of solution remains unchanged. Therefore the molarity (in mmol/L) of certain ions such as sodium will be reduced but the molality will be unaltered. This apparently low sodium concentration is known as pseudohyponatraemia.

Measured plasma osmolality

Osmometers measure changes in the properties of a solution, such as freezing-point depression or vapour pressure, which depend on the total osmolality of the solution — the osmotic effect that would be exerted by the sum of all the dissolved molecules and ions across a membrane permeable only to water. These properties are known as colligative properties. Sodium and its associated anions (mainly chloride) contribute 90 per cent or more to this measured plasma osmolality, the effect of protein being negligible. As the only major difference in composition between plasma and interstitial fluid is in protein content, the plasma osmolality is almost identical to the osmolality of the interstitial fluid surrounding cells.

Calculated plasma osmolarity

It is the osmola**l**, rather than the osmola**r**, concentration that exerts an effect across cell membranes and that is controlled by homeostatic mechanisms. However, as discussed below, the calculated plasma osmolarity is usually as informative as the measured plasma osmolality.

Although, because of the space-occupying effect of protein, the measured osmolality of plasma should be higher than the osmolarity, calculated from the sum of the molar concentrations of all the ions, there is usually little difference between the two figures. This is because there is incomplete ionization of, for example, NaCl to Na^+ and Cl^-; this reduces the osmotic effect by almost the same amount as the volume occupied by protein raises it. Consequently, the calculated plasma osmolarity is a valid approximation to the true measured osmolality. However, if there is gross hyperproteinaemia or hyperlipidaemia such that either protein or lipid contributes much more than 6 per cent to the measured plasma volume, the calculated osmolarity may be significantly lower than the true osmolality in the plasma water. A hypothetical example is shown in Fig. 2.2.

Many formulae of varying complexity have been proposed to calculate plasma osmolarity. None of them can predict the osmotic *effect*, but the following formula (in which square brackets indicate concentration) gives a close approximation to plasma osmolality:

$$\text{Plasma osmolality} = 2[Na^+] + 2[K^+] + [\text{urea}] + [\text{glucose}] \text{ in mmol/L} \quad (2.1)$$

The factor of 2, which is applied to the sodium and potassium concentrations, allows for the associated anions and assumes complete ionization. This calculation is not valid if gross hyperproteinaemia or hyperlipidaemia is present or an unmeasured osmotically active solute, such as mannitol, methanol, ethanol or ethylene glycol, is circulating in plasma.

A significant difference between measured and calculated osmolality in the absence of hyperproteinaemia or hyperlipidaemia may suggest alcohol or other poisoning. For example, a plasma alcohol concentration of 1 g/L contributes about 20 mmol/kg to the osmolality. This osmotic difference is known as the osmolar gap and can be used to assess the presence in plasma of unmeasured osmotically active particles. In such cases the plasma sodium concentration may be misleading as a measure of the osmotic effect, and plasma osmolality should be measured.

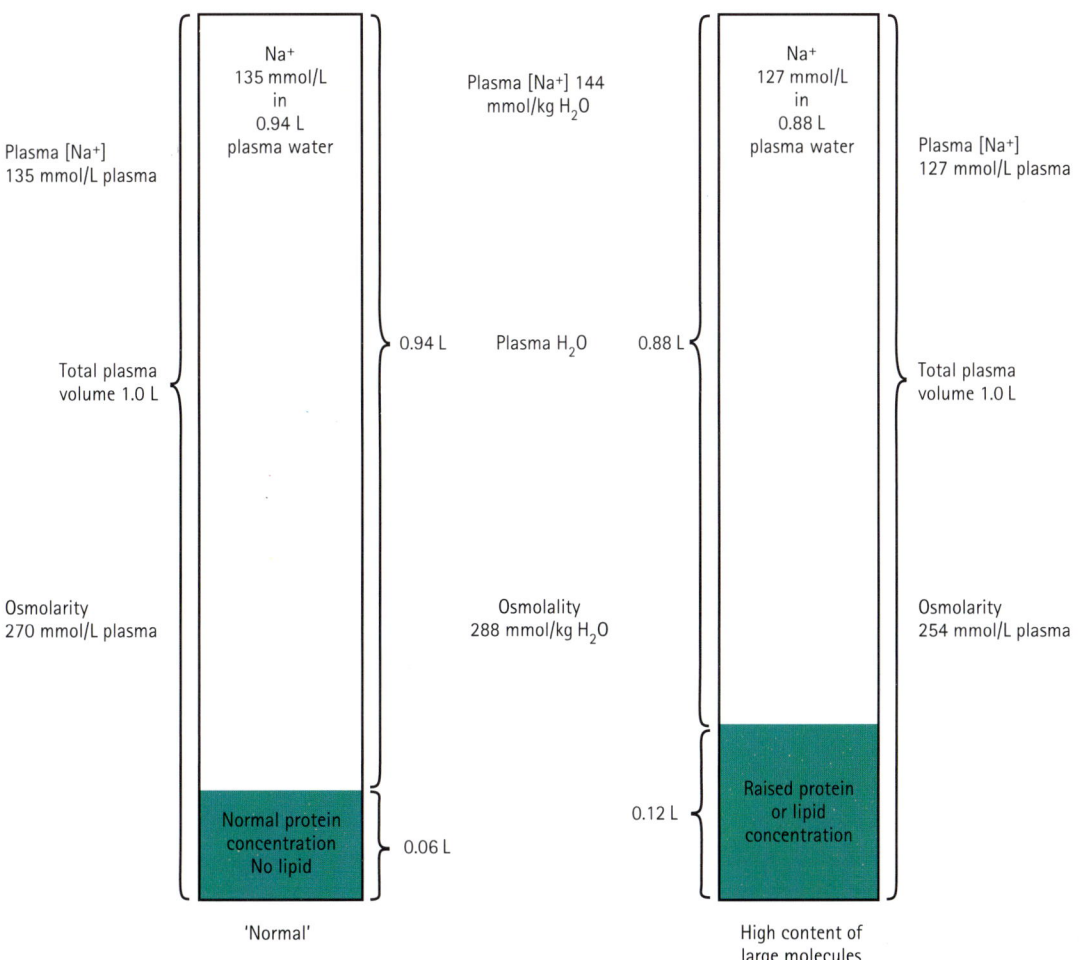

Fig. 2.2 The consequence of gross hyperproteinaemia or hyperlipidaemia on the plasma water volume and its effect on the calculated plasma osmolarity and the true plasma osmolality.

It is not possible to calculate urinary osmolarity because of the considerable variation in the concentrations of different, sometimes unmeasured, solutes; the osmotic pressure of urine can only be determined by measuring the osmolality.

Distribution of water across cell membranes

Osmotic pressure gradient

Because the hydrostatic pressure difference across the cell membrane is negligible, cell hydration depends on the effective osmotic difference between intracellular and extracellular fluids. The cell membranes are freely permeable to water and to some solutes, but different solutes diffuse (or are actively transported) across cell membranes at different rates, although always more slowly than water. In a stable state, the total intracellular osmolality, due mostly to potassium and associated anions, equals that of the interstitial fluid, due mostly to sodium and associated anions; consequently, there is no *net* movement of water into or out of cells. In some pathological states, rapid changes of extracellular solute concentration affect cell hydration; slower changes may allow time for the redistribution of solute and have little or no effect.

Sodium. In normal subjects sodium and its associated anions account for at least 90 per cent of extracellular osmolality. Rapid changes in their concentration therefore affect cellular hydration. If there is no significant change in the other solutes, a rise causes cellular dehydration and a fall causes cellular over-hydration.

Urea. Normal extracellular concentrations are so low as to contribute very little to the measured plasma osmolality. However, concentrations fifteen-fold or more above normal can occur in severe uraemia and can then make a significant contribution (see Chapter 3). However, urea does diffuse into cells very much more slowly than water. Consequently, in acute uraemia, the increased osmotic gradient alters cell hydration, but in chronic uraemia, although the measured plasma osmolality is often increased, the osmotic effect of urea is reduced as the concentrations gradually equalize on the two sides of the membrane.

Glucose. Like urea, the normally low extracellular concentration of glucose does not contribute significantly to the osmolality. However, unlike urea, glucose is actively transported into many cells, but once there it is rapidly metabolized, even at high extracellular concentrations, and the intracellular concentration remains low. Severe hyperglycaemia, whether acute or chronic, causes a marked osmotic effect across cell membranes, with movement of water from cells into the extracellular compartment causing cellular dehydration.

Although hyperglycaemia and acute uraemia can cause cellular dehydration, the contribution of normal urea and glucose concentrations to plasma osmolality is so small that reduced levels of these solutes, unlike those of sodium, do not cause cellular over-hydration.

Solutes such as potassium, calcium and magnesium are present in the ECF at very low concentrations. Significant changes in these are lethal at much lower concentrations than those that would change osmolality.

Mannitol is an example of an exogenous substance that remains in the extracellular compartment because it is not transported into cells, and may be infused to reduce cerebral oedema. Ethanol is only slowly metabolized and a high concentration in the ECF may lead to cerebral cellular dehydration; this may account for some of the symptoms of a hangover. High glucose levels account for the polyuria of severe diabetes mellitus.

Large rises in the osmotic gradient across cell membranes may result in the movement of enough water from the intracellular compartment to dilute extracellular constituents. Consequently, if the change in osmolality has not been caused by sodium and its associated anions, a fall in plasma sodium concentration is appropriate to the state of osmolality. If, under such circumstances, the plasma sodium concentration is not low, this indicates hyperosmolality.

Generally, plasma osmolarity calculated from sodium, potassium, urea and glucose concentrations is at least as clinically valuable as measured plasma osmolality. It has the advantage that the solute responsible, and therefore its likely osmotic effect, is often identified.

Distribution of water across capillary membranes

The maintenance of blood pressure depends on the retention of fluid within the intravascular compartment at a higher hydrostatic pressure than that of the interstitial space. Hydrostatic pressure in capillary lumina tends to force fluid into the extravascular space. In the absence of any effective opposing force, fluid would be lost rapidly from the vascular compartment. Unlike other cell membranes, those of the capillaries are permeable to small ions. *Therefore sodium alone exerts almost no osmotic effect and the distribution of water across capillary membranes is little affected by changes in electrolyte concentration.*

Colloid osmotic pressure

The very small osmotic effect of plasma protein molecules produces an effective osmotic gradient across capillary membranes; this is known as the colloid osmotic, or oncotic, pressure. It is the most important factor opposing the net outward hydrostatic pressure (Fig. 2.3). Albumin (molecular weight 65 kDa) is the most important protein contributing to the colloid osmotic pressure. It is present intravascularly at significant concentration but extravascularly only at a very low concentration because it cannot pass freely across the capillary wall.

The osmotic gradient across vascular walls cannot be estimated by simple means. The total plasma osmolality gives no information about this. Moreover, the plasma albumin concentration is a poor guide to the colloid osmotic pressure and its estimation for this purpose is rarely indicated. Although other proteins, such as globulins, are present in the plasma at about the same concentration as albumin, their estimation for this purpose is even less useful: their higher molecular weights mean that they have even less effect than albumin.

Relation between sodium and water homeostasis

In normal subjects, the concentrations of sodium and its associated anions are the most important osmotic factors affecting ADH secretion. Plasma volume, by its effect on renal blood flow, controls aldosterone secretion and therefore sodium balance. The homeostatic mechanisms controlling sodium and water excretion are interdependent. (A simplified scheme is shown in Fig. 2.4.) Thirst depends on a rise in extracellular osmolality, whether due to water depletion or sodium excess, and also to a very large increase in the activity of the renin–angiotensin system.

A rise in extracellular osmolality reduces water loss by stimulating ADH release and increases intake by stimulating thirst; both these actions dilute the extracellular osmolality. Osmotic balance (and therefore cellular hydration) is rapidly corrected. If the primary abnormality is in the

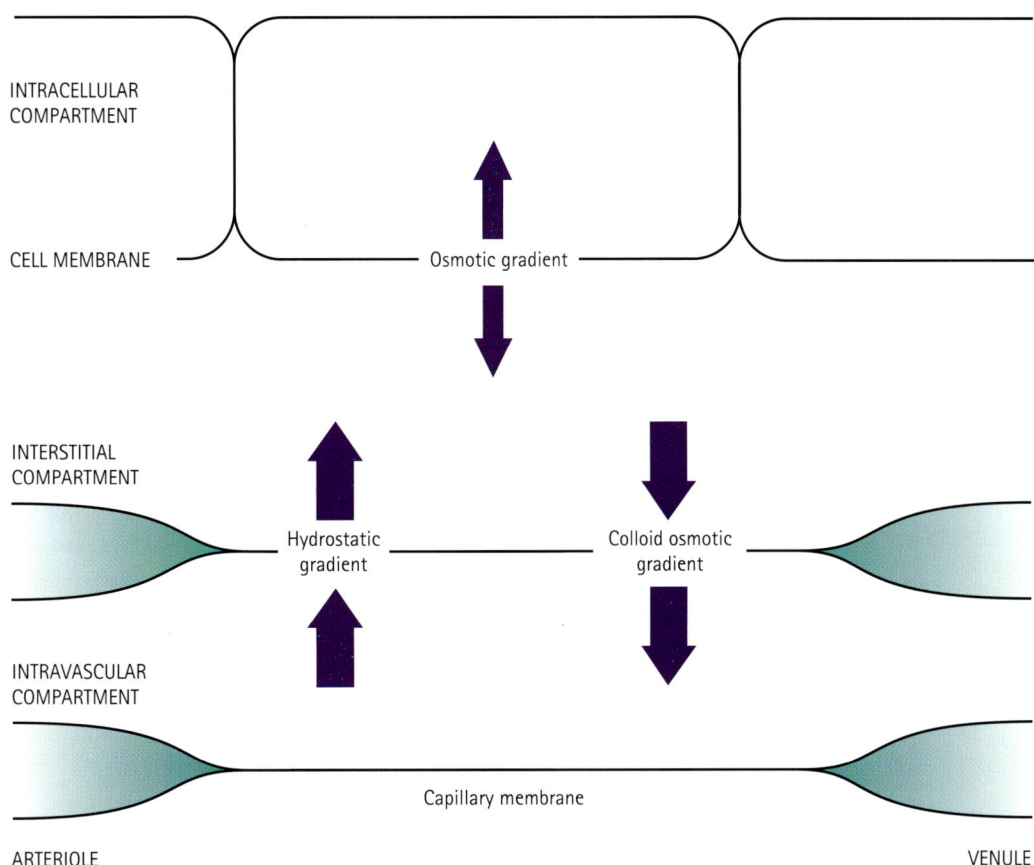

Fig. 2.3 Osmotic factors that control the distribution of water between the fluid compartments of the body.

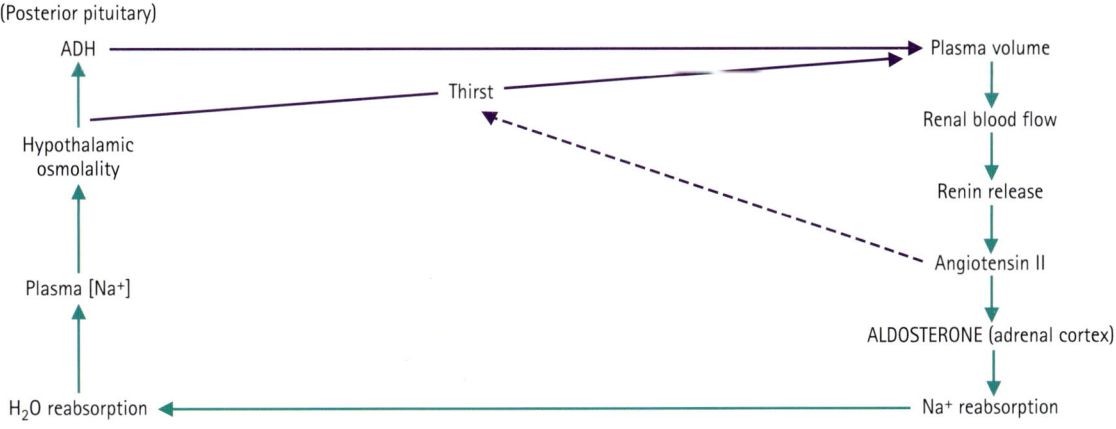

Fig. 2.4 Control of water and sodium homeostasis. (ADH = antidiuretic hormone.)

balance of sodium, rather than that of water, cellular hydration is sometimes protected at the expense of aggravating abnormalities in total body volume.

Assessment of sodium status

As already discussed, the plasma sodium concentration is important because of its osmotic effect on fluid distribution. Plasma sodium concentrations should be monitored while volume is being corrected to ensure that the distribution of fluid between the intracellular and extracellular compartments is optimal. The presence of other osmotically active solutes should be taken into account. The measurement of total body sodium is not a useful investigation.

URINARY SODIUM ESTIMATION

Urinary sodium excretion is not related to body content but to renal blood flow.

Estimation of the urinary sodium concentration in a random specimen may be of value in the diagnosis of the syndrome of inappropriate ADH secretion (SIADH) and may help to differentiate renal circulatory insufficiency (pre-renal) from intrinsic renal damage (see Chapter 3).

The fractional excretion of sodium (FENa%) may also be useful in helping to assess renal blood flow and can be measured using a simultaneous blood sample and spot urine sample.

$$\text{FENa\%} = \frac{\text{urine[sodium]}}{\text{plasma[sodium]}} \times \frac{\text{plasma[creatinine]}}{\text{urine[creatinine]}} \times 100\% \quad (2.2)$$

A value of less than 1 per cent may be found in poor renal perfusion, for example pre-renal failure, and of more than 1 per cent in intrinsic renal failure.

DISTURBANCES OF WATER AND SODIUM METABOLISM

The initial clinical consequences of primary sodium disturbances depend on changes of extracellular osmolality and hence of cellular hydration, and those of primary water disturbances depend on changes in extracellular volume.

Plasma sodium concentration is usually a substitute for measuring plasma osmolality. Plasma sodium concentrations per se are not important, but their effect on the osmotic gradient across cell membranes is, and it should be understood that one does not always reflect the other.

If the concentration of plasma sodium alters rapidly, and the concentrations of other extracellular solutes remain the same, most of the clinical features are due to the consequence of the osmotic difference across cell membranes, with redistribution of fluid between cells and the ECF. However, gradual changes, which allow time for redistribution of diffusible solute such as urea, and therefore for equalization of osmolality without major shifts of water, may produce little effect on fluid distribution.

We now discuss in some detail conditions involving water and sodium deficiency and excess. These are discussed together, as the two are so closely interrelated in vivo and can result in abnormal plasma sodium concentrations.

Water and sodium deficiency (Figs 2.5–2.7)

Apart from the loss of solute-free water in expired air, water and sodium are usually lost together from the body. An imbalance between the degrees of their deficiency is relatively common and may be due to the composition of the fluid lost or to that of the fluid given to replace it. The initial effects depend on the composition of the fluid lost compared with that of plasma.

- Isosmolar volume depletion results if the sodium concentration of the fluid lost is similar to that of plasma; changes in plasma sodium concentration are then unusual.

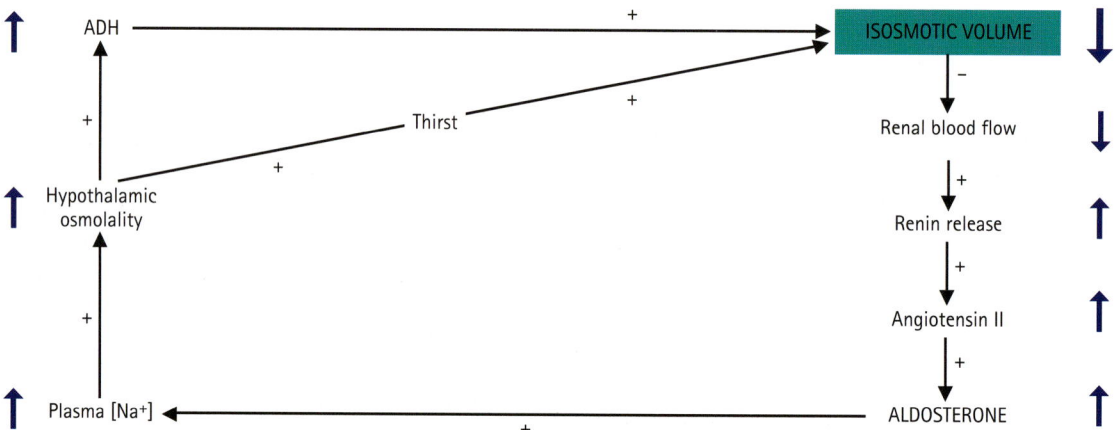

Fig. 2.5 Homeostatic correction of isosmotic volume depletion. The reduced intravascular volume impairs renal blood flow and stimulates renin and therefore aldosterone secretion. There is selective sodium reabsorption from the distal tubules and a low urinary sodium concentration. (Shaded area indicates primary change; ADH = antidiuretic hormone.)

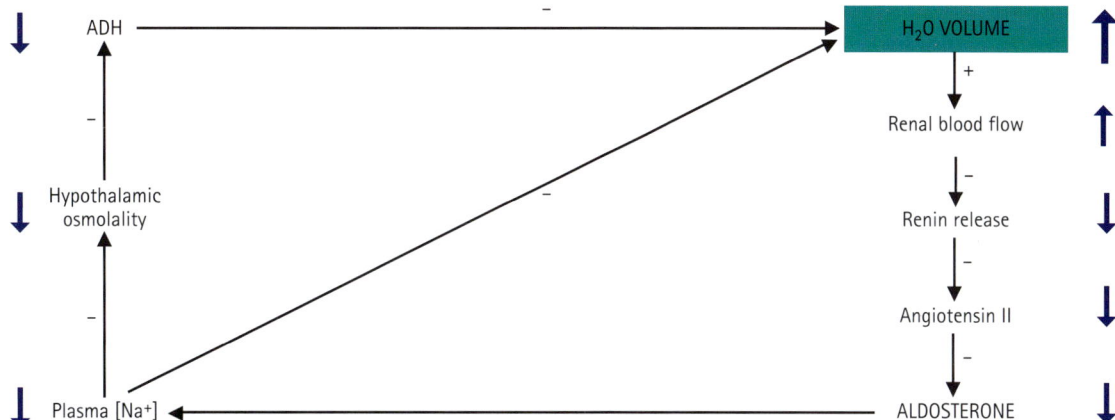

Fig. 2.6 Infusion of hypotonic fluid as a cause of predominant sodium depletion. Increased circulating volume with reduction in plasma osmolality inhibits aldosterone and antidiuretic hormone (ADH) secretion. (Shaded area indicates primary change.)

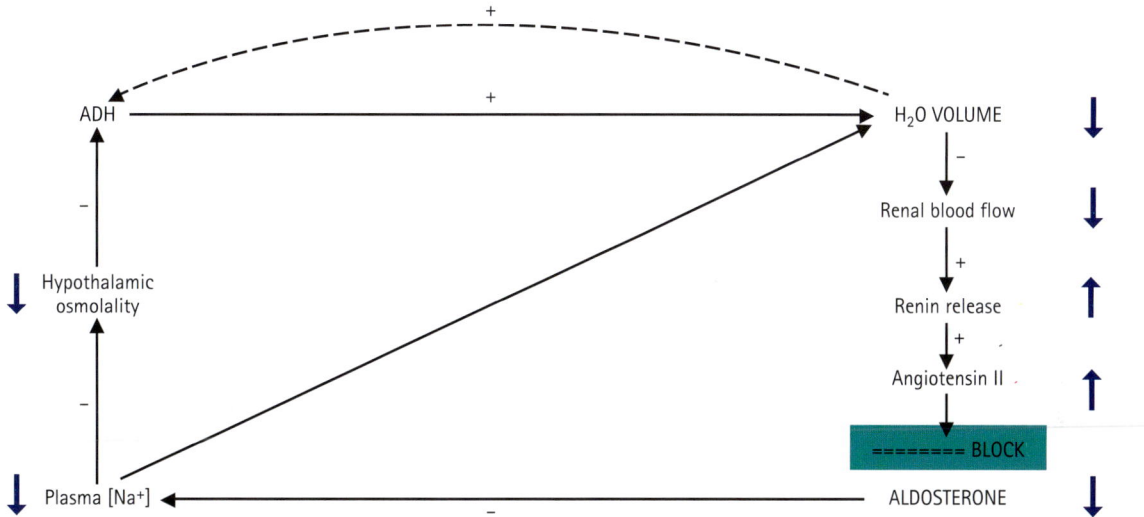

Fig. 2.7 Initial effect of aldosterone deficiency is impaired sodium retention and hypovolaemia; later, severe hypovolaemia stimulates increased antidiuretic hormone (ADH) secretion with water retention, sometimes causing a dilutional hyponatraemia. (Shaded area indicates the primary change.)

- Predominant sodium depletion is usually the result of inappropriate treatment, since only bile, secreted in small volumes, has a significantly higher sodium concentration than that of plasma. Hyponatraemia (a low plasma sodium concentration) usually results.
- Predominant water depletion results if the sodium concentration of the lost fluid is much less than that of plasma. Hypernatraemia (an abnormally high concentration of sodium) may occur and indicates loss of relatively more water than sodium, even if there is little evidence of volume depletion.

The term 'dehydration' can be misleading. It is often used interchangeably to describe the conditions listed above, although the clinical and biochemical findings are very different. The consequent confusion may lead to inappropriate and possibly dangerous treatment; therefore, an attempt should be made to assess the approximate composition of fluid lost by identifying its origin.

Isosmolar volume depletion

Causes of isosmolar fluid loss

The sodium concentrations of all small intestinal secretions and of urine when tubular function is grossly impaired are between 120 mmol/L and 140 mmol/L.

Clinical conditions causing approximately isosmolar loss are therefore:

- small intestinal fistulae and ileostomy,
- small intestinal obstruction and paralytic ileus, in which the fluid accumulating in the gut lumen has, like urine in the bladder, been lost from the ECF,
- severe renal tubular damage with minimal glomerular dysfunction, for example the recovery phase of acute oliguric renal dysfunction, or polyuric chronic renal dysfunction (see Chapter 3).

Results of isosmolar fluid loss

Hypovolaemia reduces renal blood flow and causes renal circulatory insufficiency with oliguria with uraemia. Sodium and water are lost in almost equivalent amounts and the plasma sodium concentration is usually normal; for this reason the patient may not complain of thirst despite some volume depletion.

Haemoconcentration confirms considerable loss of fluid other than blood, although its absence does not exclude such loss.

Postural hypotension (a fall in blood pressure on standing) is a relatively early sign of volume depletion, and tachycardia may also occur.

Changes produced by homeostatic mechanisms

The ability to respond to hormonal homeostatic changes depends mainly on renal tubular function and cannot occur if the isosmolar volume depletion is due to tubular damage. The reduced intravascular volume impairs renal blood flow and stimulates renin and therefore aldosterone secretion. There is selective sodium reabsorption from the distal tubules and therefore a low urinary sodium concentration.

The tendency of the retained sodium to increase plasma osmolality stimulates ADH secretion, and water is reabsorbed; this tends to correct the circulating volume and keep the plasma sodium concentration normal. Severe intravascular volume depletion may also stimulate ADH secretion and therefore water retention, causing mild hyponatraemia. This additional water is distributed throughout the total body water and moves from the depleted, and now slightly hypo-osmolar, ECF into the relatively well-hydrated intracellular compartment.

Even maximal renal water and sodium retention cannot correct extrarenal losses that exceed those of a normal urine output. Water and sodium must be replaced in adequate amounts.

Effects of intravenous volume replacement

Patients unable to absorb adequate amounts of oral fluid because of gastrointestinal loss usually need intravenous replacement.

Fluid replacement in a patient who presents with hypovolaemia can be monitored by clinical observation and by measurement of urine output, plasma electrolytes and urea.

The infusion of protein-free fluid increases the hydrostatic gradient and reduces the opposing colloid osmotic gradient by diluting plasma proteins. The desirable increase in glomerular filtration caused by the over-correction of hypovolaemia results in an increase in urine output and is a common cause of a low plasma urea concentration.

Measurement of urinary sodium concentration may sometimes help. If tubular function is adequate, a urinary sodium concentration of less than about 20 mmol/L suggests that renal blood flow is still low enough to stimulate maximal renin and aldosterone secretion, and infusion should be increased. A urinary sodium concentration greater than 20 mmol/L in a patient with adequate tubular function suggests over-correction and the need to slow the rate of infusion. In cases in which all losses, other than in sweat, faeces and expired air, can be measured, further maintenance of normal balance should be based on accurate fluid balance charts.

Predominant sodium depletion

Incorrect intravenous fluid administration

An important and common cause of sodium depletion is due to infusion of intravenous fluid of inappropriate composition. No body secretion (other than bile, which is secreted in very small amounts) has a sodium concentration significantly higher than that of plasma. The composition of the fluid is even more important than the volume.

Patients with isosmolar fluid depletion, or recovering from major surgery, may be infused with fluid such as 'dextrose saline', which contains about 30 mmol/L of sodium. Glucose in the infused fluid renders it isosmolar despite the low sodium concentration, but the glucose is metabolized, and both plasma sodium concentration and osmolality are diluted by the remaining hypo-osmolar fluid. Homeostatic mechanisms tend to correct this hypo-osmolality but may be overwhelmed if the infusion rate is high. Severe, and even life-threatening, hyponatraemia can result from the imprudent administration of hypotonic fluid, such as 5 per cent dextrose.

Excess hypo-osmolar infused fluid dilutes the plasma sodium, causing a dilutional hyponatraemia with hypo-osmolality. The homeostatic mechanisms that tend to correct this hypo-osmolality involve the inhibition of ADH secretion. The excess water is lost in the urine until the restoration of normal plasma osmolality again stimulates normal ADH secretion. Correction of osmolality may occur at the expense of intravascular volume. This would stimulate renin and aldosterone secretion and sodium would be retained, with the consequent restoration of osmolality and normal ADH secretion.

However, if intravascular volume is maintained by replacing the urinary volume with effectively hypotonic fluid, hypo-osmolality with hyponatraemia persists and sodium depletion is aggravated (Fig. 2.6). Restoration of the plasma volume inhibits renin and aldosterone secretion and sodium is lost in the urine despite hypo-osmolality. The net effect of this procedure is the restoration of circulating volume at the expense of sodium depletion and cellular over-hydration.

The findings include:

- hypo-osmolality,
- a large volume of dilute urine due to the inhibition of ADH secretion,
- hyponatraemia.

  If fluid intake is excessive, the following may also occur:

- haemodilution,
- a low plasma urea concentration due to the high GFR (excessive intravenous infusion is one of the commonest causes of a low plasma urea concentration),
- high urinary sodium concentration, due to the inhibition of aldosterone secretion.

During the immediate postoperative period, pain and stress also stimulate ADH secretion and therefore water retention; this effect is short lived. Such hyponatraemia is rarely a problem, but may become so if hypo-osmolar fluid is being infused. In rare cases it can then be lethal due to cerebral damage. In subjects with normal renal and cardiac function, alternating 'dextrose saline' and isotonic saline may maintain relatively normal plasma sodium and urea concentrations, and an adequate volume of urine is passed; the danger of overloading the circulation is minimal. Infusion should be stopped as soon as the patient can take oral fluids. Conversely, the infusion of 'dextrose saline' or 5 per cent dextrose without any other fluid in seriously ill patients whose homeostatic mechanisms may be impaired may be life threatening.

Sodium depletion due to failure of homeostatic mechanisms

Aldosterone deficiency, such as occurs in Addison's disease, is a rare cause of sodium depletion. *Initial* homeostatic reactions tend to maintain osmolality at the expense of volume (see Chapter 8).

Although less than 1.5 per cent of the filtered sodium is reabsorbed in the renal distal convoluted tubules, this is where the fine adjustment is made in the ratio of sodium to water and therefore to plasma osmolality, and thus normal cell hydration is safeguarded. If aldosterone cannot be secreted normally in response to appropriately increased amounts of renin and angiotensin, this adjustment cannot be made (Fig. 2.7). Under such circumstances, although a greater proportion of sodium may be reabsorbed from the proximal tubules, there may still be relative sodium deficiency and hypovolaemia. *Initially* plasma osmolality and therefore plasma sodium concentration are maintained by water loss; loss of relatively more sodium than water reduces plasma osmolality and cuts off ADH secretion. *Later*, hypovolaemia stimulates ADH secretion, with water retention in excess of sodium; dilutional hyponatraemia may occur despite intravascular volume depletion.

The clinical features include circulatory insufficiency with postural hypotension and the following findings:

- haemoconcentration due to fluid depletion,
- renal circulatory insufficiency with mild uraemia due to volume depletion,
- an inappropriately high urinary sodium concentration in the presence of volume depletion,
- dilutional hyponatraemia and hyperkalaemia.

Predominant water depletion

Predominant water depletion is caused by loss of water in excess of sodium. It is usually due to loss of fluid that has a sodium concentration less than that of plasma, deficient water intake, or both. The rise in extracellular osmolality stimulates both ADH secretion (which minimizes water loss) and thirst. Laboratory abnormalities are most marked if the patient is unable to respond to thirst.

The causes of predominant water depletion can be divided into the following groups.

- Predominant water depletion with normal homeostatic mechanisms (Fig. 2.8).
  - Excessive loss of fluid that has a sodium concentration less than that of plasma. The causes include: loss of excessive fluid stools of low sodium concentration, usually in infantile gastroenteritis,

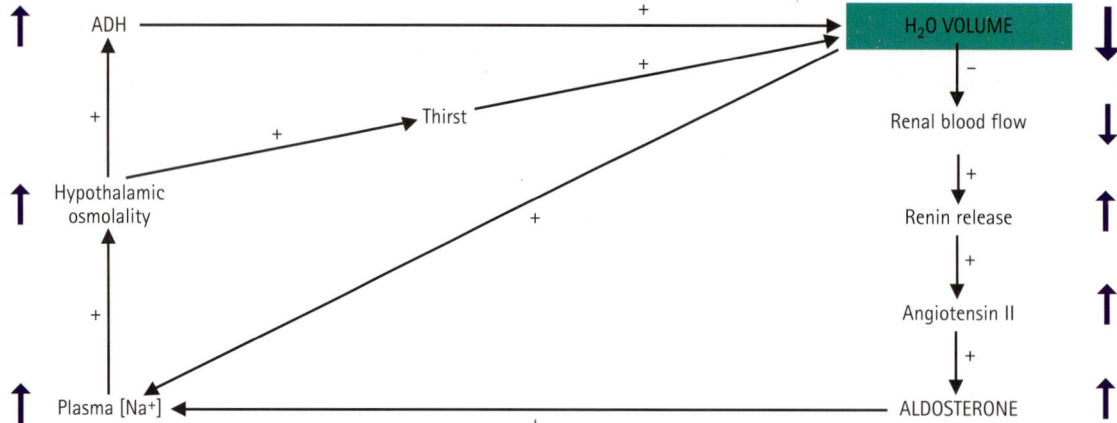

Fig. 2.8 Homeostatic correction of predominant water depletion. Reduced circulating water volume and hypernatraemia, due to water depletion, stimulate aldosterone and antidiuretic hormone (ADH) secretion. (Shaded area indicates the primary change.)

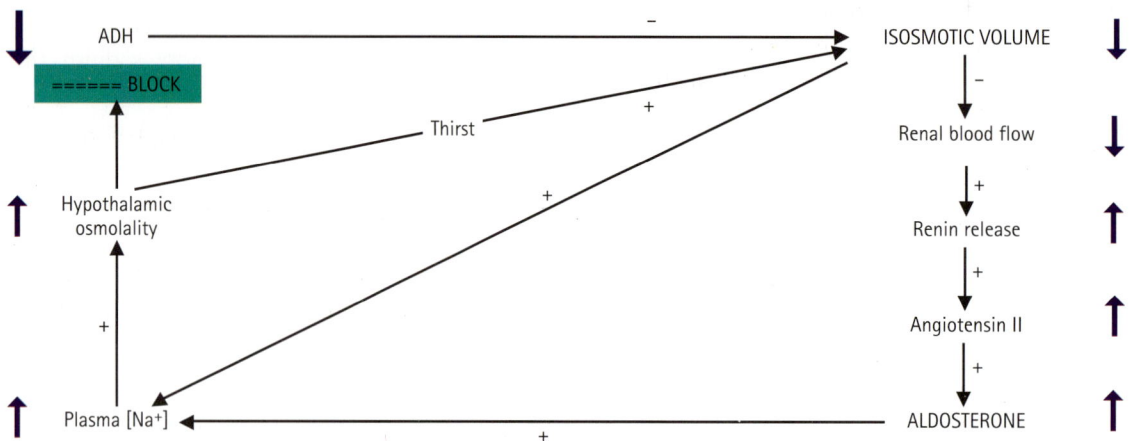

Fig. 2.9 Consequences of antidiuretic hormone (ADH) deficiency (diabetes insipidus). Impaired water retention results in an increased plasma osmolality with stimulation of thirst and hypovolaemia with increased aldosterone secretion. (Shaded area indicates the primary change.)

excessive respiratory loss due to hyperventilation in, for example, pneumonia,
loss of gastric fluid,
loss of large amounts of sweat, such as in pyrexial patients,
loss of fluid from the body surface after extensive burns.
– Deficiency of water intake as a result of inadequate water supply, or mechanical obstruction to its intake.
• Failure of homeostatic mechanisms controlling water retention.
– Inadequate response to thirst:
in comatose or confused patients,
in infants,
caused by damage to the cerebral thirst centre (rare).
– Excess water loss due to polyuria:
osmotic diuresis, which can be caused by hypertonic intravenous infusions, for example to provide nutrients (glucose or amino acids); tissue damage and hence increased production of urea from protein; and glycosuria in severe diabetes mellitus with a very high plasma glucose level.
• Failure of homeostatic mechanisms involving ADH (Fig. 2.9). These syndromes are relatively rare and include the following.
– Cranial diabetes insipidus, a syndrome associated with impairment of ADH secretion. It may be idiopathic in origin or due to either pituitary or

hypothalamic damage caused by head injury or by invasion of the region by tumour or infiltration. Diabetes insipidus following a head injury may present with polyuria and then pass through a temporary 'recovery' phase following transient release of ADH from the remaining granules in the pituitary stalk; this results in water retention and occasionally causes a dilutional hyponatraemia. Some patients with diabetes insipidus due to trauma recover partially or completely as cerebral oedema resolves.

There is a hereditary autosomal dominant form of cranial diabetes insipidus due to mutations in the arginine vasopressin-neurophysin II gene. In addition, there is the autosomal recessive form DIDMOAD (diabetes insipidus, diabetes mellitus, optic atrophy and deafness – see Chapter 12), due to mutations in the wolframin gene.

– Nephrogenic diabetes insipidus is caused by the reduced action of ADH on the renal collecting ducts. The disorder may be either familial or acquired. There is an X-linked recessive form due to mutations in the vasopressin type 2 (V2) receptor gene and also an autosomal recessive form due to mutations in the aquaporin-2 gene (chromosome 12), which codes for the vasopressin-dependent water channel in the renal collecting ducts. Causes of secondary acquired diabetes insipidus include:

drugs, such as lithium carbonate, amphotericin or demeclocycline, which interfere with the action of ADH causing the clinical picture of nephrogenic diabetes insipidus,

hypercalcaemia or hypokalaemia, both of which impair the urine-concentrating mechanism and may present with polyuria.

Water deficiency without thirst is called adipsic, or hypodipsic, hypernatraemic syndrome or essential hypernatraemia, and is thought to be due to a hypothalamic disorder. In this syndrome there is a lack of thirst without polyuria.

Features of predominant water depletion

The *immediate effects* of water depletion result in:

- loss of water in excess of sodium: the plasma sodium concentration and therefore osmolality increase,
- reduction of circulating volume, which reduces renal blood flow and stimulates aldosterone secretion; sodium is retained and hypernatraemia is aggravated.

Compensatory effects occur because the increase in the plasma osmolality stimulates:

- thirst, increasing water intake, if water is available and if the patient can respond to it,
- ADH secretion: urinary volume falls and water loss through the kidney is reduced.

If an adequate amount of water is available, depletion is rapidly corrected. If there is an inadequate intake to replace the loss, hypernatraemia may occur before clinical signs of volume depletion are detectable. The clinical features of predominant water depletion include:

- thirst,
- oliguria and concentrated urine due to ADH secretion,
- *later* – signs of volume depletion.

Conversely, the clinical features differ if there is ADH deficiency, and include polyuria and dilute urine. The laboratory findings are:

- hypernatraemia,
- haemoconcentration due to fluid depletion,
- mild uraemia due to volume depletion and therefore low GFR,
- high urinary osmolality and urea concentration due to the action of ADH,
- low urinary sodium concentration in response to high aldosterone levels stimulated by the low renal blood flow.

Water and sodium excess

An excess of water or sodium is usually rapidly corrected. Syndromes of excess are usually associated with impaired homeostatic mechanisms. These can be conveniently classified into those with:

- oedematous states;
- predominant sodium excess, which may be caused by hyperaldosteronism or, in mentally disturbed subjects, by excessive salt intake; there may be mild hypernatraemia;
- predominant water excess, which may result from excessive ADH secretion or increased water intake and usually results in hyponatraemia.

Oedematous states (increased interstitial fluid)

Volume excess not primarily due to an osmotic difference across cell membranes may cause hypertension and cardiac failure. Oedema only occurs if:

- the capillary hydrostatic pressure is increased, as in congestive cardiac failure,

- the capillary colloid osmotic pressure is reduced due to hypoalbuminaemia.

Laboratory findings are characteristic of haemodilution and, unless there is glomerular dysfunction, plasma urea concentrations tend to be low.

Some factors that increase fluid accumulation in the interstitial space are summarized in Box 2.1.

Secondary aldosteronism

By convention, the term secondary aldosteronism usually refers to the clinical condition in which longstanding aldosterone secretion is stimulated by the renin–angiotensin system following a low renal blood flow (Fig. 2.10). This may be due to local abnormalities in renal vessels or to a reduced circulating volume and is therefore usually associated with the following.

> **Box 2.1 Some factors that increase the accumulation of fluid within the interstitial space (oedema)**
>
> *Decrease in colloid osmotic pressure gradient*
> Decrease in plasma colloid osmotic pressure
> Decrease in plasma albumin concentration
> Increase in capillary permeability to albumin:
> – 'Shock' and any severe illness
> – Infection with inflammation and therefore increased permeability of the capillary endothelium
>
> *Increase in hydrostatic pressure gradient*
> Heart failure with sodium retention

- Redistribution of ECF, leading to a reduced plasma volume despite a normal or even high total ECF volume. The resulting conditions may be caused by a reduction in plasma colloid osmotic pressure and are therefore associated with low plasma albumin concentrations. Oedema is present. Persistent hypoalbuminaemia may be due to liver disease, nephrotic syndrome or protein malnutrition.
- Cardiac failure, in which two factors may reduce renal blood flow and a third factor aggravates the hyperaldosteronism:
  - a low cardiac output results in poor renal perfusion,
  - an increased capillary hydrostatic pressure in cardiac failure may cause the redistribution of fluid into the interstitial space, with oedema,
  - both impaired catabolism of aldosterone and elevated plasma atrial natriuretic peptide concentration may aggravate the condition.
- Damage to renal vessels, reducing renal blood flow. These conditions are rarely associated with oedema and include:
  - essential hypertension,
  - malignant hypertension,
  - renal hypertension, such as that due to renal artery stenosis.

The reduced renal blood flow stimulates aldosterone secretion, with enhanced sodium reabsorption from the distal convoluted tubules and subsequent water retention. These processes tend to restore the intravascular volume. If there is hypoalbuminaemia or heart failure, more fluid passes into the interstitial fluid as the retained water dilutes

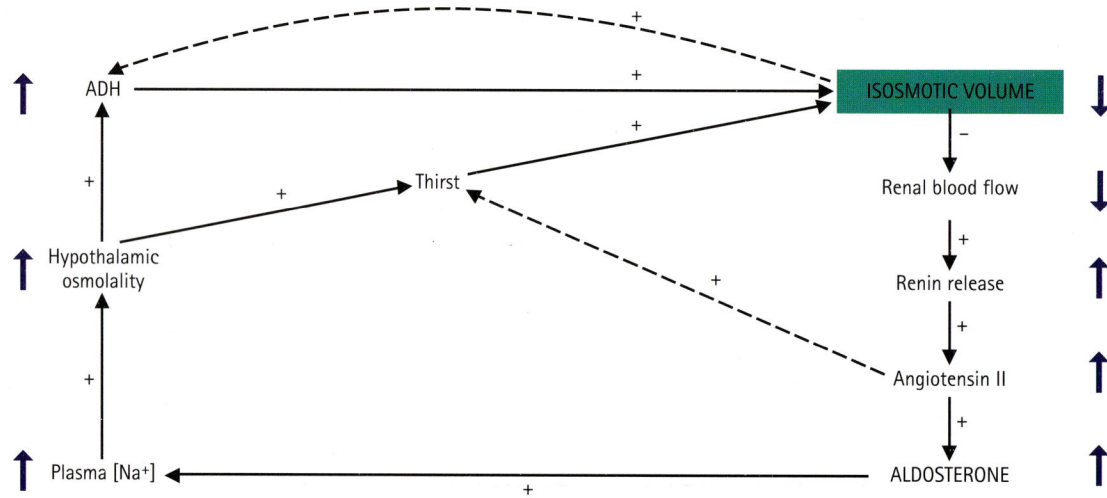

Fig. 2.10 Effect of secondary aldosterone secretion. Decreased effective intravascular volume increases renin and aldosterone secretion; if pronounced, antidiuretic hormone (ADH) secretion may be increased and thirst stimulated, resulting in hyponatraemia despite an increase in total body sodium. (Shaded area indicates the primary change.)

the plasma albumin concentration and therefore lowers the colloid osmotic pressure and raises the capillary hydrostatic pressure. The circulating volume can only be maintained by further fluid retention. A vicious cycle leads to the accumulation of excess fluid in the interstitial compartment (oedema).

Initially, this cycle stimulates a parallel increase in water and sodium retention, with normonatraemia. However, stimulation of ADH secretion by hypovolaemia, if long-standing, may cause enough sodium-free water retention to produce mild hyponatraemia despite the excess of total body sodium. Angiotensin II also stimulates thirst and therefore increases water intake.

Hypokalaemia is less common in secondary than in primary hyperaldosteronism, perhaps because the low GFR reduces the amount of sodium reaching the distal tubules and therefore the amount available for exchange with either hydrogen or potassium ions (see Chapters 4 and 5). However, if reabsorption of sodium without water is inhibited by loop diuretics, potassium depletion occurs more readily than in subjects without hyperaldosteronism.

The clinical features found in these patients are those of the underlying primary condition. Laboratory findings include:

- normonatraemia or hyponatraemia,
- a low urinary sodium concentration,
- those due to the primary abnormality, such as hypoalbuminaemia.

Predominant excess of sodium

Predominant sodium excess is rare. It is usually caused by inappropriate secretion of aldosterone, such as in primary hyperaldosteronism (Conn's syndrome), or by corticosteroids, as in Cushing's syndrome (see Chapter 8). In these syndromes, sodium retention stimulates the retention of water, minimizing changes in plasma sodium concentration. Sodium excess can also be caused by excessive sodium intake.

Primary hyperaldosteronism (Conn's syndrome)

About 50 per cent of cases of this syndrome are due to a single benign adenoma of the glomerulosa cells of the adrenal cortex, about 10 per cent of adenomas are multiple, and most of the remaining cases are associated with bilateral nodular hyperplasia of the adrenal cortex. Rarer causes include aldosterone-producing carcinoma of the adrenal gland or ectopic aldosterone-secreting tumours. Another rare form is glucocorticoid-suppressible hyperaldosteronism. In all these conditions aldosterone secretion is relatively autonomous (Fig. 2.11).

- Aldosterone excess causes urinary sodium retention.
- The rise in plasma sodium concentration stimulates ADH secretion and water retention.
- Water retention tends to restore plasma sodium concentrations to normal.
- Aldosterone secretion is not subject to normal feedback suppression. Its action causes sodium and water retention at the expense of potassium loss; hypokalaemic alkalosis is common (see Chapters 3, 4 and 5).

The typical clinical features of primary hyperaldosteronism are those of hypervolaemia (patients have mild to moderate hypertension but are rarely oedematous) and

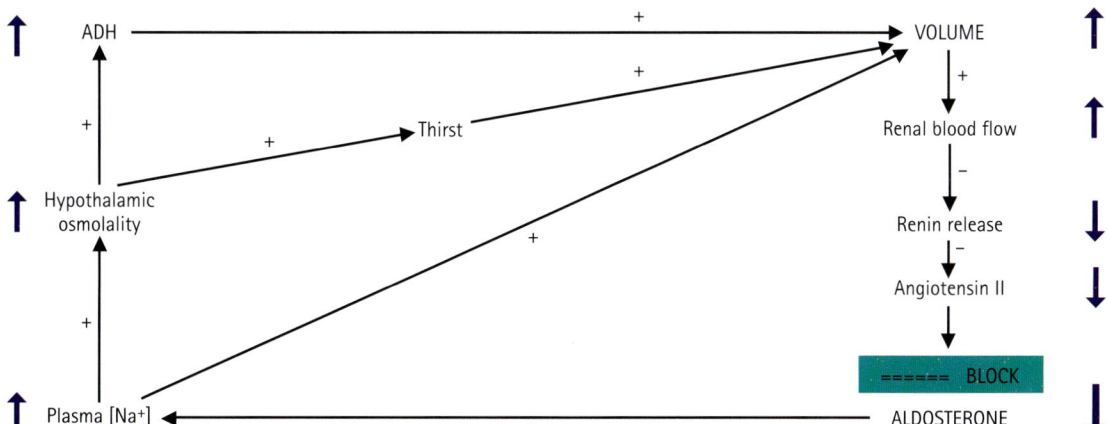

Fig. 2.11 Effect of primary aldosteronism (Conn's syndrome). Aldosterone secretion is relatively autonomous, causing sodium retention and increasing the plasma osmolality. This stimulates antidiuretic hormone (ADH) secretion. The increase in intravascular volume inhibits renin secretion. (Shaded area indicates the primary change.)

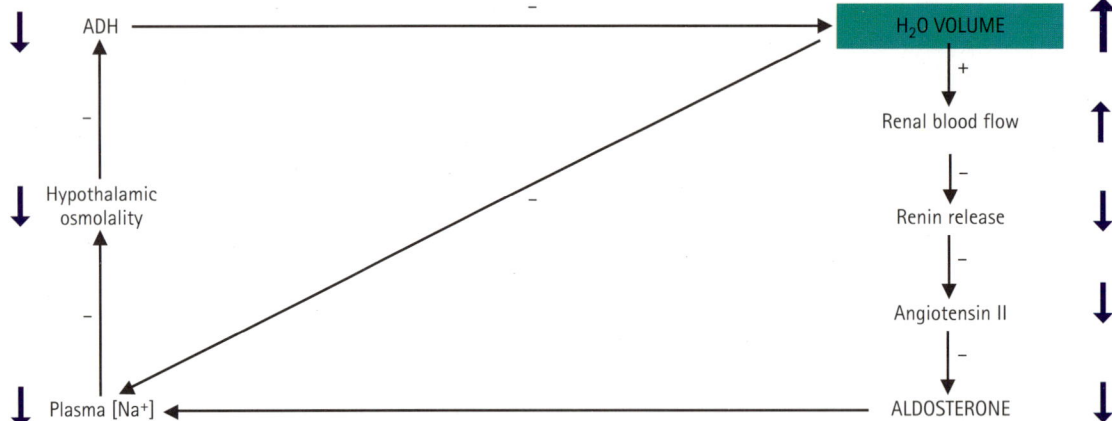

Fig. 2.12 Homeostatic correction of water excess. Increased intravascular water volume, with decreased plasma osmolality, inhibits aldosterone and antidiuretic hormone (ADH) secretion. (Shaded area indicates the primary change.)

those associated with hypokalaemia. The laboratory findings include the following.

- A plasma sodium concentration that may be within the higher reference range but may show hypernatraemia.
- Hypokalaemic alkalosis (low plasma potassium and raised plasma bicarbonate concentrations) due to excess aldosterone secretion.
  - A urinary potassium concentration greater than about 20 mmol/L, indicating kaliuria (urinary potassium loss) in the face of hypokalaemia.
  - A low urinary sodium concentration in the early stages; later, sodium excretion may rise, possibly because of hypokalaemic tubular damage.

These findings in a patient without an obvious reason for potassium loss and with mild to moderate hypertension suggest the diagnosis of primary hyperaldosteronism. The finding of high plasma aldosterone with low renin activity confirms the diagnosis; in secondary aldosteronism both the plasma aldosterone concentration and renin activity are high.

Cushing's syndrome

This results from glucocorticoid excess such as is found with adrenal or pituitary adenomas, ectopic adrenocorticotrophic hormone (ACTH) secretion or iatrogenically in patients treated with glucocorticoids (see Chapter 8).

Increased sodium intake

Sodium excess may be due to increased sodium intake, such as when excessive salt has been swallowed or overenthusiastic infusion of saline or sodium-containing solutions such as sodium bicarbonate or sodium salts of antibiotics have been infused.

Hyperosmolar saline is dangerous if used as an emetic in cases of poisoning. The movement of water into the gut along the osmotic gradient and absorption of some of the sodium can cause marked hypernatraemia. Death has occurred as a consequence of this practice, particularly when patients could not respond to hyperosmolality by drinking because of vomiting or because they were unconscious.

Predominant excess of water

Predominant water overload may occur in circumstances in which normal homeostasis has failed, for example in the following.

- If fluid of low sodium concentration, such as 5 per cent dextrose, has been infused, especially in the postoperative period or if there is glomerular dysfunction (see Fig. 2.12 and Chapter 3).
- If there is 'inappropriate' ADH secretion. Antidiuretic hormone release may be stimulated by stress, such as that due to pain, nausea, chest infection and cerebral trauma (Box 2.2).

Hormone secretion is defined as inappropriate if it continues when it should be cut off by negative feedback control, in this case by a low plasma osmolality. Like many other peptide hormones, ADH can sometimes be synthesized by non-endocrine malignant cells, such as small oat-cell carcinoma of the lung, and released ectopically. Inappropriate secretion of ADH, from the pituitary or hypothalamus and therefore not 'ectopic', is very common in many illnesses, such as disorders of the pulmonary and central nervous systems.

The diagnosis of SIADH is usually made by finding a urinary sodium concentration more than 20 mmol/L in

> **Box 2.2 Some causes of hyponatraemia due to the syndrome of inappropriate antidiuretic hormone secretion (SIADH)**
>
> Stress/nausea/vomiting/pain
> Postoperation/trauma
> Infections, e.g. pneumonia
> Ectopic secretion by tumours, e.g. oat-cell or small-cell lung carcinoma
> Central nervous system disease, e.g. meningitis or stroke
> Acute porphyria
> Drugs, e.g. vincristine, chlorpropamide, carbamazepine, non-steroidal anti-inflammatory drugs, certain antidepressants, oxytocin and opiates

the presence of euvolaemic hyponatraemia or low plasma osmolality and in the absence of hypovolaemia, oedema, impaired renal function, diuretic usage, adrenal insufficiency or hypothyroidism. According to the Bartter and Schwartz criteria for SIADH, the urinary osmolality is inappropriately concentrated in relation to the plasma osmolality, i.e. in the hypo-osmal state the urine is not maximally diluted. In SIADH, the GFR is usually high and plasma urea and urate concentrations tend to be low.

- During the intravenous administration of the posterior pituitary hormone oxytocin (Syntocinon) to induce labour (see Chapter 7). Oxytocin has an antidiuretic effect similar to that of the chemically closely related ADH. If 5 per cent dextrose saline is used as a carrier, the glucose is metabolized and the net effect is retention of solute-free water. Death from acute hypo-osmolality has resulted after prolonged infusion; oxytocin should be given in the smallest possible volume of isotonic saline and the fluid balance and plasma sodium concentrations should be monitored carefully.
- Excess water intake can also occur if water intake exceeds water clearance (about 20 L/day), for example in beer potomania (excess beer intake) or psychogenic polydipsia.

Features of water excess

In the presence of normal homeostatic mechanisms, excessive water intake:

- tends to lower plasma sodium concentration, leading to hyponatraemia,
- increases renal blood flow and cuts off aldosterone secretion, increasing urinary sodium loss and therefore further decreasing its plasma concentration,
- lowers plasma osmolality and therefore cuts off ADH secretion; a large volume of dilute urine is passed.

When glomerular function is impaired, the excretion of excess water may be limited. If there is appropriate ADH secretion, or if oxytocin is being infused, for example during labour, water retention continues despite the low plasma osmolality and compensation cannot occur.

Hyponatraemia

Hyponatraemia is usually caused by excessive water relative to sodium within the extracellular compartment or, more rarely, by sodium deficiency, and may reflect extracellular hypo-osmolality (see Box 2.3). If this is the case, it may cause cellular over-hydration. However, hyponatraemia associated with a normal plasma osmolality may occur in the following situations.

> **Box 2.3 Some causes of hyponatraemia**
>
> *Plasma osmolality normal or increased*
> Pseudohyponatraemia:
>   severe hyperlipidaemia or hyperproteinaemia
>   artefactual, e.g. drip arm
> Appropriate hyponatraemia:
>   acute uraemia
>   hyperglycaemia
>   infusion of amino acids or mannitol
>   alcohol
> Sick cell syndrome
>
> *Plasma osmolality low*
> Hypovolaemic (decreased extracellular volume):
>   non-renal losses (e.g. vomiting, diarrhoea)
>   renal losses (e.g. diuretics or salt-losing nephropathy)
>   adrenal insufficiency (Addison's disease)
> Euvolaemic:
>   excess fluid replacement, e.g. hypotonic (sodium free) 5% dextrose
>   syndrome of inappropriate antidiuretic hormone secretion (SIADH)
>   hypothyroidism
>   potomania or psychogenic polydipsia
> Hypervolaemic (increased extracellular volume):
>   congestive cardiac failure
>   nephrotic syndrome
>   cirrhosis and ascites

- *Artefactual hyponatraemia* may be due to blood being taken from the limb into which fluid of low sodium concentration, such as 5 per cent dextrose, is being infused.
- *Pseudohyponatraemia* may be due to gross hyperlipidaemia or to hyperproteinaemia. The sodium concentration in plasma water, and therefore the osmolality at cell membranes, may then be normal (see Fig. 2.2).
- *Appropriate* hyponatraemia may be due, for example, to hyperglycaemia, acute uraemia, the infusion of amino acids or mannitol, a high plasma alcohol or other solute concentrations (redistributive hyponatraemia). All these may increase extracellular osmolality; the consequent homeostatic dilution of total extracellular solute concentration towards normal causes hyponatraemia, which reflects partial or complete compensation of hyperosmolality rather than hypo-osmolality.

$$\text{Corrected plasma concentration} = \text{measured plasma sodium concentration} + \frac{\text{plasma glucose concentration}}{4 \text{ (mmol/L)}} \quad (2.3)$$

The infusion of isosmolal sodium-containing fluids with the aim of 'correcting' artefactual, appropriate or pseudo-hyponatraemia is dangerous.

When hyponatraemia reflects true hypo-osmolality, cerebral cellular over-hydration may cause headache, confusion, fits and even death. If the plasma sodium concentration falls slowly over days or weeks, the brain can compensate by the redistribution of water and solute between the intracellular and extracellular fluid. However, if the plasma sodium concentration declines rapidly over 24–48 hours, these processes are inefficient and cerebral oedema can occur. Cerebral pontine myelinolysis can occur if the plasma sodium concentration is corrected too rapidly, before redistribution can be reversed. The rapid change in osmolality causes focal demyelination in the pons and extrapontine regions, which may lead to hypotension, seizures, quadriparesis and death.

Some causes of hyponatraemia are shown in Box 2.3. These can be conveniently grouped into hypovolaemic, euvolaemic and hypervolaemic forms based on the clinical features.

- *Hypovolaemic hyponatraemia*: the total body water (TBW) decreases although the total body sodium decreases to a larger extent. Thus the ECF volume is decreased.
- *Euvolaemic hyponatraemia*: total body sodium is normal, while TBW increases. The ECF volume is slightly increased but there is no oedema. One cause is SIADH (Box 2.2).
- *Hypervolaemic hyponatraemia*: the total body sodium increases but TBW increases to a greater extent. The ECF is markedly increased and oedema is present.

Investigation of hyponatraemia (Fig. 2.13)

- Exclude artefactual hyponatraemia when blood is taken from the vein into which fluid is being infused. This occurs whether the blood is taken proximally or distally to the site of infusion, where the infused fluid is at a higher concentration than in the rest of the circulation.
- Is there hyperlipidaemia or hyperproteinaemia? Exclude pseudohyponatraemia when plasma osmolality is normal.

CASE 1

A 74-year-old retired male presented to his general practitioner with haemoptysis and weight loss. He had smoked 20 cigarettes a day for 55 years. Chest X-ray revealed a left upper lobe shadow, and bronchoscopy confirmed a primary lung carcinoma. His blood pressure was 132/80 mmHg and clinically he was euvolaemic.

There was no evidence of adrenal insufficiency or thyroid disease and he was not taking any medications.

Some results were as follows.

Plasma
Sodium 112 mmol/L (135–145)
Potassium 3.6 mmol/L (3.5–5.0)
Urea 3.6 mmol/L (2.5–7.0)
Creatinine 98 μmol/L (70–110)
Urine spot sodium: 58 mmol/L

DISCUSSION

The most likely explanation for the severe hyponatraemia is SIADH. Some lung carcinomas ectopically release ADH. Note that the patient was clinically euvolaemic and there was no other evidence of other causes of euvolaemic hyponatraemia, such as adrenal insufficiency or hypothyroidism. The urinary sodium concentration is inappropriate for the hyponatraemia (>20 mmol/L).

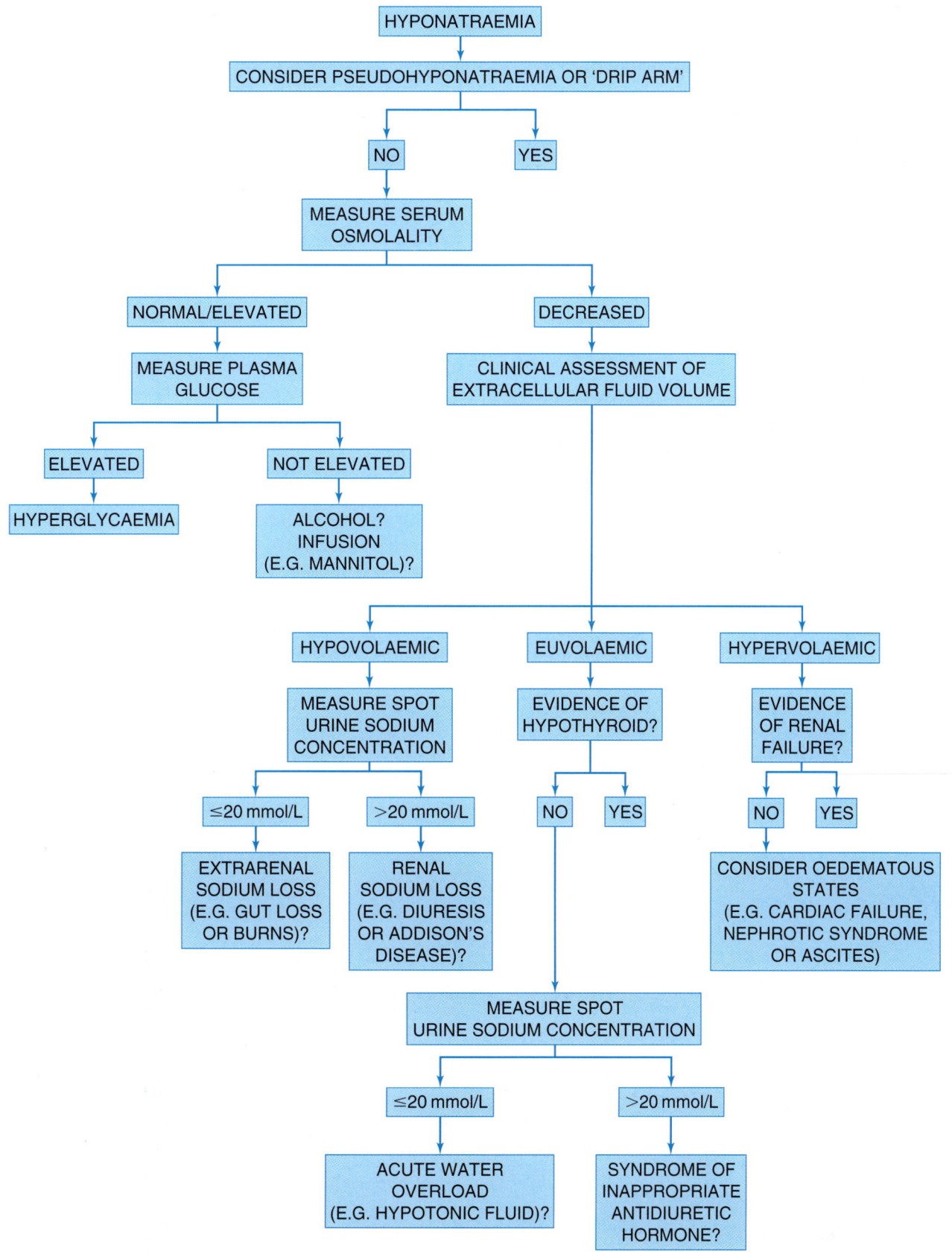

Fig. 2.13 Summary algorithm for the investigation of hyponatraemia.

- Assess the patient's medication history, including intravenous fluid therapy and also alcohol intake.
- Hyperglycaemia can result in excessive extracellular solute and water shift out of cells:

Corrected sodium concentration
$$= \frac{[glucose]}{4} + \text{measured [sodium] (mmol/L)} \quad (2.4)$$

- Abnormal electrolyte shifts may occur very rarely in critically ill patients (the sick cell syndrome).
- It is important to exclude adrenal insufficiency (Addison's disease) and hypothyroidism (see Chapters 8 and 11). These are rare causes.
- Clinically assess the state of the ECF volume; is there obvious hypovolaemia, euvolaemia or hypervolaemia?
  - If there is obvious hypovolaemia, check the sodium concentration in a random urine specimen: if it is less than or equal to 20 mmol/L, it is suggestive of extrarenal sodium loss; if it is more than 20 mmol/L, it suggests renal sodium loss.
  - If the patient is clinically euvolaemic, check a random urinary sodium concentration: if it is less than or equal to 20 mmol/L, consider acute water overload, for example due to the administration of too much fluid postoperatively; if it is more than 20 mmol/L, consider SIADH (see Box 2.2).
  - If the patient is oedematous and is not in cardiac or renal tubular failure, consider nephrotic syndrome.

See Box 2.3 for some of the other causes of hyponatraemia.

Treatment of hyponatraemia

It cannot be stressed too strongly that treatment should not be based on plasma sodium concentrations alone. Hyponatraemia per se only rarely needs to be treated. Ignorance of the causes of hyponatraemia is, unfortunately, still common. For example, iatrogenic postoperative hyponatraemia due to the injudicious use of isotonic dextrose is still encountered and can result in neurological damage or death. Menopausal women, children and the elderly are especially susceptible to mild hyponatraemia, particularly if they are taking diuretics or some antidepressant drugs. Furthermore, there is also misunderstanding about the most appropriate treatment of severe hyponatraemia: rapid correction can cause cerebral myelinolysis, and correction that is too slow may allow cerebral oedema to develop.

Severe hyponatraemia known to have been present for less than 48 hours should be treated as a medical emergency; because of the danger of brainstem herniation, the aim should be to abolish symptoms or to raise the plasma sodium concentration to about 125 mmol/L. Some people recommend infusion of sodium at the rate of 1 or 2 mmol/hour. Patients with signs of acute brainstem herniation such as coma or seizures may need twice-normal (hypertonic) saline rapidly to correct plasma sodium concentration to about 120 mmol/L; only enough should be given to stop neurological symptoms.

Conversely, similar severe degrees of hyponatraemia that are known to have been present for more than 48 hours and without clinical evidence of cerebral oedema can be treated by *slow* infusion of 0.5 mmol/hour until

CASE 2

A 74-year-old woman underwent a left total hip replacement and had received 5 L of 5 per cent dextrose intravenously over one day. She had the following postoperative results.

Plasma
Sodium 117 mmol/L (135–145)
Potassium 3.7 mmol/L (3.5–5.0)
Urea 3.4 mmol/L (2.5–7.0)
Creatinine 76 μmol/L (70–110)

The preoperative results were as follows.

Plasma
Sodium 138 mmol/L (135–145)

Potassium 4.2 mmol/L (3.5–5.0)
Urea 5.6 mmol/L (2.5–7.0)
Creatinine 90 μmol/L (70–110)

DISCUSSION

The patient was being infused with large amounts of 5 per cent dextrose intravenously. This was the most likely cause of her postoperative hyponatraemia. The administration of hypotonic and sodium-free fluid was causing a dilutional hyponatraemia. This is a particularly dangerous practice postoperatively, when ADH secretion is increased due to the stress of the operation and of nausea and pain, thus increasing the likelihood of water retention.

the plasma concentration reaches 130 mmol/L. Normal (isotonic) or hypertonic saline should be infused, and fluid restriction or administration of loop diuretics depend on the severity of the hyponatraemia. Close monitoring of plasma (hourly) and urinary sodium is required to ensure safe correction.

If the patient is not dehydrated and SIADH has been diagnosed, fluid intake restriction to 80–1000 mL/day may be indicated. Administration of demeclocycline, by antagonizing the action of ADH on renal tubules, may also help.

Remember when considering intravenous sodium treatment that:

- 0.9 per cent (normal) saline contains 154 mmol/L of sodium,
- 1.8 per cent (twice-normal) saline contains 308 mmol/L of sodium.

Sodium (Na) requirement
= total body water (TBW) × (desired [Na]   (2.5)
  − current [Na])

$$TBW = \text{body weight (kg)} \times \%\text{water} \quad (2.6)$$

Children: TBW = 0.6 × body weight.
Adults: TBW = 0.55 × body weight.
Elderly: TBW = 0.5 × body weight.

The example below shows how to calculate saline replacement in an elderly patient weighing 80 kg with symptomatic severe hyponatraemia of 110 mmol/L. The patient is euvolaemic and the aim is for plasma sodium of 125 mmol/L.

$$\text{Na requirement} = 80 \times 0.5 \times (125 - 110)$$
$$= 600 \text{ mmol} \quad (2.7)$$

If you aim to give treatment over 30 hours = 20 mmol/hour of sodium. That is 20 × 1000/154 mL of normal saline an hour = approximately 130 mL, or 65 mL/hour twice-normal saline.

Hypernatraemia (Fig. 2.14)

Hypernatraemia always reflects hyperosmolality if artefactual causes such as the use of sodium heparin as an anticoagulant in the specimen container have been excluded. Severe hypernatraemia can never be appropriate to the osmolal state; the plasma concentrations of solutes other than sodium are very low and do not contribute significantly to the plasma osmolality. For example, although hyperglycaemia can increase the plasma osmolality by as much as 50 mmol/kg in 290 mmol/kg (about

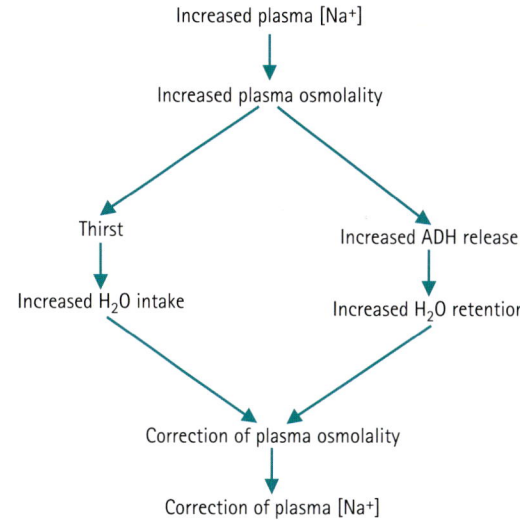

Fig. 2.14 Homeostatic mechanisms involved in the correction of hypernatraemia. (ADH = antidiuretic hormone.)

17 per cent), complete absence of glucose would only reduce it by about 5 mmol/kg (about 2 per cent).

The symptoms associated with hypernatraemia may include weakness, malaise, mental confusion, delirium and coma.

Some causes of hypernatraemia are shown in Box 2.4. These can also be grouped into euvolaemic, hypovolaemic and hypervolaemic forms based on the clinical features.

Investigation of hypernatraemia (Fig. 2.15)

- Remember that hypernatraemia is most commonly due to predominant loss of water rather than to excess of sodium.
- Is fluid of high sodium concentration being infused? Much less commonly there may be a very high oral sodium intake, but this is often deliberate. Some antibiotics have a high sodium content.
- Clinically assess the patient's state of hydration and fluid balance.
- Is there polyuria? If so, look for evidence of diabetes insipidus. Determine the ratio of urinary to plasma osmolality (see later).
- If there is mild hypernatraemia with hypokalaemia and hypertension, consider mineralocorticoid excess, due, for example, to administration of steroids or to Cushing's syndrome or primary hyperaldosteronism.

Other causes of hypernatraemia are shown in Box 2.4, and may be clinically obvious.

> **Box 2.4 Some causes of hypernatraemia**
>
> *Artefactual hypernatraemia*
> e.g. The use of sodium heparin as an anticoagulant
>
> *Water deficit greater than sodium deficit (hypovolaemic)*
> Poor intake:
>   unavailability of water
>   failure to drink
>   unconsciousness or confusion
>   infants
>   damage to thirst centre
> Renal loss:
>   osmotic diuretics, post-obstructive diuresis
> Extrarenal loss:
>   diarrhoea, fistulas, vomiting, major burns
>
> *Impaired water retention (euvolaemic)*
> Extrarenal loss:
>   increased insensible loss, e.g. hyperventilation
> Renal losses of water:
>   osmotic diuresis such as glycosuria, increased urea load
>   diabetes insipidus (cranial or nephrogenic)
>
> *Excessive sodium retention (sodium gains greater than water gains – hypervolaemic)*
> Excessive sodium intake
> Hypertonic saline
> Excess sodium bicarbonate administration
> Accidental salt ingestion
> Drugs containing sodium, e.g. carbenicillin
> Excess mineralocorticoid:
>   Conn's syndrome
>   Cushing's syndrome

> **Box 2.5 Some causes of polyuria**
>
> *Increased fluid intake (oral or intravenous)*
> Oral or intravenous therapy
> Thyrotoxicosis
> Psychogenic polydipsia
>
> *Osmotic diuresis*
> Endogenous substances:
>   glycosuria
>   uraemia
> Exogenous substances:
>   mannitol infusion (used therapeutically)
>
> *Impaired antidiuretic hormone production (cranial diabetes insipidus)*
> Congenital
> Acquired:
>   cerebral trauma
>   infection
>   cerebral tumours and other infiltrations
>   drugs and other agents, e.g. alcohol
>
> *Impaired renal tubular response to antidiuretic hormone (nephrogenic diabetes insipidus)*
> Congenital
> Acquired:
>   chronic failure
>   interstitial nephritis
>   medullary cystic disease
>   hypercalcaemia or hypokalaemia
>   drugs – lithium carbonate, demeclocycline
>   predominant tubular dysfunction
>
> *Other drugs*
> Diuretics

Treatment of hypernatraemia

If the hypernatraemia is due to water depletion, oral repletion is the treatment of choice. If this is not possible, fluid of low sodium concentration should be infused *slowly*. The aim should be to lower the plasma sodium concentration at no more than 1–2 mmol/L per hour or less, especially if the hypernatraemia is of long standing.

In hypervolaemic hypernatraemia, the hypernatraemia may improve if patients reduce their salt intake. The management of primary hyperaldosteronism (Conn's syndrome) and Cushing's syndrome is discussed in Chapter 8.

Cranial diabetes insipidus is usually treated with desmopressin. Hereditary nephrogenic diabetes insipidus can be difficult to treat, although thiazide diuretics or prostaglandin inhibitors such as indometacin have been used.

Investigation of polyuria (Fig. 2.16)

The causes of polyuria are given in Box 2.5. Polyuria is usually defined as more than 3 L of urine per day. The causes and investigation of anuria (no urine) or oliguria (less than 400 mL/day) are discussed in Chapter 3.

- Take a clinical history and examine the patient.
  – Distinguish between true polyuria (check 24-hour urinary volume) and frequency (a normal 24-hour volume but abnormally frequent micturition).

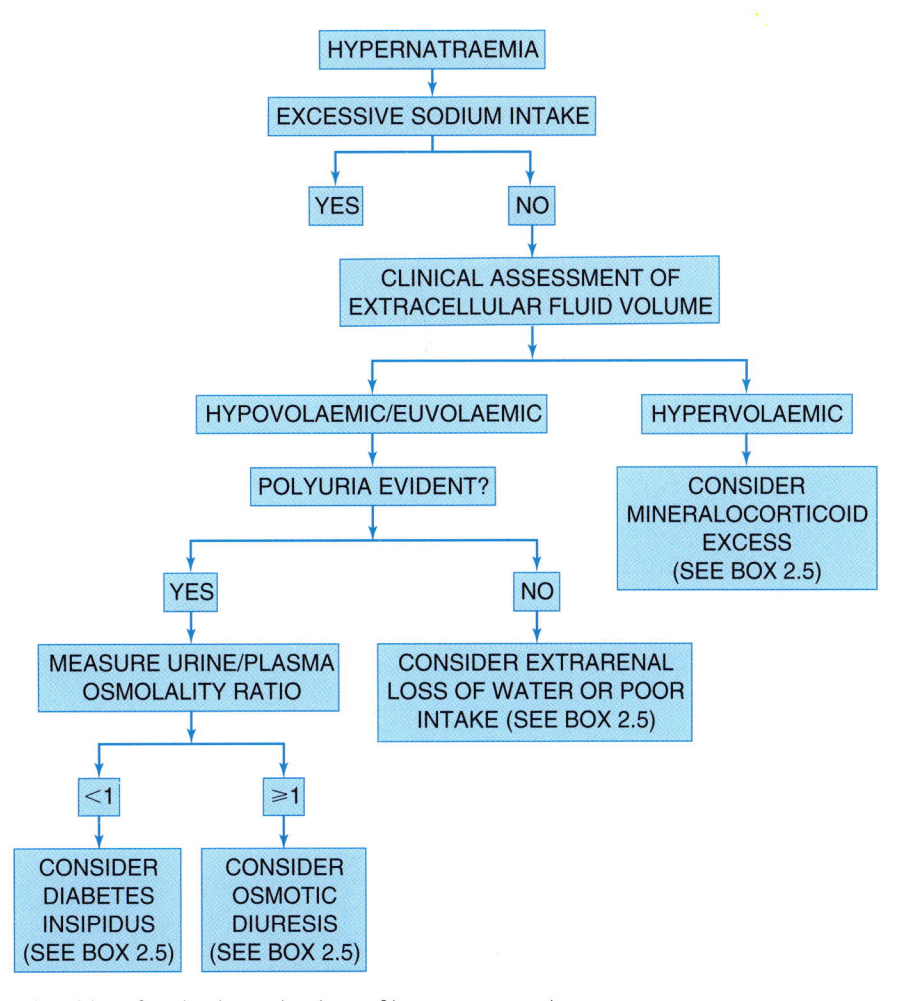

Fig. 2.15 Summary algorithm for the investigation of hypernatraemia.

CASE 3

A 5-year-old girl was admitted to hospital because of a 4-day history of diarrhoea and vomiting. On examination she was found to be clinically 'dehydrated' with loss of skin turgor; her pulse was 120 beats/minute and her blood pressure 74/50 mmHg.

Her admission results were as follows.

Plasma
Sodium 167 mmol/L (135–145)
Potassium 3.0 mmol/L (3.5–5.0)
Urea 19 mmol/L (2.5–7.0)
Creatinine 110 µmol/L (70–110)
Urine spot sodium: <10 mmol/L

DISCUSSION

The severe hypernatraemia is in keeping with hypotonic fluid loss due to the diarrhoea and vomiting. The loss of skin turgor, tachycardia and hypotension suggest hypovolaemia. The low urinary sodium concentration indicates renal sodium conservation. Children are particularly susceptible to hypernatraemia induced by hypotonic fluid loss.

A midstream urine specimen may be useful to exclude urinary tract infection as a cause of urinary frequency.
- Is the patient taking diuretics? Consider other drugs, for example lithium or demeclocycline.
- If there is a recent history of oliguric renal failure, the patient has probably entered the polyuric phase, and should be treated accordingly (see Chapter 3).
- Exclude chronic renal failure, hypokalaemia, hypercalcaemia, adrenal insufficiency and thyrotoxicosis.

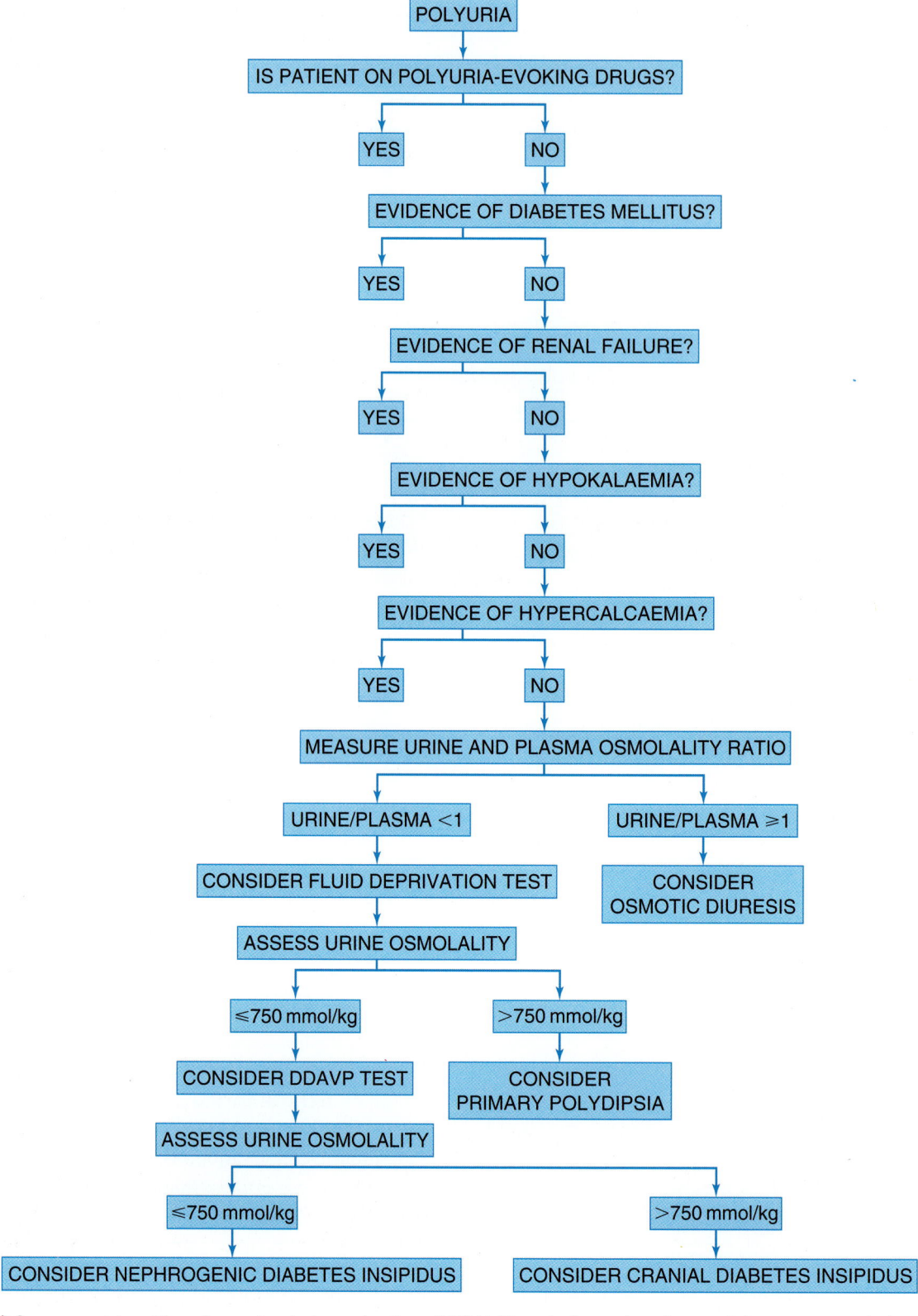

Fig. 2.16 Summary algorithm for polyuria investigation. (DDAVP = 1-desamino-8-D-arginine vasopressin.)

- Check for causes of an osmotic diuresis such as:
  - severe glycosuria due to diabetes mellitus or infusion of dextrose,
  - tissue damage, leading to a high urea load,
  - infusion of amino acids, for example during parenteral nutrition,
  - in infants, consider inborn errors of metabolism (see Chapter 27),
  - osmotic diuretics, for example mannitol.
- Accurately monitor fluid intake and output. The patient should be carefully watched for secret fluid ingestion (psychogenic polydipsia). Some patients may even add fluid to their urine.
- Measure plasma urea and creatinine and electrolyte concentrations.
  - Elevated plasma urea and/or creatinine concentrations suggests renal impairment.
  - Low or low-normal plasma urea or creatinine concentrations, especially if there is mild hyponatraemia, suggest that polydipsia is the primary cause and that the polyuria is appropriate. Question the patient about his/her intake in relation to true thirst. Patients with true psychogenic polydipsia may give misleading answers.
- Measure the urinary and plasma osmolality. In an osmotic diuresis the urine:plasma osmolality ratio is usually more than 1.
- If urinary osmolality is more than 750 mmol/kg, a water deprivation test is not usually indicated.
- If it is still not possible to distinguish between psychogenic polydipsia and diabetes insipidus, contact the laboratory to arrange a water deprivation test, if necessary by administering 1-desamino-8-D-arginine vasopressin (DDAVP) (see below). This may help distinguish cranial diabetes insipidus from nephrogenic diabetes insipidus (see below).
- In difficult cases when diabetes insipidus is suspected and the water deprivation test has not been helpful, a hypertonic saline test may be indicated (see below).
- In cases of cranial diabetes insipidus, a neurological opinion may be necessary. Is there a possible obvious cause for diabetes insipidus, such as a head injury? (See Chapter 7.) Consider brain imaging such as computerized tomography or magnetic resonance imaging.

The causes of nephrogenic diabetes insipidus are given in Box 2.5 (see also Chapter 3).

Water deprivation test

This section should be read in conjunction with Chapter 7, in which pituitary hormonal function is discussed. The restriction of water intake for some hours should stimulate posterior pituitary ADH secretion. Solute-free water is reabsorbed from the collecting ducts and concentrated urine is passed. Maximal water reabsorption is impaired if:

- the countercurrent multiplication mechanism is impaired,
- ADH activity is low.

If the feedback mechanism is intact, plasma ADH levels are already high and the administration of exogenous hormone will not improve the renal concentrating power. If diabetes insipidus is the cause, tubular function is normal and

---

CASE 4

Below are the preoperative blood results of a 44-year-old male. The sample was reported by the laboratory to be grossly 'lipaemic'.

Plasma
Sodium 118 mmol/L (135–145)
Potassium 4.0 mmol/L (3.5–5.0)
Urea 6.0 mmol/L (2.5–7.0)
Creatinine 95 μmol/L (70–110)
Glucose 4.0 mmol/L (3.5–5.5)
Cholesterol 17.3 mmol/L (3–5)
Triglycerides 68 mmol/L (<1.5)
Osmolality 290 mmol/kg (275–295)

Further tests excluded other common causes of hyponatraemia.

DISCUSSION

The plasma osmolality was not low despite hyponatraemia, suggesting pseudohyponatraemia. This is probably due to the gross lipaemia when measured by indirect sodium-ion-detecting electrodes (direct electrodes do not usually detect pseudohyponatraemia). Note that calculated plasma osmolality is 2[118 + 4] + 6.0 + 4.0 mmol/L = 254 mmol/kg, which differs markedly from the measured value of 290 mmol/kg.

therefore the administration of ADH will increase the renal concentrating ability and increase the urinary osmolality.

Warning. The test should not be performed if the patient is volume depleted or has even mild hypernatraemia. In such cases the finding of a low urinary to plasma osmolality ratio (see below) should be diagnostic, and further fluid restriction may be dangerous. If the test is necessary, it must be stopped if:

- the patient becomes distressed;
- the plasma osmolality (or sodium concentration) rises to high or high-normal concentrations – usually taken as more than 300 mmol/kg; urine and blood specimens should be collected at once;
- the patient loses more than 3 per cent of their body weight.

Procedure

Always contact the laboratory *before* starting the test, both to ensure efficient and speedy analysis and to check local variations in the protocol.

Patients are not allowed food or water after about 20.00 hours on the night before the test. *They must be in hospital and closely observed* during the period of fluid restriction. The duration of water deprivation depends on the clinical presentation and the degree of polyuria.

On the day of the test

08.00 hours The bladder is emptied. Blood and urine are collected and plasma and urinary osmolalities are measured. If the plasma osmolality is low-normal or low, water depletion is unlikely and polyuria is probably due to an appropriate response to a high intake. If the plasma osmolality is high-normal or high and the urinary osmolality is more than 750 mmol/kg, the test should be stopped.

09.00 hours Blood and urine are again collected and the plasma and urinary osmolalities are measured.

Interpretation (Table 2.5)

The duration of the test depends on changes in the urinary osmolalities.

- If the urinary osmolality is more than 750 mmol/kg, neither significant tubular disease nor diabetes insipidus is likely and the test may be stopped.
- If the urinary osmolality is less than 750 mmol/kg, and plasma osmolality is normal, fluid restriction should be continued and the estimations repeated at hourly intervals. The test should be stopped as soon as the urinary osmolality exceeds 750 mmol/kg.

Table 2.5 Summary of the results of water deprivation/DDAVP tests

Post-water restriction		Post-DDAVP	
Plasma osmolality (mmol/kg)	Urine osmolality (mmol/kg)	Urine osmolality (mmol/kg)	Interpretation
285–295	>750	>750	Normal
>295	<300	>750	Cranial diabetes insipidus
>295	<300	<300	Nephrogenic diabetes insipidus

DDAVP = 1-desamino-8-D-arginine vasopressin.

- Failure of concentration of three consecutive urine specimens indicates either tubular disease or diabetes insipidus. If the diagnosis of diabetes insipidus is considered, continue with the DDAVP test.

DDAVP test

DDAVP is a potent synthetic analogue of vasopressin.

Procedure

Give 2 µg DDAVP intramuscularly; continue to collect urine and plasma samples.

Interpretation

If there is tubular dysfunction or nephrogenic diabetes insipidus, there will be no change in the urinary osmolality, but the plasma osmolality may increase due to water loss during the test. In cranial diabetes insipidus the urinary osmolality increases, usually to a value more than 750 mmol/kg.

After prolonged over-hydration, usually due to psychogenic polydipsia, concentrating power may be impaired, even after the administration of exogenous hormone. This is due to 'washing out' of medullary hyperosmolality. The test should be repeated after several days of relative water restriction. The patient should be kept under close observation, both for signs of genuine distress associated with a rise in plasma osmolality and for surreptitious drinking.

Hypertonic saline test

In some cases in which there is diagnostic difficulty with the fluid deprivation test, the hypertonic saline test is used, but expert advice should be sought. This test is sometimes used to make a diagnosis of cranial diabetes insipidus in patients with polyuria but normal plasma osmolality. It is potentially dangerous, as fluid overload can occur, and therefore should not be used in patients with cardiac or cerebral disease, or epilepsy.

The test is based on the principle that the infusion of 5 per cent hypertonic saline, by raising plasma osmolality, normally causes maximal ADH secretion. It can be summarized as follows.

- The patient fasts from midnight.
- 5 per cent saline is infused (0.06 mL/kg per minute for 2 hours).
- Blood samples are taken at baseline and 30-minute intervals.
- Plasma ADH is measured before and after the test along with urine and plasma osmolality.
- The patient must be closely monitored during the test and the blood pressure and weight recorded.

Patients with cranial diabetes insipidus have little or no ADH rise. Conversely, in nephrogenic diabetes insipidus there is ADH release during the test.

CONCLUSIONS

- Water and sodium homeostasis are intimately related and essential for doctors to understand when investigating and managing hyponatraemia and hypernatraemia. Summary algorithms for the investigation of hyponatraemia and hypernatraemia are depicted in Figs 2.13 and 2.15.
- Patient fluid balance must be monitored carefully, with attention to the input and output, particularly for those on 'drip' therapy.
- Sodium is the main ECF cation and is controlled by adrenal aldosterone (renal sodium retention if ECF falls) and atrial natrial peptides.
- Body water excretion is controlled by ADH (vasopressin). Decreased ECF volume and increased ECF osmolality stimulate ADH release from post-pituitary gland.
- Polyuria (daily urine output more than 3 L) may be due to failures of renal concentrating ability or lack of ADH (Fig. 2.16).

3 THE KIDNEYS

Renal glomerular function	37	Nephrotic syndrome	49
Renal tubular function	37	Diagnosis of renal dysfunction	50
Water reabsorption: urinary concentration and dilution	38	Urinary sodium and osmolality	52
Biochemistry of renal disorders	42	Biochemical principles of the treatment of renal dysfunction	53
Syndromes reflecting predominant tubular damage – renal tubular acidosis	49	Renal calculi	54

In this chapter kidney function and how it can be altered in disease states is also discussed. It is best read in conjunction with Chapters 2, 4 and 5. Interpretation of renal function tests is also discussed.

The kidneys excrete metabolic waste products and have an essential homeostatic function by controlling the body solute and water status and the acid–base balance. There are about one million nephrons per kidney, each of which is made up of five main functional segments (Fig. 3.1).

The *glomeruli*, in the cortex of the kidney, are invaginated and surround a capillary network of blood vessels derived from the afferent, and draining into the efferent, arterioles. Small molecules and water are passively filtered during the passage of blood through these capillaries, the ultrafiltrate passing through the vessel walls and the glomerular membranes into the glomerular spaces (Bowman's capsules).

The *proximal convoluted tubules*, also in the cortex, receive filtrate from the glomerular spaces. Convolution increases the tubular length and therefore contact between the luminal fluid and the proximal tubular cells.

The *loops of Henle* extend down into the renal medulla and ascend again after forming the loop.

The *distal convoluted tubules*, situated in the cortex, are important for fine adjustment of luminal fluid. They lie

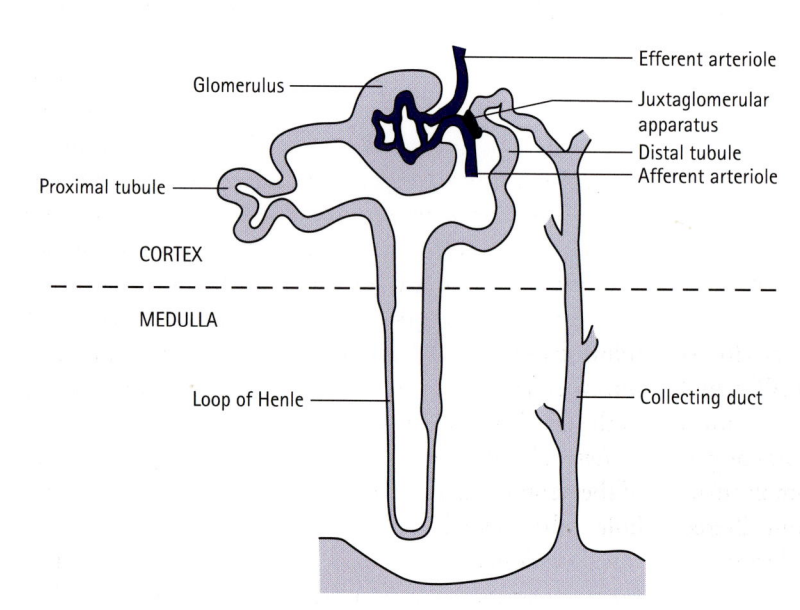

Fig. 3.1 The anatomical relation between the nephron and the juxtaglomerular apparatus.

near the afferent arterioles with the juxtaglomerular apparatus between them. The peptide hormone renin is produced by the latter and its release is controlled by local blood flow.

The *collecting ducts* start as the distal tubules lead down into the medulla and end by opening into the renal pelvis. The modified fluid from the original filtrate flows from the collecting ducts into the renal tract.

Normal function of the kidneys depends on the following:

- An adequate blood supply, which under normal circumstances is about 20 per cent of the cardiac output, flowing through the kidneys.
- Normal secretion and feedback control of hormones acting on the kidney.
- The integrity of the glomeruli and the tubular cells.

In addition to the excretory function and acid–base control, the kidneys have important endocrine functions, including:

- 1,25-dihydroxyvitamin D is the active metabolite of vitamin D. It is produced following hepatic hydroxylation of 25-hydroxyvitamin by the renal enzyme 1-hydroxylase.
- Erythropoietin, which stimulates erythropoiesis.
- Renin is produced by the juxtaglomerular apparatus.

RENAL GLOMERULAR FUNCTION

About 200 L of plasma ultrafiltrate usually enter the tubular lumina daily, mainly by glomerular filtration into glomerular capsules but also through the spaces between cells lining the tubules (tight junctions). Production of ultrafiltrate depends on the blood flow through normal glomeruli and on the difference between the hydrostatic pressure gradient and the plasma effective colloid osmotic (oncotic) pressure gradient across the membranes (Fig. 3.2) and tight junctions. The colloid osmotic effect is weak relative to the hydrostatic gradient but does facilitate some reabsorption of fluid from the proximal renal tubules.

The filtrate contains diffusible constituents at almost the same concentrations as in plasma. About 30 000 mmol of sodium, 800 mmol of potassium, 800 mmol of urea, 300 mmol of free-ionized calcium and 1000 mmol of glucose are filtered daily. Proteins (mainly low-molecular-weight proteins) and protein-bound substances are filtered in only small amounts by normal glomeruli and most are reabsorbed. The huge volume of filtrate allows adequate

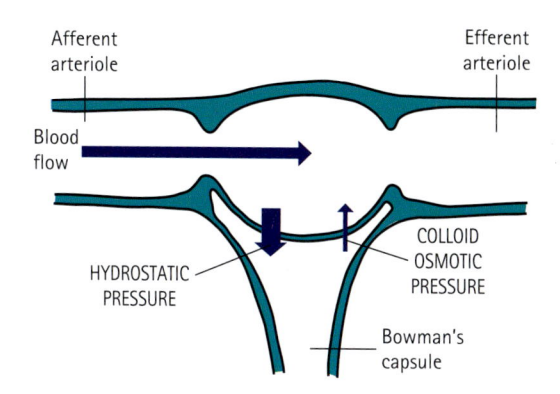

Fig. 3.2 The relationship between flow of blood through the glomerulus and the factors that affect the rate of filtration across the glomerular basement membrane.

elimination of waste products such as urea; death from water and electrolyte depletion would occur within a few hours unless the bulk of this water containing essential solutes were reclaimed.

RENAL TUBULAR FUNCTION

Changes in filtration rate alter the total amount of water and solute filtered, but not the composition of the filtrate. From the 200 L of plasma filtered daily, only about 2 L of urine are formed. The composition of urine differs markedly from that of plasma, and therefore of the filtrate. The tubular cells use adenosine triphosphate-dependent active transport, sometimes selectively, against physicochemical gradients. Transport of charged ions tends to produce an electrochemical gradient that inhibits further transport. This is minimized by two processes.

Isosmotic transport: this occurs mainly in the proximal tubules and reclaims the bulk of filtered essential constituents. Active transport of one ion leads to passive movement of an ion of the opposite charge in the same direction, along the electrochemical gradient. For instance, isosmotic reabsorption of sodium (Na^+) depends on the availability of diffusible negatively charged ions, such as chloride (Cl^-). The process is 'isosmotic' because the active transport of solute causes equivalent movement of water in the same direction. Isosmotic transport also occurs to a lesser extent in the distal part of the nephron.

Ion exchange: this occurs mainly in the more distal parts of the nephrons and is important for fine adjustment after bulk reabsorption has taken place. Ions of the same charge, usually cations, are exchanged and neither electrochemical nor osmotic gradients are created. Therefore, during cation exchange there is insignificant net movement of anion or water. For example, Na$^+$ may be reabsorbed in exchange for potassium (K$^+$) or hydrogen (H$^+$) ions. Na$^+$ and H$^+$ exchange also occurs proximally, but at that site it is more important for bicarbonate reclamation than for fine adjustment of solute reabsorption (see Chapter 4).

In the cells lining the renal tubules, the intestine and many secretory organs, the pumps are located on the membrane on one side of the cell only and therefore solute flows in one direction.

Other substances, such as phosphate and urate, are secreted into, as well as reabsorbed from, the tubular lumen. The tubular cells do not deal actively with waste products such as urea and creatinine to any significant degree. Most filtered urea is passed in urine, but some diffuses back passively from the collecting ducts with water; by contrast, some creatinine is secreted into the tubular lumen.

Reclamation of solute from the proximal tubule

Almost all the potassium is actively reabsorbed from the proximal tubules, as is more than 70 per cent of the filtered sodium, free ionized calcium and magnesium.

Some free ionized calcium is reabsorbed at more distal sites, possibly from the loops of Henle. This reabsorption may be stimulated by parathyroid hormone (PTH) and inhibited by loop diuretics such as furosemide. Only about 2 per cent of filtered calcium appears in the urine.

Many inorganic anions follow an electrochemical gradient; the reabsorption of sodium is limited by the availability of chloride, the most abundant diffusible anion in the filtrate. Bicarbonate is almost completely recovered following exchange of sodium and hydrogen ions (Fig. 3.3; see also Chapters 2 and 4). Specific active transport mechanisms result in the almost complete reabsorption of glucose, urate and amino acids. Some urate is secreted into the lumina, mainly in the proximal tubules, but most of this is reabsorbed.

Phosphate reabsorption is incomplete; phosphate in tubular fluid is important for buffering hydrogen ions. Inhibition of phosphate reabsorption by PTH occurs in both the proximal and distal convoluted tubules and accounts for the hypophosphataemia of PTH excess. Thus almost all the re-usable nutrients and the bulk of electrolytes are reclaimed from the proximal tubules, with fine homeostatic adjustment taking place more distally. Almost all the filtered metabolic waste products, such as urea and creatinine, which cannot be re-used by the body, remain in the luminal fluid.

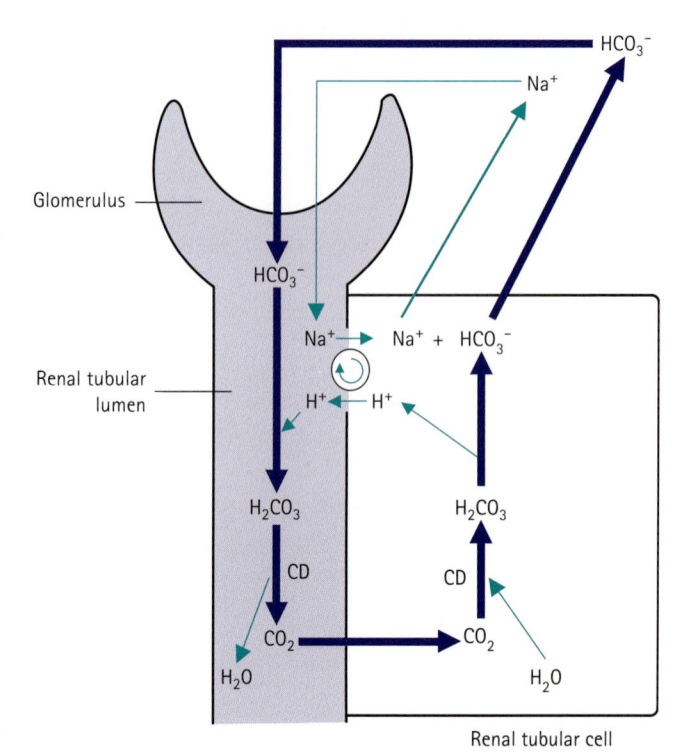

Fig. 3.3 'Reclamation' of filtered bicarbonate by the renal tubular cell. See text for explanation. (CD = carbonate dehydratase.)

WATER REABSORPTION: URINARY CONCENTRATION AND DILUTION

Water is always reabsorbed passively along an osmotic gradient. However, active solute transport is necessary to produce this gradient (see also Chapter 2). Two main processes are involved in water reabsorption.

- Isosmotic reabsorption of water from the proximal tubules. The nephrons reabsorb 99 per cent of the filtered water, about 70–80 per cent (140–160 L/day) of which is returned to the body from the proximal tubules. Active solute reabsorption from the filtrate is accompanied by passive reabsorption of an osmotically equivalent amount of water. Therefore, fluid entering the lumina of the loops of Henle, although much reduced in volume, is still almost isosmotic.
- Dissociation of water reabsorption from that of solute in the loops of Henle, distal tubules and collecting ducts. Normally between 40 L and 60 L of water enter the loops of Henle daily. This volume is reduced to about 2 L as varying amounts of water are reabsorbed,

helping to correct for changes in extracellular osmolality. At extremes of water intake, urinary osmolality can vary from about 40 to 1400 mmol/kg. The proximal tubules cannot dissociate water and solute reabsorption, and the adjustment must occur between the end of the proximal tubule and the end of the collecting duct.

Two mechanisms are involved.

- *Countercurrent multiplication* is an active process occurring in the loops of Henle whereby a high osmolality is created in the renal medulla and urinary osmolality is reduced. This can occur in the absence of antidiuretic hormone (ADH) and a dilute hypo-osmolal urine is produced.
- *Countercurrent exchange* is a passive process, only occurring in the presence of ADH. Water without solute is reabsorbed from the collecting ducts into the ascending vasa recta along the osmotic gradient created by countercurrent multiplication and by the high osmolality in the medulla, producing a concentrated urine.

Countercurrent multiplication

This occurs in the loops of Henle. It depends on the close apposition of the descending and ascending limbs of the loops to the vasa recta. The vasa recta make up a capillary network derived from the efferent arterioles and, like the loops of Henle, pass deep into the medulla. The descending limbs are permeable to water but the thick ascending limbs are impermeable to water and solute. Chloride is probably actively pumped from the thick ascending to the descending limbs as fluid flows through the lumina of the loops; positively charged sodium ions follow along the electrochemical gradient. Thus the osmolality progressively increases in the descending limbs and renal medullary interstitium; it decreases in the ascending limbs, but as these are impermeable to water, this change is not transmitted to the interstitium.

The almost isosmolal fluid enters the descending limbs having the same osmolality as the plasma, just under 300 mmol/kg. If the fluid in the loops were stationary and no pumping had taken place, the osmolality throughout the loops and the adjacent medullary tissue would be about 300 mmol/kg (Fig. 3.4a).

Suppose the fluid column remained stationary and 1 mmol of solute per kilogram were pumped from the ascending into the descending limb, the result would be as in Figure 3.4b.

If this pumping continued and there were no flow, the fluid in the descending limb would become hyperosmolal and that in the ascending limb correspondingly hypo-osmolal.

Suppose that the fluid flowed so that each figure 'moved two places' (Fig. 3.4c). As this happened, more solute would be pumped from the ascending to the descending limbs (Fig. 3.4d). If the fluid again flowed 'two places', the situation would be as shown in Figure 3.4e.

If these steps occurred simultaneously and continuously, the consequences would be as follows.

- Increasing osmolality in the tips of the loops of Henle: because the walls of most of the loops are permeable to water and solute, osmotic equilibrium would be reached with the surrounding tissues in the deeper layers of the medulla, including the plasma within the vasa recta.
- Hypo-osmolal fluid leaving the ascending limbs (Fig. 3.4f): in the absence of ADH, the walls of the collecting ducts are impermeable to water, and therefore no further change in osmolality occurs and hypo-osmolal urine would be passed.

Countercurrent exchange (Fig. 3.5)

Countercurrent exchange is essential, together with multiplication, for the osmolal concentration of urine. It can only occur in the presence of ADH and depends on the 'random' apposition of the collecting ducts and the ascending vasa recta. Antidiuretic hormone increases the permeability of the cell membranes lining the distal parts of the collecting ducts to water, which then moves passively along the osmotic gradient created by multiplication. Consequently luminal fluid is concentrated as the collecting ducts pass into the increasingly hyperosmolal medulla.

The increasing concentration of the fluid would reduce the osmotic gradient as it passes down the ducts if it did not meet even more concentrated plasma flowing in the opposite (countercurrent) direction. The gradient is thus maintained, and water continues to be reabsorbed until the fluid reaches the deepest layers, where the osmolality is about four or five times that of plasma (Fig. 3.4f). The low capillary hydrostatic pressure at this site and the osmotic effect of plasma proteins ensure that much of the reabsorbed water within the interstitium enters the vascular lumina. The diluted blood is carried towards the cortex and ultimately enters the general circulation and helps to dilute the extracellular fluid.

The osmotic action of urea in the medullary interstitium may potentiate the countercurrent multiplication. As water is reabsorbed from the collecting ducts under

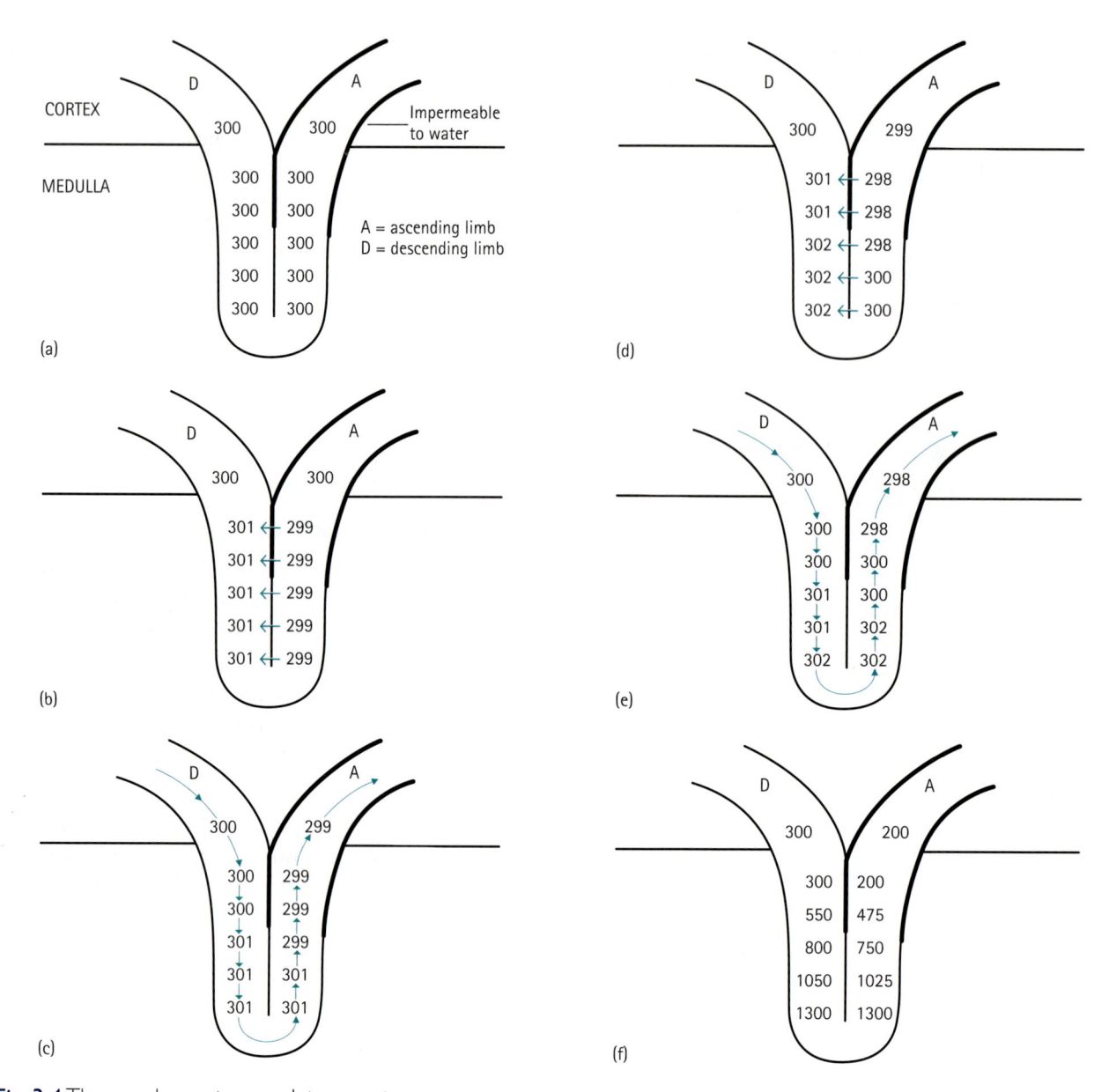

Fig. 3.4 The renal counter-regulatory system.

the influence of ADH, the luminal urea concentration increases. Because the distal collecting ducts are permeable to urea, it enters the deeper layers of the medullary interstitium, increasing the osmolality and drawing water from the lower parts of the descending limbs of the loops. The amount of urea reabsorbed depends on:

- the amount filtered,
- the rate of flow of tubular fluid: as much as 50 per cent of filtered urea may be reabsorbed when flow is significantly reduced.

In summary, both concentration and dilution of urine depend on active processes, which may be impaired if tubules are damaged.

Renal homeostatic control of water excretion

In this section, the mechanisms involved in the normal homeostatic control of urinary water excretion in the extremes of water intake are discussed. It may be helpful to read it in conjunction with Chapter 2, which deals with sodium and water balance.

Water restriction

By increasing the plasma osmolality, water restriction increases ADH secretion and allows countercurrent exchange with enhanced water reabsorption. Reduced

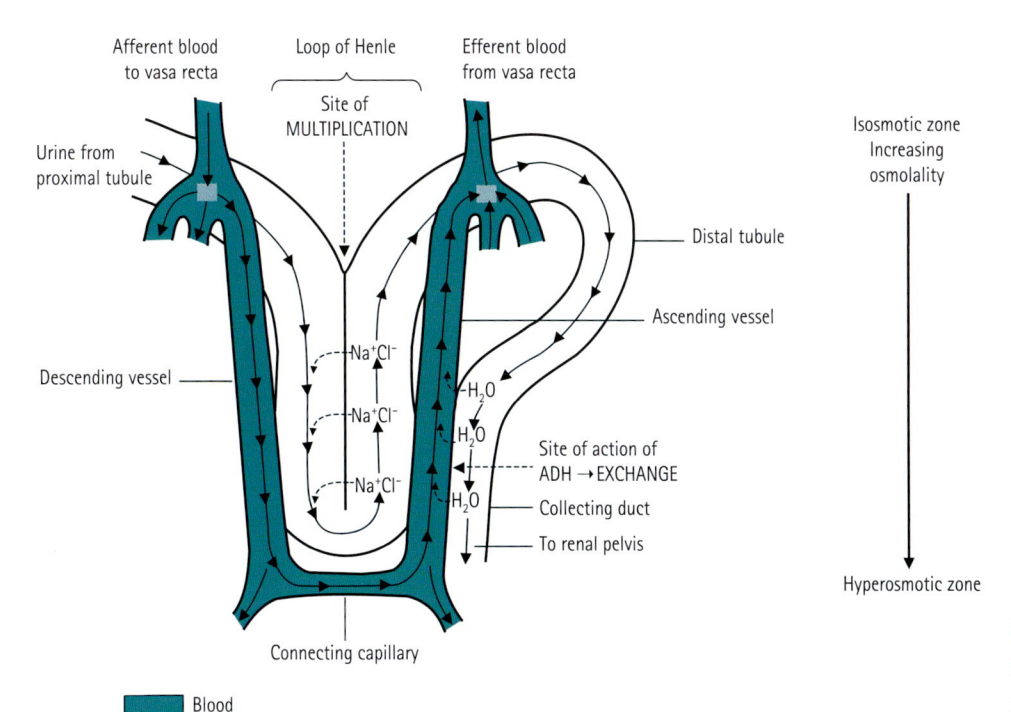

Fig. 3.5 The countercurrent mechanism, showing the relationship between the renal tubules and the vasa recta. (ADH = antidiuretic hormone.)

circulatory volume results in a sluggish blood flow in the vasa recta and increased urea reabsorption, allowing a build-up of the medullary hyperosmolality produced by multiplication. This potentiates water reabsorption in the presence of ADH. The reduced capillary hydrostatic pressure and increased colloid osmotic pressure, due to the haemoconcentration following non-protein fluid loss, ensure that much of the reabsorbed water enters the vascular compartment.

Water load

A high water intake dilutes the extracellular fluid and the consequent fall in plasma osmolality reduces ADH secretion. The walls of the collecting ducts therefore remain impermeable to water and the countercurrent multiplication produces a dilute urine and a high osmolality within the medulla and medullary vessels. Blood from the latter flows into the general circulation, so helping to correct the fall in systemic osmolality.

During maximal water diuresis the osmolality at the tips of the medullary loops may be 600 mmol/kg or less, rather than the maximum of about 1400 mmol/kg. Increasing the circulating volume increases renal blood flow; the rapid flow in the vasa recta 'washes out' medullary hyperosmolality, returning some of the solute, without extra water, to the circulation. Thus not only is more water than usual lost in the urine, more solute is 'reclaimed'. Because medullary hyperosmolality, and therefore the ability to concentrate the urine maximally, is dependent on medullary blood flow, under normal circumstances urinary osmolality will only be fully restored several days after a prolonged water load has stopped (see Chapter 2).

Osmotic diuresis

An excess of filtered solute in the proximal tubular lumina impairs the bulk water reabsorption from this site by its osmotic effect. Unabsorbed solute concentration rises progressively as water is reabsorbed with other solute during passage through the proximal tubules and this opposes further water reabsorption. Thus a larger volume than usual reaches the loops of Henle. Moreover, fluid leaving the proximal tubules, although still isosmotic with plasma, has a lower sodium concentration than plasma. The relative lack of the major cation (sodium) to accompany the anion chloride along the electrochemical gradient inhibits the pump in the loops. The resulting impairment of build-up of medullary osmolality inhibits distal water reabsorption, under the influence of ADH from the collecting ducts, resulting in a diuresis (see Chapter 2).

The most effective osmotic diuretics are substances that cannot cross cell membranes to any significant degree; therefore, they must be infused, as they cannot be absorbed from the gut. One example is mannitol, a sugar alcohol, which is sometimes used therapeutically as a diuretic.

Normally most filtered water leaves the proximal tubular lumina with reabsorbed solute. For example glucose (with an active transport system) and urea (which diffuses back passively) are sometimes filtered at high enough concentration to exceed the proximal tubular reabsorptive capacity. They too can then act as osmotic diuretics and cause water depletion. This is important, for example, in diabetes mellitus or in uraemia.

Homeostatic solute adjustment in the distal tubule and collecting duct

Sodium reabsorption in exchange for hydrogen ions occurs throughout the nephrons. In the proximal tubules the main effect of this exchange is on reclamation of filtered bicarbonate. In the distal tubules and collecting ducts, the exchange process is usually associated with net generation of bicarbonate to replace that lost in extracellular buffering. Potassium and hydrogen ions compete for secretion in exchange for sodium ions. The possible mechanism stimulated by aldosterone is discussed in Chapter 2. The most important stimulus to aldosterone secretion is mediated by the effect of renal blood flow on the release of renin from the juxtaglomerular apparatus; this method of reabsorption is part of the homeostatic mechanism controlling sodium and water balance.

BIOCHEMISTRY OF RENAL DISORDERS

Pathophysiology

Different parts of the nephrons are in close anatomical association and are dependent on a common blood supply. Renal dysfunction of any kind affects all parts of the nephrons to some extent, although sometimes either glomerular or tubular dysfunction is predominant. The net effect of renal disease on plasma and urine depends on the proportion of glomeruli to tubules affected and on the number of nephrons involved.

To understand the consequences of renal disease it may be useful to consider the *hypothetical* individual nephrons, first with a low glomerular filtration rate (GFR) and normal tubular function, and then with tubular damage but a normal GFR. It should be emphasized that these are hypothetical examples, as in clinical reality a combination of varying degree may exist.

Uraemia is the term used to describe a raised plasma urea concentration and is almost always accompanied by an elevated creatinine concentration: in North America this is usually referred to as azotaemia (a raised nitrogen concentration).

Reduced glomerular filtration rate with normal tubular function

The total amounts of urea and creatinine excreted are affected by the GFR. If the rate of filtration fails to balance that of production, plasma concentrations will rise.

Phosphate and urate are released during cell breakdown. Plasma concentrations rise because less than normal is filtered. Most of the reduced amount reaching the proximal tubule can be reabsorbed, and the capacity for secretion is impaired if the filtered volume is too low to accept the ions; these factors further contribute to high plasma concentrations.

A large proportion of the reduced amount of filtered sodium is reabsorbed by isosmotic mechanisms; less than usual is then available for exchange with hydrogen and potassium ions distally. This has two main outcomes:

- reduced hydrogen ion secretion throughout the nephron: bicarbonate can only be reclaimed if hydrogen ion is secreted; plasma bicarbonate concentrations will fall;
- reduced potassium secretion in the distal tubule, with potassium retention (potassium can still be reabsorbed proximally).

If there is a low GFR accompanied by a low renal blood flow:

- systemic aldosterone secretion will be maximal: in such cases, any sodium reaching the distal tubule will be almost completely reabsorbed in exchange for H^+ and K^+, and the urinary sodium concentration will be low;
- ADH secretion will be increased: ADH acting on the collecting ducts allows water to be reabsorbed in excess of solute, further reducing urinary volume and increasing urinary osmolality well above that of plasma. This high urinary osmolality is mainly due to substances not actively dealt with by the tubules. For example, the urinary urea concentration will be well above that of plasma. This distal response will only occur in the presence of ADH; in its absence, normal nephrons will form a dilute urine.

If the capacity of the proximal tubular cells to reabsorb solute, and therefore water, is normal, a larger proportion than usual of the reduced filtered volume will be reclaimed by isosmotic processes, thus further reducing urinary volume.

In summary, the findings in venous plasma and urine from the affected nephrons will be as follows.

Plasma

- High urea (uraemia) and creatinine concentrations.
- Low bicarbonate concentration, with low pH (acidosis).
- Hyperkalaemia.
- Hyperuricaemia and hyperphosphataemia.

Urine

- Reduced volume (oliguria).
- Low (appropriate) sodium concentration – only if renal blood flow is low, stimulating aldosterone secretion.
- High (appropriate) urea concentration and therefore a high osmolality – only if ADH secretion is stimulated.

Reduced tubular function with normal glomerular filtration rate

Damage to tubular cells impairs adjustment of the composition and volume of the urine. Impaired solute reabsorption from proximal tubules reduces isosmotic water reabsorption. Counter-current multiplication may also be affected, and therefore the ability of the collecting ducts to respond to ADH is reduced. A large volume of inappropriately dilute urine is produced.

The tubules cannot secrete hydrogen ions and therefore cannot reabsorb bicarbonate normally or acidify the urine.

The response to aldosterone and therefore the exchange mechanisms involving reabsorption of sodium are impaired; the urine contains an inappropriately high concentration of sodium for the renal blood flow.

Potassium reabsorption from the proximal tubule is impaired and plasma potassium concentrations may be low.

Reabsorption of glucose, phosphate, magnesium, urate and amino acids is impaired. Plasma phosphate, magnesium and urate concentrations may be low.

Thus, the findings in venous plasma and urine from the affected nephrons will be as follows.

Plasma

- Normal urea and creatinine concentrations (normal glomerular function).
- Due to proximal or distal tubular failure:
  - low bicarbonate concentration and low pH,
  - hypokalaemia.
- Due to proximal tubular failure:
  - hypophosphataemia, hypomagnesaemia and hypouricaemia.

Urine

- Due to proximal and/or distal tubular failure:
  - increased volume,
  - pH inappropriately high compared with that in plasma.
- Due to proximal tubular failure:
  - generalized aminoaciduria,
  - phosphaturia
  - glycosuria.

  There may also be tubular proteinuria.

- Due to distal tubular failure:
  - even if renal blood flow is low, an inappropriately high sodium concentration (inability to respond to aldosterone),
  - even if ADH secretion is stimulated, an inappropriately low urea concentration and therefore osmolality (inability of the collecting ducts to respond to ADH).

Clinical features of renal disease

The biochemical findings and urine output in renal disease depend on the relative contributions of glomerular and tubular dysfunction.

When the GFR falls, substances that are little affected by tubular action (such as urea and creatinine) are retained. Although their plasma concentrations start rising above the baseline for that individual soon after the GFR falls, they seldom rise above the reference range for the population until the GFR is below about 60 per cent of normal, although in individual patients they do rise above baseline.

Plasma concentrations of urea and creatinine depend largely on glomerular function (Fig. 3.6). By contrast, urinary concentrations depend almost entirely on tubular function. However little is filtered at the glomeruli, the concentrations of substances in the initial filtrate are those of a plasma ultrafiltrate. Any difference between these concentrations and those in the urine is due to tubular activity. The more the tubular function is impaired, the nearer the plasma concentrations will be to those of urine. Urinary concentrations *inappropriate to the state of hydration* suggest tubular damage, whatever the degree of glomerular dysfunction.

The plasma sodium concentration is not primarily affected by renal disease. The urinary volume depends on the balance between the volume filtered and the proportion reabsorbed by the tubules. Since 99 per cent of filtered water is normally reabsorbed, a very small impairment of reabsorption causes a large increase in urine volume. Consequently, if tubular dysfunction predominates, impairment of water reabsorption causes polyuria, even though glomerular filtration is reduced (see Chapter 2).

The degree of potassium, phosphate and urate retention depends on the balance between the degree of glomerular retention and the loss due to a reduced proximal tubular reabsorptive capacity. If glomerular dysfunction predominates, so little is filtered that plasma concentrations rise despite the failure of reabsorption. Conversely, if tubular dysfunction predominates, glomerular retention is more than balanced by impaired reabsorption of filtered potassium, urate and phosphate, and therefore plasma concentrations may be normal or even low. A low plasma bicarbonate concentration is found in association with metabolic acidosis, which may worsen the hyperkalaemia.

Acute renal dysfunction (or failure)

In adults, oliguria is defined as a urine output of less than 400 mL/day, or less than 15 mL/hour; it usually indicates a low GFR and acute renal failure. Oliguria may be caused by the factors discussed below.

Acute oliguria with reduced GFR (pre-renal)

This is caused by factors that reduce the hydrostatic pressure gradient between the renal capillaries and the tubular lumen. A low intracapillary pressure is the most common cause. It is known as *renal circulatory insufficiency* ('pre-renal uraemia') and may be due to:

- intravascular depletion of whole blood (haemorrhage) or plasma volume (usually due to gastrointestinal loss), or reduced intake;
- reduced pressure as a result of the vascular dilatation caused by 'shock', causes of which include myocardial infarction, cardiac failure and intravascular haemolysis, including that due to mismatched blood transfusion.

The patient is usually hypotensive and clinically volume depleted. If renal blood flow is restored within a few

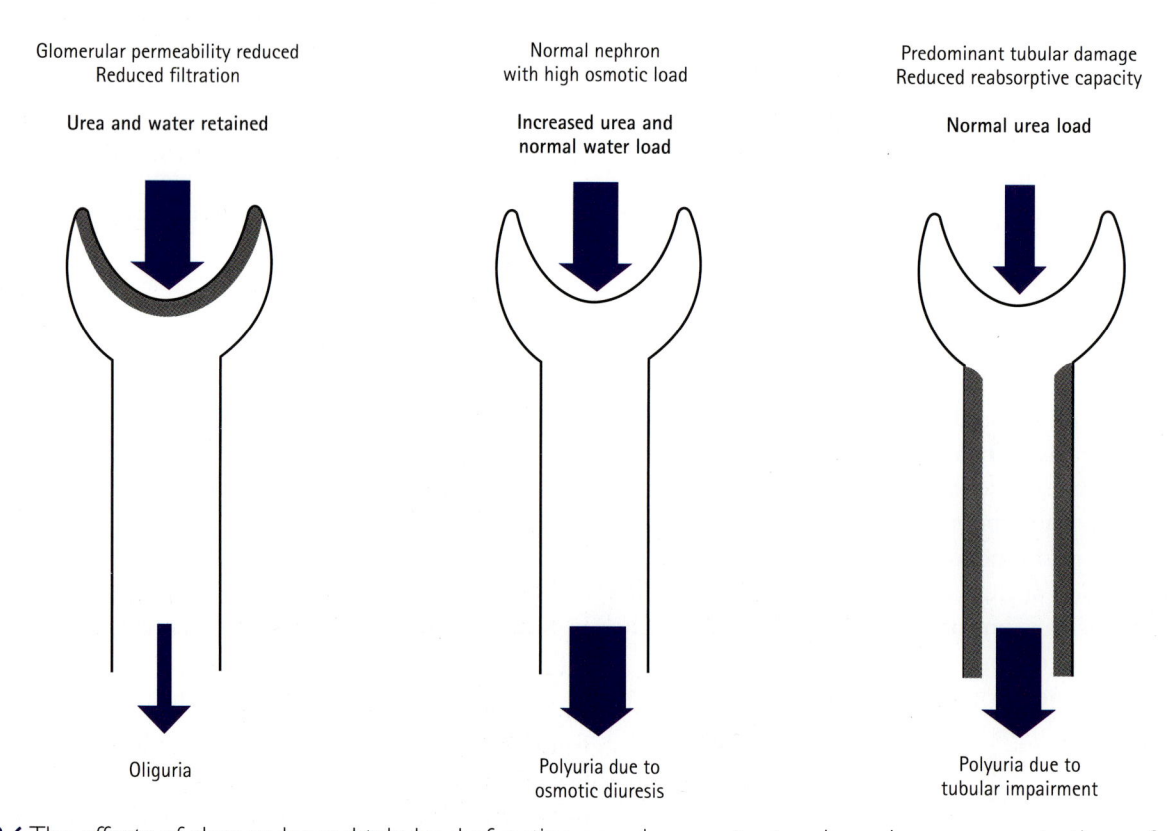

Fig. 3.6 The effects of glomerular and tubular dysfunction on urinary output and on plasma concentrations of retained 'waste' products of metabolism, the volume depending on the proportion of nephrons involved.

hours, the condition is reversible, but the longer it persists, the greater the danger of intrinsic renal damage.

Since most glomeruli are involved and tubular function is relatively normal, the biochemical findings in plasma and urine are those described earlier. Uraemia due to renal dysfunction may be aggravated if there is increased protein breakdown as a result of tissue damage, a large haematoma or the presence of blood in the gastrointestinal lumen. Intravenous amino acid infusion may have the same effect because the urea is derived, by hepatic metabolism, from the amino groups of amino acids. Increased tissue breakdown may also aggravate hyperkalaemia, hyperuricaemia and hyperphosphataemia.

Acute oliguria due to intrinsic renal damage

This may be due to:

- prolonged renal circulatory insufficiency;
- acute glomerulonephritis, usually in children – the history of a sore throat and the finding of red cells in the urine usually make the diagnosis obvious;
- septicaemia, which should be considered when the cause of oliguria is obscure;
- ingestion of a variety of poisons or drugs;
- myoglobulinuria (see Chapters 18 and 19);
- Bence-Jones proteinuria (see Chapter 19).

One problem in the differential diagnosis of acute oliguria is to distinguish between renal circulatory insufficiency and intrinsic renal damage that may have followed it. Acute oliguric renal dysfunction often follows a period of reduced GFR and renal circulatory insufficiency. The oliguria is due to reduced cortical blood flow with glomerular damage, aggravated by back-pressure on the glomeruli due to obstruction to tubular flow by oedema. At this stage, the concentrations of many constituents in plasma, such as urea and creatinine, are raised with hyperkalaemia; tubular damage results in an inappropriately dilute urine for the degree of hypovolaemia. Fluid must be given with caution, and only until volume depletion has been corrected; there is a danger of overloading the circulation.

During recovery, oliguria is followed by polyuria. When cortical blood flow increases, and as tubular oedema resolves, glomerular function recovers before that of the tubules. The biochemical findings gradually progress to those of tubular dysfunction until they approximate those for 'pure' tubular lesions. Urinary output is further increased by the osmotic diuretic effect of the high load of urea. The polyuria may cause water and electrolyte depletion. The initial hyperkalaemia may be followed by hypokalaemia. Mild acidosis (common to both glomerular and tubular disorders) persists until late. Recovery of the tubules may restore full renal function.

Acute oliguria due to renal outflow obstruction (post-renal)

Oliguria or anuria (absence of urine) may occur in post-renal failure. The cause is usually, but not always, clinically obvious and may be due to the following.

- *Intrarenal obstruction*, with blockage of the tubular lumina by haemoglobin, myoglobin and, very rarely, urate or calcium. Obstruction caused by casts and oedema of tubular cells is usually the result of true renal damage.
- *Extrarenal obstruction*, due to calculi, neoplasms, e.g. prostate or cervix, urethral strictures or prostatic

CASE 1

A 19-year-old male was involved in a road traffic accident. Both femurs were fractured and his spleen was ruptured. Two days after surgery and transfusion of 16 units of blood, the following results were found:

Plasma
Sodium 136 mmol/L (135–145)
Potassium 6.1 mmol/L (3.5–5.0)
Urea 20.9 mmol/L (2.5–7.0)
Creatinine 190 μmol/L (70–110)
'Corrected' calcium 2.40 mmol/L (2.15–2.55)
Phosphate 2.8 mmol/L (0.80–1.35)
Bicarbonate 17 mmol/L (24–32)

The patient was producing only 10 mL of urine per hour and a spot urinary sodium was 8 mmol/L.

DISCUSSION
The results are compatible with pre-renal dysfunction or failure secondary to massive blood loss. Note the oliguria, low urinary sodium concentration, hyperkalaemia, hyperphosphataemia and also low plasma bicarbonate concentration, suggestive of a metabolic acidosis.

hypertrophy, any of which may cause sudden obstruction. The finding of a palpable bladder indicates urethral obstruction and in males is most likely to be due to prostatic hypertrophy, although there are other, rarer, causes.

Early correction of outflow obstruction may rapidly increase the urine output. The longer it remains untreated, the greater the danger of ischaemic or pressure damage to renal tissue. Imaging studies such as abdominal X-ray or renal tract ultrasound may be useful to confirm post-renal obstruction (Box 3.1).

Investigation of acute renal dysfunction

- A careful clinical history, especially of taking nephrotic drugs, and examination may give clues as to the cause of acute renal failure. It is essential to exclude reversible causes of pre-renal failure, including hypovolaemia or hypotension, and also post-renal urinary tract obstruction (renal tract imaging may be useful – see Box 3.1).
- Monitor urine output, plasma urea and creatinine and electrolytes as well as acid–base status.

Box 3.1 Some causes of acute renal failure

Pre-renal
Hypotension
Hypovolaemia
Renal artery stenosis + angiotensin-converting enzyme inhibitor
Hepatorenal syndrome

Renal or intrinsic renal disease
Acute tubular necrosis, e.g. hypotension, toxins, myoglobinuria, sepsis, drugs, sustained pre-renal oliguria
Vasculitis
Glomerulonephritis
Drugs that are nephrotoxic
Sepsis
Thrombotic microangiopathy
Hypercalcaemia
Hyperuricaemia
Bence-Jones proteinuria

Post-renal
Calculi
Retroperitoneal fibrosis
Prostate hypertrophy/malignancy
Carcinoma of cervix or bladder

- Hyperkalaemia, hypermagnesaemia, hyperphosphataemia, hyperuricaemia and metabolic acidosis may occur in the oliguric phase of acute renal failure.
- Urine microscopy may show granular casts supportive of the diagnosis of acute tubular necrosis.
- The urinary to plasma urea ratio can be useful and when more than 10:1 is suggestive of pre-renal problems. The urinary to plasma creatinine or osmolality ratio may also be useful (Table 3.1).
- The fractional excretion of sodium (FENa%) is also useful diagnostically and can be measured using a simultaneous blood sample and spot urine (see above and Fig. 3.7).

$$FENa\% = \frac{urine[sodium]}{plasma[sodium]} \times \frac{plasma[creatinine]}{urine[creatinine]} \times 100\% \quad (3.1)$$

An FENa% of less than 1% is typical of pre-renal failure, as is a urinary sodium concentration more than 20 mmol/L.

- Blood may be necessary for full blood count, coagulation screen and blood cultures. Also exclude myeloma and look for Bence-Jones proteinuria and cryoglobulins. Autoantibody screen, including ANCA, ANA, ENA and double-stranded DNA, myoglobin, plasma calcium may also be indicated depending on the clinical situation.
- In obscure cases, renal biopsy may be necessary to establish a diagnosis.

Table 3.1 Some laboratory tests used to investigate acute renal failure

	Pre-renal failure	Intrinsic renal failure/acute tubular necrosis
Urine sodium (mmol/L)	<20	>40
FENa%	<1	>1
Urine:plasma creatinine ratio	>40	<20
Urine:plasma osmolality ratio	>1.2	<1.2
Urine:plasma urea ratio	>10	<10

Note that in post-renal failure there is usually anuria.
FENa% = percentage fractional excretion of sodium.

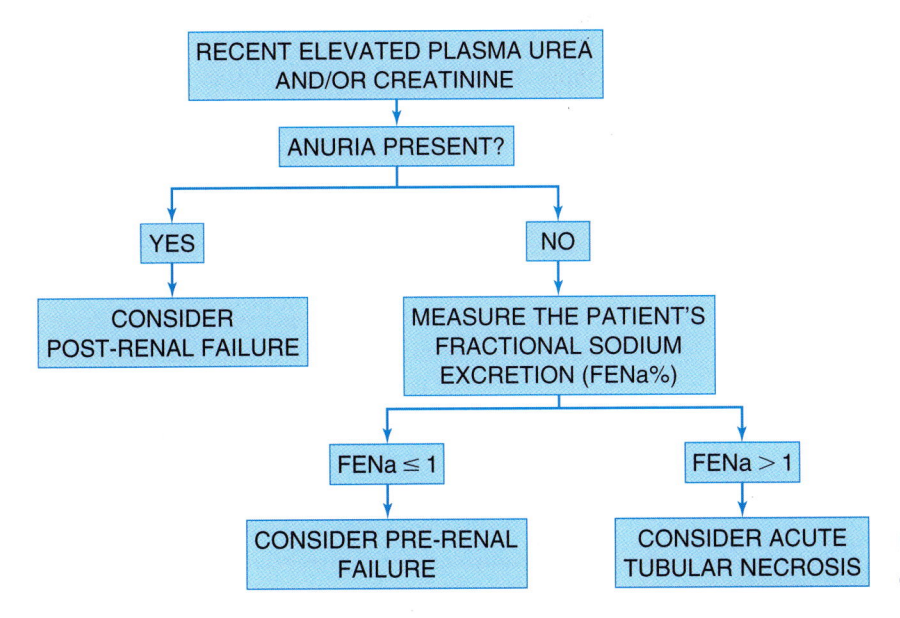

Fig. 3.7 Algorithm for the investigation of acute renal failure.

Chronic renal dysfunction (or failure)

Chronic renal dysfunction (defined as being of more than 3 months' duration) is usually the end result of conditions such as diabetes mellitus, hypertension, primary glomerulonephritis, autoimmune disease, obstructive uropathy, polycystic disease, renal artery stenosis, infections and tubular dysfunction and the use of nephrotoxic drugs (Box 3.2).

In most cases of acute oliguric renal disease there is diffuse damage involving the majority of nephrons. A patient who survives long enough to develop chronic renal disease must have some functioning nephrons.

Histological examination shows that not all nephrons are equally affected: some may be completely destroyed and others almost normal. Also, some segments of the nephrons may be more affected than others. The effects of chronic renal disease can be explained by this patchy distribution of damage; acute renal disease may sometimes show the same picture.

In chronic renal failure the functional adaptive effects can be divided into three main categories: diminished renal reserve, renal insufficiency, and end-stage uraemia. This helps to explain why the loss of 75 per cent of renal tissue produces a fall of GFR by 50 per cent.

Although there is a loss of renal function, homeostasis is initially preserved at the expense of various adaptations such as glomerulotubular changes and secondary hyperparathyroidism.

Chronic renal dysfunction may pass through two main phases:

- an initially polyuric phase,
- subsequent oliguria or anuria, sometimes needing dialysis or renal transplantation.

Polyuric phase

At first, glomerular function may be adequate to maintain plasma urea and creatinine concentrations within the reference range. As more glomeruli are involved, the rate of urea excretion falls and the plasma concentration rises. This causes an osmotic diuresis in functioning nephrons; in other nephrons the tubules may be damaged out of proportion to the glomeruli. Both tubular dysfunction in nephrons with functioning glomeruli and the osmotic diuresis through intact nephrons contribute to the polyuria, other causes of which should be excluded (see Chapter 2).

Box 3.2 Some causes of chronic renal dysfunction or failure

Diabetes mellitus
Nephrotoxic drugs
Hypertension
Glomerulonephritis
Chronic pyelonephritis
Polycystic kidneys
Urinary tract obstruction
Severe urinary infections
Amyloid and paraproteins
Progression from acute renal dysfunction

During the polyuric phase, the plasma concentration of many substances, other than urea and creatinine, may be anywhere between the glomerular and tubular ends of the spectrum, although metabolic acidosis is usually present.

Oliguric phase

If nephron destruction continues, the findings become more like those of pure glomerular dysfunction. Glomerular filtration decreases significantly and urine output falls; oliguria precipitates a steep rise in plasma urea, creatinine and potassium concentrations; and the metabolic acidosis becomes more severe.

The diagnosis of chronic renal failure is usually obvious. In the early phase, before plasma urea and creatinine concentrations have risen significantly, there may be microscopic haematuria or proteinuria. However, haematuria may originate from either the kidney or urinary tract and may therefore indicate the presence of other conditions, such as urinary tract infections, renal calculi or tumours (see Box 3.2).

Other abnormal findings in chronic renal failure

Apart from uraemia, hyperkalaemia and metabolic acidosis, other abnormalities that may occur in chronic renal failure include the following.

- Plasma phosphate concentrations rise and plasma total calcium concentrations fall. The increased hydrogen ion concentration increases the proportion of free ionized calcium, the plasma concentration of which does not fall in parallel with the fall in total calcium concentration. Impaired renal tubular function and the raised phosphate concentration inhibit the conversion of vitamin D to the active metabolite and this contributes to the fall in plasma calcium concentration. Usually, *hypocalcaemia should only be treated after correction of hyperphosphataemia*. After several years of chronic renal failure, secondary hyperparathyroidism (see Chapter 6) may cause decalcification of bone, with a rise in the plasma alkaline phosphatase activity. Some of these features of chronic renal failure can also evoke renal osteodystrophy associated with painful bones. The increase in plasma PTH occurs early when the GFR falls below 60 mL/min.
- Plasma urate concentrations rise in parallel with plasma urea. A high plasma concentration does not necessarily indicate primary hyperuricaemia; clinical gout is rare unless hyperuricaemia is the cause of the renal damage.
- Hypermagnesaemia can also occur (see Chapter 6).
- Normochromic, normocytic anaemia due to erythropoietin deficiency is common and, because haemopoiesis is impaired, does not respond to iron therapy; this can be treated with recombinant erythropoietin.
- One of the commonest causes of death in patients with chronic renal failure is cardiovascular disease, in part explained by a dyslipidaemia of hypertriglyceridaemia and low high-density lipoprotein cholesterol. Some of these effects may be due to reduced lipoprotein lipase activity.
- Abnormal endocrine function, such as hyperprolactinaemia, insulin resistance, low plasma testosterone and abnormal thyroid function, may also be seen in chronic renal dysfunction.
- Some of the features of chronic renal failure may be explained by the presence of 'middle molecules' – compounds that the kidneys would normally excrete. These compounds, of relatively small molecular weights, can exert toxic effects upon body tissues.

CASE 2

A 56-year-old male attended renal out-patients because of polycystic kidneys, which had been diagnosed 20 years previously. He was hypertensive and the following blood results were returned.

Plasma
Sodium 136 mmol/L (135–145)
Potassium 6.2 mmol/L (3.5–5.0)
Urea 23.7 mmol/L (2.5–7.0)
Creatinine 360 μmol/L (70–110)
'Corrected' calcium 1.80 mmol/L (2.15–2.55)
Phosphate 2.6 mmol/L (0.80–1.35)
Bicarbonate 13 mmol/L (24–32)

DISCUSSION

These results are typical of a patient with chronic renal failure with raised plasma urea and creatinine concentrations.

The patient has hyperkalaemia and a low plasma bicarbonate concentration, suggestive of a metabolic acidosis. The hypocalcaemia and hyperphosphataemia are also in keeping with chronic renal failure.

- The presence of increasing proteinuria may be the best single predictor of disease progression.

Irreversible but potentially modifiable complications such as anaemia, metabolic bone disease, malnutrition and cardiovascular disease occur early in the course of chronic renal failure. A summary of the clinical features of chronic renal failure is shown in Table 3.2.

Mild 'uraemia' with normal urinary volume

A slight rise of plasma urea and creatinine concentrations is a common incidental finding, especially in elderly subjects. It almost certainly indicates some degree of renal damage which, unless progressive, is unlikely to need treatment. Congestive cardiac failure may impair renal circulation enough to cause mild uraemia.

SYNDROMES REFLECTING PREDOMINANT TUBULAR DAMAGE – RENAL TUBULAR ACIDOSIS

There is a group of conditions that primarily affect tubular function more than the function of the glomeruli. However, scarring involving whole nephrons may eventually cause chronic renal dysfunction. Impaired function may involve a single transport system, particularly disorders associated with amino acid or phosphate transport, or may affect multiple transport systems. Conditions associated with multiple transport defects may cause renal tubular acidoses – renal tubular disorders associated with a systemic metabolic acidosis because of impaired reclamation of bicarbonate or excretion of H^+ (see Chapter 4).

Disorders affecting the urine-concentrating mechanism and causing nephrogenic diabetes insipidus but which rarely in themselves cause a metabolic acidosis are discussed elsewhere (see Chapter 4).

NEPHROTIC SYNDROME

The nephrotic syndrome is caused by increased glomerular basement membrane permeability, resulting in protein loss, usually more than 3 g a day, with consequent hypoproteinaemia, hypoalbuminaemia and peripheral oedema. All but the highest molecular weight plasma proteins can pass through the glomerular basement membrane. The main effects are on plasma proteins and are associated with hyperlipidaemia and hyperfibrinoginaemia. (This is discussed more fully in Chapter 19.) Uraemia only occurs in late stages of the disorder, when many glomeruli cease to function.

Table 3.2 Stages of renal dysfunction[a]

Stage	Description	GFR (mL/min per 1.73 m^2)	Metabolic features
1	Normal or increased GFR	>90	Normal
2	Early renal insufficiency	60–89	Plasma urea and creatinine rise PTH starts to rise
3	Chronic renal failure	30–59	Calcium absorption decreased Lipoprotein lipase decreased Malnutrition Anaemia – erythropoietin decreased
4	Severe renal failure (pre-end stage)	15–29	Hypertriglyceridaemia Hyperphosphataemia Metabolic acidosis Hyperkalaemia
5	End-stage renal failure	<15	Marked elevation of urea (uraemia) and creatinine

[a]National Kidney Foundation.
GFR = glomerular filtration rate; PTH = parathyroid hormone.

DIAGNOSIS OF RENAL DYSFUNCTION

Glomerular function tests

As glomerular function deteriorates, substances that are normally cleared by the kidneys, such as urea and creatinine, accumulate in plasma.

Measurement of plasma concentrations of urea and creatinine

Urea is derived in the liver from amino acids and therefore from protein, whether originating from the diet or from tissues. The normal kidney can excrete large amounts of urea. If the rate of production exceeds the rate of clearance, plasma concentrations rise. The rate of production is accelerated by:

- a high-protein diet;
- absorption of amino acids and peptides from digested blood after haemorrhage into the gastrointestinal lumen or soft tissues;
- increased catabolism due to starvation, tissue damage, sepsis or steroid treatment.

In catabolic states, glomerular function is often impaired due to circulatory factors and this contributes more to the uraemia than does increased production. An elevated plasma urea concentration above about 15 mmol/L usually indicates impaired glomerular function, which can be confirmed by measurement of plasma creatinine.

Conversely, the plasma urea concentration may be lower than 1.0 mmol/L, the causes of which include the following.

- Those due to increased GFR (common):
  - pregnancy (the commonest cause in young women),
  - over-enthusiastic intravenous infusion (the commonest cause in hospital patients),
  - 'inappropriate' ADH secretion (syndrome of inappropriate ADH secretion).
- Those due to decreased synthesis:
  - use of amino acids for protein anabolism during growth, especially in children,
  - low protein intake,
  - very severe liver disease (low amino acid deamination),
  - inborn errors of the urea cycle are rare and usually only occur in infants.

Creatinine is largely derived from endogenous sources by tissue creatine breakdown. Plasma creatinine is usually related to muscle mass. The plasma creatinine concentration varies more than that of urea during the day due to protein intake in meals. However, sustained high-protein diets and catabolic states probably affect the plasma concentration of creatinine less than that of urea. Many laboratories prefer to measure the plasma creatinine concentration to assess renal function. However, its assay may be less precise than that of urea, and is prone to analytical interference by substances such as bilirubin, ketone bodies and certain drugs.

If the plasma concentration of either urea or creatinine is significantly raised, and especially if it is rising, impaired glomerular function is likely. Serial changes may be used to monitor changes in the GFR.

In renal dysfunction caused by a reduced GFR, plasma urea concentrations tend to rise faster than those of creatinine and tend to be disproportionately higher with respect to the upper reference limit. The rate at which urea is reabsorbed from the collecting ducts is dependent on the amount filtered by the glomerulus and by the rate of luminal fluid flow (see Table 3.2).

Clearance as an assessment of glomerular filtration rate (Fig. 3.8)

For a substance (S) that is filtered by the glomerulus, but not reabsorbed from or secreted into the tubules, the amount filtered (GFR $\times$ plasma[S]) must equal the amount excreted in the urine (urinary[S] $\times$ volume per unit time):

$$\text{GFR} \times \text{plasma[S]} = \text{urinary[S]} \times \text{urine volume per unit time} \quad (3.2)$$

Thus, rearranging gives:

$$\text{GFR} = \frac{\text{urinary[S]} \times \text{urine volume per unit time}}{\text{plasma[S]}} \quad (3.3)$$

The GFR thus measured is referred to as the *clearance* – the volume of plasma that could theoretically be completely cleared of a substance in 1 minute.

Only substances freely filtered by glomeruli and not acted on by the tubules can be used to give true measurement of GFR. There is no such endogenous substance, but inulin, a polysaccharide, fulfils the criteria closely. Inulin is not produced by the body; it must be given either by constant infusion in order to maintain steady plasma

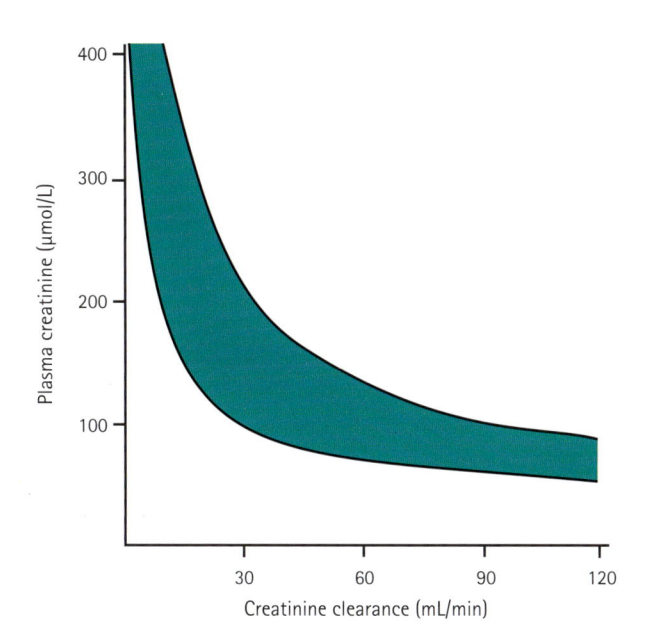

Fig. 3.8 The inverse relationship between plasma creatinine and creatinine clearance. (Shaded area is approximate 95 per cent confidence intervals.)

concentrations during the period of the test, or by a single injection followed by serial blood sampling to enable the concentration at the midpoint of the collection to be calculated.

Radiochromium-labelled EDTA is another exogenous compound that some consider the 'gold standard' for calculating patient GFR, although this requires the use of nuclear medicine tests and is rarely used.

For endogenously produced substances such as creatinine, the following equation can be used to calculate a clearance that acts as an approximation for GFR:

$$\text{Creatinine clearance (mL/min)} = \frac{\text{urinary[creatinine]} \times \text{urine volume (mL)}}{\text{plasma[creatinine]} \times \text{collection period (min)}} \quad (3.4)$$

The Cockcroft–Gault equation can also be used to assess GFR indirectly. It avoids the need for urine collection, but patient weight and age are required to calculate it (see Equations 3.5 and 3.6). There are also other similar equations for estimating GFR (eGFR).

In men:

$$\text{Creatinine clearance (mL/min)} = \frac{(140 - \text{age[years]}) \times \text{weight (kg)}}{72 \times \text{plasma creatinine (}\mu\text{mol/L)}} \quad (3.5)$$

In women:

$$\text{Creatinine clearance (mL/min)} = \frac{(140 - \text{age[years]}) \times \text{weight (kg)}}{72 \times \text{plasma creatinine (}\mu\text{mol/L)}} \times 0.85 \quad (3.6)$$

The reciprocal of the plasma creatinine concentration is called the *renal index*.

Creatinine clearance is higher than inulin clearance because some creatinine is secreted by the tubules. Urea clearance is lower than inulin clearance as some urea is reabsorbed into the tubules. However, there are various factors that make the measurement of creatinine clearance inaccurate.

- All laboratory assays have an inherent imprecision. The combined imprecision of two assays is greater than that of one. Urine as well as plasma is assayed for clearance measurements.
- The most significant error of any method depending on a timed urine collection is in the measurement of urine volume. Inaccurate urine collection may yield misleading results. The difficulties are increased in infants and young children, and in patients who have difficulty in bladder emptying or are incontinent. Unlike analytical imprecision, the probable magnitude of these errors cannot be estimated; it is likely to be much larger than those of laboratory assays.
- Both creatinine and urea may be partly destroyed by bacterial action in infected or old urine.

For an individual patient, plasma creatinine concentrations may rise above the baseline level but remain within the population reference range despite a deterioration in glomerular function. The plasma creatinine concentration may not exceed the upper limit of the reference range until the GFR, and therefore the creatinine clearance, has been reduced by approximately 60 per cent (see Fig. 3.8). Thus the measurement of creatinine clearance should be a more sensitive but is a less accurate indicator of early glomerular dysfunction than that of plasma creatinine concentration.

Clearance values will be low whether the reduced GFR is due to renal circulatory insufficiency, intrinsic renal damage or 'post-renal' causes, and cannot distinguish between them. Creatinine clearance has been said to be useful in deciding the dose of a renally excreted drug.

Cystatin C

Another endogenous substance that can be used as a marker of GFR is plasma cystatin C (Cys C) and its use may alleviate some of the problems associated with creatinine clearance determinations. This is a 13-kDa protein that is a member of the family of cysteine proteinase inhibitors. Unlike other endogenous compounds such as creatinine, Cys C is not secreted by the renal tubules and does not return to the bloodstream after glomerular filtration. It has been suggested that plasma Cys C may approximate to the 'ideal' endogenous marker for GFR, as blood concentrations are independent of patient age and sex.

Renal tubular function tests

Reduced tubular function, with normal glomerular function, impairs the adjustment of the composition and volume of the urine with minimal effect on the plasma urea or creatinine concentration. The investigations used to diagnose tubular disorders can be divided into those that predominantly identify proximal tubular dysfunction and those that predominantly identify distal tubular dysfunction.

Proximal tubular function tests

Impaired solute reabsorption from the proximal tubules reduces isosmotic water reabsorption. Countercurrent multiplication may also be affected, and hence the ability to respond to ADH is reduced. A large volume of inappropriately dilute urine is produced.

The tubules cannot secrete hydrogen ions and so *cannot reabsorb bicarbonate normally* and therefore the urine is inappropriately alkaline for the degree of acidosis in the blood.

The reabsorption of potassium, phosphate, magnesium, urate, glucose and amino acids is impaired. The following findings may be present, and measurement may occasionally be useful.

- *Plasma*:
  - normal urea and creatinine concentrations (normal glomerular function),
  - low bicarbonate concentration with low pH (metabolic acidosis),
  - hypokalaemia, hypophosphataemia, hypomagnesaemia and hypouricaemia.
- *Urine*:
  - increased volume (polyuria),
  - pH high compared with plasma,
  - phosphaturia, glycosuria, uricosuria,
  - generalized aminoaciduria.

Tubular proteinuria can be diagnosed by measuring specific low-molecular-weight proteins such as retinol-binding protein, N-acetyl-β-D-glucosaminidase or α_1-microglobulin.

If there is detectable glycosuria, phosphaturia and non-selective aminoaciduria, the condition is known as the Fanconi syndrome.

Distal tubular function tests

Impaired distal tubular function primarily affects urine acidification, with a failure to excrete hydrogen ions; the urinary pH rarely falls below 5.5. There is an impaired response to aldosterone involving reabsorption of sodium, and the urine contains an inappropriately high concentration of sodium for the renal blood flow. The associated findings may include the following.

- *Plasma*:
  - low bicarbonate and high chloride concentration with low pH (hyperchloraemic acidosis),
  - hypokalaemia.
- *Urine*:
  - increased volume,
  - pH high compared with plasma,
  - an inappropriately high sodium concentration, even if renal blood flow is low (inability to respond to aldosterone),
  - an inappropriately low urea concentration, and therefore osmolality, even if ADH secretion is stimulated.

The *water deprivation test* may be used if tubular damage is suspected (see Chapter 2). The ability to form concentrated urine in response to fluid deprivation depends on normal tubular function (countercurrent multiplication) and on the presence of ADH. Failure of this ability is usually due to renal disease, but if there is any suspicion of cranial diabetes insipidus, the test can be repeated after giving 1-desamino-8-D-arginine-vasopressin, the synthetic analogue of ADH (see Chapter 2). The investigation of renal tubular acidosis is covered in Chapter 4.

URINARY SODIUM AND OSMOLALITY

Urinary sodium estimation

Urinary sodium estimation may be used to differentiate acute oliguria due to renal damage from that due to renal circulatory insufficiency. *Aldosterone secretion will only be maximal if renal blood flow is reduced*; in such circumstances, functioning tubules respond appropriately by selectively reabsorbing sodium by distal tubular exchange mechanisms. A urinary sodium concentration of less than about 20 mmol/L, although not strictly normal if there is a very low renal blood flow, is usually taken to indicate that tubular function is not significantly impaired.

Measurement of urinary osmolality

Measurement of urinary osmolality or other indicators of selective water reabsorption, such as urinary urea or creatinine concentrations, is less valuable than assaying urinary sodium concentration, since ADH secretion is not invariably stimulated (see Table 3.1).

BIOCHEMICAL PRINCIPLES OF THE TREATMENT OF RENAL DYSFUNCTION

Acute renal failure

Careful attention should be given to nephrotoxic drugs in acute renal failure.

In oliguric acute renal failure, fluid intake is usually restricted to a volume equal to urine output plus measured extrarenal losses plus 500 mL/day for insensible loss. Dialysis may improve fluid and electrolyte imbalances (see below). It is important to prevent dangerous hyperkalaemia. A polyuric phase may occur, particularly on relief of urinary obstruction with excretion of potassium and magnesium, and this can result in hypovolaemia, hypokalaemia and hypomagnesaemia, which may need correcting.

Pre-renal acute renal failure can sometimes be reversed by careful control of fluid balance and prompt treatment of hypovolaemia. Sometimes furosemide with mannitol or dopamine infusion may re-establish normal urine flow.

If oliguria is due to parenchymal/intrinsic damage, some clinicians may restrict fluid and sodium intake, giving only enough fluid to replace losses and provide an adequate low-protein energy intake to minimize aggravation of uraemia. If possible, the cause of the intrinsic renal failure should be treated.

In post-renal failure, prompt relief of the obstruction may reverse the situation.

Chronic renal failure

Dietary modification may help in chronic renal failure. Increased caloric intake along with reduced dietary protein intake may slow the decline in GFR by reducing protein catabolism. Nevertheless, it is also important to ensure that the patient is well nourished.

Careful control of fluid and electrolyte balance is important; water intake is usually only restricted if the plasma sodium concentration is not maintained. Similarly, sodium intake should be unrestricted unless contraindications such as hypertension or oedema exist. Plasma potassium monitoring is essential and potassium restriction is necessary if there is hyperkalaemia, which may need specific therapy and can be life threatening (see Chapter 5).

Tissue precipitation of calcium:phosphate may occur early in renal disease and is related to hyperphosphataemia and the calcium phosphate product (calcium concentration $\times$ phosphate concentration). This precipitation can be reduced by adequate fluid intake. Dietary phosphate restriction is used in the early stages of chronic renal dysfunction. If the plasma phosphate concentration is raised, phosphate-binding agents such as calcium acetate or carbonate may be indicated. Oral calcitriol can sometimes also be used to treat hypocalcaemia, suppress plasma PTH concentrations and help avoid renal osteodystrophy.

Recombinant erythropoietin can be used to treat anaemia when haemoglobin is less than 11 g/dL; this may slow progression of chronic renal disease. Optimization of glycaemic control if the patient has diabetes mellitus and treating hypertension are also important.

Dialysis removes urea and other toxic substances from the plasma and corrects electrolyte balance by dialysing the patient's blood against fluid containing no urea and appropriate concentrations of electrolytes, free ionized calcium and other plasma constituents. The following are the principal forms of dialysis.

- Haemofiltration is a form of haemodialysis in which large volumes of fluid and solute can be removed through a highly permeable membrane; dialysis is dependent primarily on the blood pressure. Fluid is replaced intravenously.
- In haemodialysis, blood is passed through an extracorporeal circulation and dialysed across an artificial membrane with a solution of low solute concentration before being returned to the body. Negative pressure on the dialysate side of the membrane can be varied to adjust the amount of water removed.
- In intermittent and continuous ambulatory peritoneal dialysis, the folds of the peritoneum are used as the dialysing membrane with capillaries on one side, and an appropriate fluid of higher osmolality is

infused into the peritoneal cavity on the other. After a suitable time to allow for equilibration of diffusible solutes, depending on the type of peritoneal dialysis, the peritoneal cavity is drained and the cycle is repeated.

Dialysis is used in some cases of acute renal failure until renal function improves, or as a regularly repeated procedure in suitable cases of chronic renal failure. It may also be used to prepare patients for renal transplantation.

RENAL CALCULI

Renal calculi are usually composed of products of metabolism present in normal glomerular filtrate, often at concentrations near their maximum solubility (Fig. 3.9).

Conditions favouring renal calculus formation

- A high urinary concentration of one or more constituents of the glomerular filtrate, due to:
  - a low urinary volume with normal renal function, because of restricted fluid intake or excessive fluid loss over a long period of time; this is particularly common in hot climates; this favours formation of most types of calculi, especially if one of the other conditions listed below is also present;
  - a high rate of excretion of the metabolic product forming the stone, due either to high plasma and therefore filtrate levels or to impairment of normal tubular reabsorption from the filtrate.
- Changes in pH of the urine, often due to bacterial infection, which favour precipitation of different salts at different hydrogen ion concentrations.

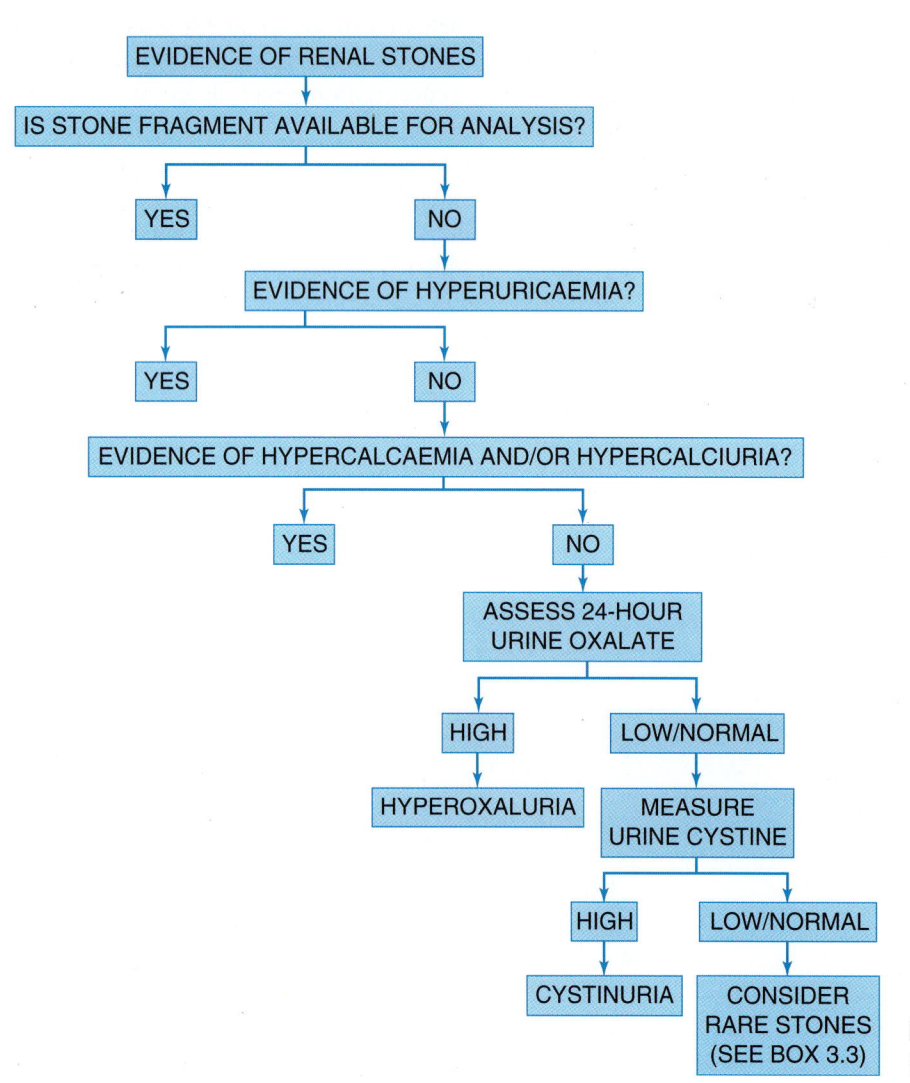

Fig. 3.9 Algorithm for the investigation of renal calculi.

- Urinary stagnation due to obstruction to urinary outflow.
- Lack of normal inhibitors: urine normally contains inhibitors, such as citrate, pyrophosphate and glycoproteins, which inhibit the growth of calcium phosphate and calcium oxalate crystals respectively. Hypocitraturia may partly explain the renal calculi found in distal or type 1 renal tubular acidosis (see Chapter 4).

Constituents of urinary calculi

Renal calculi may consist of the following (Box 3.3).

- Calcium-containing salts:
  – calcium oxalate,
  – calcium phosphate.
- Urate.
- Cystine.
- Xanthine.

Calculi composed of calcium salts

About 80 per cent of all renal stones contain calcium. Precipitation is favoured by hypercalciuria, and the type of salt depends on urinary pH and on the availability of oxalate. Any patient presenting with calcium-containing calculi should have plasma calcium and phosphate estimations performed, and if the results are normal, they should be repeated at regular intervals to exclude primary hyperparathyroidism.

Hypercalcaemia causes hypercalciuria if glomerular function is normal. The causes and differential diagnosis of hypercalcaemia are discussed in Chapter 6. In many subjects with calcium-containing renal calculi the plasma calcium concentration is normal. Any increased release of calcium from bone (as in actively progressing osteoporosis, in which loss of matrix causes secondary decalcification, or in prolonged acidosis, in which ionization of calcium is increased) causes hypercalciuria; hypercalcaemia is unusual in such cases. In distal renal tubular acidosis there is an increased calcium load and, because of the relative alkalinity of the urine, calcium precipitation in the kidney and renal tract may occur – nephrocalcinosis. Hypercalciuria has been defined as a daily urinary calcium excretion of more than 6.2 mmol in adult females and 7.5 mmol in adult males.

A significant proportion of cases remain in which there is no apparent cause for calcium precipitation. A common cause is hypercalciuria despite normocalcaemia (see Chapter 6).

Hyperoxaluria favours the formation of the very poorly soluble calcium oxalate, even if calcium excretion is normal. The source of the oxalate may be derived exogenously from the diet. Oxalate absorption is increased by fat malabsorption: calcium in the bowel is bound to fat instead of precipitating with oxalate, which is then free to be absorbed. Foods rich in oxalate include rhubarb, chocolate, beetroot, spinach, nuts and tea. Primary hyperoxaluria, a rare inborn error, should be considered if renal calculi occur in childhood. There are two main types, 1 and 2, the former being more common. Type 1 is due to deficiency of alanine glyoxylate aminotransferase, and type 2 is due to deficient D-glycerate dehydrogenase. Hyperoxaluria (urinary oxalate greater than 400 μmol/24 hours) is a more important risk factor for formation of renal stones than hypercalciuria.

Calcium-containing calculi are usually hard, white and radio-opaque. Calcium phosphate may form 'staghorn' calculi in the renal pelvis, while calcium oxalate stones tend to be smaller and to lodge in the ureters, where they are compressed into a fusiform shape. Alkaline conditions favouring calcium phosphate precipitation and stone formation are particularly common in patients with chronic renal infection.

The treatment of calcium-containing calculi depends on the cause. Urinary calcium concentration should be reduced:

- by treating the primary condition, such as urinary infection or hypercalcaemia;
- if this is not possible, by reducing dietary calcium and oxalate intake;
- by maintaining a high fluid intake, unless there is glomerular failure.

Thiazide diuretics reduce urinary calcium excretion.

Struvite (magnesium ammonium phosphate)

These stones (about 10 per cent of all renal calculi) are associated with chronic urinary tract infections by organisms

---

Box 3.3 Some causes of renal calculi

Calcium phosphate or oxalate
Triple phosphate stones
Urate
Cystine
Complex/mixture stones
Rarities, e.g. xanthine, dihydroxyadenine or indinavir
Artefacts, e.g. fibrin/clots/Munchausen's syndrome

such as *Proteus* species capable of splitting ammonium. The urinary pH is usually greater than 7. These urease-containing bacteria convert urea to ammonia and bicarbonate.

Uric acid stones

About 8 per cent of renal calculi contain uric acid; these are sometimes associated with hyperuricaemia, with or without clinical gout. In most cases, no predisposing cause can be found. Precipitation is favoured in an acid urine.

Uric acid stones are usually small, friable and yellowish-brown, but can occasionally be large enough to form 'staghorn' calculi. They are radiolucent but may be visualized by ultrasound or by an intravenous pyelogram.

The treatment of hyperuricaemia is discussed in Chapter 20. If the plasma urate concentration is normal, fluid intake should be kept high and the urine alkalinized. A low-purine diet may help to reduce urate production and excretion.

Cystine stones

Cystine stones are rare. In normal subjects the concentration of cystine in urine is soluble, but in homozygous cystinuria this may be exceeded and the patient may present with radio-opaque renal calculi. Like urate, cystine is more soluble in alkaline than in acidic urine; the principles of treatment are the same as for uric acid stones. Penicillamine can also be used to treat the condition (see Chapter 27).

Miscellaneous stones

Xanthine stones

Xanthine stones are very uncommon and may be the result of the rare inborn error xanthinuria.

Indinavir stones

These are seen in patients with human immunodeficiency virus infection who have been treated with the protease inhibitor indinavir. The stones are composed of pure protease inhibitor.

Other rare stones may consist of dihydroxyadenine (due to adenine phosphoribosyltransferase deficiency) or poorly calcified mucoproteinaceous material associated with chronically infected kidneys (matrix stone). Some stones may be factitious, as sometimes found in patients with Munchausen's syndrome, who may add stones to their urine.

Investigation of a patient with renal calculi

- If the stone is available, send it to the laboratory for analysis.
- Exclude hypercalcaemia (see Chapter 6) and hyperuricaemia (see Chapter 20).
- Collect a 24-hour specimen of urine for urinary volume, calcium and oxalate estimations. These tests will help to detect hypercalciuria or hyperoxaluria.
- If all these tests are negative, and especially if there is a family history of calculi, screen the urine for cystine. If the qualitative test is positive, the 24-hour excretion of cystine and basic amino acids should be estimated.
- If fresh uninfected urine is alkaline despite a systemic metabolic acidosis, the diagnosis of renal tubular acidosis is likely (see Chapter 4). A pH more than 8 is suggestive of a urinary infection with a urea-splitting organism such as *Proteus vulgaris*, in which case consider struvite calculi. A midstream urine specimen is useful to exclude infection before diagnosing renal tubular acidosis.
- Low plasma urate and high urinary xanthine concentrations suggest xanthinuria, particularly in a child.
- Determination of urinary citrate (an inhibitor of some renal calculi) concentrations may sometimes be useful, as low concentrations may be found.
- If the cause is still unclear, consider the rare causes of renal calculi shown in Box 3.3.
- Renal tract imaging techniques to clarify the anatomy, such as ultrasound or intravenous pyelogram, may also be necessary.

Treatment of renal calculi

Apart from specific treatments, patients with a tendency to form calculi are generally advised to drink more water. The aim is usually to increase the urinary volume to about 2–3 L in 24 hours. Reducing calcium intake may not be advisable, as it may increase oxalate absorption and excretion. Calculi removal by fragmentation using extracorporeal shock wave lithotripsy has in some cases reduced the need for surgical intervention.

CASE 3

A 21-year-old male presented to the urology out-patient department because of renal calculi. There was also a family history of renal calculi.

Plasma
Sodium 137 mmol/L (135–145)
Potassium 4.2 mmol/L (3.5–5.0)
Urea 5.9 mmol/L (2.5–7.0)
Creatinine 108 µmol/L (70–110)
'Corrected' calcium 2.43 mmol/L (2.15–2.55)
Phosphate 1.1 mmol/L (0.80–1.35)
Bicarbonate 27 mmol/L (24–32)

Urate 0.33 mmol/L (0.20–0.43)

Urinary excretion of both calcium and oxalate fell within the laboratory reference ranges. However, cystine was detected in the urine.

DISCUSSION

In conjunction with the family history and relatively young age of presentation, the results are suggestive of cystinuria manifesting cystine stones. This is one of the commonest aminoacidurias and is treated by increasing fluid intake and alkalinizing the urine.

CONCLUSIONS

- The kidneys are vital organs for the excretion of various waste products as well as for acid–base balance, fluid volume control, hormone production and metabolic function, such as calcium homeostasis.
- Plasma creatinine determination is a useful test of renal function but plasma creatinine concentration can still remain within the reference range in the presence of a significant decline in renal function.
- Acute renal failure can be due to pre-renal, renal or post-renal causes. Raised plasma urea and creatinine concentrations occur along with fluid retention, anuria or oligouria, hyperkalaemia, hyperphosphataemia and metabolic acidosis.
- Chronic renal failure implies slow, irreversible renal disease. Raised plasma urea and creatinine concentrations occur initially and as renal reserve declines, there is further hyperkalaemia, hyperphosphataemia, metabolic acidosis, hypocalcaemia and anaemia.
- Renal calculi can be the result of urinary stasis or infection associated with urinary supersaturation. The commonest calculi are calcium containing.
- Nephrotic syndrome is defined as gross proteinuria associated with oedema and hypoproteinaemia (discussed further in Chapter 19). This is a disorder of the renal glomerular membrane.
- Renal tubular disease can result in Fanconi's syndrome associated with acid–base and potassium disturbance, glycosuria and hypophosphataemia.

4 ACID–BASE DISTURBANCES

Definitions	58	Blood gases	77
Acid–base control systems	59	Investigation of hydrogen ion disturbances	80
Acid–base disorders	64		

The importance of acid–base homeostasis cannot be overstated because of its importance in keeping hydrogen ion (H^+) balance under control. Acid–base abnormalities are relatively common medically and it is therefore essential for clinicians to be fully conversant with their interpretation.

Our cells release between 50 mmol and 100 mmol of H^+ into the extracellular fluid daily. Despite this, the extracellular H^+ concentration ($[H^+]$) is maintained at about 40 nmol/L (pH 7.4).

The predominant sources of H^+ are:

- Anaerobic carbohydrate metabolism produces lactate, and anaerobic metabolism of fatty acids and of ketogenic amino acids produces acetoacetate, which releases equimolar amounts of H^+. Lactic acidosis or ketoacidosis can occur if the release of H^+ by these reactions exceeds the compensatory capacity.
- Release of H^+ can occur during conversion of amino nitrogen to urea in the liver, or of the sulphydryl groups of some amino acids to sulphate.

Hydrogen ion balance is largely dependent upon the secretion of H^+ from the body into the urine due to renal tubular action. Aerobic metabolism of the carbon skeletons of organic compounds converts carbon, hydrogen and oxygen into carbon dioxide and water. Carbon dioxide is an essential component of the extracellular buffering system. Thus the body is dependent upon healthy function of the kidneys and the lungs for normal acid–base homeostasis.

DEFINITIONS

Acids can dissociate to produce H^+ (protons), which can be accepted by a base. An alkali dissociates to produce hydroxyl ions (OH^-). Acidosis is commoner than alkalosis because metabolism tends to produce H^+ rather than OH^-.

A strong acid is almost completely dissociated in aqueous solution, and so produces many H^+. For example, hydrochloric acid is a strong acid and is almost entirely dissociated in water to form H^+ and chloride (Cl^-). Weak acids dissociate less, although very small changes in $[H^+]$ may have important consequences.

Buffering is a process by which a strong acid (or base) is replaced by a weaker one, with a consequent reduction in the number of free H^+, and therefore the change in pH, after addition of acid, is less than it would be in the absence of the buffer. For example:

$$H^+Cl^- + NaHCO_3 \leftrightarrow H_2CO_3 + NaCl$$
$$\text{(strong acid)} \quad \text{(buffer)} \quad \text{(weak acid)} \quad \text{(neutral salt)}$$
(4.1)

The pH is a measure of H^+ activity. It is log 10 of the reciprocal of $[H^+]$ in mol/L. The log 10 of a number is the power to which 10 must be raised to produce that number:

$$\log 100 = \log 10^2 = 2, \text{ and } \log 10^7 = 7 \quad (4.2)$$

If $[H^+]$ is 10^{-7} (0.0000001) mol/L, then $-\log[H^+] = 7$. But:

$$pH = \log \frac{1}{[H^+]} = -\log[H^+] \quad (4.3)$$

Therefore pH = 7.

A change of 1 pH unit represents a tenfold change in $[H^+]$. Changes of this magnitude do not normally occur in tissues. However, in pathological conditions the blood pH can change by more than 0.3 of a unit; a decrease of pH by 0.3, from 7.4 to 7.1, represents a doubling of the [H^+] from 40 to 80 nmol/L. Thus, the use of the pH notation makes a very significant change in [H^+] appear deceptively small.

A blood pH of 7.0 indicates a severe acidosis. A blood pH of 7.7 similarly indicates a severe alkalosis. Urinary pH is much more variable than that of blood, where [H^+] can vary 1000-fold (a change of 3 pH units).

The Henderson–Hasselbalch equation expresses the relation between pH and a buffer pair – that is, a weak acid and its conjugate base. The equation is valid for any buffer pair, the pH being dependent on the ratio of the concentration of base to acid. Note that pK_a is the negative logarithm of the acid dissociation constant (K_a).

$$pH = pK_a + \log \frac{[base]}{[acid]} \quad (4.4)$$

In this equation the base is bicarbonate (HCO_3^-) and the acid is carbonic acid (H_2CO_3). It is not possible to measure the latter directly; however, it is in equilibrium with dissolved CO_2, of which the partial pressure ($P{CO_2}$) can be estimated. The concentration of H_2CO_3 is derived by multiplying this measured value by the solubility constant (S) for CO_2. Thus:

$$pH = pK_a + \log \frac{[HCO_3^-]}{P_{CO_2} \times S} \quad (4.5)$$

If the P_{CO_2} is expressed in kilopascals (kPa), S = 0.23, or in mmHg, S = 0.03.

The overall pK_a of the bicarbonate system is 6.1. Therefore if P_{CO_2} is in kPa:

$$pH = 6.1 + \log \frac{[HCO_3^-]}{P_{CO_2} \times 0.23} \quad (4.6)$$

Plasma [HCO_3^-] is controlled largely by the kidneys and P_{CO_2} by the lungs. In acid–base disturbances due to respiratory problems the kidneys are essential for compensation and, conversely, in metabolic (non-respiratory) causes of acid–base imbalance the compensation is due mainly to changes in pulmonary function.

Despite considerable fluctuations in the rate of release of H^+ into the extracellular fluid, the [H^+], and therefore pH, is relatively tightly controlled in blood by the following mechanisms.

- H^+ can be incorporated into water:

$$H^+ + HCO_3^- \leftrightarrow H_2CO_3 \leftrightarrow CO_2 + H_2O \quad (4.7)$$

This mechanism occurs during oxidative phosphorylation. The reaction is reversible, and H^+ combines with HCO_3^- only if the reaction is driven to the right by the removal of CO_2. By itself this would cause HCO_3^- depletion.

- Buffering of H^+ is a temporary measure, as the H^+ has not been excreted from the body. The production of the weak acid of the buffer pair causes only a small change in pH (see Henderson–Hasselbalch equation). If H^+ are not completely neutralized or eliminated from the body and if production continues, buffering power will eventually be so depleted that the pH will change significantly.
- There are two main ways by which H^+ can be lost from the body: through the kidneys or some of the intestine, mainly the stomach. This mechanism is coupled with the generation of HCO_3^-. In the kidney this is the method by which secretion of excess H^+ ensures regeneration of buffering capacity.

ACID–BASE CONTROL SYSTEMS

Carbon dioxide and H^+ are potentially toxic products of aerobic and anaerobic metabolism respectively. Most CO_2 is lost through the lungs, but some is converted to HCO_3^-, thus contributing important extracellular buffering capacity; inactivating one toxic product provides a means of minimizing the effects of the other.

A buffer pair is most effective at maintaining a pH near its pK_a, i.e. when the ratio of the concentrations of base to acid is close to 1. However, the optimum pH of the extracellular fluid is about 7.4 and the pK_a of the bicarbonate system is 6.1. Although this may seem to be disadvantageous, the bicarbonate system is the most important buffer in the body because:

- it accounts for more than 60 per cent of the blood buffering capacity,
- H^+ secretion by the kidney depends on it,
- it is necessary for efficient buffering by haemoglobin (Hb), which provides most of the rest of the blood buffering capacity.

The control of carbon dioxide by the lungs

The partial pressure of CO_2 (P_{CO_2}) in plasma is normally about 5.3 kPa (40 mmHg) and depends on the balance between the rate of production by metabolism and the loss through the pulmonary alveoli. The sequence of events is as follows.

(1) Inspired oxygen (O_2) is carried from the lungs to the tissues by Hb.
(2) The tissue cells use the O_2 for aerobic metabolism; some of the carbon in organic compounds is oxidized to CO_2.
(3) CO_2 diffuses along a concentration gradient from the cells into the extracellular fluid and is returned by the blood to the lungs, where it is eliminated in expired air.
(4) The rate of respiration, and therefore the rate of CO_2 elimination, is controlled by chemoreceptors in the respiratory centre in the medulla of the brainstem and by those in the carotid and aortic bodies. The receptors respond to changes in the [CO_2] or [H^+] of plasma or of the cerebrospinal fluid. If the $P{CO_2}$ rises much above 5.3 kPa, or if the pH falls, the rate of respiration increases.

Normal lungs have a very large reserve capacity for elimination of CO_2. Not only is there a plentiful supply of CO_2, the denominator in the Henderson–Hasselbalch equation, but the normal respiratory centre and lungs can control its concentration within narrow limits by responding to changes in the [H^+] and therefore compensate for changes in acid–base disturbances.

Bicarbonate generation

The control of bicarbonate by the kidneys and erythrocytes

The erythrocytes and renal tubular cells generate HCO_3^-, the buffer base in the bicarbonate system, from CO_2. Under physiological conditions:

- the erythrocyte mechanism makes fine adjustments to the plasma [HCO_3^-] in response to changes in $P{CO_2}$ in the lungs and tissues;
- the kidneys play the major role in maintaining the circulating [HCO_3^-] and in eliminating H^+ from the body.

The carbonate dehydratase system

Bicarbonate is produced following the dissociation of carbonic acid formed from CO_2 and H_2O. This is catalysed by carbonate dehydratase (CD; carbonic anhydrase), which is present in high concentrations in erythrocytes and renal tubular cells.

$$CO_2 + H_2O \underset{CD}{\leftrightarrow} H_2CO_3 \leftrightarrow H^+ + HCO_3^-$$

(4.8)

Erythrocytes and renal tubular cells have high concentrations of CD, but also have means of removing one of the products, H^+; thus both reactions continue to the right and HCO_3^- is formed. One of the reactants (water) is freely available and one of the products (H^+) is removed. Bicarbonate ion generation is therefore accelerated if the concentration of:

- CO_2 rises,
- HCO_3^- falls,
- H^+ falls because it is either buffered by erythrocytes or excreted from the body by renal tubular cells.

Therefore, an increase of intracellular $P{CO_2}$ or a decrease in intracellular [HCO_3^-] in the erythrocytes and renal tubular cells maintains the extracellular [HCO_3^-] by accelerating the production of HCO_3^-. This minimizes changes in the ratio of [HCO_2^-] to $P{CO_2}$ and therefore changes in pH.

In the normal subject, at a plasma $P{CO_2}$ of 5.3 kPa (a [CO_2] of about 1.2 mmol/L), erythrocytes and renal tubular cells maintain the extracellular HCO_3^- at about 25 mmol/L. The extracellular ratio of [HCO_3^-] to [CO_2] (both in mmol/L) is just over 20:1. It can be calculated from the Henderson–Hasselbalch equation, and with a pK_a of 6.1 this represents a pH very near 7.4. An increase of intracellular $P{CO_2}$, or a decrease in intracellular [HCO_3^-], accelerates HCO_3^- production and minimizes changes in the ratio and therefore in pH.

Bicarbonate generation by the erythrocytes
(Fig. 4.1)

Haemoglobin is an important blood buffer. However, it only works effectively in cooperation with the bicarbonate system.

$$pH = pK_a + \log \frac{[Hb^-]}{[HHb]}$$

(4.9)

Erythrocytes produce little CO_2 as they lack aerobic pathways. Plasma CO_2 diffuses along a concentration gradient into erythrocytes, where CD catalyses its reaction with water to form carbonic acid (H_2CO_3), which then dissociates. Much of the H^+ is buffered by Hb and the HCO_3^- diffuses out into the extracellular fluid along a concentration gradient.

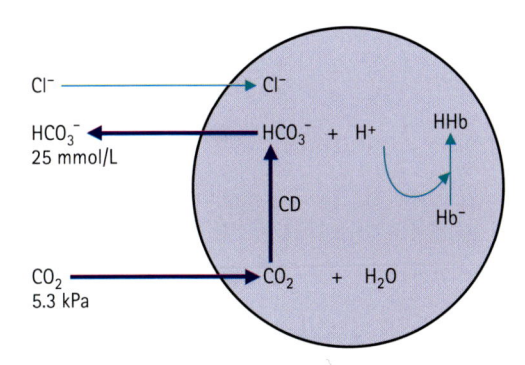

Fig. 4.1 Generation of bicarbonate by erythrocytes, showing the chloride shift. (CD = carbonate dehydratase; Hb = haemoglobin.)

Electrochemical neutrality is maintained by diffusion of Cl^- in the opposite direction into cells. This movement of ions is known as the 'chloride shift'.

Under normal circumstances the higher $P\text{CO}_2$ in the blood leaving tissues stimulates erythrocyte HCO_3^- production; consequently the arteriovenous difference in the ratio $[HCO_3^-]:[CO_2]$, and therefore the pH, is kept relatively constant.

Extracellular and intracellular buffers other than HCO_3^- and Hb do not contribute significantly to blood buffering. They include:

- phosphate, which has a plasma concentration of about 1 mmol/L, but a higher concentration in bone and inside cells where buffering capacity is of more importance;
- proteins, which, because of their low concentrations in plasma, also have little blood buffering capacity.

The kidneys

Carbonate dehydratase is also of central importance in the mechanisms involved in H^+ secretion and in maintaining the HCO_3^- buffering capacity in the blood. Hydrogen ions are secreted from renal tubular cells into the lumina, where they are buffered by constituents of the glomerular filtrate. Unlike Hb in erythrocytes, urinary buffers are constantly being replenished by continuing glomerular filtration. For this reason, and because most of the excess H^+ can only be eliminated from the body by the renal route, the kidneys are of major importance in compensating for chronic acidosis. Without them, the Hb buffering capacity would soon become saturated.

Two renal mechanisms control $[HCO_3^-]$ in the extracellular fluid:

- *Bicarbonate reclamation* ('reabsorption'), the predominant mechanism in maintaining the steady state.

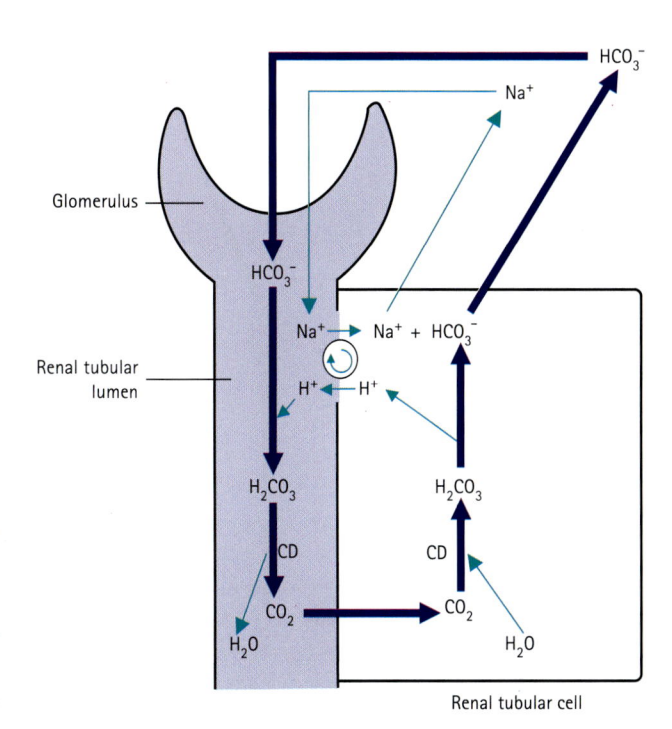

Fig. 4.2 Normal reabsorption of filtered bicarbonate from the renal tubules. (CD = carbonate dehydratase.)

The CO_2 driving the CD mechanism in renal tubular cells is derived from filtered HCO_3^-. There is no net loss of H^+ (Fig. 4.2).

- *Bicarbonate generation*, a very important mechanism for correcting acidosis, in which the levels of CO_2 or $[HCO_3^-]$ affecting the CD reaction in renal tubular cells reflect those in the extracellular fluid. There is a net loss of H^+ (Fig 4.3).

Bicarbonate reclamation

Normal urine is nearly HCO_3^- free. An amount equivalent to that filtered by the glomeruli is returned to the body by the tubular cells. The luminal surfaces of renal tubular cells are impermeable to HCO_3^-. Thus, HCO_3^- can only be returned to the body if first converted to CO_2 in the tubular lumina, and an equivalent amount of CO_2 is converted to HCO_3^- within tubular cells. The mechanism depends on the action of CD, both in the brush border on the luminal surfaces and within tubular cells, and on H^+ secreted into the lumina in exchange for sodium (Na^+). This occurs predominantly in the proximal tubules but also in the first part of the distal tubules.

- Bicarbonate is filtered through the glomeruli at a plasma concentration of about 25 mmol/L.

ACID–BASE DISTURBANCES

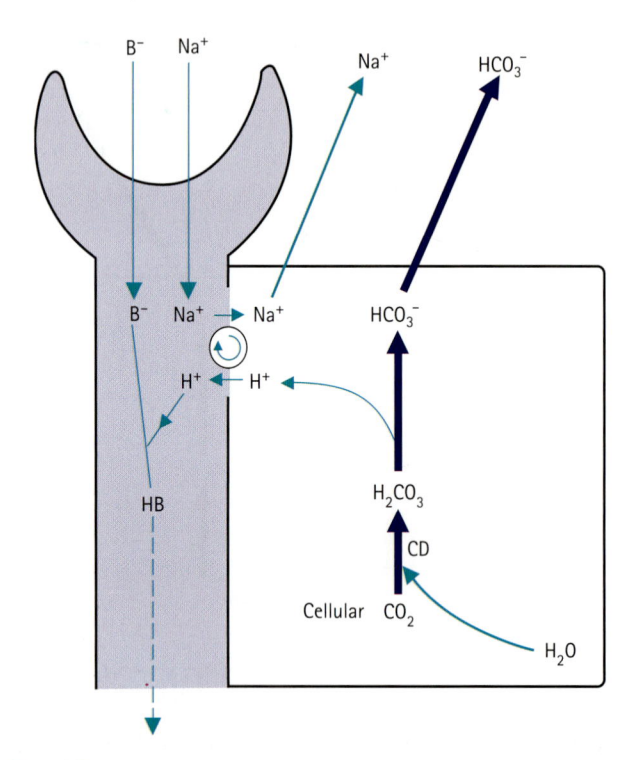

Fig. 4.3 Net generation of bicarbonate by renal tubular cells with excretion of hydrogen ions. (B^- = non-bicarbonate base; CD = carbonate dehydratase.)

- Filtered HCO_3^- combines with H^+, secreted by tubular cells, to form H_2CO_3.
- The H_2CO_3 dissociates to form CO_2 and water. In the proximal tubules this reaction is catalysed by CD in the brush border. In the distal tubules, where the pH is usually lower, H_2CO_3 probably dissociates spontaneously.
- As the luminal $P{CO_2}$ rises, CO_2 diffuses into tubular cells along a concentration gradient, and as the intracellular concentration of CO_2 rises, CD catalyses its combination with water to form H_2CO_3, which dissociates into H^+ and HCO_3^-.
- Hydrogen ions are secreted in the tubular lumina in exchange for Na^+ and so the HCO_3^- generating reactions start again from the second stage. As the intracellular concentration of HCO_3^- rises, HCO_3^- diffuses into the extracellular fluid accompanied by Na^+, which has been reabsorbed in exchange for H^+.

This self-perpetuating cycle reclaims buffering capacity that would otherwise have been lost from the body by glomerular filtration. The secreted H^+ is derived from cellular water, and is incorporated into water in the lumina. Because there is no net change in H^+ balance and no net gain of HCO_3^-, this mechanism cannot correct an acidosis but can maintain a steady state.

Bicarbonate generation

The mechanism in renal tubular cells for generating HCO_3^- is identical to that of HCO_3^- reabsorption, but there is net loss of H^+ from the body as well as a net gain of HCO_3^-. Therefore this mechanism is well suited to correcting any type of acidosis.

Within tubular cells, CD may be stimulated by the following.

- A rise in $P{CO_2}$. In this case, the rise in $[CO_2]$ is the indirect result of a rise in the extracellular $P{CO_2}$. Renal tubular cells, unlike erythrocytes with anaerobic pathways, constantly produce CO_2 aerobically. This diffuses out of cells into the extracellular fluid along a concentration gradient. An increase in extracellular $P{CO_2}$, by reducing the gradient, slows this diffusion and the intracellular $P{CO_2}$ rises.
- A fall of $[HCO_3^-]$. Reduction of extracellular $[HCO_3^-]$, by increasing the concentration gradient across renal tubular cell membranes, increases the loss of HCO_3^- from cells.

Normally almost all the filtered HCO_3^- is reabsorbed. Once the luminal fluid is HCO_3^- free, continued secretion of H^+ and the intracellular generation of HCO_3^- depend on the presence of other filtered buffer bases (B^-). In their absence, the luminal acidity would increase so much that further H^+ secretion would be inhibited. These buffers, unlike HCO_3^-, do not form compounds capable of diffusing back into tubular cells, nor is H^+ incorporated into water. There is net loss of H^+ in urine as HB. The HCO_3^- formed in the cell is derived from cellular CO_2 and therefore represents a net gain in HCO_3^-.

Whenever 1 mmol of H^+ is secreted into the tubular lumen, 1 mmol of HCO_3^- passes into the extracellular fluid with Na^+. The mechanism of HCO_3^- generation is very similar to that in erythrocytes. However, unlike red cells, renal tubular cells are exposed to a relatively constant $P{CO_2}$. Bicarbonate generation, coupled with H^+ secretion, becomes very important in acidosis, when it is stimulated by either a fall in extracellular $[HCO_3^-]$ (metabolic acidosis) or a rise in extracellular $P{CO_2}$ (respiratory acidosis).

Urinary buffers

Apart from HCO_3^-, the two other major urinary buffers are phosphate and ammonia (NH_3); they are also involved in HCO_3^- generation.

Phosphate buffer pair

At pH 7.4, most of the phosphate in plasma, and also in the glomerular filtrate, is monohydrogen phosphate (HPO_4^{2-}), which can accept H^+ to become dihydrogen phosphate ($H_2PO_4^-$). Bicarbonate can continue to be generated within tubular cells, with H^+, and to be returned to the body after all that in the filtrate has been reabsorbed. Therefore it can help to replace that used in extracellular buffering. The pK_a of this buffer pair is about 6.8.

$$pH = 6.8 + \log \frac{[HPO_4^{2-}]}{[H_2PO_4^-]} \quad (4.10)$$

Phosphate is normally the most important buffer in the urine because its pK_a is relatively close to the pH of the glomerular filtrate and because the concentration of phosphate increases 20-fold, to nearly 25 mmol/L, as water is reabsorbed from the tubular lumen.

Even in a mild acidosis, more phosphate ions are released from bone than at normal pH; the need for increased urinary H^+ secretion is linked with increased buffering capacity in the glomerular filtrate due to the increase of phosphate. At a urinary pH below 5.5, most of the filtered phosphate is converted to dihydrogen phosphate. Therefore at low pH urinary phosphate cannot maintain the essential buffering of continued H^+ secretion. The predominant urinary anion is Cl^-, but, because hydrochloric acid is almost completely ionized in aqueous solution, it cannot act as a buffer.

The role of ammonia

As the urine becomes more acid, it can be shown to contain increasing amounts of ammonium ion (NH_4^+). Urinary ammonia probably allows H^+ secretion, and therefore HCO_3^- formation, to continue after other buffers have been depleted.

Ammonia, produced by hepatic deamination of amino acids, is rapidly incorporated into urea, with a net production of H^+. However, as the systemic $[H^+]$ increases, there is some shift from urea to glutamine ($GluCONH_2$) synthesis, with a slight fall in hepatic H^+ production. Glutamine is taken up by renal tubular cells, where it is hydrolysed by glutaminase to glutamate ($GluCOO^-$) and NH_4^+.

$$H_2O + GluCONH_2 \rightarrow GluCOO^- + NH_4^+ \quad (4.11)$$

Ammonia and NH_4^+ form a buffer pair with a pK_a of about 9.8.

$$pH = 9.8 + \log \frac{[NH_3]}{[NH_4^+]} \quad (4.12)$$

Because of the very high pK_a, at pH 7.4 and below the equilibrium is overwhelmingly in favour of NH_4^+ production. Ammonia can diffuse out of the cell into the tubular lumen much more rapidly than NH_4^+. If the luminal fluid is acidic, NH_3 will be retained within the lumen by avid combination with H^+ derived from the CD mechanism. This allows H^+, produced in the kidneys, to be excreted as ammonium chloride ($NH_4^+Cl^-$); thus in severe acidosis, HCO_3^- formation can continue even when phosphate buffering power has been exhausted. There is a net gain of HCO_3^-. However, H^+ as well as NH_3 is released in renal tubular cells when NH_4^+ dissociates; this is maintained by passive diffusion of NH_3 into the luminal fluid (Fig. 4.4).

On the face of it there seems no advantage in buffering one H^+ secreted into the lumen if, at the same time, another is produced within the cell.

Explanations for the role of NH_3 in the correction of acidosis include the following.

- The fate of the $GluCOO^-$ produced at the same time as the NH_4^+. After further deamination to 2-oxoglutarate, it can be converted to glucose; gluconeogenesis uses an equivalent amount of H^+ to the generation of NH_4^+ produced from glutamine. Therefore, the H^+ liberated into the cell may be incorporated into glucose.
- A shift from urea synthesis to glutamine production in the liver with a fall in systemic H^+ production in the presence of an acidosis. This is a minor factor.

The rate of gluconeogenesis and glutamine synthesis and glutaminase activity all increase in an acidosis.

Bicarbonate formation in the gastrointestinal tract

Carbonate dehydratase also catalyses the formation of HCO_3^- in intestinal mucosal cells. The HCO_3^- may pass either into the extracellular fluid or into the intestinal lumen – a mechanism that can only continue if H^+ is pumped in the opposite direction. Electrochemical neutrality is maintained by one of two mechanisms:

- Na^+ exchange for H^+, by a mechanism that is the opposite of that in renal tubular cells,
- passage of Cl^- with H^+.

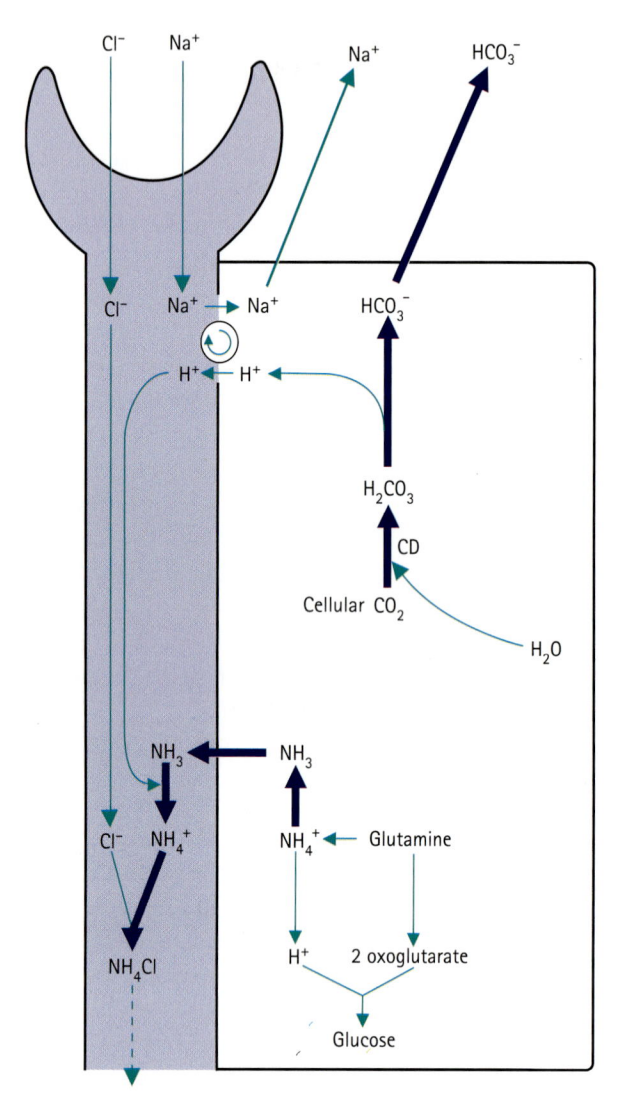

Fig. 4.4 The role of ammonia in the generation of bicarbonate by renal tubular cells. (CD = carbonate dehydratase). (Modified with kind permission from Williams DL, Marks V, eds. *Biochemistry in clinical practice*, London: Heinemann Medical Books, 1983.)

Acid secretion by the stomach

The parietal cells of the stomach secrete H^+ into the lumen together with Cl^-. As H^+Cl^- enters the gastric lumen, HCO_3^- diffuses into the extracellular fluid, thus accounting for the postprandial 'alkaline tide'. In the normal subject this is rapidly corrected by HCO_3^- secretion, mainly by the pancreas, as food passes down the intestinal tract. This mechanism explains the metabolic alkalosis that occurs in pyloric stenosis.

Sodium bicarbonate secretion by pancreatic and biliary cells

Sodium bicarbonate secretion by the pancreatic and biliary cells in response to stimulation by secretin accounts for the alkalinization of the duodenal fluid and occurs by the reverse process of $NaHCO_3$ reabsorption in renal tubular cells. The pancreatic and biliary mechanisms are accelerated by the local rise in $P\text{CO}_2$ that results when H^+ is pumped into the extracellular fluid and reacts with the HCO_3^- generated by gastric parietal cells. This is analogous to the stimulation of renal HCO_3^- formation by the rise in luminal $P\text{CO}_2$. Loss of large amounts of duodenal fluid may cause HCO_3^- depletion.

Bicarbonate secretion and chloride reabsorption by intestinal cells

As fluid passes down the intestinal tract, HCO_3^- enters and Cl^- leaves the lumen by a reversal of the gastric mucosal mechanism. Therefore the gastric loss of Cl^- and the gain of HCO_3^- are finally corrected. Preferential reabsorption of urinary Cl^- by this mechanism after ureteric transplantation into the ileum, ileal loops or the colon explains the hyperchloraemic acidosis (normal anion-gap acidosis) associated with this operation (Fig. 4.5).

ACID–BASE DISORDERS

Disturbances of H^+ homeostasis always involve the bicarbonate buffer pair. In respiratory disturbances abnormalities of CO_2 are primary, whereas in so-called metabolic or non-respiratory disturbances $[HCO_3^-]$ is affected early and changes in CO_2 are secondary.

Acid blood pH is known as acidaemia, and alkaline blood pH is called alkaemia. Abnormal processes, either respiratory or metabolic, generate abnormal amounts of acid or base – acidosis or alkalosis respectively. The blood pH may or may not be abnormal because of the compensatory mechanisms.

Acidosis

Acidosis occurs if there is a fall in the ratio $[HCO_3^-]:P\text{CO}_2$ in the extracellular fluid. It may be due to:

- *metabolic (non-respiratory) acidosis*, in which the primary abnormality in the bicarbonate buffer system is a reduction in $[HCO_3^-]$;
- *respiratory acidosis*, in which the primary abnormality in the bicarbonate buffer system is a rise in $P\text{CO}_2$.

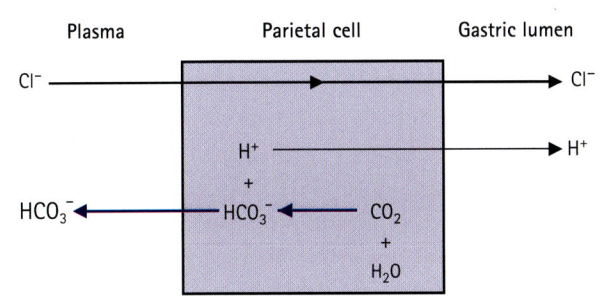

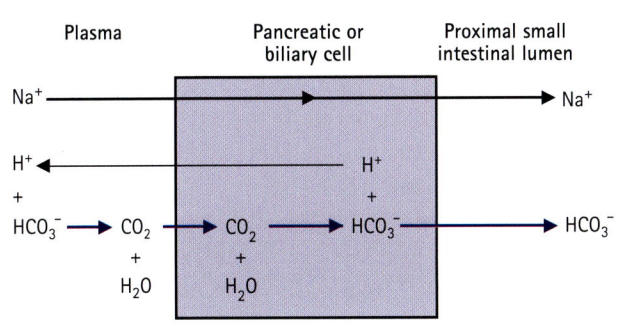

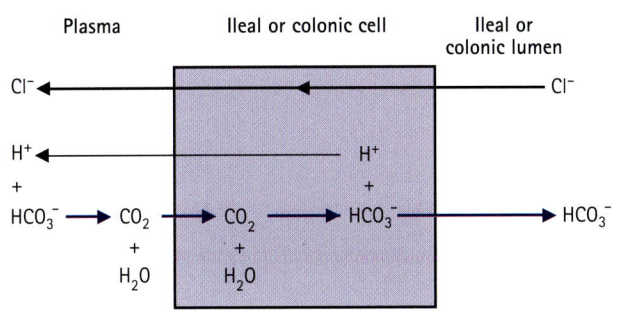

Fig. 4.5 Acid–base balance in intestinal cells.

Metabolic acidosis

The primary disorder in the bicarbonate buffer system in a metabolic acidosis is a reduction in $[HCO_3^-]$, resulting in a fall in blood pH. The reduction in the HCO_3^- may be due to:

- its use in buffering H^+ more rapidly than it can be generated by normal homeostatic mechanisms,
- loss in the urine or gastrointestinal tract more rapidly than it can be generated by normal homeostatic mechanisms,
- impaired production.

> **Box 4.1 Some causes of a metabolic acidosis**
>
> *High plasma anion gap*
> Acute or chronic renal failure
> Ketosis (diabetes mellitus [commonest]); also ethanol or starvation
> Lactic acidosis (see Box 4.2)
> Intoxicants:
>   salicylates (can cause other acid–base disturbances)
>   methanol
>   ethanol
>   ethylene glycol (anti-freeze)
>   paraldehyde
>   paracetamol
> Massive rhabdomyolysis (muscle release of H^+ and organic anions)
> Organic acidurias
>
> *Normal plasma anion gap*
> Hyperchloraemic acidosis (see Box 4.3)

The causes of a metabolic acidosis are shown in Box 4.1 and can be divided into those with a high and those with a normal plasma anion gap.

Concept of plasma anion gap

One negative charge balances one positive charge, and some substances are multivalent, having more than one charge per mole. If the molecular weight is divided by the valency, the charges on each resulting equivalent will be the same as those on an equivalent of any other chemical. Most of the ions in the following discussion are monovalent, and hence the number of millimoles is numerically the same as that of milliequivalents (mEq). However, when calculating ion balance, the latter notation should strictly be used, i.e. concentration of charges.

Sodium and potassium (K^+) provide more than 90 per cent of plasma cation concentration in the normal subject; the balance includes low concentrations of calcium (Ca^{2+}) and magnesium (Mg^{2+}), which vary only by small amounts.

More than 80 per cent of plasma anions are accounted for by Cl^- and HCO_3^-; the remaining 20 per cent or so (sometimes referred to as unmeasured anion) is made up of protein, and the normally low concentrations of urate, phosphate, sulphate, lactate and other organic anions. The protein concentration remains relatively constant, but the concentrations of other unmeasured anions can vary considerably in disease.

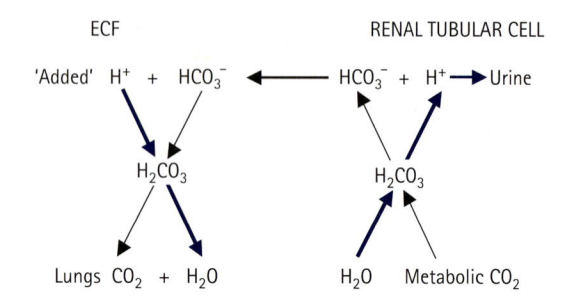

Fig. 4.6 Hydrogen ion 'shuttle' between the site of production and buffering and the site of elimination in the kidneys. (ECF = extracellular fluid.)

The anion gap, represented as A^- in the following equations, is the difference between the total concentration of measured cations (Na^+ and K^+) and measured anions (Cl^- and HCO_3^-); it is normally about 15–20 mEq/L. Therefore:

$$[Na^+] + [K^+] = [HCO_3^-] + [Cl^-] + [A^-]$$
$$140 + 4 = 25 + 100 + 19 \text{ mEq/L}$$

(4.13)

It is worth noting that the plasma anion gap can be decreased by an increase in unmeasured cations, e.g hyperkalaemia, hypercalcaemia, hypermagnesaemia, high immunoglobulin G (IgG), bromide or lithium intoxication, or by a decrease in unmeasured anions, for example hypoalbuminaemia.

As we will see later, the urinary anion gap can also be measured and is useful in the diagnosis of renal tubular acidosis (Fig. 4.6).

High anion gap acidosis

A useful mnemonic to help remember some of the causes of a high anion gap metabolic acidosis is DR MAPLES: D = **d**iabetic ketoacidosis, R = **r**enal, M = **m**ethanol, A = **a**lcoholic ketoacidosis, P = **p**aracetamol, L = **l**actic acidosis, E = **e**thylene glycol, S = **s**alicylates.

If the number of negatively charged ions (in this case HCO_3^-) is reduced, electrochemical neutrality is maintained by replacing them with an equivalent number of other anion(s), such as Cl^-, or with ketone bodies (acetoacetate and 3-hydroxybutyrate) in ketoacidosis or lactate in lactic acidosis. Other causes of unmeasured anion (A^-) are salicylate in aspirin overdose and metabolites from methanol, paracetamol or ethylene glycol poisoning.

In renal glomerular dysfunction (see Chapter 3), even if tubular function is normal, HCO_3^- generation is impaired because the amount of Na^+ available for exchange with H^+ and the amount of filtered buffer A^- available to accept H^+, are both reduced. These buffer anions contribute to the unmeasured A^-. For each milliequivalent of buffer A^- retained, 1 mEq fewer H^+ can be secreted, and therefore 1 mEq fewer HCO_3^- is generated. The retained A^- therefore replaces HCO_3^-.

In the following example, the plasma $[HCO_3^-]$ will be assumed to have fallen by 10 mmol(mEq)/L.

$$[Na^+] + [K^+] = [HCO_3^-] + [Cl^-] + [A^-]$$
$$140 + 4 = 15 + 100 + 29 \text{ mEq/L}$$

(4.14)

The $[HCO_3^-]$ has fallen from 25 to 15 mEq/L and the anion gap, entirely due to $[A^-]$, has risen by the same

---

CASE 1

A 7-year-old boy was admitted unconscious to a casualty department. On examination he was found to be hyperventilating. He had inadvertently consumed ethylene glycol anti-freeze, which he had found in his parents' garage stored in a lemonade bottle.

Blood results were as follows.

Plasma
Sodium 134 mmol/L (135–145)
Potassium 6.0 mmol/L (3.5–5.0)
Bicarbonate 10 mmol/L (24–32)
Chloride 93 mmol/L (95–105)
Glucose 5.3 mmol/L (3.5–6.0)

Arterial blood gases
pH 7.2 (7.35–7.45)
$PaCO_2$ 3.18 kPa (4.6–6.0)
PaO_2 13.1 kPa (9.3–13.3)

DISCUSSION
The results show a high anion gap, normally about 15–20 mmol/L, but in this case 37 mmol/L, with metabolic acidosis, the anion gap being raised at 37, i.e. (134 + 6) − (10 + 93). Hyperkalaemia is present due to the movement of intracellular K^+ out of cells because of the acidosis. The compensatory mechanism of hyperventilation aims to 'blow off' volatile acid in the form of CO_2, hence the low PCO_2.

amount, from 19 to 29 mEq/L, i.e. a high anion gap. If renal HCO_3^- generation is so impaired that it cannot keep pace with its peripheral utilization, the pH will fall.

Lactic acidosis

Lactic acidosis is a form of high anion gap metabolic acidosis; some of the causes are shown in Box 4.2. One definition used is an arterial pH of less than 7.2 with a plasma lactate concentration greater than 5.0 mmol/L. The normal fasting blood lactate is between 0.4 and 1.0 mmol/L, which can rise to 1.5 mmol/L on prolonged exercise (hyperlactataemia).

Most forms of lactic acidosis are due to increased L-lactate, although in some malabsorption states, with bacterial overgrowth, D-lactic acidosis may occur.

The Cohen and Woods classification of lactic acidosis is as follows. The commonest type of lactic acidosis is Type A, due to poor tissue perfusion or hypoxia. Type B1 is due to various miscellaneous conditions, including severe hepatic disturbances as the liver is involved in lactate metabolism. Metastatic malignant disease can also evoke a lactic acidosis, probably because the carcinoma tissue produces lactic acid. Many drugs and toxins can rarely cause lactic acidosis (B2). A number of metabolic or inborn errors of the metabolism of enzymes involved in glycolysis can also lead to lactic acidosis, as in B3.

Hyperchloraemic acidosis or normal anion gap metabolic acidosis

The combination of a low plasma $[HCO_3^-]$ and a high $[Cl^-]$, known as hyperchloraemic acidosis, is rare. The anion gap in such cases is normal.

$$[Na^+] + [K^+] = [HCO_3^-] + [Cl^-] + [A^-]$$
$$140 \;\; + \;\; 4 \;\; = \;\; 15 \;\; + 110 \;\; + 19 \text{ mEq/L}$$

(4.15)

The causes, which can usually be predicted on clinical grounds, include HCO_3^- loss in a one-to-one exchange for Cl^-. This occurs if the ureters are transplanted into the ileum or colon, usually after cystectomy for carcinoma of the bladder. If Cl^--containing fluid such as urine enters the ileum, ileal loops or colon, the cells exchange some of the Cl^- for HCO_3^-.

Duodenal fluid, with a $[HCO_3^-]$ about twice that of plasma, is alkaline. If the rate of loss (for example through small intestinal fistulae) exceeds that of the renal ability to regenerate HCO_3^-, the plasma $[HCO_3^-]$ may fall enough to cause acidosis.

Over enthusiastic infusion of saline can also be associated with a hyperchloraemic acidosis.

Acetazolamide therapy is used to treat glaucoma. By inhibiting CD activity in the eye, it reduces the formation of aqueous humour. Inhibition of the enzyme in renal tubular cells and erythrocytes impairs H^+ secretion and HCO_3^- formation. Hyperchloraemic acidosis sometimes complicates treatment with acetazolamide and can be associated with hypokalaemia.

Another cause of hyperchloraemic acidosis is impaired H^+ secretion, and therefore HCO_3^- production, due to renal tubular acidosis.

In normal tubules, most filtered Na^+ is reabsorbed with Cl^-; the rest is exchanged for secreted H^+ or K^+. If H^+ secretion is impaired, and yet the same amount of Na^+ is reabsorbed, Na^+ must be accompanied by Cl^- or exchanged for K^+. This type of hyperchloraemic acidosis is therefore often accompanied by hypokalaemia – like acetazolamide

---

Box 4.2 Some causes of lactic acidosis

Type A: hypoxic/poor circulation
Cardiovascular shock
Hypoxia
Severe anaemia
Carbon monoxide poisoning
Asphyxia
Respiratory/cardiac failure
Sepsis

Type B1: miscellaneous diseases
Cirrhosis
Fulminant hepatic failure
Widespread malignant disease, e.g. breast carcinoma or haematological malignancies

Type B2: drugs and toxins
Biguanides
Salicylate
Ethanol
Methanol
Ethylene glycol
High-dose fructose or xylitol
Iron overdose
Human immunodeficiency virus retroviral therapy

Type B3: metabolic disorders and inborn errors
Glucose-6-phosphatase deficiency
Pyruvate dehydrogenase/carboxylase deficiency
Fructose 1,6-diphosphate deficiency
Mitochondrial defects
Beri-beri (thiamine deficiency)

treatment. This is an unusual finding in acidosis, which is usually associated with hyperkalaemia (Box 4.3).

Renal tubular acidosis

There are various forms of renal tubular acidosis, which can present as a hyperchloraemic metabolic acidosis. (See Box 4.4 for some causes.)

The commoner, sometimes called classical, renal tubular acidosis (type I) is due to a distal tubular defect. The urinary pH cannot fall much below that of plasma, even in severe acidosis. The distal luminal cells are abnormally permeable to H^+ and this impairs the ability of distal tubules to build up a $[H^+]$ gradient between the tubular lumina and cells. The re-entry of H^+ into distal tubular cells inhibits CD activity at that site; proximal HCO_3^- reabsorption is normal. The inability to acidify the urine normally can be demonstrated by using the furosemide test or an NH_4Cl load.

In renal tubular acidosis type II there is impairment of HCO_3^- reabsorption in the proximal tubule. Loss of HCO_3^- may cause systemic acidosis, but the ability to form acid urine when acidosis becomes severe is retained; the response to NH_4Cl loading may therefore be normal. Type II renal tubular acidosis is also associated with aminoaciduria, phosphaturia and glycosuria, as in Fanconi's syndrome.

Renal tubular acidosis type IV is thought to be due to hyporeninism hypoaldosteronism (see Chapter 8) and is associated with a hyperkalaemic hyperchloraemic acidosis.

Investigation of renal tubular acidosis

- Measure the urinary anion gap and pH in a fresh spot urine sample along with the plasma anion gap. In practice, the urinary anion gap is the difference between

---

Box 4.3 Some causes of a hyperchloraemic acidosis (normal anion gap acidosis)

Ingestion of ammonium chloride, arginine, lysine, sulphur or hydrochloric acid
Drugs such as acetazolamide or anion-binding resins, e.g. cholestyramine
Renal tubular acidosis (see Box 4.4)
Gastrointestinal disease, e.g. fistula or diarrhoea
Ureteric diversion, e.g. ileal bladder or ureterosigmoidostomy

---

Box 4.4 Some causes of type 1 and type 2 renal tubular acidosis

Type I (failure of distal tubule secretion of hydrogen ions)
Primary: sporadic/hereditary
Genetic: Wilson's disease
Dysproteinaemia: amyloidosis, cryoglobulinaemia
Renal diseases: chronic pyelonephritis, renal transplants
Autoimmune: Sjögren's syndrome, chronic active hepatitis
Hyperparathyroidism
Drugs/toxins: lithium, amphotericin

Type II (defect of proximal tubule bicarbonate reabsorption)
Primary: familial
Secondary
   Myeloma
   Amyloidosis
   Heavy metal poisons

CASE 2

A 52-year-old woman with Sjögren's syndrome and distal or type 1 renal tubular acidosis attended a renal out-patient department.
Her blood results were as follows.

Plasma
Sodium 144 mmol/L (135–145)
Potassium 3.0 mmol/L (3.5–5.0)
Bicarbonate 13 mmol/L (24–32)
Chloride 118 mmol/L (95–105)

DISCUSSION

The results are suggestive of a normal anion gap metabolic acidosis or hyperchloraemic acidosis. Hypokalaemia is unusual in the face of an acidosis, one of the exceptions being renal tubular acidosis type I or II. Note the anion gap here is $(144 + 3) - (13 + 118) = 16$ mmol/L (mEq/L), which is normal with high plasma $[Cl^-]$ and low $[HCO_3^-]$.

the sum of the urinary [Na$^+$] and [K$^+$] minus the urinary [Cl$^-$].

- A urinary anion gap less than 100 mmol/L implies low urinary [NH$_4^+$].
  In such cases a urinary pH more than 5.5 in the presence of a hyperchloraemic metabolic acidosis and hypokalaemia is suggestive of type I, or distal, renal tubular acidosis. Conversely, a urinary pH less than 5.5 in the presence of hyperchloraemic metabolic acidosis and hyperkalaemia is suggestive of renal tubular acidosis type IV. Plasma aldosterone and renin concentrations may show hyporeninism hypoaldosteronism in renal tubular acidosis type IV (Table 4.1).
- A urinary anion gap more than 100 mmol/L implies high urinary [NH$_4^+$].
- Measure fractional excretion of HCO$_3^-$ (FE% HCO$_3^-$), which equals:

$$\frac{\text{urine}[\text{HCO}_3^-] \times \text{plasma}[\text{creatinine}]}{\text{plasma}[\text{HCO}_3^-] \times \text{urine}[\text{creatinine}]} \times 100\% \tag{4.16}$$

which is normally less than 5 per cent.
If the fractional excretion of HCO$_3^-$ is increased, this is suggestive of renal tubular acidosis type II, particularly if glycosuria, hypophosphaturia and hypophosphataemia are also present.
- Sometimes a diagnosis of acidosis is difficult to establish and additional tests are indicated.

Ammonium chloride load test for type I renal tubular acidosis

This test is not necessary if the pH of a urinary specimen, collected overnight, is already less than 5.5.

The NH$_4^+$ is potentially acid because it can dissociate to NH$_3$ and H$^+$. After ingestion of ammonium chloride, the kidneys usually secrete the H$^+$, and the urinary pH falls.

Procedure
- No food or fluid is taken after midnight.
- 08.00 hours: ammonium chloride is given orally in a dose of 0.1 g/kg body weight.
- Urine specimens are collected hourly and the pH of each is measured immediately in the laboratory.

Interpretation
In normal subjects, the urinary pH falls to 5.5 or below between 2 and 8 hours after the dose. In generalized tubular disease there may be a sufficient number of functioning nephrons to achieve a normal level of acidification. In distal renal tubular acidosis this degree of acidification does not occur. Urinary acidification is normal in proximal tubular acidosis.

This test can cause nausea and vomiting and is contraindicated in liver disease.

Furosemide test

The test relies on the fact that increased Na$^+$ delivery to the distal tubules results in exchange for H$^+$ and K$^+$, resulting in a decrease in urinary pH to less than 5.5 under normal conditions.

Furosemide 40 mg is given orally and urine is collected for pH every half-hour. However, like the ammonium chloride test, a urinary pH less than 5.5 usually precludes its need. Generally this is simpler and safer than the ammonium chloride test and may be preferable, assuming there are no contraindications to the use of furosemide.

Management of metabolic acidosis

The biochemical findings in plasma in a metabolic acidosis are:

- plasma [HCO$_3^-$] is always low,
- $P\text{CO}_2$ is usually low (compensatory change),
- the pH is low (uncompensated or partly compensated) or near normal (fully compensated),
- plasma [Cl$^-$] is unaffected in most cases unless there is hyperchloraemic acidosis, for example it is raised after ureteric transplantation, saline excess, diarrhoea/

Table 4.1 Biochemical features of renal tubular acidosis (RTA)

	Classic dRTA Type I	Proximal RTA Type II	Type IV RTA
Urine pH	>5.5	<5.5	<5.5
Urine anion gap	Positive	Negative	Positive
FE% HCO$_3^-$	<5–10%	>15%	5–15%
Furosemide test	Abnormal	Normal	Normal
Urine calcium	Normal/high	Normal	Normal
Urine citrate	Low	Normal	Normal
Nephrocalcinosis	Common	Rare	Rare
Metabolic bone disease	Rare	Common	Rare
Other tubular defects	Rare	Common	Rare
Plasma potassium	Normal/low	Normal/low	High

FE% HCO$_3^-$ = fractional excretion of bicarbonate.
dRTA = distal renal tubular acidosis.

fistulae, in renal tubular acidosis or during acetazolamide treatment.

In many cases the diagnosis may be obvious from the clinical history (particularly drug history) and examination (Fig. 4.7).

Tests that may help to elucidate the cause of the metabolic acidosis are:

- plasma urea and creatinine estimation,
- determination of plasma anion gap,
- plasma glucose estimation,
- blood lactate determination,
- tests for ketones in urine,
- tests for blood gases,
- tests for drugs or poisons, for example ethanol, paracetamol, salicylate (if indicated),
- specialized tests for renal tubular acidosis.

Treatment of a metabolic acidosis is usually that of the underlying condition. Dialysis may be necessary in the face of uraemia. Overdoses may also require dialysis, for example ethylene glycol, methanol and salicylate. Infusion of sodium bicarbonate (usually small boluses containing about 50–100 mmol) is only rarely indicated in severe metabolic acidosis of pH less than 7.1 and can cause complications such as hypernatraemia, volume overload, hypokalaemia, 'overshoot' alkalosis and paradoxical central nervous system acidosis.

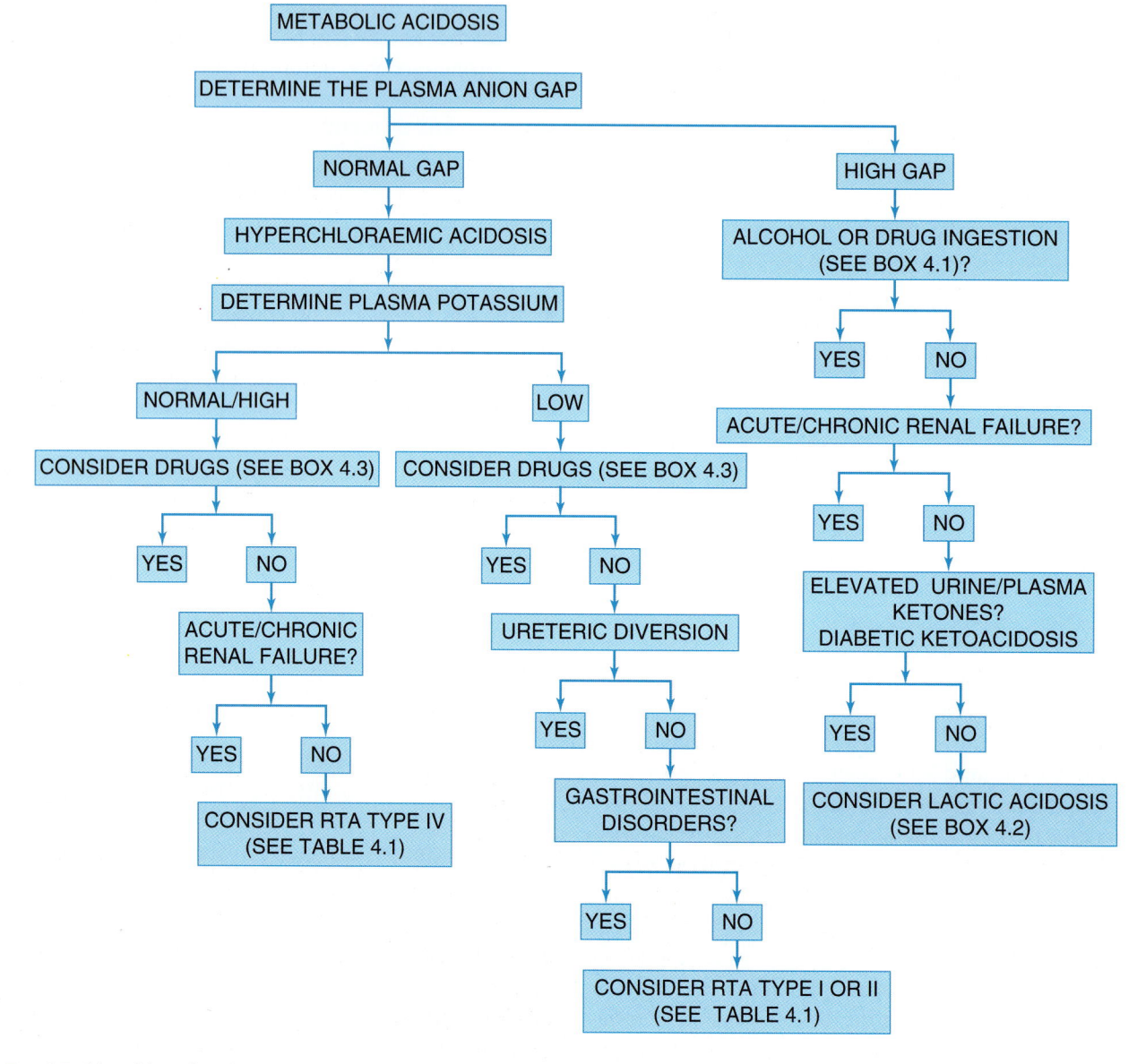

Fig. 4.7 Algorithm for the investigation of a metabolic acidosis. (RTA = renal tubular acidosis.)

In distal type I and type II renal tubular acidosis, oral HCO_3^- therapy may be necessary. In type IV, if due to hyporeninism hypoaldosteronism, fludrocortisone (sometimes in conjunction with furosemide) may be useful.

Respiratory acidosis

The findings in respiratory acidosis differ significantly from those in non-respiratory disturbances. Some of the causes of respiratory acidosis are given in Box 4.5.

The primary abnormality in the bicarbonate buffer system is CO_2 retention, usually due to impaired alveolar ventilation with a consequent rise in PCO_2. As in the metabolic disturbance, the acidosis is accompanied by a fall in the ratio $[HCO_3^-]:PCO_2$.

In acute respiratory failure, for example due to bronchopneumonia or status asthmaticus, both the erythrocyte and renal tubular mechanisms increase the rate of generation as soon as the PCO_2 rises. In the short term, renal contribution to HCO_3^- production is limited by time. A relatively large proportion of the slight rise in plasma $[HCO_3^-]$ is derived from erythrocytes because, in normal circumstances, the Hb buffering mechanism is not saturated. This degree of compensation is rarely adequate to prevent a fall in pH.

In chronic respiratory failure, for example due to chronic obstructive pulmonary disease (COPD), the renal tubular mechanism is of great importance. Haemoglobin buffering power is of limited capacity, but as long as the glomerular filtrate provides an adequate supply of Na^+ for exchange with H^+ and buffers to accept H^+, tubular cells continue to generate HCO_3^- until the ratio $[HCO_3^-]:PCO_2$ is normal. In stable chronic respiratory failure the pH may be normal despite a very high PCO_2, because of an equally high plasma $[HCO_3^-]$.

Management of respiratory acidosis

The blood findings in a respiratory acidosis are as follows.

- PCO_2 is always raised.
- In acute respiratory failure:
  - pH is low,
  - $[HCO_3^-]$ is high-normal or slightly raised.
- In chronic respiratory failure:
  - pH is normal or low, depending upon chronicity (allowing time for compensation to occur),
  - $[HCO_3^-]$ is raised.

In many cases the cause of the respiratory acidosis can be deduced from the clinical history and examination in conjunction with a chest X-ray and lung function tests, if indicated (Fig. 4.8).

Treatment of a respiratory acidosis is usually of the underlying disorder. Sodium bicarbonate infusion (see above) is rarely indicated, except perhaps if the pH is less than 7.1, such as in cardiopulmonary arrest. In cases of bronchospasm or COPD, bronchodilators such as β-agonists (for example salbutamol), anticholinergic agents (for example ipratropium) or methylxanthines (for example theophylline) may be useful. Sedative drugs should be avoided and naloxone may reverse the actions of opiates and flumazenil the effects of benzodiazepines.

Mechanical ventilation may be needed. Respiratory stimulants such as doxapram or nikethamide are not

CASE 3

A 67-year-old retired printer presented to casualty because of increasing breathlessness. He had smoked 20 cigarettes a day for 50 years. On examination he was found to be centrally cyanosed and coughing copious green phlegm.

His arterial blood results were as follows.

pH 7.31 (7.35–7.45)
$PaCO_2$ 9.3 kPa (4.6–6.0)
PaO_2 6.9 kPa (9.3–13.3)
Bicarbonate 37 mmol/L (24–32)

DISCUSSION

The patient had chronic obstructive airways disease and the blood gases show a respiratory acidosis with hypercapnia and hypoxia. The latter has resulted in central cyanosis. Compensation is via the kidneys, with increased acid excretion and HCO_3^- reclamation. Chronic cases of respiratory acidosis are usually almost totally compensated as there is time for the kidneys and buffer systems to adapt. This is unlike an acute respiratory acidosis due to bilateral pneumothorax, in which the rapid acute changes do not give sufficient time for the compensatory mechanisms to take place. This patient had an acute exacerbation of his lung disease and the CO_2 retention exceeded the compensatory mechanisms.

> **Box 4.5 Some causes of a respiratory acidosis**
>
> *Suppression of respiratory centre*
> Opiates, benzodiazepines, anaesthetic agents
> Head injury, cerebral tumours, central nervous system infection
>
> *Upper airways obstruction*
> Foreign body, tumour, aspiration
> Bronchospasm, asthma
> Obstructive sleep apnoea
> Laryngospasm
>
> *Respiratory muscle disease*
> Muscle-relaxing drugs, e.g. pancuronium or amino glycosides
> Severe hypophosphataemia or hypokalaemia
> Muscular dystrophy
> Myasthenia gravis
>
> *Disorders affecting nerves supplying respiratory muscles*
> Polio
> Spinal cord injury
> Botulinism
> Guillain–Barré syndrome
>
> *Disorders affecting mechanics of chest wall*
> Pneumothorax
> Flail chest
> Diaphragm paralysis
> Severe kyphoscoliosis
> Pickwickian syndrome due to severe obesity
>
> *Diseases of the lungs*
> Severe asthma
> Pneumonia
> Large pulmonary embolus
> Chronic obstructive pulmonary disease
> Pulmonary fibrosis
> Acute respiratory distress syndrome

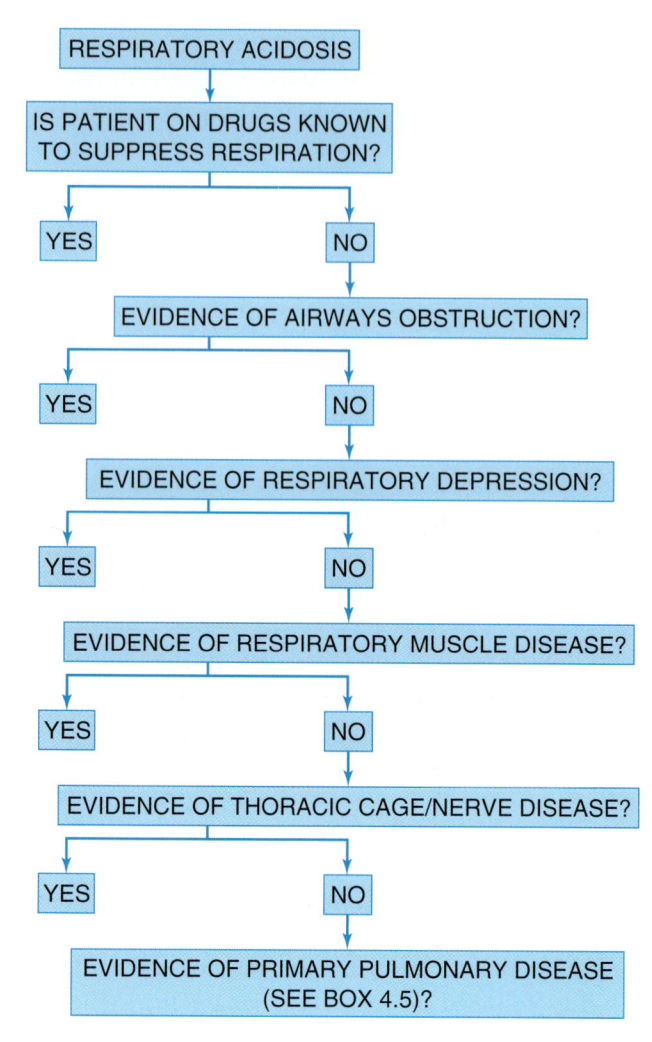

Fig. 4.8 Algorithm for the investigation of a respiratory acidosis.

without side-effects, for example they may lower the epilepsy threshold. Medroxyprogesterone can increase respiratory drive and has been used in pickwickian syndrome (obesity–hypoventilation). Oxygen therapy may be indicated if the patient is hypoxic and, in patients with COPD who fulfil the criteria for O_2 therapy, this may decrease mortality and reduces pulmonary hypertension. However, as discussed later, O_2 therapy should be used with caution if there is hypercapnia (raised $P\text{CO}_2$), which may aggravate the acidosis.

Alkalosis

Alkalosis occurs if there is a rise in the ratio $[\text{HCO}_3^-]:P\text{CO}_2$ in the extracellular fluid.

In metabolic alkalosis the primary abnormality in the bicarbonate buffer system is a rise in $[\text{HCO}_3^-]$. There is little compensatory change in $P\text{CO}_2$.

In respiratory alkalosis the primary abnormality is a fall in the $P\text{CO}_2$. The compensatory change is a fall in $[\text{HCO}_3^-]$.

As the primary products of metabolism are H^+ and CO_2, not OH^- and HCO_3^-, alkalosis is less common than acidosis. The presenting clinical symptom of alkalosis may be tetany despite a normal plasma total calcium concentration; this is due to a fall in the free ionized calcium fraction.

Metabolic alkalosis

A primary rise in plasma $[\text{HCO}_3^-]$ may occur in the following situations.

- Bicarbonate administration, such as the ingestion of large amounts of HCO_3^- to treat indigestion (milk-alkali syndrome, which is rare) or during intravenous HCO_3^- infusion. Usually both the cause and the treatment are obvious.
- Severe K^+ depletion with the generation of HCO_3^- by the kidney. This is one of the commonest causes (discussed in the next chapter). Here, H^+ shifts into the intracellular space. As the extracellular $[K^+]$ decreases, K^+ flow out of the cells and, to maintain electrical neutrality, H^+ move into the intracellular space.
- Loss of H^+. If a H^+ is excreted, a HCO_3^- is gained in the extracellular space. The most likely loss of H^+ is through either the kidneys or the gastrointestinal tract. In the case of the former, renal losses occur when the distal tubule $[Na^+]$ increases in the presence of excessive aldosterone, which stimulates the electrogenic epithelial Na^+ channel in the collecting duct. As this channel reabsorbs Na^+, the tubular lumen becomes more negative, resulting in H^+ and K^+ secretion into the lumen. In the case of the gastrointestinal tract, nasogastric suction or vomiting causes loss of gastric secretions, which are rich in hydrochloric acid.
- Contraction alkalosis. Thiazide or loop diuretic use or Cl^--losing diarrhoea results in the loss of HCO_3^--poor, Cl^--rich extracellular fluid. This results in a contraction of extracellular fluid volume and, because the original HCO_3^- is now dissolved in a smaller fluid volume, a slight (2–4 mmol/L) increase in $[HCO_3^-]$ occurs.

Box 4.6 shows some of the causes of metabolic alkalosis.

Compensation for metabolic alkalosis is relatively ineffective. Although acidosis stimulates the respiratory centre, alkalosis cannot usually depress it sufficiently to bring the pH back to normal; respiratory inhibition not only leads to CO_2 retention but also causes hypoxia, which can override the inhibitory effect of alkalosis on the respiratory centre. Consequently CO_2 may not be retained in adequate amounts to compensate for the rise in plasma $[HCO_3^-]$.

Two factors may impair the ability to lose HCO_3^- in the urine and so may aggravate a metabolic alkalosis.

- A reduced glomerular filtration rate due to volume depletion limits the total amount of HCO_3^- that can be lost.
- The $[Cl^-]$ in the glomerular filtrate may be reduced if there is severe hypochloraemia due to gastric Cl^- loss. Isosmotic Na^+ reabsorption in proximal tubules depends on passive reabsorption of Cl^- along the electrochemical gradient. A reduction in available Cl^- limits isosmotic reabsorption, and more Na^+ becomes available for exchange with H^+ and K^+. The urine becomes inappropriately acid, and H^+ secretion stimulates inappropriate HCO_3^- reabsorption. The increased K^+ loss aggravates the hypokalaemia due to alkalosis. Thus prolonged vomiting such as pyloric stenosis vomiting or gastric aspiration may cause:
  - hypochloraemic alkalosis,
  - hypokalaemia,
  - mild uraemia and haemoconcentration due to volume depletion.

> **Box 4.6 Some causes of metabolic alkalosis**
>
> *Saline responsive (urine chloride < 20 mmol/L)*
> Consider volume-depleted states
> Ingestion of exogenous alkalis, e.g. milk-alkali syndrome (rare) or salts of strong acids, previous diuretic use or poorly reabsorbable anions, e.g. penicillin
> Chloride loss from gastrointestinal tract, e.g. vomiting, gastric suction, chloride-losing diarrhoea
> Chloride loss from skin, e.g. cystic fibrosis
>
> *Saline unresponsive (urine chloride > 20 mmol/L)*
> Certain drugs such as current diuretic therapy or exogenous mineralocorticoids, e.g. liquorice or carbenoxolone
> Severe hypokalaemia
> Severe hypomagnesaemia
> Endogenous mineralocorticoid excess, e.g. Cushing's syndrome, primary hyperaldosteronism (Conn's syndrome), Liddle's syndrome, 11-hydroxylase and 17-hydroxylase deficiencies, Bartter's or Gitelman's syndrome

The hypokalaemia may become apparent only when the plasma volume has been restored, but it should be anticipated. Pyloric stenosis is usually treated before severe hypochloraemic alkalosis develops. Nevertheless, the typical changes in plasma HCO_3^- and Cl^- may indicate the diagnosis. Chronic vomiting due to pyloric stenosis is one of the commonest causes of hypochloraemia. If the pylorus is patent, the fluid vomited is mixed with alkaline intestinal fluid and does not cause this syndrome.

Management of a metabolic alkalosis

The arterial blood findings in metabolic alkalosis are:

- blood pH high,
- $[H^+]$ low,
- $[HCO_3^-]$ raised,
- $P\text{CO}_2$ raised in compensation.

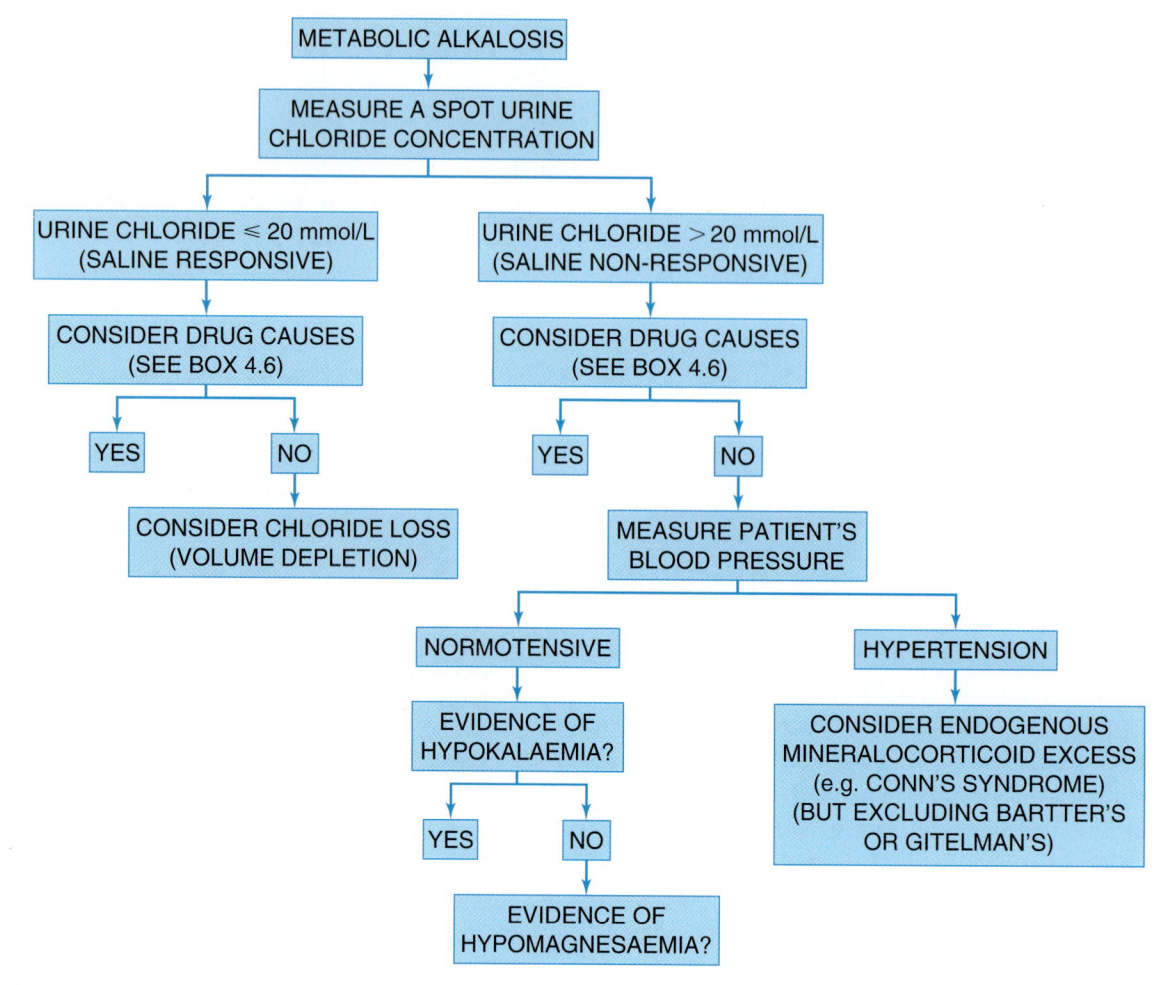

Fig. 4.9 Algorithm for the investigation of a metabolic alkalosis.

A clinical and drug history and physical examination may reveal the cause of the metabolic alkalosis (Fig. 4.9). Useful laboratory investigations in a metabolic alkalosis may include:

- plasma Na^+, K^+, Cl^-, Mg^{2+} urea and creatinine,
- blood gases,
- spot urine $[Cl^-]$ less than 20 mmol/L suggests the saline-responsive form of metabolic alkalosis, and more than 20 mmol/L the saline-non-responsive form.

Other tests are indicated according to the clinical situation, for example if primary hyperaldosteronism (Conn's syndrome) or Cushing's syndrome is suspected (mineralocorticoid excess syndromes) (see Chapter 8).

Hypokalaemia should be investigated and treated (see Chapter 5). If the patient is on a thiazide or loop diuretic, this may need to be reduced or stopped. Anti-emetics may help stop vomiting, and proton pump inhibitors may reduce gastric acid secretion.

If a saline-responsive alkalosis occurs with volume depletion, intravenous infusion of isotonic saline may help. The saline non-responsive form is often due to mineralocorticoid excess.

Respiratory alkalosis

The primary abnormality in the bicarbonate buffer system in respiratory alkalosis is a fall in $P\text{CO}_2$. This is due to abnormally rapid or deep respiration when the CO_2 transport capacity of the pulmonary alveoli is relatively normal. The fall in $P\text{CO}_2$ reduces the CD activity in renal tubular cells and erythrocytes. The compensatory fall in plasma $[HCO_3^-]$ tends to correct the pH.

It may be difficult to distinguish clinically between the over-breathing due to metabolic acidosis, in which the fall in plasma $[HCO_3^-]$ is the primary biochemical abnormality, and that due to respiratory alkalosis, in which it is compensatory. In doubtful cases, estimation of arterial pH and $P\text{CO}_2$ is indicated.

CASE 4

A baby girl a few days old had had projectile vomiting since birth due to pyloric stenosis.

Her blood results were as follows.

Plasma
Sodium 137 mmol/L (135–145)
Potassium 3.0 mmol/L (3.5–5.0)
Bicarbonate 40 mmol/L (24–32)
Chloride 82 mmol/L (95–105)

Arterial blood gases
pH 7.52 (7.35–7.45)
$Pa\text{CO}_2$ 6.2 kPa (4.6–6.0)
$Pa\text{O}_2$ 12.9 kPa (9.3–13.3)

DISCUSSION

The results are suggestive of a metabolic alkalosis due to the severe vomiting. Note also the low plasma $[Cl^-]$ due to loss of hydrochloric acid in vomit, and hypokalaemia resulting from K^+ movement into cells due to the alkalosis.

Compensation is by hypoventilation and retention of CO_2.

CASE 5

A 20-year-old woman presented to casualty with a panic attack. She had noticed peri-oral paraesthesia and was found on examination to be hyperventilating.

Her arterial blood results were as follows.

pH 7.61 (7.35–7.45)
$Pa\text{CO}_2$ 2.7 kPa (4.6–6.0)
$Pa\text{O}_2$ 13.3 kPa (9.3–13.3)
Bicarbonate 18 mmol/L (24–32)

DISCUSSION

The patient is showing a respiratory alkalosis. The panic attack had resulted in hyperventilation. The peri-oral paraesthesia is due to a lowering of plasma ionized calcium concentration as a result of the alkalosis. Compensation is by the kidneys, which increase HCO_3^- excretion and reduce acid excretion.

The arterial blood findings in respiratory alkalosis are:

- $P\text{CO}_2$ is always reduced,
- $[HCO_3^-]$ is low-normal or low,
- pH is raised (uncompensated or partly compensated) or near normal (fully compensated).

Acute hypocapnia (low $P\text{CO}_2$) can cause hypokalaemia due to increased intracellular uptake of K^+. A reduction in free or ionized calcium can lead to tetany and paraesthesiae.

The causes of respiratory alkalosis are shown in Box 4.7. One of the commonest causes is anxiety-induced hyperventilation. Salicylates stimulate the respiratory centre directly, and over-dosage initially causes respiratory alkalosis. They also uncouple oxidative phosphorylation, and may evoke a lactic acidosis. Both these effects lower plasma $[HCO_3^-]$, but the pH may be high if respiratory alkalosis is predominant, normal if the two cancel each other out, or low if metabolic acidosis is predominant.

Management of respiratory alkalosis

The cause of the hyperventilation may be obvious from the clinical history and examination (Fig. 4.10). A chest X-ray and lung function tests may be indicated.

> **Box 4.7 Some causes of a respiratory alkalosis**
>
> Hyperventilation, e.g. anxiety states, increased mechanical ventilation
> Exogenous agents that increase respiratory drive, e.g. salicylates, theophylline, catecholamines, nikethamide, doxapram, thyroxine and progestogens
> Hypoxaemia due to early and non-severe pulmonary disease (e.g. asthma, pulmonary embolus, pneumonia) or high attitude
> Increased cerebral respiratory centre drive, e.g. head injury, cerebral tumour, meningitis, cerebrovascular accidents
> Increased non-cerebral causes of respiratory centre drive, e.g. pregnancy, heat exposure, hepatic failure, septicaemia

Laboratory tests could include:

- blood gases,
- plasma $[K^+]$ and ionized $[Ca^{2+}]$ may be low,

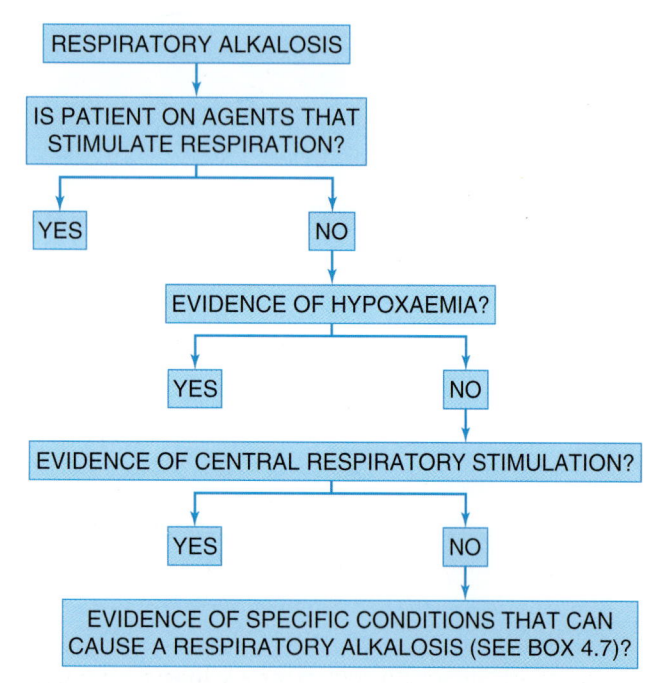

Fig. 4.10 Algorithm for the investigation of a respiratory alkalosis.

- elevated white cell count and relevant cultures may point to sepsis as a cause of hyperventilation,
- full blood count to exclude anaemia,
- liver function tests when hepatic failure is suspected,
- exclude salicylate overdose and respiratory stimulants.

Treatment is usually of the underlying condition, which is rarely life threatening unless arterial pH is more than 7.5. During hyperventilation syndrome, patients may benefit from reassurance, the treatment of underlying psychological stress and re-breathing into a paper bag during acute episodes.

Compensatory changes in acid–base disturbances

In either metabolic or respiratory acidosis the ratio of $[HCO_3^-]:P_{CO_2}$, and therefore the pH, can be corrected by a change in concentration of the other member of the buffer pair in the same direction as the primary abnormality. This compensation may be either partial or complete, but never over-compensates, i.e. there is no pH overshoot.

The compensatory change in a metabolic acidosis is a reduction in P_{CO_2} by hyperventilation whilst in a respiratory acidosis it is a rise in plasma $[HCO_3^-]$ by the action of the renal tubules.

In a metabolic alkalosis, compensation by hypoventilation results in an elevation of P_{CO_2}, whilst in a respiratory alkalosis the kidneys increase HCO_3^- excretion, thereby lowering plasma $[HCO_3^-]$.

The pH in a fully compensated acidosis is normal. However, the concentrations of the other components of the Henderson–Hasselbalch equation are abnormal. All parameters can only return to normal if the primary abnormality is corrected: if normalization occurs, this removes the 'drive' of the compensation.

See Table 4.2 for a summary of acid–base disorders and their respective compensations. These are simplifications as in practice mixed acid–base disturbances may occur (e.g. in metabolic acidosis with respiratory acidosis).

In an uncomplicated metabolic acidosis with a high anion gap the change in $[HCO_3^-]$ is equimolar with the change in the $[A^-]$. Deviations from this relationship

Table 4.2 Summary of findings in arterial blood in disturbances of hydrogen ion homeostasis

	pH	P_{CO_2}	$[HCO_3^-]$	Plasma $[K^+]$
Acidosis				
Metabolic				
Acute state	↓	N	↓	Usually ↑ (↓ in RTA I or II or acetazolamide)
Compensation	N	↓*	↓	↑
Respiratory				
Acute change	↓	↑	N or ↑	↑
Compensation	N	↑	↑↑*	↑
Alkalosis				
Metabolic				
Acute state	↑	N	↑	↓
Compensation	N	↑*	↑	↓
Respiratory				
Acute change	↑	↓	N or ↓	↓
Compensation	N	↓	↓*	↓

Arrows = primary change; *arrows = compensatory change; N = normal.
RTA = renal tubular acidosis.
Potassium depletion can cause alkalosis, or alkalosis can cause hypokalaemia. The clinical history may differentiate the cause of the combination of hypokalaemia and alkalosis.
Overbreathing causes a low $[HCO_3^-]$ in respiratory alkalosis.
Metabolic acidosis, with a low $[HCO_3^-]$, causes overbreathing. Only measurement of blood pH and P_{CO_2} can differentiate these two.

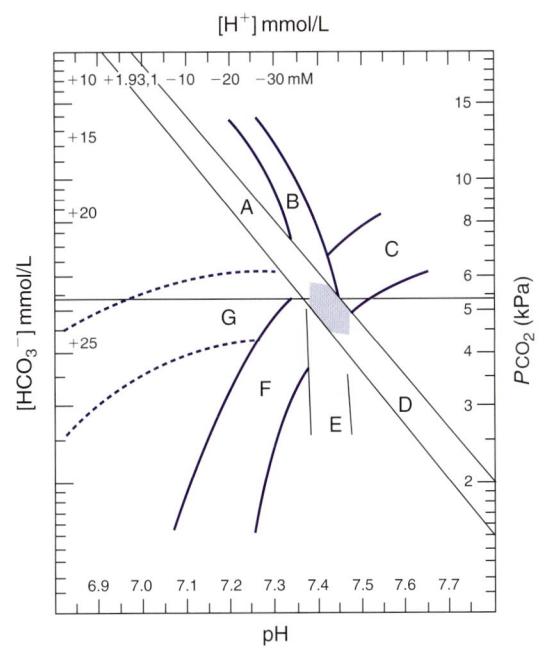

A – Acute respiratory acidosis
B – Chronic respiratory acidosis
C – Chronic metabolic alkalosis
D – Acute respiratory alkalosis
E – Chronic respiratory alkalosis
F – Chronic metabolic acidosis
G – Acute metabolic acidosis
Central shaded area = Normal

Fig. 4.11 Siggaard-Andersen acid–base chart for arterial blood. Copyright Radiometer Medical Aps. Adapted with permission.

indicate a mixed acid–base disturbance, for example a metabolic acidosis and respiratory acidosis (Fig. 4.11).

BLOOD GASES

The amount of O_2 in blood is determined by the amount dissolved, the Hb concentration and the affinity of Hb for O_2. Haemoglobin consists of four subunits, each made up of a haem, a porphyrin ring containing iron, and a polypeptide. As a haem takes up an O_2 molecule, there is a rearrangement of the subunits that facilitates the uptake of additional O_2. This accounts for the shape of the oxyhaemoglobin dissociation curve (see Fig. 4.12). Factors that affect the affinity of haem for oxygen include the following.

- pH of blood: as the pH falls, the affinity for O_2 decreases. This is known as the Bohr effect. Deoxygenated Hb binds H^+ more avidly and accounts for the increased buffering capacity of Hb in venous blood.

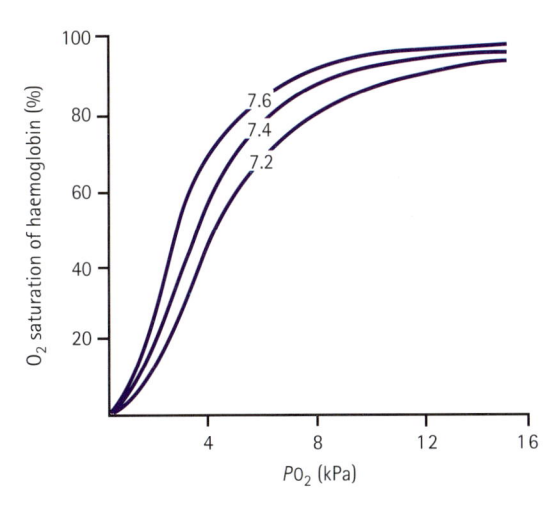

Fig. 4.12 The oxyhaemoglobin dissociation curve showing the effect of pH (Bohr effect) on oxygen saturation.

- 2,3-diphosphoglycerate (DPG) is formed during glycolysis and is plentiful within the erythrocyte. It binds to Hb, liberating more O_2, so that the dissociation curve shifts to the right. A fall in pH decreases DPG levels, thus potentially reducing tissue oxygenation. Erythrocyte levels of DPG increase in anaemia and in some conditions associated with chronic hypoxia.
- Fetal Hb has a greater affinity for O_2 than adult Hb, thus facilitating the transfer of O_2 across the placenta.

Factors affecting blood gas results

In respiratory acidosis it is often important to know the partial pressure of oxygen (P_{O_2}) as well as the pH, P_{CO_2} and $[HCO_3^-]$.

Normal gaseous exchange across the pulmonary alveoli involves loss of CO_2 and gain of O_2. However, in disease a fall in P_{O_2} and a rise in P_{CO_2} do not always coexist. The reasons for this are as follows.

- Carbon dioxide is much more soluble in water than O_2 and its rate of diffusion is about 20 times as high. For example, in pulmonary oedema, diffusion of O_2 across alveolar walls is hindered by oedema fluid and arterial P_{O_2} falls. The hypoxia and alveolar distension stimulate respiration and CO_2 is excreted. However, the rate of O_2 transport through the fluid cannot be increased enough to restore normal arterial P_{O_2}. This results in a low or normal P_{CO_2} and a low P_{O_2}. Only in very severe cases is the P_{CO_2} raised.
- Haemoglobin in arterial blood is normally 95 per cent saturated with O_2, and the small amount of O_2 in simple solution in the plasma is in equilibrium

with oxyhaemoglobin. Increased air entry at atmospheric P_{O_2} cannot significantly increase O_2 carriage in blood leaving normal alveoli, but can reduce the P_{CO_2}. Breathing pure O_2 increases arterial P_{O_2}, but not Hb saturation.

- In conditions such as lobar pneumonia, pulmonary collapse and pulmonary fibrosis or infiltration, not all alveoli are affected equally. At first the gaseous composition of blood leaving them is normal. Increasing the rate or depth of respiration may later lower the P_{CO_2} considerably, but does not alter either the P_{O_2} or the Hb saturation.
- Obstruction of small airways means that air cannot reach those alveoli supplied by them; the composition of blood leaving them will be near that of venous blood and there is a ventilation/perfusion mismatch with a right-to-left shunt. Only if gaseous flow due to increased respiratory exertion can overcome the obstruction will it help to correct the low P_{O_2} and high P_{CO_2}.
- Some alveoli may have normal air entry, but much reduced blood supply. This is 'dead space'. Increased ventilation will have no effect, because there is little blood to interact with the increased flow of gases.

Blood from unaffected alveoli and from those with obstructed airways mixes in the pulmonary vein before entering the left atrium. The high P_{CO_2} and low P_{O_2} stimulate respiration and, if there are enough unaffected alveoli, the very low P_{CO_2} in blood leaving them may compensate for the high P_{CO_2} in blood from poorly aerated alveoli. By contrast, neither the P_{O_2} nor the Hb saturation will be significantly altered by mixing. The systemic arterial blood will then have a low or normal P_{CO_2} with a low P_{O_2}.

If the proportion of affected to normal alveoli is very high, P_{CO_2} cannot adequately be corrected by hyperventilation and there will be a high arterial P_{CO_2} with a low P_{O_2}.

If there are mechanical or neurological lesions impairing respiratory movement or obstruction of large, or most of the small, airways as in an acute asthmatic attack, almost all alveoli will have a normal blood supply; the poor aeration will cause a high P_{CO_2} and low P_{O_2} in the blood draining them, and therefore in systemic arterial blood. Occasionally, stimulation of respiration by alveolar stretching can maintain a normal, or even low, P_{CO_2} early in an acute asthmatic attack. A raised P_{CO_2} in an asthmatic indicates a severe attack (Box 4.8).

Respiratory failure

Respiratory failure can be classified as either hypoxaemic or hypercapnic.

Box 4.8 Blood gases and respiratory disease

In the list of examples given below the conditions marked * may fall into either group, depending on the severity of the disease.

Low arterial P_{O_2} with low or normal P_{CO_2} (hypoxia)
  Pulmonary oedema (diffusion defect)
  Lobar pneumonia
  Pulmonary collapse*
  Pulmonary fibrosis or infiltration*

Low arterial P_{O_2} with a high P_{CO_2} (hypoxia and hypercapnia)
  Impairment of movement of the chest
  Chest injury
  Gross obesity
  Ankylosing spondylitis
  Neurological conditions affecting the respiratory drive
  Neurological conditions, e.g. poliomyelitis, affecting innervation of respiratory muscles
  Extensive airway obstruction: chronic obstructive pulmonary disease; severe asthma; laryngeal spasm
  Bronchopneumonia
  Pulmonary collapse*
  Pulmonary fibrosis or infiltration*

Reference ranges for blood gases being:
pH = 7.35–7.45
$PaCO_2$ = 4.6–6.0 kPa
PaO_2 = 9.3–13.3 kPa
Bicarbonate = 24–32 mmol/L

- *Hypoxaemic respiratory failure* (type 1) is defined as hypoxaemia with a normal or low $PaCO_2$. This is the commonest form of respiratory failure and is associated with most forms of pulmonary disease, particularly when there is collapse of or fluid in the alveoli. Examples are pulmonary oedema or pneumonia. It may be difficult to determine from blood gases whether hypoxaemic failure is acute or chronic, although in chronic failure polycythaemia or cor pulmonale may occur.
- *Hypercapnic respiratory failure* (type II) is characterized by both hypoxaemia and hypercapnia. Hypoxaemia may occur, particularly if the patient is breathing room air. Common causes include chest wall abnormalities,

neuromuscular disease, drug overdose or severe airway disease, for example asthma or COPD. This may be acute (within a few hours), when pH may be less than 7.3, because there is not time for renal compensation to take place, or chronic, when arterial pH is only slightly low.

As well as treatment for the cause of the condition, some patients may need mechanical ventilation. It is important to remember that CO_2 narcosis can occur in some patients with hypercapnia who are given O_2. This is because they may lose their hypoxic respiratory drive, which can lead to rapid increases in $P\text{CO}_2$.

Pulse oximeters

Pulse oximeters give non-invasive estimation of the arterial Hb O_2 saturation. They are useful in anaesthesia, recovery or intensive care (including neonatal units) and during patient transport. There are two main principles involved:

- differential light absorption by Hb and oxyhaemoglobin,
- identification of pulsatile blood component of signal.

Oximetry gives a good estimation of adequate oxygenation, but no direct information about ventilation, including CO_2 status.

Inaccuracies of oximetry

Bright overhead lighting may give pulsatile waveforms and saturation values when there is no pulse. Dyes and pigments, including nail varnish, may give artificially low values. Abnormal haemoglobins, such as methaemoglobinaemia, cause readings to tend towards 85 per cent. Furthermore, carboxyhaemoglobin, caused by carbon monoxide (CO) poisoning, causes saturation values to tend towards 100 per cent. A pulse oximeter is thus misleading in cases of CO poisoning for this reason and should not be used. Oxygen saturation values less than 70 per cent can be inaccurate.

Cardiac arrhythmias may interfere with the oximeter picking up the pulsatile signal properly and with calculation of the pulse rate. Vasoconstriction and hypothermia cause reduced tissue perfusion and failure to register a signal. Cardiac valve defects may cause venous pulsation and therefore venous O_2 saturation is recorded by the oximeter.

Collection of specimens for blood gas estimations

- Arterial specimens are preferable to capillary specimens.
- The heparin and specimen in the syringe must be well mixed. *Warning* Excess heparin may dilute the specimen and cause haemolysis.
  If sodium heparin is used, do not estimate $[Na^+]$ using the same specimen as a resultant factitious hypernatraemia can occur.
- Expel any air bubbles at once. The nozzle should then be stoppered. Leaving the specimen in the syringe should minimize gas exchange with the atmosphere.
- Performing the assay as soon as possible should minimize the effect on pH of anaerobic erythrocyte metabolism. The specimen should be kept cool.

In newborn infants, arterial puncture may have to be used or capillary samples taken as an alternative. However, the following precautions are essential.

- In order for the composition of the blood to be as near arterial as possible, the area from which the specimen is taken should be warm and pink. If there is peripheral cyanosis, results may be dangerously misleading.
- The blood should flow freely. Squeezing the skin while sampling may dilute the specimen with interstitial fluid.
- The capillary tubes must be heparinized, and mixing with the blood must be complete (see above).
- The tubes must be completely filled with blood. Air bubbles invalidate the results.
- The ends of the tubes should be sealed immediately.

Indications for arterial blood gas determination

Arterial blood gas estimations may be indicated in the following situations.

- There is doubt about the cause of the abnormal plasma HCO_3^- (for example to differentiate metabolic acidosis from respiratory alkalosis or metabolic alkalosis from respiratory acidosis).
- An acid–base disturbance is suspected, for example after cardiopulmonary arrest, in renal failure complicated by lung disease or in salicylate overdose. In such conditions, the estimations are required only if the results will influence treatment.

- There is an acute exacerbation of COPD or acute, potentially reversible, lung disease. In such cases, vigorous therapy or artificial respiration may tide the patient over until lung function improves; more precise information than the plasma $[HCO_3^-]$ is needed to monitor and control treatment.
- If blood is being taken for estimation of Po_2 and to guide O_2 therapy or artificial ventilation.
- To complement oximetry, particularly if low saturations are found or hypercapnia is suspected.

INVESTIGATION OF HYDROGEN ION DISTURBANCES

Measurements that may be used to assess acid–base disturbances in patients. (See Fig. 4.11.)

Blood gases

Measurement of blood pH

Measurement of blood pH determines whether there is an acidosis or alkalosis. If the pH is abnormal, the primary abnormality may be in the control of CO_2 by the lungs or respiratory centre, or in the balance between HCO_3^- utilization in buffering and its reabsorption and regeneration by renal tubular cells and erythrocytes. However, a normal pH does not exclude a disturbance of these pathways: compensatory mechanisms may be maintaining it. Assessment of these factors can only be made by measuring components of the bicarbonate buffer system.

Measurement of blood $[HCO_3^-]$

There are two methods that may be used to estimate the circulating $[HCO_3^-]$, although it can of course be measured directly.

- Plasma total CO_2 (TCO_2). The plasma $[HCO_3^-]$ is probably the most commonly measured index of H^+ homeostasis. If pH and Pco_2 estimations are not needed, the assay has certain advantages: venous blood can be used and it can be performed together with assays for urea and electrolytes. It is an estimate of the sum of plasma HCO_3^-, carbonic acid and dissolved CO_2. At pH 7.4 the ratio of $[HCO_3^-]$ to the other two components is about 20 to 1, and at pH 7.1 it is still 10 to 1. Thus, if the TCO_2 were 21 mmol/L, $[HCO_3^-]$ would contribute 20 mmol/L at pH 7.4 and just over 19 mmol/L at pH 7.1. Only 1 mmol/L and just under 2 mmol/L, respectively, would be due to H_2CO_3 and CO_2 respectively. Thus TCO_2 is effectively a measure of the plasma $[HCO_3^-]$.
- The $[HCO_3^-]$ is calculated from the Henderson–Hasselbalch equation, using the measured values of pH and Pco_2 (in kPa) in whole arterial blood. It is a measure of the whole blood $[HCO_3^-]$ and, for the reasons discussed above, usually agrees well with plasma TCO_2. It is the estimate of choice if the other two parameters are being measured.

Concentration of dissolved CO_2

The concentration of dissolved CO_2 is calculated by multiplying the measured Pco_2 by the solubility constant of the gas: 0.23 if Pco_2 is in kPa or 0.03 if it is in mmHg.

Indications for plasma and urinary chloride estimation

Hyperchloraemia occurs in a normal anion gap metabolic acidosis. Conversely, hypochloraemia is seen in the metabolic alkalosis of pyloric stenosis or chronic vomiting.

Plasma $[Cl^-]$ estimation may help in two main situations.

- If a patient who is vomiting has a high plasma $[HCO_3^-]$, the finding of a low $[Cl^-]$ favours the diagnosis of pyloric stenosis or chronic vomiting.
- If there is a low plasma $[HCO_3^-]$, the finding of a high plasma $[Cl^-]$ (and therefore a normal anion gap) strengthens the suspicion of hyperchloraemic acidosis. In metabolic acidosis due to most other causes the plasma $[Cl^-]$ is normal and the anion gap is increased.

A spot urinary $[Cl^-]$ can be useful in determining the cause of a metabolic alkalosis. A $[Cl^-]$ less than 20 mmol/L is indicative of a saline-responsive metabolic alkalosis, for example chronic vomiting, and urinary $[Cl^-]$ more than 20 mmol/L of a saline-non-responsive form of metabolic alkalosis, for example as in mineralocorticoid excess syndromes such as Bartters' syndrome.

CONCLUSIONS

- Tight homeostatic control of acid–base balance is essential, otherwise cell malfunction and death can occur. The kidneys excrete non-volatile acid via the renal tubules into the urine, whilst the lungs excrete volatile acid as CO_2.
- The major extracellular buffer system involves HCO_3^-.
- Blood pH is inversely proportional to the P_{CO_2} and directly to the $[HCO_3^-]$.
- Respiratory acidosis results from disorders of the respiratory system and is caused by CO_2 retention. Conversely, respiratory alkalosis is due to excess CO_2 loss, as in hyperventilation. In the case of the former, compensation is by the renal excretion of non-volatile acid and reclamation of HCO_3^-. In the latter, the kidneys compensate by losing HCO_3^-.
- Metabolic (non-respiratory) acidosis results from increased non-volatile acid such as lactic acid or certain ketones. Compensation is by the lungs, which increase CO_2 excretion by hyperventilation. Metabolic (non-respiratory) alkalosis is caused by HCO_3^- excess and acid loss, such as in prolonged vomiting, and its compensation is via the lungs, which hypoventilate, thereby retaining volatile acid as CO_2.

5 POTASSIUM

| Potassium homeostasis | 82 | Abnormalities of plasma potassium | 85 |

There is an important inter-relationship between the processes of potassium metabolism and those of water and sodium balance, renal function and acid–base disorders (discussed in the preceding chapters). Abnormalities of potassium homeostasis such as plasma concentrations that are too low (hypokalaemia) or too high (hyperkalaemia) are also relatively common in clinical practice and important to know about, as they may become life threatening.

POTASSIUM HOMEOSTASIS

The total amount of potassium in the body is about 3000 mmol, of which about 98 per cent is intracellular. For this reason the plasma potassium concentration is a poor indicator of the total body content.

Factors affecting plasma potassium concentration

The intracellular potassium ion concentration ($[K^+]$) is large and provides a reservoir for the extracellular compartment. Consequently changes in water balance have little direct effect on the plasma $[K^+]$, unlike sodium (Na^+).

The normal potassium intake is about 60–100 mmol/day. Potassium enters and leaves the extracellular compartment by three main routes:

- the intestine,
- the kidneys,
- the membranes of all other cells.

The intestine

Potassium is principally absorbed in the small intestine. Dietary intake replaces net urinary and faecal loss. Prolonged starvation can cause or aggravate potassium depletion leading to hypokalaemia.

Dried figs, molasses and seaweed are rich in potassium (more than 25 mmol/100 g). Foods with a high content (more than 12.5 mmol/100 g) include dried fruits (dates and prunes), nuts, avocados and bran/wheat grain.

Potassium leaves the extracellular compartment in all intestinal secretions, usually at concentrations near to or a little above that in plasma. A total of about 60 mmol/day is lost into the intestinal lumen, most of which is reabsorbed. Less than 10 mmol/day is present in formed faeces. Excessive intestinal potassium loss can occur in diarrhoea, ileostomy fluid or through fistulae.

The kidneys

Glomerular filtrate

Potassium is filtered by the glomeruli and, due to the huge volume of the filtrate, about 800 mmol (about a quarter of the total body content) would be lost daily if there were no tubular regulation. The net loss is about 10 per cent of that filtered.

The tubules

Potassium is normally almost completely reabsorbed in the proximal tubules. Damage to these may cause potassium depletion. Potassium is secreted in the distal tubules and collecting ducts in exchange for Na^+; hydrogen ions (H^+) compete with potassium ions (K^+). Aldosterone stimulates both exchange mechanisms. If the proximal tubules are functioning normally, potassium loss in the urine depends on three factors.

- The amount of sodium available for exchange: this depends on the glomerular filtration rate, filtered sodium load, and sodium reabsorption from the proximal tubules and loops of Henle. As discussed later, reabsorption in the loops is inhibited by many diuretics, as discussed later.

- The circulating aldosterone concentration: this is increased following fluid loss, with volume contraction, which usually accompanies intestinal loss of potassium, and in most conditions receiving diuretic therapy. Hyperkalaemia stimulates aldosterone release in synergy with angiotensin II, while hypokalaemia inhibits it.
- The relative amounts of H^+ and K^+ in the cells of the distal tubules and collecting ducts, and the ability to secrete H^+ in exchange for Na^+: this may be impaired during treatment with carbonate dehydratase (CD) inhibitors and in some types of renal tubular acidosis (Chapter 4).

The cell membranes

The Na^+/K^+-adenosine triphosphatase 'pump' on cell surfaces maintains a high intracellular $[K^+]$. This exchanges three Na^+ ions from cells in exchange for two K^+ ions in the extracellular fluid (ECF), thus establishing an electrochemical gradient across the cell membrane, with a net positive charge in the ECF. The loss of K^+ from cells down the concentration gradient is opposed by this electrochemical gradient. Potassium is also exchanged for H^+ (Fig. 5.1).

A small shift of K^+ out of cells may cause a significant rise in plasma concentrations, whether in vivo or in vitro. In the latter situation, the artefactual hyperkalaemia due to haemolysed or old specimens may be misinterpreted and should be avoided. Usually the shift of K^+ across cell membranes is accompanied by a shift of Na^+ in the opposite direction, but the percentage change in extracellular $[Na^+]$ is much less than that of K^+.

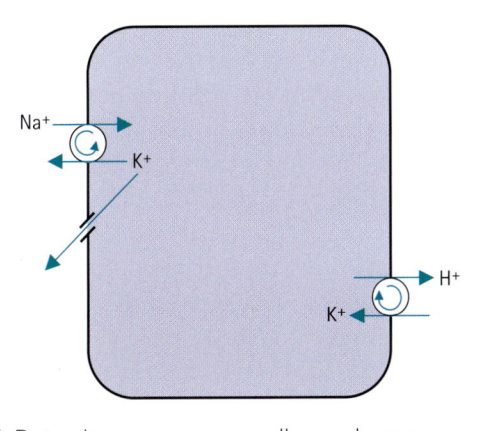

Fig. 5.1 Potassium pumps on cell membranes

Increased uptake and net gain of K^+ by cells may occur in alkalosis due to increased uptake by cells and increased urinary loss. Insulin enhances the cellular uptake of glucose and potassium. Hyperkalaemia stimulates insulin secretion and hypokalaemia inhibits it. This effect may be used to treat hyperkalaemia by giving exogenous insulin/glucose infusion (see p. 92). It is the main cause of the change from hyperkalaemia to hypokalaemia during the treatment of diabetic ketoacidosis.

Catecholamines have a similar action, and it has been suggested that this may contribute to the hypokalaemia sometimes found after the stress of myocardial infarction. Beta-adrenergic stimulation increases cellular potassium uptake by stimulating the Na^+/K^+-ATPase. Beta-blockade increases plasma potassium concentration and β-agonists decrease it, an effect that is independent of body potassium stores.

Synthesis of Na^+/K^+-ATPase is stimulated by thyroxine, which may contribute to the hypokalaemia sometimes associated with hyperthyroidism.

Relationship between hydrogen and potassium ions (Fig 5.2)

The extracellular $[H^+]$ affects the entry of potassium into all cells. Changes in the relative proportions of K^+ and H^+ in distal renal tubular cells affect the urinary loss of potassium. There is a reciprocal relationship between K^+ and H^+.

- In *acidosis*, increased loss of potassium from cells into the ECF coupled with reduced urinary secretion of potassium causes hyperkalaemia.
- In *alkalosis*, net increased uptake of potassium into cells and increased urinary potassium loss cause hypokalaemia.

In the kidney, Na^+ derived from the luminal fluid is pumped through the cell in exchange for either K^+ or H^+. If K^+ is lost from the ECF, it passes down the increased concentration gradient, so reducing its intracellular content. Unless there is renal tubular cell damage, Na^+ is reabsorbed in exchange for less K^+ and more H^+ than usual. For each H^+ formed within the tubular cell by the CD mechanism, one bicarbonate ion (HCO_3^-) is produced:

$$H_2O + CO_2 \underset{CD}{\rightarrow} H^+ + HCO_3^- \quad (5.1)$$

As more H^+ is secreted into the urine, the reaction is increased and more HCO_3^- is generated, passing into

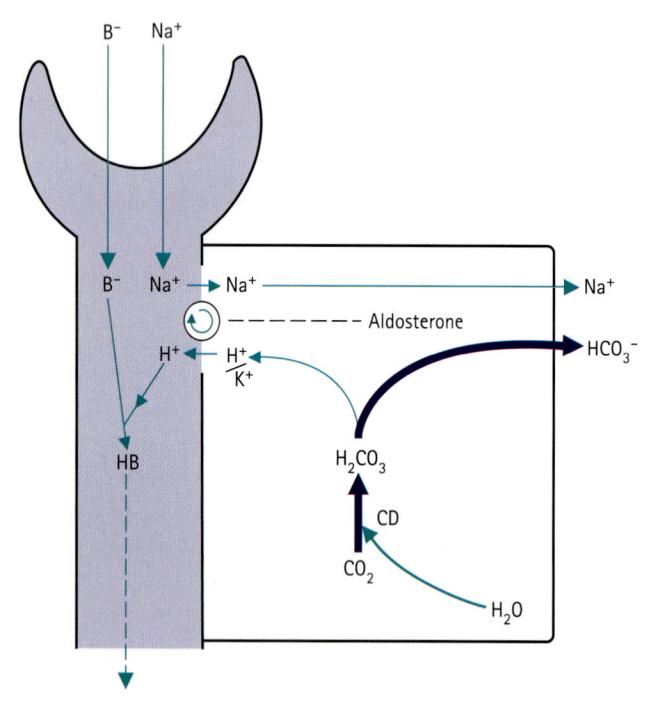

Fig. 5.2 Exchange of Na^+ for either K^+ or H^+ in the renal tubules. (B^- = non-bicarbonate base; CD = carbonate dehydratase.)

the ECF accompanied by the reabsorbed Na^+. The result is an extracellular alkalosis and acid urine. Therefore, chronic potassium depletion is usually accompanied by a high plasma bicarbonate concentration.

The combination of hypokalaemia and a high plasma bicarbonate concentration is more likely to be due to K^+ depletion than to metabolic alkalosis.

Potassium and diuretic therapy

Diuretics may be used to treat hypertension as well as oedema, for example in cardiac failure. They can be divided into two principal groups, based upon their site of action.

- *Potassium-losing diuretics* increase the sodium load on the distal tubules and collecting ducts with enhanced Na^+/K^+ exchange. This may result in hypokalaemia.
  - Loop diuretics, such as furosemide or bumetanide inhibit sodium reabsorption from the ascending limb of the loops of Henle.
  - Thiazides act at the junction of the loops and the distal tubules, which are sometimes called the 'cortical diluting segments'.
  - Carbonate dehydratase inhibitors, such as acetazolamide are rarely used as diuretics but are still used to treat glaucoma. They may cause a hypokalaemic hyperchloraemic acidosis.

- *Potassium-sparing diuretics.*
  - Diuretics that inhibit either aldosterone directly or the exchange mechanisms in the distal tubules and collecting ducts cause potassium retention and may lead to hyperkalaemia, especially if glomerular function is impaired. Potassium-sparing/retaining diuretics include spironolactone, a competitive aldosterone antagonist.
  - Other potassium-sparing diuretics include amiloride and triamterene, which are direct inhibitors of the Na^+/K^+ exchange mechanism in the distal tubules.

Potassium-sparing diuretics can be used together with those causing potassium loss when hypokalaemia cannot be controlled by potassium supplementation. Used alone, they have only a weak diuretic action. Beware of giving potassium supplements to patients taking potassium-sparing diuretics or angiotensin-converting enzyme (ACE) inhibitors or angiotensin receptor blockers because of the risk of hyperkalaemia.

Measurement of plasma and urinary potassium

In rapidly changing clinical states frequent estimation of plasma potassium is the best way of assessing therapy. Plasma potassium is best measured in a freshly collected, unhaemolysed venous sample and is lower than corresponding serum concentrations. In chronic potassium depletion, measurement of the plasma bicarbonate concentration ($[HCO_3^-]$) may help to indicate the state of cellular repletion.

Urinary potassium (kaluria) estimations to determine the primary cause of potassium depletion may be useful diagnostically to help find the cause of hypokalaemia. Most extrarenal causes of potassium loss are associated with volume depletion and therefore with secondary hyperaldosteronism. Excretion of less than about 20 mmol/day can only be expected in the well-hydrated hypokalaemic patient with extrarenal losses in whom aldosterone secretion is inhibited. Therefore a low potassium excretion confirms extrarenal loss, but a high one does not prove that it is the primary cause. High urinary potassium concentration (for example more than 20 mmol/L) in the face of hypokalaemia suggests inappropriate K^+ renal loss as a cause of the hypokalaemia, for example due to renal tubular problems or mineralocorticoid excess syndromes.

The transtubular potassium gradient (TTKG) is an estimate of the potassium concentration at the end of the cortical collecting duct beyond the site where aldosterone

Table 5.1 Some causes of hypokalaemia classified into predominantly non-renal and renal causes

Renal causes	Non-renal causes	Combined causes

Increased Na^+/K^+ exchange
   primary hyperaldosteronism (Conn's syndrome)
   secondary hyperaldosteronism
   Cushing's syndrome
   steroid therapy
   'ectopic' ACTH secretion
   Bartter's syndrome or Gitelman's syndrome
   carbenoxolone therapy
   liquorice excess
   Liddle's syndrome
   11-hydroxylase and 17-hydroxylase deficiencies (rare)
 	
 Excess Na^+ available for exchange
   infusion of saline
   diuretics ('loop' diuretics)
 Decreased Na^+/H^+ exchange
   carbonate dehydratase inhibitors
   renal tubular acidosis (types I and II)
 	
 Impaired proximal tubular reabsorption
   renal tubular dysfunction
   Fanconi syndrome
   hypomagnesaemia
	Redistribution
	   glucose and insulin
	   catecholamines
	   familial hypokalaemic periodic paralysis (rare)
	   barium intoxication (rare)
	   vitamin B_{12} therapy
	   certain rapidly growing tumours
	
	 Intestinal loss
	   prolonged vomiting
	   diarrhoea
	   loss through intestinal fistula
	   purgative abuse
	
	 Reduced intake
	   poor diet
	   Geophagia (rare)
		alkalosis
		 pyloric stenosis

influences potassium secretion. This can be calculated on a spot urine (which should have an osmolality greater than that of the plasma) and plasma samples from the following equation:

$$\frac{\text{urinary}[K^+] \times \text{plasma osmolality}}{\text{plasma}[K^+] \times \text{urine osmolality}} \quad (5.2)$$

The TTKG may be useful diagnostically in the investigation of hyperkalaemia, when a TTKG less than 3 implies the kidneys are not excreting potassium appropriately (i.e. a lack of aldosterone effect).

ABNORMALITIES OF PLASMA POTASSIUM

Hypokalaemia

Hypokalaemia is often the result of potassium depletion, but if the rate of loss of potassium from cells equals or exceeds that from the ECF, potassium depletion may exist without hypokalaemia. Hypokalaemia can also occur without depletion if there is a shift of K^+ into cells.

The causes of hypokalaemia (summarized in Table 5.1) may be classified according to the predominant cause as either renal or non-renal. Pseudohypokalaemia is defined as the in-vitro uptake of K^+ from the plasma into blood cells, primarily erythrocytes. This sometimes occurs if the blood sample is kept in a warm environment. This contrasts with the more usual hyperkalaemia found in specimens stored in the refrigerator.

Renal causes of hypokalaemia

- Enhanced renal secretion of potassium due to increased activity of the pump in distal renal tubules by mineralocorticoid activity. This is associated with a hypokalaemic alkalosis.
  - Primary hyperaldosteronism (Conn's syndrome) due to adrenal adenoma or hyperplasia (see Chapter 8).
  - Secondary hyperaldosteronism often aggravates other causes of potassium depletion (see Chapter 2).

- Cushing's syndrome and steroid therapy. Patients secreting excess of, or on prolonged therapy with, glucocorticoids tend to become hypokalaemic due to the mineralocorticoid effect on the distal renal tubules (see Chapter 8).
- 'Ectopic' adrenocorticotrophic hormone (ACTH) secretion, which stimulates cortisol secretion (see Chapter 8).
- Bartter's syndrome is a rare autosomal recessive condition in which there is hyperplasia of the renal juxtaglomerular apparatus with increased renin and therefore aldosterone secretion. Angiotensin II activity is impaired and therefore there is no vasoconstriction; consequently the patient is normotensive. This latter finding helps to distinguish the syndrome from that of primary hyperaldosteronism, in which there can also be a hypokalaemic alkalosis. Individuals may have polyuria, polydipsia, short stature, learning difficulties and maternal polyhydramnios. The defect is in the epithelial ion channels of the ascending limb. The biochemical features mimic those of high-dose loop diuretic intake. Treatment consists of potassium supplementation, often with a potassium-sparing diuretic such as spironolactone or amiloride. By suppressing prostaglandin-stimulated renin release, non-steroidal anti-inflammatory drugs may also improve the condition.
- The very rare Gitelman's syndrome, in contrast to Bartter's syndrome, is often asymptomatic until adulthood. It is an autosomal recessive condition due to a mutation in the thiazide-sensitive Na^+/Cl^- co-transporter in the distal convoluted tubules. Unlike Bartter's, there is more severe hypomagnesaemia and hypocalciuria. Once thiazide use has been excluded, a hypokalaemic hypomagnesaemic alkalosis in the presence of a urinary calcium:creatinine molar ratio less than 0.2 is suggestive of Gitelman's syndrome.
- Liddle's syndrome, also very rare, is an autosomal dominant condition with hypertension and hypokalaemic metabolic alkalosisis, in which suppressed plasma aldosterone and renin concentrations are associated with cerebrovascular disease. Mutations in the selective sodium channels cause increased sodium reabsorption through the collecting duct epithelial sodium channel, causing hypertension. Treatment involves sodium restriction and potassium-sparing diuretics such as amiloride or triamterene; spironolactone is ineffective.
- Carbenoxolone therapy is occasionally used to accelerate the healing of peptic ulcers. It potentiates the action of aldosterone and can cause hypokalaemia by inhibiting the enzyme 11-β-hydroxysteroid dehydrogenase. (See Chapter 8.)
- Liquorice and tobacco contain glycyrrhizinic acid, which also inhibits the enzyme 11-β-hydroxysteroid dehydrogenase. Over-indulgence in liquorice-containing sweets or habitual tobacco chewing can rarely cause hypokalaemia. (See Chapter 8.)

- Increased renal potassium loss may also result from impaired proximal tubular potassium reabsorption as in:
  - Renal tubular dysfunction (for example the recovery phase of acute oliguric renal failure).
  - Fanconi's syndrome (see Chapter 3).
  - Hypercalcaemia, which may impair the reabsorption of potassium even if there is no renal damage.
  - Hypomagnesaemia can also reduce the intracellular potassium concentration and causes renal potassium wasting. It may be a cause of a refractory hypokalaemia unless the plasma magnesium is corrected.
  - A number of drugs can cause increased renal loss of potassium, including diuretics (non-potassium sparing) cisplatin, aminoglycosides, amphotericin and foscarnet, and CD inhibitors, e.g. acetazolamide.

- Decreased renal Na^+/H^+ exchange because of impaired generation of H^+ within the renal tubular cells, which favours Na^+/K^+ exchange associated with a hypokalaemia. Causes include renal tubular acidosis types I and II (see Chapter 4).

- Excess sodium available for exchange in the distal renal tubules can also increase renal potassium loss. These include:
  - Prolonged infusion of saline.
  - Diuretics inhibiting the pump in the loops of Henle. The activity of the distal pump is enhanced by secondary hyperaldosteronism.

Non-renal causes of hypokalaemia

- Redistribution within the body, by entry into cells.
  - Glucose and insulin therapy. This may be used to treat severe hyperkalaemia.
  - Increased secretion of catecholamines, such as may occur due to the stress of myocardial infarction. The use of β-agonists such as salbutamol in inhalers may also stimulate this secretion.

- Rapidly growing tumours, such as certain leukaemias, can evoke hypokalaemia, presumably by potassium uptake into the proliferating cells.
- Familial hypokalaemic periodic paralysis is rare and is an autosomal dominant defect of the dihydropyridine receptor, a voltage-gated calcium channel. In this condition episodic paralysis is associated with entry of potassium into cells, which can be provoked by a high carbohydrate intake. Thyrotoxic periodic paralysis is a similar condition, but genetically different, that is found in hyperthyroidism.
- Barium ingestion blocks potassium exit from cells.
- Treatment of pernicious anaemia with vitamin B_{12}, by rapid cellular uptake of potassium into cells (see Chapter 15).
- Reduced potassium intake.
  - Chronic starvation. If water and salt intake are also reduced, secondary hyperaldosteronism may aggravate the hypokalaemia.
  - Inadequate potassium replenishment in patients receiving intravenous fluid replacement or total parenteral nutrition.
- Loss from the ECF into intestinal secretions.
  - Prolonged vomiting.
  - Diarrhoea, whether due to infections, malabsorption states, radiation or chemotherapy.
  - Loss through intestinal fistulae.
  - Habitual purgative users may present with hypokalaemia. It may be possible to detect laxatives in the stools to confirm this.
  - The concentration of potassium in fluid from a recent ileostomy and in diarrhoea stools may be five to ten times that of plasma, but a prolonged drain of any intestinal secretion, even if its potassium concentration is not very high, causes depletion, especially if urinary loss is increased by secondary hyperaldosteronism.
  - Mucus-secreting villous adenomas of the intestine are very rare but may cause considerable potassium loss. Zollinger–Ellison syndrome and vipomas are other rare causes.
  - Rare chloride-losing diarrhoea (intestinal ion transport defect) (see Chapter 16).
  - The unusual habit of geophagia (earth eating) can also cause hypokalaemia, possibly by chelating K^+.

Clinical features of hypokalaemia

The clinical features of disturbances of potassium metabolism are due to changes in the extracellular concentration of the ion. Hypokalaemia, by interfering with neuromuscular transmission, causes muscular weakness, hypotonia and cardiac arrhythmias, and may precipitate digoxin toxicity. Patients with mild hypokalaemia (3.0–3.5 mmol/L) may have no symptoms, although those in which it is more severe may show generalized weakness, lassitude and constipation. If the K^+ is below 2.5 mmol/L, muscle necrosis and rhabdomyolysis may rarely occur. Hypokalaemia may also aggravate paralytic ileus and hepatic encephalopathy.

Cardiac symptoms depend on the rate of change of potassium loss and also on the state of the heart. Hypokalaemia can increase the risk of digoxin toxicity and causes prolongation of the P–R interval, flattening of the T waves and prominent U waves on the electrocardiogram (ECG).

Intracellular potassium depletion causes extracellular alkalosis. This reduces the plasma free ionized calcium concentration and, in long-standing depletion of gradual onset, the presenting symptoms may be muscle cramps and even tetany. This syndrome is accompanied by high plasma bicarbonate concentrations. Prolonged potassium depletion impairs the renal concentrating mechanism and may cause polyuria with further potassium depletion.

Investigation of hypokalaemia (Fig. 5.3)

The following procedure should help elucidate the cause of the hypokalaemia in conjunction with plasma potassium and bicarbonate determinations (see Table 5.1). Raised plasma bicarbonate concentration, in the absence of chronic pulmonary disease, is indicative of a metabolic alkalosis, and low plasma bicarbonate concentration is suggestive of a metabolic acidosis. Therefore hypokalaemia can be divided into alkalosis and acidosis groups.

Hypokalaemic alkalosis

Diuretic therapy is the commonest cause of hypokalaemic alkalosis in hypertensive patients. Primary hyperaldosteronism and ectopic ACTH production are very rare.

- Take a careful drug history, with special reference to potassium-losing diuretics, purgatives and steroids. Rare causes of a steroid-like effect are ingestion of carbenoxolone or liquorice.
- Check the potassium concentration in a spot urine sample. If less than or equal to 20 mmol/L, it is suggestive of gastrointestinal loss or transcellular potassium shift or poor potassium intake. If it is more than 20 mmol/L, it is indicative of renal potassium loss

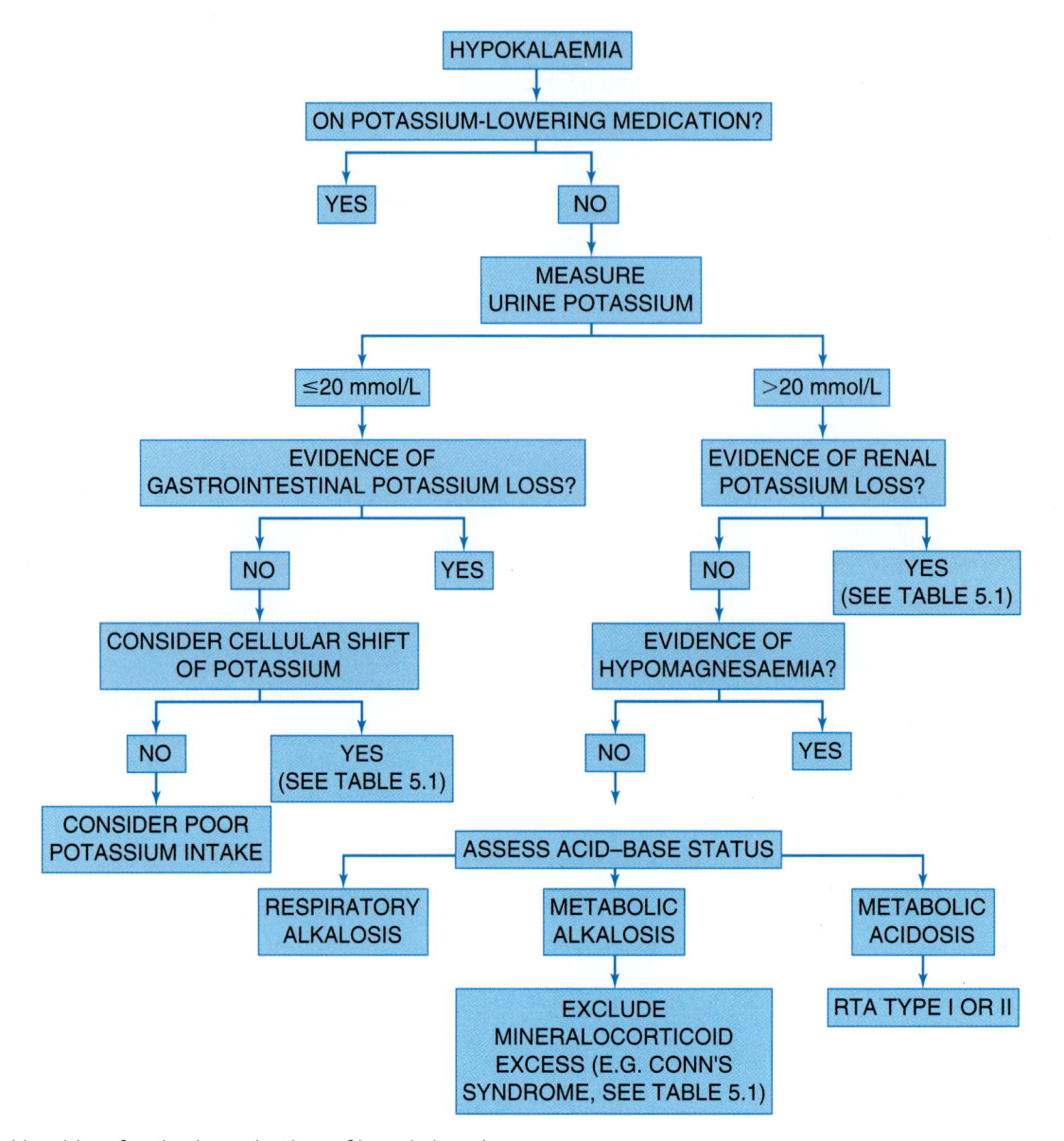

Fig. 5.3 Algorithm for the investigation of hypokalaemia

such as occurs in the very rare Bartter's and Gitelman's syndromes and other mineralocorticoid excess disorders.
- The urinary chloride concentration is usually more than 20 mmol/L in Bartter's or Gitelman's syndrome. This is useful diagnostically to distinguish them from other causes of hypokalaemia such as gastrointestinal loss of potassium, for example vomiting or diarrhoea in which urinary chloride is usually less than 20 mmol/L. If purgative abuse is suspected, an estimation of the drug levels in stool samples may be indicated.
- Exclude hypomagnesaemia, which may be associated with hypokalaemia (see Chapter 6).
- For the investigation of primary hyperaldosteronism (Conn's syndrome), Cushing's syndrome and other mineralocorticoid excess syndromes see Chapter 8.

Hypokalaemic acidosis

Hypokalaemic acidosis, which may be associated with hyperchloraemia (hyperchloraemic acidosis), is relatively rare and the cause is usually obvious (see Chapter 4). Having checked plasma potassium, chloride and bicarbonate concentrations, consider the following.

- Loss of potassium through fistulae in the proximal small intestine may be accompanied by significant bicarbonate loss.

CASE 1

A 17-year-old student presented to her general practitioner with generalized muscle weakness and tiredness. Her blood pressure was 116/70 mmHg. The following biochemical results were obtained.

Plasma
Sodium 135 mmol/L (135–145)
Potassium 2.0 mmol/L (3.5–5.0)
Urea 2.3 mmol/L (2.5–7.0)
Creatinine 79 μmol/L (70–110)
Bicarbonate 38 mmol/L (24–32)
Chloride 80 mmol/L (95–105)

Urine
Chloride <20 mmol/L

DISCUSSION
The results suggest a hypokalaemic metabolic alkalosis. There is also hypochloraemia, due to chloride loss from chronic vomiting. It transpired that the patient had anorexia nervosa with bulimia and had been self-inducing vomiting for many months. This had resulted in a metabolic alkalosis and severe hypokalaemia. The low urinary chloride concentration helps distinguish this from the much rarer Bartter's syndrome, in which the urinary chloride concentration would be expected to be more than 20 mmol/L.

- Certain drugs should be considered. These include azetazolamide, a carbonic dehydratase inhibitor sometimes used in the treatment of glaucoma and altitude sickness or as a diuretic.
- If neither of these causes is present, a diagnosis of renal tubular acidosis should be considered (see Chapter 4).

Treatment of hypokalaemia

Mild hypokalaemia can be treated with oral potassium supplements, which can be continued until plasma potassium concentrations have returned to normal. The normal subject loses about 60 mmol of potassium daily in the urine, much larger amounts being excreted during diuretic therapy. By the time hypokalaemic alkalosis is present, the total deficit is probably 100–200 mmol. A patient with hypokalaemia should usually be given about 80 mmol/day, but more may be needed if plasma potassium concentrations fail to rise.

It may sometimes be dangerous to give potassium, especially intravenously, if there is renal impairment. One of the most common forms of hyperkalaemia in hospital patients results from supplemental potassium administration. Generally the plasma potassium decreases by 0.3 mmol/L for each 100 mmol reduction in total body stores. Typically, 40–100 mmol of supplemental potassium are needed per day to maintain potassium concentrations within the reference range in most patients receiving diuretics.

The commonly used oral potassium supplements are:

- potassium chloride effervescent tablets, containing 6.5 mmol K^+ per tablet,
- slow K: 8 mmol K^+ per tablet (as chloride),
- Sando K: 12 mmol K^+ per tablet (as bicarbonate and chloride).

Oral therapy may be safer, as potassium enters the circulation more slowly. However, oral potassium salts can cause gastrointestinal upset and are not adequate if there is life-threatening hypokalaemia (for example less than 2.0 mmol/L or clinical symptoms and signs). The slow-release forms may be better tolerated but may cause gastrointestinal ulceration.

In severe hypokalaemia, particularly if the patient is unable to take oral supplements, intravenous potassium should be given cautiously. Diarrhoea not only reduces the absorption of oral potassium supplements, but may also be aggravated by them; this too may be an indication for intravenous therapy.

Intravenous potassium should only be used if there is significant depletion or if oral potassium cannot be taken or retained. In most cases, oral potassium treatment is preferable. Intravenous potassium should be given with care, especially in the presence of poor glomerular function; ECG monitoring is wise. Potassium chloride is the usual intravenous form. The following rules should be observed.

- Unless the deficit is unequivocal and severe, intravenous potassium should not be given if there is oliguria.
- Potassium in intravenous fluid should not usually exceed a concentration of 40 mmol/L.
- Intravenous potassium should not usually be given at a rate of more than 20 mmol/hour and ideally should

be given by infusion pump. In very severe depletion this dose may have to be exceeded; in such cases frequent plasma potassium estimations *must* be performed.
- Twenty millimoles of potassium chloride can be added to a full bag (500 mL) of intravenous fluid and mixed well. Potassium chloride solution should never be given undiluted.
- Always check the labelling of vials carefully when giving potassium, as fatalities have occurred due to errors in administration.

If hypomagnesaemia is present, this should also be treated, as it can be a cause of refractory hypokalaemia.

Hyperkalaemia

Pseudohyperkalaemia

Plasma potassium results should not be reported if the specimen is haemolysed or if plasma was not separated from cells within a few hours after the blood was taken. Pseudohyperkalaemia, due to in-vitro leakage of potassium from cells into plasma, is often misinterpreted, sometimes with dangerous consequences. This may occur if there has been a delay in separating the plasma from the cells, particularly if the blood sample has been refrigerated, when activity of the pump is slowed. A rare familial form of pseudohyperkalaemia is thought to be due to defective red cell membranes. Thrombocytosis and leucocytosis can also result in pseudohyperkalaemia. Also, beware of potassium-EDTA (ethylenediamine tetra-acetic acid) contaminated blood tubes: blood samples for potassium assay should usually be collected in lithium heparin tubes.

The causes of hyperkalaemia are summarized in Table 5.2, and can be classified into renal and non-renal causes.

Renal causes of hyperkalaemia

- Drugs.
  - Angiotensin-converting enzyme inhibitors, such as captopril and enalapril (which are used to treat hypertension), inhibit the conversion of angiotensin I to angiotensin II and therefore aldosterone secretion. They may cause hyperkalaemia, especially if glomerular function is impaired.
  - Angiotensin II receptor blockers, for example losartan, and diuretics that either act on the distal tubules and antagonize aldosterone activity (spironolactone) or inhibit the pump (amiloride). Non-steroidal anti-inflammatory drugs may also cause hyperkalaemia, as can heparin.
- Acute or chronic renal failure involves impaired renal secretion of potassium and decreases the activity of

Table 5.2 Some causes of hyperkalaemia classified into predominantly renal and non-renal causes

Renal causes	Non-renal causes
Insufficient Na$^+$ exchange	*In vitro effects* or pseudohyperkalaemia
renal glomerular dysfunction (e.g. acute or chronic renal failure)	haemolysis
sodium depletion	leukocytosis
	thrombocytosis
	delayed separation of plasma
Decreased Na$^+$/K$^+$ exchange	
mineralocorticoid deficiency	*Increased input*
hypoaldosteronism (Addison's disease)	dietary source
congenital adrenal hyperplasia (21-hydroxylase deficiency)	intravenous/oral potassium
hyporeninaemic hypoaldosteronism (Type IV renal tubular acidosis)	
pseudohypoaldosteronism	*Redistribution*
Drugs e.g.	acidosis
angiotensin converting enzyme inhibitors	hypoxia
spironolactone	severe tissue damage
potassium sparing diuretics	haemolysis (in vivo)
angiotensin receptor blockers	familial hyperkalaemic periodic paralysis (rare)
	drugs e.g. digoxin

the Na^+/K^+-ATPase pump in the distal renal tubules. This is especially true when the glomerular filtration rate (GFR) is less than 25 per cent of normal (see Chapter 3).
- Another mechanism is gain of K^+ by ECF via more than one route with reduced renal excretion.
  - Acidosis. In diabetic ketoacidosis in poorly controlled type 1 diabetes mellitus (Chapter 12), potassium enters the ECF from cells because normal action of the pump depends on the energy supplied by glucose metabolism. If glomerular function is relatively normal, urinary potassium loss is increased, resulting in total body potassium depletion. Loss from the plasma into the urine rarely keeps pace with the gain from cells, and mild hyperkalaemia is common. As the condition progresses, two other factors contribute to hyperkalaemia: namely volume depletion causing a reduced GFR and ketoacidosis.

All these factors are reversed during insulin and fluid therapy. As potassium re-enters cells, extracellular potassium concentrations fall and the depletion is revealed. Plasma potassium concentrations must be monitored regularly during therapy and potassium must be given as soon as the concentration begins to fall.

- Hypoxia causes impairment of the pump in all cells, with a net gain of potassium within the ECF. Such impairment in the distal tubules causes potassium retention. If hypoxia is severe, lactic acidosis aggravates hyperkalaemia (see Chapter 4).
- Mineralocorticoid deficiency. Mineralocorticoids such as aldosterone have a sodium-retaining and potassium-losing action (see Chapter 2). Thus deficiency of these hormones can cause hyperkalaemia. This is dealt with in more detail in Chapter 8, but examples include:
  - adrenal insufficiency (Addison's disease) due to absence of or damage to the adrenal glands;
  - congenital adrenal hyperplasia such as C21-hydroxylase deficiency (rare);
  - hyporeninaemic hypoaldosteronism, a very rare disorder presenting in the elderly, often with renal impairment and glucose intolerance or type 2 diabetes mellitus; it is associated with hyperkalaemia and type IV renal tubular acidosis (see Chapter 4);
  - rare causes include pseudohypoaldosteronism (discussed in Chapter 8).

Non-renal causes of hyperkalaemia

These are due to the gain of potassium by the body from the intestine or by the intravenous route.

- Excess potassium therapy, especially in patients with impaired glomerular function, either orally as potassium supplementation or, more commonly, intravenously, for example with potassium-chloride-containing fluids.
- Redistribution within the body or loss from cells.
  - Severe tissue damage, for example haemolysis, burns, crush injury, tumour lysis syndrome, rhabdomyolysis and severe exercise. In these cases intracellular potassium moves out of cells.
  - Familial hyperkalaemic periodic paralysis is exceedingly rare and is associated with release of potassium from cells.
  - Various drugs, such as digoxin, β-adrenergic blockers and succinylcholine, can cause hyperkalaemia by reducing the entry of potassium into cells (see Table 5.2).

CASE 2

A 64-year-old patient was being treated for hypertension. Her medications were enalapril and amiloride. The results were:

Plasma
Sodium 143 mmol/L (135–145)
Potassium 6.2 mmol/L (3.5–5.0)
Urea 9.3 mmol/L (2.5–7.0)
Creatinine 159 mmol/L (70–110)

DISCUSSION
The hyperkalaemia was eventually found to be due to the injudicious use of an ACE inhibitor and potassium-sparing diuretic. This drug combination can lead to severe hyperkalaemia, especially in someone with impaired renal function.

Clinical features of hyperkalaemia

Hyperkalaemia, particularly if severe, carries the danger of cardiac arrest. Changes are also seen on ECG, such as widening of the QRS complex and tall, 'tented' T waves.

Investigation of hyperkalaemia (Fig. 5.4)

- Exclude artefactual (pseudohyperkalaemia) causes of hyperkalaemia such as haemolysis, thrombocytosis, leucocytosis or delayed separation of plasma from blood cells or potassium-EDTA-contaminated tubes.
- Is the patient taking drugs, such as:
  - potassium supplements?
  - potassium-retaining diuretics?
  - an ACE inhibitor or angiotensin II receptor antagonist?
- Is there a cause for cell damage or transcellular potassium shifts, such as hypoxia, rhabdomyolysis or severe trauma?
- What are the plasma urea and creatinine concentrations? Severe renal glomerular dysfunction is a common cause of hyperkalaemia.
- Measure the plasma bicarbonate concentration. An acidosis, whether metabolic (with a low plasma bicarbonate concentration) or respiratory (with a normal or high plasma bicarbonate concentration), may cause mild hyperkalaemia even if glomerular function is normal. A cause of respiratory acidosis is usually obvious clinically (see Chapter 4).
- Measurement of the TTKG (described above) may help to determine whether there is a potassium renal excretory effect.
- Is there evidence of mineralocorticoid deficiency? This should not be forgotten, as adrenal insufficiency can be life threatening. If there is any doubt, consider performing a short Synacthen test (see Chapter 8 for details of the investigation of adrenal insufficiency).
- Rare causes of hyperkalaemia, such hyporeninaemic hypoaldosteronism, pseudohypoaldosteronism and type IV renal tubular acidosis, are shown in Table 5.2. The investigation of renal tubular acidosis is described in Chapter 4.

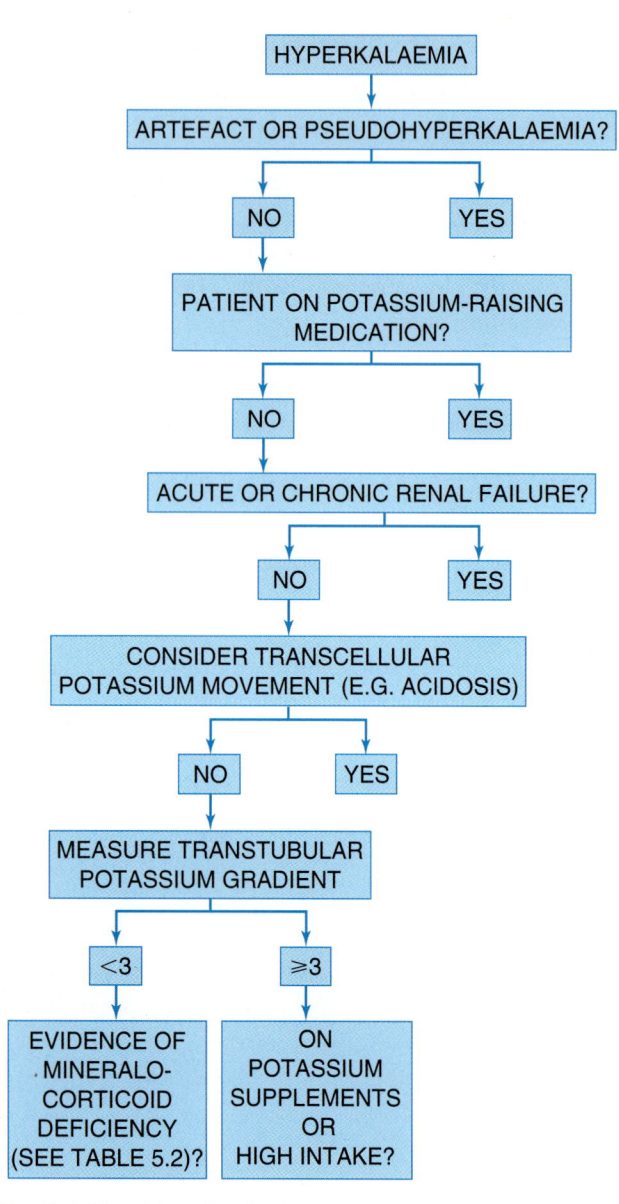

Fig. 5.4 Algorithm for the investigation of hyperkalaemia

Treatment of hyperkalaemia

Emergency treatment

Emergency treatment may be necessary if there is life-threatening hyperkalemia, for example more than 7.0 mmol/L or significant ECG changes.

Calcium gluconate, 10 mL of a 10 per cent solution, is given slowly intravenously with ECG monitoring. This antagonizes the effect of hyperkalaemia on heart muscle but does not alter potassium concentrations. However, calcium should never be added to bicarbonate solutions because calcium carbonate is poorly soluble in water. If too much calcium is given, hypercalcaemia may cause cardiac arrest.

Intravenous 50 mL glucose 50 per cent with 10 units of soluble insulin by intravenous injection over 15–30 minutes starts to lower plasma potassium concentrations for a couple of hours by increasing potassium entry into cells. Insulin enhances the activity of the pump and must be given with glucose to prevent hypoglycaemia.

More rarely, 50–100 mL of 8.4 per cent sodium bicarbonate, usually via a central line, may be infused over 30 minutes if a severe acidosis (for example pH less than 7.1) is present, or 1.26 per cent solution in isotonic saline if the situation is less urgent. Remember that 8.4 per cent sodium bicarbonate is hyperosmolar. Infusing bicarbonate increases the rate of potassium entry into cells.

Sometimes, if the hyperkalaemia is not too severe, nebulized salbutamol (5–10 mg) is used to treat hyperkalaemia by causing redistribution of potassium into cells. Reductions in plasma potassium of 0.5–1.0 mmol/L can occur and last for 2–3 hours.

Long-term treatment of chronic hyperkalaemia

Sodium or calcium polystyrene sulphonate (Resonium-A or Calcium Resonium) 15 g orally three or four times a day can remove potassium from the body but may take at least 24 hours to work.

CONCLUSIONS

- Disorders of potassium homeostasis are common in clinical practice and can be life threatening.
- Potassium is a predominant intracellular cation and thus plasma levels do not adequately reflect total body potassium stores.
- Potassium ions are controlled by renal excretion, which is increased by aldosterone and reduced by H^+.
- Hypokalaemia can cause weakness, paralytic ileus and ECG changes; common causes are potassium loss from the kidneys or gastrointestinal tract, cellular redistribution and poor intake.
- Hyperkalaemia can cause lethal cardiac arrhythmias and is commonly due to renal retention, movement out of cells or increased intake.

6 CALCIUM, PHOSPHATE AND MAGNESIUM

Calcium metabolism	94	Abnormalities of plasma phosphate concentration	111
Total body calcium	94	**Magnesium metabolism**	112
Concept of plasma calcium and albumin correction	94	Plasma magnesium and its control	112
Disorders of calcium metabolism	98	Clinical effects of abnormal plasma magnesium concentrations	112
Phosphate metabolism	110		
The function of phosphate in vivo	111		

Disorders of calcium metabolism are common in clinical practice and may result in hypocalcaemia or hypercalcaemia as well as bone abnormalities. Intimately associated with calcium disorders are disorders involving phosphate and magnesium metabolism.

CALCIUM METABOLISM

TOTAL BODY CALCIUM

The total body calcium depends upon the calcium absorbed from dietary intake and that lost from the body (Fig. 6.1). Ninety-eight per cent of body calcium is found in the skeleton. The extra-osseous fraction, although amounting to only 1 per cent of the total, is essential because of its effect on neuromuscular excitability and cardiac muscle. An important mediator of intracellular calcium is calmodulin, a calcium-binding regulatory protein.

Factors affecting calcium intake

About 25 mmol (1 g) of calcium is ingested per day, of which there is a net absorption of 6–12 mmol (0.25–0.5 g). The active metabolite of vitamin D, 1,25-dihydroxycholecalciferol (1,25-$(OH)_2D_3$, also called calcitriol), is needed for calcium absorption.

Factors affecting calcium loss

Calcium is lost in urine and faeces. Urinary calcium excretion depends on the amount of calcium reaching the glomeruli, the glomerular filtration rate (GFR) and renal tubular function. Parathyroid hormone and 1,25-dihydroxyvitamin D increase urinary calcium reabsorption.

Faecal calcium is derived from the diet and that portion of the large amount of intestinal secretions that has not been reabsorbed. Calcium in the intestine may form insoluble, poorly absorbed complexes with oxalate, phosphate or fatty acids. An excess of fatty acids in the intestinal lumen in steatorrhoea may contribute to calcium malabsorption.

CONCEPT OF PLASMA CALCIUM AND ALBUMIN CORRECTION

The mean plasma calcium concentration in healthy subjects is tightly controlled, at around 2.15–2.55 mmol/L, and is present in two main forms.

- *Calcium bound to proteins*, mainly albumin: this accounts for a little less than half the total calcium concentration as measured by routine analytical methods and is the physiologically inactive form.

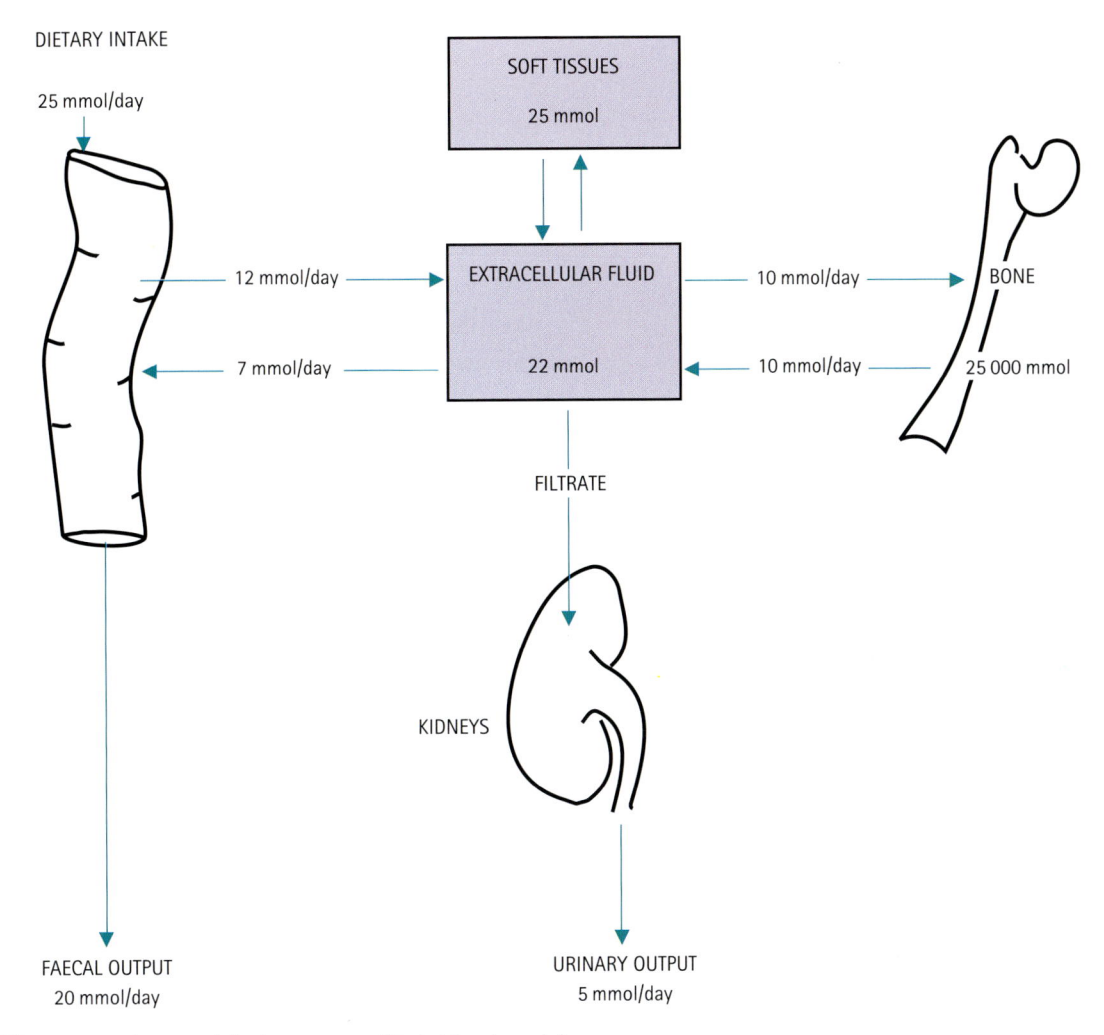

Fig. 6.1 The approximate daily turnover of total body calcium.

- *Free ionized calcium* (Ca^{2+}), which comprises most of the rest. This is the physiologically active fraction.

Changes in plasma protein concentration, particularly of albumin, the principal plasma protein, alter the most commonly measured concentration, that of plasma total calcium, but not that of the free ionized fraction. The plasma total (but not free ionized) calcium concentration is lower in the supine than in the erect position because of the effect of posture on fluid distribution and therefore on plasma protein concentration. The direct measurement of the physiologically active free calcium ionized fraction is, for technical reasons, confined to special cases such as acid–base disturbance.

Formulae incorporating the albumin concentration have been devised in an attempt to calculate the active fraction of the plasma total calcium concentration, but, because binding is not simple, these are not always reliable, particularly if extremes of plasma albumin concentration occur. The following is a commonly used formula:

plasma albumin adjusted or 'corrected' calcium (mmol/L)
 = plasma measured calcium
 + (40 − plasma[albumin]) (g/L)
 × 0.02   (6.1)

Changes in plasma hydrogen ion concentration ([H$^+$]) affect the binding of calcium to plasma proteins because H$^+$ competes with Ca^{2+} for binding sites. The plasma total calcium concentration is unaltered by changes in [H$^+$]. If [H$^+$] falls, as in an alkalosis, tetany may occur despite a normal plasma total calcium concentration. Conversely, an acidosis decreases binding and so increases the proportion of plasma calcium in the free ionized form. Also, by increasing calcium solubility, it increases the rate of release of calcium from bones into the extracellular fluid (ECF).

> **CASE 1**
>
> A 45-year-old male was in the intensive care unit for multiple trauma following a road traffic accident. Some of his biochemistry results were as follows.
>
> *Plasma*
> Calcium 1.98 mmol/L (2.15–2.55)
> Albumin 30 g/L (35–45)
> Phosphate 0.92 mmol/L (0.80–1.35)
> What is the albumin-adjusted or corrected calcium?
>
> **DISCUSSION**
>
> $$\text{Corrected calcium} = 1.98 + (40 - 30) \times 0.02$$
> $$= 1.98 + 0.20 = 2.18 \text{ mmol/L}$$
>
> (6.2)
>
> Note that the plasma calcium now corrected falls within the reference range and does not require specific treatment. Remember this if the patient has hypoalbuminaemia.

The increased load reaching the kidneys increases the renal calcium loss. Prolonged acidosis may cause osteomalacia, partly due to the buffering effect of bone.

Control of plasma calcium

There are a number of mechanisms by which plasma calcium concentrations are controlled. Calcium homeostasis follows the general rule that extracellular concentrations are controlled rather than the total body content. The effectiveness of this control depends upon:

- an adequate supply of:
  - calcium
  - vitamin D,
- normal functioning of the:
  - intestine
  - parathyroid glands
  - kidneys.

If any one of these factors is impaired, calcium leaves bone by passive physicochemical diffusion, and plasma concentrations may be maintained at the expense of bone calcification.

Parathyroid hormone

Parathyroid hormone (PTH) is a single-chain polypeptide containing 84 residues, with its 34 N-terminal amino acids largely determining its biological activity. It is metabolized by renal, hepatic and bone cells. Renal clearance from plasma of the physiologically inert C-terminal fragment is slower than that of the N-terminal fragment. The C-terminal fragment may accumulate in plasma in renal glomerular dysfunction and this may complicate the interpretation of results of some PTH assays, although many now measure only the intact active form. The biological actions of PTH include:

- stimulation of osteoclastic bone resorption, so releasing both free ionized calcium and phosphate into the ECF; this action increases the plasma concentrations of both calcium and phosphate;
- decreased renal tubular reabsorption of phosphate, causing phosphaturia and increased reabsorption of calcium; this action tends to increase the plasma calcium concentration but to decrease the phosphate.

The control of PTH secretion depends on the concentration of free ionized calcium in blood circulating through the parathyroid glands. A fall increases the rate of PTH secretion, which, under physiological conditions, continues until the calcium concentration returns to normal. The secretion of PTH is also affected by the extracellular magnesium concentration, being decreased by severe, chronic hypomagnesaemia.

Detectable plasma PTH, even if the concentration is within the reference range, is inappropriate in the presence of hypercalcaemia and is consistent with primary or, more rarely, tertiary hyperparathyroidism.

Parathyroid hormone-related protein

Parathyroid hormone-related protein (PTHRP) is a peptide hormone that has a similar amino acid sequence at the biologically active end of the peptide, therefore activating the same receptors as PTH. The function of PTHRP is uncertain, but it may be important in calcium metabolism in the fetus. The gene that codes for PTHRP is widely distributed in body tissues but is normally repressed. However, it may become derepressed in certain tumours, causing humoral hypercalcaemia of malignancy.

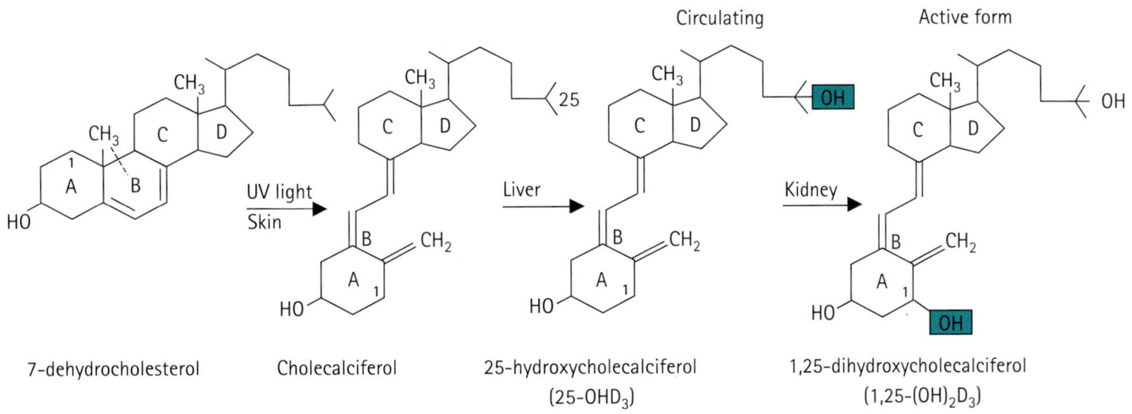

Fig. 6.2 Formation of the active vitamin D metabolite from 7-dehydrocholesterol. (UV = ultraviolet.)

Calcitonin

Calcitonin (produced in the C-cells of the thyroid gland) decreases osteoclastic activity, slows calcium release from bone and has the opposite effect on plasma concentrations of PTH. It is probably less important than PTH in physiological homeostasis. Plasma concentrations may be very high in patients with medullary carcinoma of the thyroid, although hypocalcaemia is not usually reported in this condition. However, exogenous calcitonin has been used to treat hypercalcaemia and Paget's disease of bone.

Metabolism and action of vitamin D

Vitamin D is derived from:

- ergocalciferol (vitamin D_2), obtained from plants in the diet,
- cholecalciferol (vitamin D_3), formed in the skin by the action of ultraviolet light on 7-dehydrocholesterol (Fig. 6.2); this is the form found in animal tissues, especially the liver.

In normal adults, much more cholecalciferol is derived from the action of sunlight on skin than from food. Dietary sources are important when requirements are high, such as during growth or pregnancy, or in those elderly or chronically sick individuals who are confined indoors and not exposed to the sun.

Vitamin D is transported in plasma bound to specific carrier proteins. It is inactive until metabolized. In the liver, cholecalciferol is hydroxylated to 25-hydroxycholecalciferol (25-OHD$_3$) by the enzyme 25-hydroxylase. The rate of formation of 25-OHD$_3$ is affected by the supply of substrate in the form of calciferol, whether derived from the skin or from the diet. It is the main circulating form and store of the vitamin. Other hydroxylated metabolites are found, such as 24,25-$(OH)_2D_3$.

In the proximal renal tubular cells of the kidney, 25-OHD$_3$ undergoes a second hydroxylation, catalysed by the enzyme 1-α-hydroxylase to form the active metabolite 1,25-$(OH)_2D_3$.

The activity of 1-α-hydroxylase, and hence the production of 1,25-$(OH)_2D_3$, may be stimulated by:

- a low plasma phosphate concentration,
- an increase in plasma PTH concentration, possibly because of its phosphate-lowering effect.

Its activity is inhibited by:

- hyperphosphataemia,
- high levels of free ionized calcium.

The kidney is an endocrine organ, synthesizing and releasing the hormone 1,25-$(OH)_2D_3$; impairment of the final hydroxylation helps explain the hypocalcaemia of renal disease. This hormone increases calcium absorption by intestinal mucosal cells. In conjunction with PTH, it stimulates osteoclastic activity, releasing calcium from bone.

The action of PTH on bone is impaired in the absence of 1,25-$(OH)_2D_3$. A fall in plasma free ionized calcium concentration stimulates PTH secretion. The PTH enhances 1-α-hydroxylase activity and therefore stimulates 1,25-$(OH)_2D_3$ synthesis. The two hormones act synergistically on the osteoclasts of bone, releasing calcium into the circulation; 1,25-$(OH)_2D_3$ also increases calcium absorption from the intestinal lumen. In the short term, the homeostatic mechanisms involving the effects on bone are the more important; if hypocalcaemia is prolonged, more efficient absorption becomes important. Once the plasma free ionized calcium concentration is corrected, the secretion of both PTH and 1,25-(OH)$_2$D$_3$ is suppressed.

Thus, 25-OHD$_3$ is the circulating, inactive form of vitamin D and plasma concentrations fall in deficiency states. The measurement of the biologically active metabolite, 1,25-(OH)$_2$D$_3$, which circulates in plasma in very low concentrations, is rarely indicated unless a defect in the vitamin metabolic pathway is suspected, as it does not reflect body stores.

Calcium-sensing receptor

The calcium-sensing receptor (CaSR) is a G protein-coupled receptor. This allows the parathyroid cells and the ascending loop of Henle epithelial cells to respond to changes in extracellular calcium. The parathyroid cell surface is rich in CaSR, which allows PTH secretion to be adjusted rapidly depending on the calcium concentration.

Defects in the CaSR gene are responsible for various rare defects of calcium homeostasis. Inactivating mutations include familial benign hypocalciuric hypercalcaemia and neonatal severe hyperparathyroidism; activating mutations include autosomal dominant hypocalcaemia with hypercalciuria. Calcimetric agents have been devised that bind and activate the CaSR, resulting in decreased PTH release and reduced plasma calcium concentrations.

Miscellaneous mechanisms of calcium control

Thyroid hormone excess may be associated with the histological appearance of osteoporosis and with increased faecal and urinary excretion of calcium, probably following its release from bone. Hypercalcaemia is a very rare complication of severe hyperthyroidism. Unless there is gross excess of thyroid hormone, the effects on plasma calcium are overridden by homeostatic reduction of PTH secretion and by urinary loss.

Other hormones influencing calcium metabolism include oestrogens, prolactin and growth hormone. These may increase 1,25-(OH)$_2$D$_3$ production and increase calcium absorption during pregnancy, lactation and growth.

DISORDERS OF CALCIUM METABOLISM

The consequences of most disturbances of calcium metabolism can be predicted from knowledge of the actions of PTH on bone and on renal tubular cells, and from plasma concentrations of calcium and phosphate. A low plasma free ionized calcium concentration normally stimulates PTH secretion, which results in phosphaturia; the loss of urinary phosphate overrides the tendency to hyperphosphataemia due to the action of PTH on bone. Consequently, the plasma phosphate concentration is usually low when the plasma PTH concentration is increased. Conversely, a high plasma free ionized calcium concentration, unless due to inappropriate excess of PTH, inhibits PTH secretion and causes a high plasma phosphate concentration. Therefore plasma calcium and phosphate concentrations usually vary in the same direction unless:

- renal glomerular dysfunction is severe enough to impair the phosphaturic (and therefore hypophosphataemic) effect of PTH or PTHRP,
- there is inappropriate excess or deficiency of PTH due to a primary disorder of the parathyroid gland or to secretion of PTHRP; in such cases calcium and phosphate vary in opposite directions.

Hypercalcaemia

Clinical effects of an increased plasma corrected calcium concentration

- Renal effects.
  - *Renal damage* is one of the most serious clinical consequences of prolonged hypercalcaemia. Due to the high plasma free ionized calcium concentration, the solubility of calcium phosphate may be exceeded and precipitate in extra-osseous sites such as the kidneys (see Chapter 3).
  - *Polyuria*, characteristic of chronic hypercalcaemia, may result from impairment of renal concentrating ability due to calcification of the tubular cells; acute hypercalcaemia may cause reversible inhibition of the tubular response to antidiuretic hormone rather than to cell damage. These effects can lead to dehydration.
  - *Renal calculi*, without significant parenchymal damage, may be caused by precipitation of calcium salts in the urine if the free ionized calcium concentration is high in the glomerular filtrate due to hypercalcaemia (see Chapter 3).
  - *Hypokalaemia*, often with a metabolic alkalosis, is a common finding in association with hypercalcaemia. Calcium may directly inhibit potassium reabsorption from the tubular lumen (see Chapter 5).
- High extracellular free ionized calcium concentrations can depress neuromuscular excitability in both voluntary and involuntary muscle. There may also be muscular hypotonia.

- Depression, anorexia, nausea and vomiting, associated with high plasma calcium concentrations, are probably caused by an effect on the central nervous system.
- Calcium stimulates gastrin (and therefore gastric acid) secretion. There is an association between chronic hypercalcaemia and peptic ulceration. The patient may complain of constipation and abdominal pain. Hypercalcaemia may also present as an acute abdomen.
- Some patients with hypercalcaemia may be hypertensive. If renal damage is not severe, the hypertension may respond to reducing the plasma calcium concentration.
- Severe hypercalcaemia causes characteristic changes in the electrocardiogram (ECG), with shortening of the Q–T interval and broadening of the T waves. If plasma concentrations exceed about 3.5 mmol/L, there is a risk of sudden cardiac arrest or ventricular arrhythmias. For this reason severe hypercalcaemia should be treated as a matter of urgency.
- Hypercalcaemia is also associated with bone and joint pain.

'Bones, moans, groans and stones' is a useful mnemonic to remember some of these clinical consequences of hypercalcaemia.

Causes of hypercalcaemia (Box 6.1)

Overall, thiazides are one of the commonest causes of mild hypercalcaemia. However, most causes of severe hypercalcaemia are related to either primary hyperparathyroidism or malignancy. In the case of the latter, 80 per cent are due to bony metastases, with the remainder being mainly due to ectopic PTHRP. Some causes of hypercalcaemia are depicted in Box 6.1.

True free ionized or albumin corrected hypercalcaemia with hypophosphataemia is usually caused by inappropriate secretion of PTH or PTHRP. The term 'inappropriate secretion' is used in this book to indicate that the release of hormone into the circulation is not adequately inhibited by negative feedback control. Inappropriate PTH secretion occurs in the following clinical situations.

- Production of PTH by the parathyroid glands due to:
  - primary hyperparathyroidism,
  - tertiary hyperparathyroidism.
- Production of PTHRP by non-parathyroid tissue.

If renal glomerular function is adequate, the high circulating PTH or PTHRP concentrations cause hypercalcaemia, which is associated with a low-normal or low plasma phosphate concentration in relation to GFR, and to phosphaturia. If glomerular damage develops due to

> **Box 6.1 Some causes of hypercalcaemia**
>
> *Malignancy*
> Bony metastases, e.g. breast, lung, prostate, kidney, thyroid
> Solid tumours with humoral effects
> Haematological tumours, e.g. myeloma
>
> *Parathyroid hormone abnormalities*
> Primary hyperparathyroidism (adenoma, hyperplasia or associated with multiple endocrine neoplasias)
> Tertiary hyperparathyroidism
> Lithium-induced hyperparathyroidism
>
> *High bone turnover*
> Thyrotoxicosis
> Immobilization, e.g. with Paget's disease
>
> *High levels of vitamin D*
> Vitamin D toxicity
> Granulomatous disease, e.g. sarcoidosis, tuberculosis
>
> *Drugs*
> Thiazides (reduced renal calcium excretion)
> Vitamin A toxicity
> Milk-alkali syndrome
>
> *Familial hypocalciuric hypercalcaemia*
>
> *Other endocrine causes*
> Adrenal insufficiency
> Acromegaly
>
> *Rarer causes, e.g.*
> Williams' syndrome
> Human immunodeficiency virus infection
> Leprosy
> Histoplasmosis
> Berylliosis

hypercalcaemia, the kidneys cannot respond normally to the phosphaturic effect of PTH and, because of impaired hydroxylation of 25-OHD$_3$, plasma calcium concentrations may fall towards or within the reference range as renal failure progresses. Because plasma phosphate concentrations tend to rise, diagnosis may be difficult at this stage.

The clinical features of PTH-induced or PTHRP-induced hypercalcaemia are due to:

- excess circulating concentration of free ionized calcium that is the direct consequence of increased osteoclastic activity and release of calcium from bone, and enhanced

absorption of calcium from the intestinal lumen by vitamin D; PTH increases the formation of 1,25-$(OH)_2D_3$;
- the effects of persistent PTH or PTHRP activity on bone in the presence of a normal supply of vitamin D and calcium (see Fig. 6.1).

The differences between the clinical presentations associated with inappropriately high plasma PTH concentrations depend on the duration of the disease. The following effects on bone only become evident in long-standing cases. Prolonged decalcification of bone causes a secondary increase in osteoblastic activity. Alkaline phosphatase-rich osteoblasts release the enzyme into the circulation and if the number of cells is greatly increased, plasma alkaline phosphatase activity rises.

Primary hyperparathyroidism

This is caused by inappropriate secretion of PTH by the parathyroid glands, causing hypercalcaemia. It is usually due to one or more parathyroid adenomas, but occasionally to hyperplasia of all four parathyroid glands or to carcinoma of one of the glands. Ectopic parathyroid tumours do also occur. Primary hyperparathyroidism may be associated with other multiple endocrine neoplasias (MENs), such as pituitary and pancreatic adenomas (MEN Type I), or with phaeochromocytomas and medullary carcinoma of the thyroid (MEN Type II).

The incidence of primary hyperparathyroidism increases with age, being most common in elderly females.

The majority of cases of primary hyperthyroidism are diagnosed after the chance finding of high plasma calcium, usually with low plasma phosphate concentrations.

Where there are clinical symptoms and signs at presentation, these are due to hypercalcaemia and include the following.

- *Generalized ill-health*: depression, nausea, anorexia and abdominal pain and polyuria.
- *Renal calculi*: about 10 per cent of patients who present with renal calculi have primary hyperparathyroidism.
- *Bone pain*: in most patients, subperiosteal bone erosions or cysts may be seen on X-ray of the terminal phalanges. However, extensive, severe bone disease, osteitis fibrosa cystica, is now a rare presenting feature, as patients are usually diagnosed before the disorder is extensive and consequently plasma alkaline phosphatase activity is usually normal or only slightly increased. There are increased numbers of osteoclasts and an increased risk of bone fracture.
- *Medical emergency*: occasionally patients are admitted as an emergency with abdominal pain, vomiting and constipation. Severe hypercalcaemia is a recognized cause of acute pancreatitis and should be considered as one cause of an 'acute abdomen'.

Recently, it has been reported that an incipient form of primary hyperparathyroidism exists in which there is initially normal plasma calcium but elevated PTH.

The treatment of primary hyperparathyroidism is often surgical, with removal of the parathyroid gland(s). However, this can render the patient hypocalcaemic, and asymptomatic patients are sometimes treated conservatively.

Tertiary hyperparathyroidism

This may occur if the parathyroid glands have been subjected to long-standing and sustained positive feedback by low plasma free ionized calcium concentrations (hypocalcaemia) of secondary hyperparathyroidism which has been subsequently corrected. The parathyroid glands hypertrophy; PTH secretion becomes partly autonomous and is not suppressed by negative feedback by the hypercalcaemia. The diagnosis is usually made when the cause of the original hypocalcaemia is removed, for example by renal

---

CASE 2

A 53-year-old male saw his general practitioner because of bone pain and constipation. A number of laboratory tests were requested, the results for the most relevant of which were as follows.

Plasma
Corrected calcium 2.96 mmol/L (2.15–2.55)
Phosphate 0.62 mmol/L (0.80–1.35)
Parathyroid hormone 157 ng/L (20–65)

DISCUSSION
The patient has hypercalcaemia. Note also the hypophosphataemia and inappropriately raised PTH concentration. The diagnosis was subsequently found to be primary hyperparathyroidism due to an adenoma. His symptoms are typical of chronic hypercalcaemia.

transplantation or correction of long-standing calcium or vitamin D deficiency as in malabsorption. A history of previous hypocalcaemia and the finding of a very high plasma alkaline phosphatase activity due to the prolonged osteomalacia distinguish it from primary hyperparathyroidism. In some cases, the glandular hypertrophy gradually regresses and the plasma calcium concentration returns to normal.

Unlike primary or tertiary hyperparathyroidism, in which plasma PTH concentration is increased, there are other causes of hypercalcaemia where plasma levels of PTH are reduced or suppressed. These are now discussed.

Hypercalcaemia of malignancy

Malignant disease of bone

Some patients with multiple bony metastases (for example breast, lung, prostate, kidney and thyroid tumours) or with myelomatosis show hypercalcaemia. Here there is usually a parallel rise of plasma phosphate. The hypercalcaemia is caused by direct bone breakdown due to the local action of malignant deposits.

Malignant deposits in bone stimulate a local osteoblastic reaction and hence a rise in plasma alkaline phosphatase activity. This osteoblastic reaction does not occur in bone eroded by the marrow expansion of myelomatosis. Therefore in the latter condition the plasma concentration of alkaline phosphatase of bony origin is relatively normal, despite extensive bone involvement with osteolytic lesions.

Humoral hypercalcaemia of malignancy

Parathyroid hormone-related protein is synthesized by some malignant tumours of non-endocrine tissues and is not subject to normal feedback control by the high plasma free ionized calcium concentration. Bony lesions due to circulating PTHRP are not normally present because the underlying disease is usually either fatal or successfully treated in a relatively short time. However, the plasma alkaline phosphatase activity may be raised because of secondary deposits in bone or the liver, or both. In humoral hypercalcaemia of malignancy, the plasma calcium concentration may rise from normal to dangerously high very rapidly, in contrast to primary hyperparathyroidism. Ectopic hormone production is discussed more fully in Chapter 24.

Drugs/medications

Various medications can evoke hypercalcaemia, such as thiazides (decreases renal excretion), lithium, and vitamin A excess.

Milk-alkali syndrome

This rare condition occurs with the excessive use of calcium-containing antacids for dyspepsia. It is also associated with a metabolic alkalosis. Milk-alkali is now rarely seen since the advent of proton-pump inhibitors and H2 antagonists for the treatment of dyspepsia.

Vitamin D excess

Vitamin D excess may be caused by over-vigorous treatment of hypocalcaemia. Increased intestinal calcium absorption may cause dangerous hypercalcaemia. Vitamin D therapy, with either ergocalciferol or the active metabolite 1,25-dihydroxyvitamin D, should always be monitored by frequent estimation of plasma calcium concentrations and, if there is osteomalacia, by measuring plasma alkaline phosphatase activity. If the cause of hypercalcaemia is obscure, a careful drug history should be taken. Occasionally patients inadvertently overdose themselves with vitamin D, which is available in many countries without prescription.

Sarcoidosis

Hypercalcaemia is a rare complication. 1,25-Dihydroxycholecalciferol is synthesized in the granuloma tissue and

---

CASE 3

A 76-year-old female with known breast carcinoma was admitted to hospital drowsy, with weight loss and back ache. The following results were returned.

Plasma
Corrected calcium 3.96 mmol/L (2.15–2.55)
Phosphate 1.12 mmol/L (0.80–1.35)
Parathyroid hormone less than 10 ng/L (20–65)

DISCUSSION

A bone scan subsequently showed the patient to have widespread bone metastases. Note the severe hypercalcaemia and the appropriately suppressed plasma PTH, suggesting a non-parathyroid source of the hypercalcaemia. Various tumours are associated with bone metastases, including breast tumours.

increases calcium absorption from the intestinal tract. Chronic beryllium poisoning produces a granulomatous reaction very similar to that of sarcoidosis and may also be associated with hypercalcaemia. The same is possibly also true of histoplasmosis and leprosy.

Hypercalcaemia of hyperthyroidism

Prolonged excess of thyroid hormone in severe hyperthyroidism may be associated with the histological appearance of osteoporosis and a consequent increase in urinary calcium excretion. Hypercalcaemia is a very rare complication.

Other endocrine causes of hypercalcaemia

These include acromegaly (see Chapter 7), Addison's disease (see Chapter 8) and phaeochromocytoma (see Chapter 24).

Familial hypocalciuric hypercalcaemia

Hypercalcaemia with an inappropriately high plasma PTH concentration in the presence of hypocalciuria has been reported in some families, in none of whom was a parathyroid adenoma found at operation. The condition is inherited as an autosomal dominant trait. The aetiology of the condition is thought to be due a defect on the CaSR (see above). Low urinary calcium concentration in the face of hypercalcaemia points to the diagnosis. A useful test is the calcium excreted per litre of glomerular filtrate (CAE):

$$CAE = \frac{urinary[calcium] \times plasma[creatinine]}{urinary[creatinine]} \quad (6.3)$$

Hypocalciuric hypercalcaemia is likely if this is less than 0.015 (in mmol/L). It is important to exclude this condition, as it can mimic primary hyperparathyroidism.

Hypercalcaemia of infancy

Idiopathic hypercalcaemia of infancy includes a number of conditions that cause hypercalcaemia during the first year of life. Excessive vitamin D supplementation of cow's milk is now a very uncommon cause. Williams' syndrome is a rare familial disorder associated with increased intestinal calcium absorption and hypercalcaemia. Clinical features include growth retardation, mental deficiency and characteristic 'elfin' facies. Congenital heart disease may also be present (see Chapter 26).

Investigation of hypercalcaemia (Fig. 6.3)

Establish whether the high plasma total calcium concentration is due only to a high protein-bound fraction. Two groups of causes should be differentiated for raised corrected plasma calcium concentration:

- raised albumin corrected calcium concentration due to inappropriately high PTH and usually hypophosphataemia,
- raised albumin corrected calcium concentration due to other causes and associated with low PTH concentrations and often hyperphosphataemia.

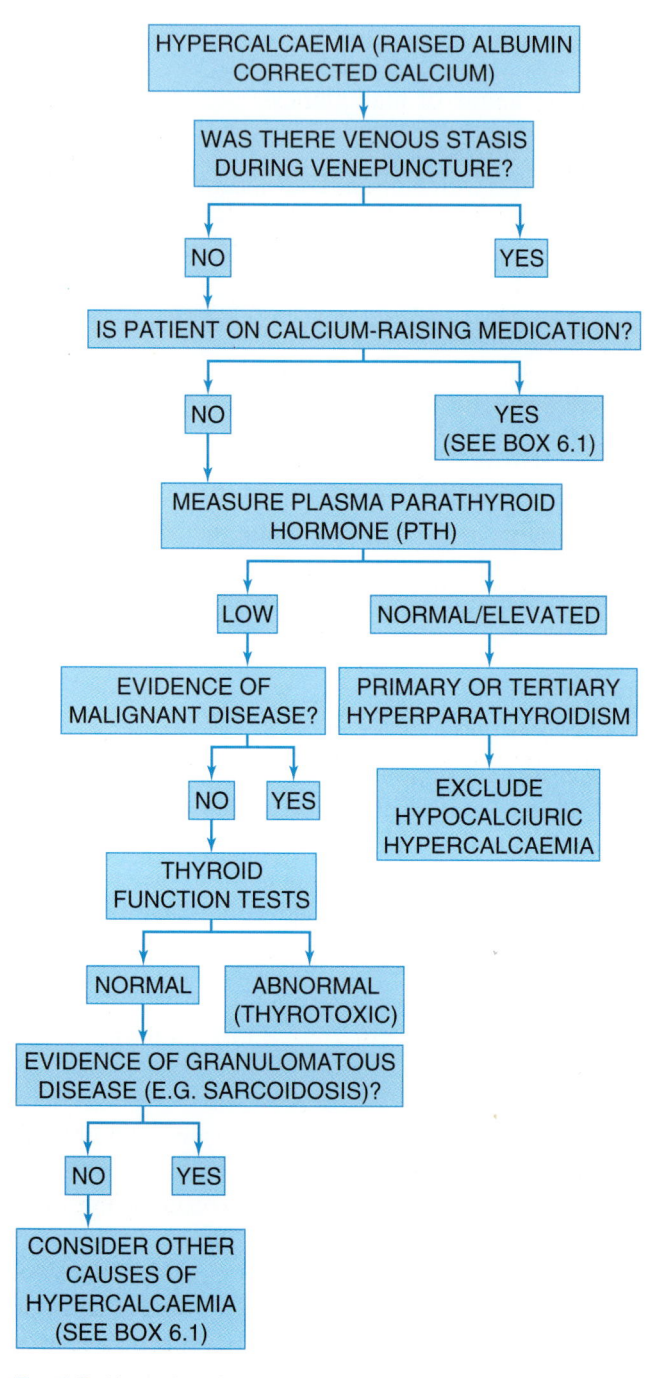

Fig. 6.3 Algorithm for the investigation of hypercalcaemia.

The following procedure may be useful to find the cause of hypercalcaemia, although the diagnosis may be obvious before all the steps have been followed.

- Establish the plasma albumin concentration.
- Check the albumin corrected calcium. Take a specimen without venous stasis (preferably without a tourniquet) to eliminate artefactual haemoconcentration and repeat the plasma calcium and albumin assays. If true hypercalcaemia is confirmed, a cause must be sought.
- Take a careful history, with special reference to the drug history, such as vitamin-D-containing preparations and thiazide diuretics. Is there evidence of milk-alkali syndrome? If so, check acid–base status.
- Is the plasma phosphate concentration low in relation to the renal function? Hypophosphataemia suggests the diagnosis of primary hyperparathyroidism.

Apart from thiazide usage, the most common causes of hypercalcaemia are either primary hyperparathyroidism or malignancy; the latter may be obvious following clinical examination and radiological and haematological tests, for example anaemia, and raised erythrocyte sedimentation rate (ESR) and biochemical investigations.

It is essential that primary hyperparathyroidism and malignant hypercalcaemia are distinguished. In the case of malignancy, pay special attention for breast, lung or prostate carcinoma.

A raised plasma PTH concentration is usually seen in primary hyperparathyroidism; conversely, suppressed levels are found in malignant states and indeed in hypercalcaemia of many other causes. Sometimes PTHRP can be measured if ectopic secretion of this is suspected, for example by a tumour.

If primary hyperparathyroidism due to an adenoma is found, exclude MEN syndrome (see Chapter 24). Imaging of the parathyroid glands is often needed to distinguish adenoma from hyperplasia of the parathyroid glands.

Very high plasma alkaline phosphatase activity is unlikely to be due to uncomplicated primary hyperparathyroidism; near-normal activity is usual, although it may be raised if there is radiological evidence of bone involvement. If it is very high, it suggests either malignancy or some concurrent disease such as Paget's disease.

Perform serum and urinary protein electrophoresis if a myeloma is suspected (see Chapter 19).

If all the findings are negative, particularly if the blood haemoglobin concentration and ESR are normal, and especially if there is a history of, for example, peptic ulceration or renal calculi, this suggests chronic hypercalcaemia.

Primary hyperparathyroidism is by far the most likely cause. Of course either of these complications may occur without hypercalcaemia. Isotope subtraction scanning or ultrasound of the neck may help to localize the adenoma, as may venous sampling for PTH levels.

- Look for evidence of sarcoidosis; plasma angiotensin-converting enzyme (ACE) concentration is often raised (see Chapter 18) and a chest X-ray may be useful.
- Is there acromegaly, Addison's disease or thyrotoxicosis (see Chapters 7, 8 and 11)?
- A urinary calcium determination (CAE) is useful to help exclude hypocalciuric hypercalcaemia.
- Rarer causes of hypercalcaemia are listed in Box 6.1.

A steroid suppression test is rarely necessary to identify the cause of hypercalcaemia because of the development of robust PTH assays. Briefly, this test relied on the fact that hypercalcaemia of primary hyperparathyroidism is not usually suppressed by steroids, unlike many of the other causes of a raised calcium concentration such as malignant disease.

Treatment of hypercalcaemia

Mild to moderate hypercalcaemia

If the plasma corrected calcium concentration is below about 3.5 mmol/L, and if there are no significant clinical symptoms or signs such as ECG changes attributable to hypercalcaemia, there is no need for urgent treatment. However, therapy should be started as soon as the abnormality is found and preliminary investigations have been performed because of the danger of renal damage. If possible, the primary cause should also be diagnosed and treated.

The patient should be fluid-volume repleted, if necessary by intravenous infusion of saline. The plasma total calcium concentration will often fall as the plasma albumin concentration is diluted, but the plasma free ionized calcium concentration is probably little affected. Correcting haemoconcentration enables a more realistic assessment to be made of the degree of true hypercalcaemia.

Bisphosphonates are first-line agents in the medical management of hypercalcaemia. These are structurally similar to pyrophosphate. They bind to hydroxyapatite in bone, thus inhibiting bone turnover and the mobilization of calcium. They are poorly absorbed from the intestinal tract and may have to be given intravenously to patients with severe hypercalcaemia. Cyclical administration may prevent the long-term complication of osteomalacia.

The management of apparently asymptomatic mild hypercalcaemia due to primary hyperparathyroidism is controversial. It has been suggested that prolonged hypercalcaemia does not always cause obvious renal dysfunction and that the risk of parathyroidectomy (e.g. rendering the patient hypocalcaemic) may be greater than that of mild hypercalcaemia. The decision as to whether to operate must be made on clinical grounds; of particular importance are the fitness of the patient for operation, plasma calcium concentration greater than 3.0 mmol/L, deteriorating renal function, renal calculi, poor bone mineral density or 24-hour urinary calcium concentration greater than 10 mmol/L.

Severe hypercalcaemia

The plasma corrected calcium concentration at which urgent treatment is indicated because of the danger of cardiac arrest is usually about 3.5 mmol/L. If in doubt, abnormalities associated with hypercalcaemia should be sought on the ECG. Consider the following.

- *Rehydration.* The patient should be volume repleted, intravenously with saline if necessary. Furosemide may also be given in an attempt to increase urinary calcium clearance and avoid fluid overload. Check electrolytes and renal function carefully.
- *Bisphosphonates.* After rehydration and correction of any electrolyte abnormalities, bisphosphonates such as pamidronate are the treatment of choice. They are probably the most effective and have the least toxic side-effects.
- *Steroids* may sometimes lower the plasma calcium concentration in malignancy and almost always in cases of sarcoidosis and vitamin D intoxication.
- *Calcitonin* is sometimes used to treat severe hypercalcaemia. The effect lasts about 3 days; repeated doses are often less successful in maintaining a 'normal' plasma calcium concentration.

Steroids and calcitonin usually have no significant effect for about 24 hours.

As with most other extracellular constituents, rapid changes in plasma calcium concentration may be dangerous because time is not allowed for equilibration across cell membranes. The aim of emergency treatment should be to lower the plasma concentration to one that is not immediately dangerous, while initiating treatment for mild hypercalcaemia as outlined above. Too rapid a reduction, even to only normal or slightly raised concentrations, may cause tetany.

Hypocalcaemia

Clinical effects of a reduced corrected plasma calcium concentration

Low plasma corrected calcium concentrations, including those associated with a normal total calcium concentration of alkalosis, cause increased neuromuscular activity eventually leading to tetany and carpopedal spasm, generalized seizures, laryngospasm, hyper-reflexia, paraesthesiae and hypotension.

Prolonged hypocalcaemia, even when mild, interferes with the metabolism of the lens in the eye and may cause cataracts. Because of this, asymptomatic hypocalcaemia should be sought when there has been a known risk of parathyroid damage, such as after partial or total thyroidectomy, and, if found, treated. Hypocalcaemia may also cause depression and other psychiatric symptoms as well as cardiac arrhythmias, including prolonged Q–T interval on ECG.

Latent neuromuscular hyperactivity, carpopedal spasm and tetany (Trousseau's sign) can be evoked by inflating a blood pressure cuff to 10–20 mmHg above systolic blood pressure for 3–5 minutes. Chvostek's sign can be elicited by tapping the facial nerve anterior to the ear, when ipsilateral facial muscle contraction may occur, although this can also occur in about 10 per cent of individuals without hypocalcaemia.

It is sometimes useful to divide hypocalcaemia into those cases with a low plasma phosphate concentration (hypophosphataemia) and those with high plasma phosphate concentration (hyperphosphataemia), although not all cases of hypocalcaemia fall neatly into this classification. The causes of hypocalcaemia are given in Box 6.2.

Hypocalcaemia with hypophosphataemia

High plasma PTH concentrations cause phosphaturia with hypophosphataemia if glomerular function is normal.

Secondary hyperparathyroidism ('appropriate' secretion of PTH) occurs in response to a low plasma free ionized calcium concentration. The parathyroid glands respond with appropriate secretion of PTH. If the response is effective, the plasma calcium concentration returns to normal, the stimulus to secretion is removed and hormone production is then inhibited by negative feedback. Preservation of plasma calcium concentrations occurs at the expense of bone mineralization and therefore decalcification may result. Parathyroid hormone cannot act effectively on bone in the absence of $1,25\text{-}(OH)_2D_3$. In cases of vitamin D

> **Box 6.2 Some causes of hypocalcaemia**
>
> Exclude hypoalbuminaemic states
>
> *Drugs and chemicals*
> Furosemide
> Enzyme-inducing drugs, e.g. phenytoin
> Ethylene glycol overdose (rare)
>
> *Causes of hypocalcaemia usually with hypophosphataemia*
> Vitamin D deficiency
>   Rickets
>   Osteomalacia
> Malabsorption states
>
> *Causes of hypocalcaemia usually with hyperphosphataemia*
> Chronic renal failure
> Hypoparathyrodism (low PTH levels)
>   Idiopathic or autoimmune
>   Surgical removal of parathyroids
>   Congenital absence of parathyroids, e.g. DiGeorge's syndrome
>   Infiltration of parathyroids, e.g. tumours, haemochromatosis
> Pseudohypoparathyroidism (rare)
> PTH resistance (raised PTH levels)
>
> *Miscellaneous causes of hypocalcaemia (rarer causes)*
> Acute pancreatitis
> Sepsis
> High calcitonin levels
> Rhabdomyolysis
> Severe hypomagnesaemia
> Autosomal dominant hypercalciuric hypocalcaemia
>
> PTH = parathyroid hormone.

deficiency with hypocalcaemia, plasma PTH concentrations may be very high.

Without an adequate supply of calcium and phosphate, osteoid cannot be calcified despite marked osteoblastic proliferation. The histological finding of uncalcified osteoid is characteristic of osteomalacia in adults or rickets in children. Osteomalacia, before fusion of the epiphyses, may present with a slightly different clinical, radiological and histological picture and is called rickets. Plasma alkaline phosphatase activity is increased because of osteoblastic proliferation.

Disorders of bone disease associated with secondary hyperparathyroidism may present:

- *With osteomalacia* in adults, or *rickets* in children, presenting before fusion of the epiphyses and is due to long-standing deficiency of calcium, phosphate and vitamin D. Predisposing factors include:
  - reduced dietary intake of vitamin D, calcium and phosphate in malnutrition,
  - impaired absorption of vitamin D in steatorrhoea after gastrectomy,
  - impaired metabolism of vitamin D to $1,25\text{-}(OH)_2 D_3$ due to renal disease,
  - increased inactivation of vitamin D due to anticonvulsant therapy,
  - renal tubular disorders of phosphate reabsorption.
- *Without osteomalacia or rickets.* If PTH action is inadequate to correct the abnormality, the plasma calcium concentration remains low and bone disorders are not present. Predisposing factors include:
  - early calcium and vitamin D deficiency,
  - the rare pseudohypoparathyroidism.

In secondary hyperparathyroidism the plasma calcium concentration is never high and usually the plasma calcium and phosphate concentrations tend to be low. High-normal or high plasma calcium concentrations in renal

CASE 4

A 72-year-old female presented to her general practitioner with tiredness, muscle aches and difficulty standing up. The following test results were found.

Plasma
Corrected calcium 1.76 mmol/L (2.15–2.55)
Phosphate 0.52 mmol/L (0.80–1.35)
Parathyroid hormone 138 ng/L (20–65)
25-hydroxyvitamin D 5 µg/L (10–35)

DISCUSSION
The patient has osteomalacia, as evidenced by the low plasma 25-hydroxyvitamin D concentration. Note also the hypocalcaemia with hypophosphataemia and secondary appropriate elevation of PTH. The symptoms are typical of osteomalacia, which can lead to proximal myopathy and bone pain. The elderly are particularly prone to osteomalacia.

glomerular dysfunction suggest either that primary hyperparathyroidism has caused the renal disease or that prolonged calcium deficiency has led to the development of tertiary hyperparathyroidism.

Reduced intake and absorption of calcium and vitamin D

In steatorrhoea, fat (and therefore vitamin D) absorption is impaired; this malabsorption may be aggravated if calcium combines with unabsorbed fatty acids to form insoluble soaps in the lumen. Deficiency due to malnutrition is more commonly caused by deficiency of vitamin D than of calcium.

In relatively affluent countries, malabsorption is the commonest cause of calcium and vitamin D deficiencies. Worldwide dietary deficiency is important. The following groups are at risk of developing osteomalacia or rickets:

- children and pregnant women, in whom increased needs may not be met by the normal supply from the skin,
- people such as the elderly and chronically sick who are not exposed to sunlight because they are confined indoors.

There is a relatively high incidence of osteomalacia and rickets amongst the Asian community in some urban Western societies. The causes are unclear but probably include dietary habits, relative lack of sunlight and possibly genetic factors.

Impaired metabolism of vitamin D

Chronic liver disease may occasionally be associated with mild osteomalacia, especially if there is cholestasis causing malabsorption due, for example, to primary biliary cirrhosis. However, it is unlikely that significant impairment of vitamin D hydroxylation is the cause.

Prolonged anticonvulsant therapy, especially if both barbiturates and phenytoin are taken, may be associated with hypocalcaemia and even osteomalacia. These drugs probably induce the synthesis of hepatic enzymes which catalyse the conversion of vitamin D to inactive metabolites.

In all these conditions, the low plasma free ionized calcium concentration stimulates PTH secretion; the plasma phosphate concentration tends to be low *relative to the GFR*. However, if there is renal glomerular dysfunction, the plasma phosphate concentration may be increased but tends to be lower than in those cases with the same concentration of plasma urea but normal plasma PTH concentrations. In chronic cases a rising plasma alkaline phosphatase activity indicates the onset of the bone changes of osteomalacia or rickets.

Type 1 vitamin-D-dependent rickets is due to 1-α-hydroxylase deficiency. It is an autosomal recessive disorder and results in low $1,25\text{-}(OH)_2D_3$ concentrations.

Type 2 vitamin-D-dependent rickets is also an autosomal recessive disorder and causes a vitamin D resistance and is a defect of the $1,25\text{-}(OH)_2D_3$ receptor. Thus plasma $1,25\text{-}(OH)_2D_3$ concentrations are elevated.

Hypocalcaemia with hyperphosphataemia

Renal dysfunction

One of the commonest causes of hyperphosphataemia is acute or chronic renal failure (dysfunction) (see Chapter 3).

Renal disease such as chronic renal failure causes relative resistance to vitamin D because of the direct effect of the disease on the functioning renal tubular cells and therefore on 1-α-hydroxylation of $25\text{-}OHD_3$ and inhibition of 1-α-hydroxylation by hyperphosphataemia associated with the low GFR of renal glomerular dysfunction.

Hypocalcaemia may develop within a few days of the onset of renal damage. Low plasma protein concentrations often contribute to the reduction in the total calcium concentration. Tetany is rare in renal disease, probably because the accompanying acidosis increases the plasma free ionized calcium concentration above tetanic concentrations. Treatment of the metabolic acidosis with bicarbonate is usually contraindicated because a rise in blood pH may cause precipitation of calcium phosphate in extra-osseous sites. In the kidney it may aggravate renal dysfunction.

Primary hypoparathyroidism

Hypoparathyroidism is usually caused by surgical damage to the parathyroid glands, either directly or indirectly by impairment of their blood supply during partial thyroidectomy. Total thyroidectomy or laryngectomy is often associated with removal or damage to the parathyroid glands and it is important to monitor plasma calcium concentrations. Post-thyroidectomy hypocalcaemia is not always due to damage to the glands and may be transient.

Parathyroidectomy, carried out to treat primary or tertiary hyperparathyroidism, also carries a risk of damage to the remaining parathyroid tissue. However, there are several causes of temporary hypocalcaemia.

If the hypercalcaemia has been severe and prolonged, the remaining parathyroid tissue may have been suppressed by negative feedback for so long that there may be true hypoparathyroidism evidenced by a rising plasma phosphate concentration, which usually recovers within a few days. Unless persistent, it should be treated if symptomatic.

In rare cases of primary hyperparathyroidism with overt bone disease, rapid entry of calcium into bone, when plasma PTH concentrations fall, may cause true, but temporary, postoperative hypocalcaemia.

Although early postoperative parathyroid insufficiency may recover, a low plasma calcium concentration persisting for more than a few weeks should usually be treated.

Autoimmune hypoparathyroidism is rare. It may occur as a *familial disorder*, presenting either during childhood or in adults or an *autoimmune disorder*, with antibodies against parathyroid tissue and sometimes other tissues. The MEDAC syndrome is associated with candida infections and other autoimmune disorders.

Congenital absence of the parathyroid glands is also rare, associated with impaired cellular immunity, a characteristic facial appearance and cardiac abnormalities known as the DiGeorge's syndrome.

Pseudohypoparathyroidism

This is a very rare inborn error associated with an impaired response of both kidneys and bone to PTH, i.e. end-organ resistance to circulating PTH. Thus plasma PTH concentration is raised with hypocalcaemia. Type 1 is a defect proximal to cyclic adenosine monophosphate (cAMP) tissue generation and thus urinary cAMP is low; type 2 pseudohypoparathyroidism is due to a defect distal to cAMP production, so urinary cAMP levels are normal. The associated phenotype shows short stature, obesity, mental retardation and short third and fourth metacarpals.

Pseudo-pseudohypoparathyroidism shows the same phenotype but normal plasma calcium concentration.

Box 6.2 shows some miscellaneous causes of hypocalcaemia that do not necessarily present with either hypophosphataemia or hyperphosphataemia.

Investigation of hypocalcaemia (Fig. 6.4)

As in the case of hypercalcaemia, the causes of hypocalcaemia fall into two main groups:

- reduced albumin corrected calcium concentration due to primary PTH deficiency and associated with hyperphosphataemia,
- reduced albumin corrected calcium concentration due to other causes and associated with appropriately high PTH concentrations and usually hypophosphataemia.

Determine first if the fall in plasma total calcium concentration (albumin corrected or adjusted calcium) is due to a low protein-bound fraction.

Patients with a low albumin concentration should not be given calcium and/or vitamin D unless there is clinical evidence of a low albumin corrected calcium concentration.

- Is the patient on drugs or chemicals that may cause hypocalcaemia (see Box 6.2)?
- Is the plasma phosphate concentration high? If the plasma urea and/or creatinine concentration is high, renal dysfunction is the likely cause (see Chapter 3).
- Is the plasma phosphate concentration low? If so, calcium deficiency with normal secretion of PTH in response to feedback is likely. At this point a plasma PTH assay may be useful. Is the plasma alkaline phosphatase activity high? This finding may suggest prolonged secondary hyperparathyroidism due to calcium deficiency.
- If indicated, do relevant bone X-rays show signs of rickets or osteomalacia? These may confirm prolonged calcium deficiency. Check plasma 25-hydroxyvitamin D levels; if the plasma levels are low, look for causes of malnutrition and malabsorption states.

In the rare hypocalcaemia of type 1 vitamin-D-dependent rickets there are low plasma $1,25-(OH)_2D_3$ concentrations, whereas type 2 vitamin-D-dependent rickets causes a vitamin D resistance and plasma $1,25-(OH)_2D_3$ concentrations are elevated.

Raised plasma phosphate in the face of hypocalcaemia and low plasma PTH concentration suggests hypoparathyroidism.

Is there a history of neck surgery which has led to hypoparathyroidism? Hypoparathyroidism may also be of autoimmune origin and associated with other autoimmune disorders. It needs to be distinguished from the even more rare 'pseudohypoparathyroidism' by measuring plasma PTH concentrations. Parathyroid hormone concentrations will be low in true hypoparathyroidism but high if there is the end-organ unresponsiveness of pseudohypoparathyroidism.

Check plasma magnesium, as severe hypomagnesaemia can cause hypocalcaemia by reducing the action of PTH.

A raised urinary calcium concentration may help diagnose the rare autosomal dominant hypercalciuric hypocalcaemia.

Treatment of hypocalcaemia

Asymptomatic hypocalcaemia

Apparent hypocalcaemia, due to low plasma albumin concentrations, should not be treated. Always look at the albumin corrected calcium value.

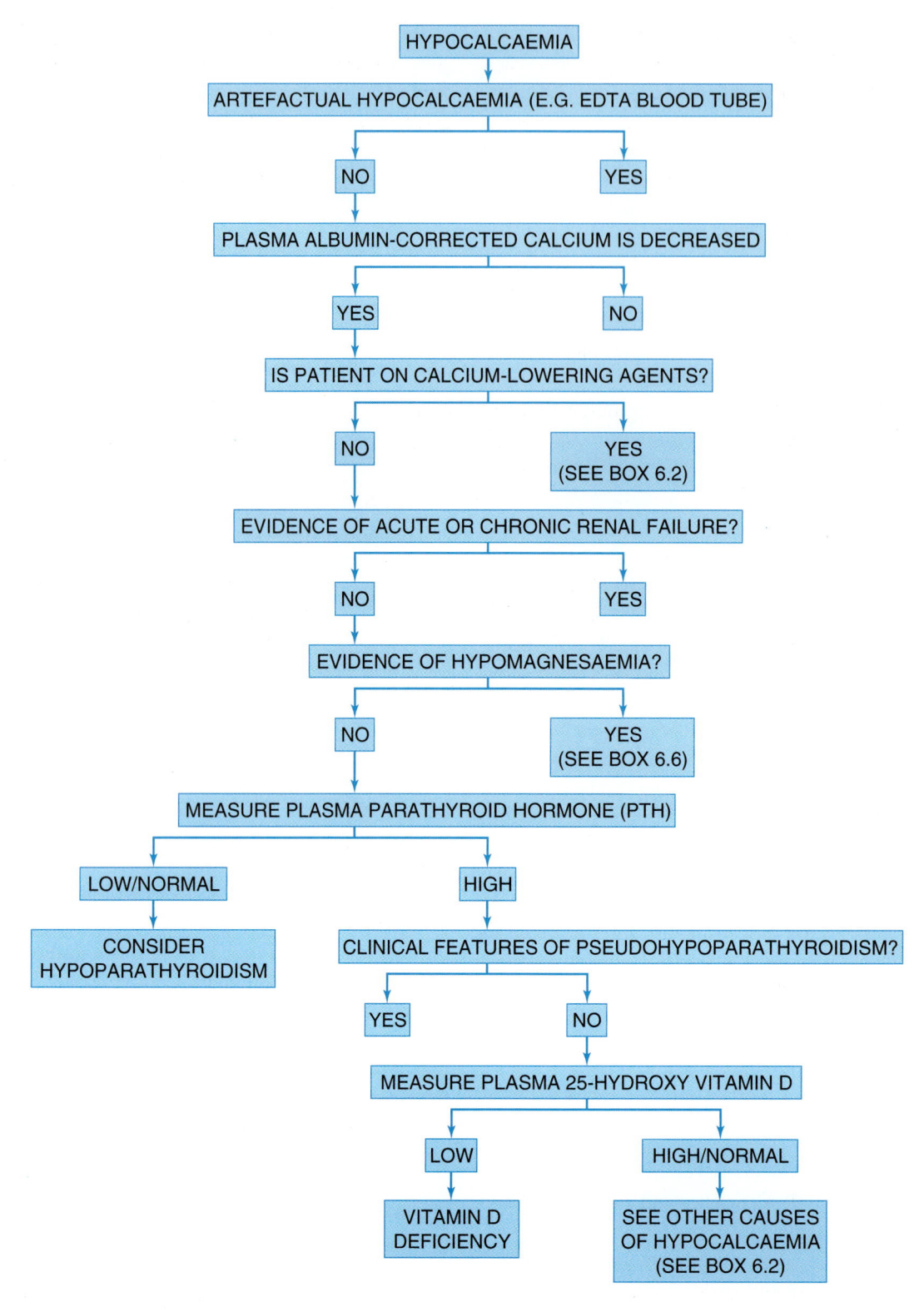

Fig. 6.4 Algorithm for the investigation of hypocalcaemia. (EDTA = ethylenediamine tetra-acetate.)

Asymptomatic true hypocalcaemia, or that causing only mild clinical symptoms, can usually be treated effectively with oral calcium supplements and vitamin D supplements. It is difficult to give enough oral calcium by itself to make a lasting and significant difference to plasma calcium concentrations. If a normal diet is being taken, vitamin D, by increasing the absorption of calcium from the intestine, is usually adequate without calcium supplements.

1,25-Dihydroxycholecalciferol and alfacalcidol (1-α-hydroxycholecalciferol) are most commonly used as they have short half-lives, particularly if there is hypoparathyroidism or a defect in vitamin D metabolism. It is important to monitor the plasma calcium closely to avoid inducing hypercalcaemia and hypercalciuria by ensuring a normal urinary excretion of calcium.

Due to the danger of ectopic calcification by precipitation of calcium phosphate, hypocalcaemia with hyperphosphataemia in renal disease should be treated cautiously. The plasma phosphate concentration should first be lowered by giving a phosphate-binding agent that binds phosphate in the intestinal lumen. 1,25-Dihydroxycholecalciferol and alfacalcidol, the active vitamin D metabolites, have been used to treat hypocalcaemia in renal disease.

Hypocalcaemia with life-threatening symptoms

If there are cardiac arrhythmias, seizures or severe tetany including laryngospasm shown to be due to hypocalcaemia, intravenous calcium, usually as 10 mL of 10 per cent calcium gluconate, should be given over about 5 minutes. Treatment can then begin as above, depending upon the aetiology of the hypocalcaemia.

Postoperative hypocalcaemia

Hypocalcaemia during the first week after a thyroidectomy or parathyroidectomy should only be treated if there is tetany, and usually with calcium replacement, which, unlike vitamin D supplements, has a rapid effect and a short half-life. Persistent hypocalcaemia may indicate that the parathyroid glands are permanently damaged and that long-standing, or even life-long, vitamin D supplementation is necessary. Parathyroid bone disease may result in 'hungry bones' and prolonged postoperative hypocalcaemia.

Hypercalciuria

Hypercalciuria in the absence of hypercalcaemia (hypercalciuria normocalcaemia) may predispose to the formation of renal calculi (see Chapter 3) and may occur in:

- some cases of osteoporosis in which calcium cannot be deposited in normal amounts because the bone matrix is reduced,
- acidosis, in which the release of free ionized calcium from bone is increased.

Hypercalciuria can broadly be divided into absorptive hypercalciuria, type I (hyperabsorption of calcium), type II (diet-responsive hypercalciuria) and type III (renal phosphate leak resulting in decreased calcium resorption) and renal hypercalciuria (decreased renal calcium resorption). These can be distinguished by tests of oral calcium absorption.

Hypercalciuria can, of course, also occur in the face of hypercalcaemia, such as resorptive hypercalciuria associated with primary hyperparathyroidism.

Estimation of urinary CAE is rarely diagnostic in the differential diagnosis of hypercalcaemia except familial hypocalciuric hypercalcaemia. If glomerular function is normal, all other causes of hypercalcaemia increase the calcium load on the glomeruli and evoke hypercalciuria. If renal glomerular function is impaired, calcium excretion is low even if there is hypercalcaemia.

Disorders of bone not usually affecting the plasma calcium concentration

Some disorders of bone rarely alter plasma calcium concentrations but are important in the differential diagnosis of changes in mineral metabolism.

Osteoporosis

Osteoporosis is not a primary disorder of calcium metabolism. The reduction of bone mass is due to thinning of the protein on which the calcium is usually deposited. A slight increase in urinary calcium loss is secondary to this. Disorders associated with an increased incidence include the following.

- Low plasma oestrogen concentrations, such as after the female menopause (the most common cause) and prolonged amenorrhoea; also low testosterone concentrations in males.
- Elderly subjects in whom there may also be mild osteomalacia because of impaired renal production of 1,25-$(OH)_2D_3$.
- Other endocrine disorders and other miscellaneous causes:
  - hypercortisolism, hyperthyroidism, long-term glucocorticoid use,
  - drugs such as heparin, anticonvulsants such as phenytoin, carbamazepine,
  - prolonged immobilization,
  - smoking, alcohol abuse,
  - calcium deficiency,
  - gastrointestinal causes, including malabsorption, anorexia nervosa.

In osteoporosis plasma calcium and phosphate concentrations do not fall and, because there is no increase in osteoblastic activity, the plasma total alkaline phosphatase activity does not rise. These findings are invaluable in distinguishing between osteomalacia and osteoporosis.

Concentrations of new bone markers, such as bone-specific alkaline phosphatase (bone formation), plasma osteocalcin (bone formation), type 1 procollagen peptides (bone formation), urinary deoxypyridinoline and cross-linked N-telopeptide and C-telopeptide of type 1 collagen (bone resorption), urinary hydroxyproline (bone resorption) and bone-resistant or tartrate-resistant acid phosphatase (bone resorption) are raised in osteoporosis and may be useful markers of the disease process. However, these bone markers do not give information about exact bone anatomy, for which imaging studies are necessary. Sometimes X-rays are useful, especially if fractures are suspected. Bone mineral density (BMD) is often used and reported as a T-score that compares the patient's BMD with that of a healthy control. Normal BMD is within -1 standard deviations (SD) from this, whereas osteopenia is defined as between -1 and -2.5 SD and osteoporosis has a T-score of less than -2.5 SD.

Treatment consists of adequate calcium and vitamin D intake. The bisphosphonates increase BMD and inhibit bone resorption, probably by inhibiting osteoclast activity. In women, hormone replacement therapy is also used if indicated, but this may have side-effects.

Paget's disease of bone

Paget's disease is more common in the elderly, possibly being present in about 5 per cent of over-60 year olds. There is increased bone turnover and remodelling due to increased osteoclastic and osteoblastic function. It may be asymptomatic or may present with bone pain, pathological fractures, deafness (due to bone overgrowth) and high-output cardiac failure due to increased vascularity within the bone. Enlargement of bones such as the skull (osteoporosis circumscripta), femur and tibia (sabre tibia) can occur.

Diagnosis may necessitate X-rays and/or bone scanning. Plasma calcium and phosphate concentrations are rarely affected unless the patient is immobilized, in which case the plasma calcium concentrations may rise. Plasma alkaline phosphatase activity is typically very high. Less than 1 per cent of patients may develop osteosarcomas and this complication may be associated with rapidly rising plasma alkaline phosphatase activity. Bisphosphonates are often used to treat Paget's disease; although calcitonin has been tried, it is probably less effective.

Rickets or osteomalacia caused by renal tubular disorders of phosphate reabsorption

In a group of inborn errors of renal tubular function, less phosphate than normal is reabsorbed from the glomerular filtrate. The consequent rickets or osteomalacia, unlike the usual form, responds poorly to vitamin D therapy. The syndrome has therefore been called 'resistant rickets'. Familial hypophosphataemia is an X-linked dominant trait; the syndrome may also be part of a more generalized reabsorption defect in the Fanconi's syndrome (see Chapter 3).

In these disorders, failure to calcify bone is probably due to phosphate deficiency, although impaired vitamin D metabolism may also be present. Plasma phosphate concentrations are usually very low and fail to rise when vitamin D is given; there is phosphaturia inappropriate to the plasma concentration. The high plasma alkaline phosphatase activity reflects increased osteoblastic activity. The usually normal plasma calcium concentrations differ from the findings in the 'classical' syndrome. As the free ionized calcium concentration is normal, the parathyroid glands are not over-stimulated and therefore evidence in the bone of high PTH concentrations is rare. The conditions respond to large doses of oral phosphate and to a small dose of the active metabolite of vitamin D.

PHOSPHATE METABOLISM

Phosphate is a divalent anion approximately 80 per cent of which is found in the bony skeleton and 20 per cent is distributed in the soft tissues and muscle. Phosphate is the major intracellular anion and shifts between the intracellular and extracellular compartments. Such transcellular movement can result from the ingestion of carbohydrate or lipid as well as from acid–base alterations, for example acidosis can result in shifts of phosphate out of cells into the plasma.

The daily phosphate intake is about 30 mmol, with approximately 80 per cent being absorbed in the jejunum. Protein-rich food is a major source of phosphate intake, as are cereals and nuts. The output is largely renal, with more than 90 per cent being excreted by this route. Most of the phosphate filtered at the glomeruli is reabsorbed by the proximal tubules. Gastrointestinal loss of phosphate accounts for only 10 per cent of the body's phosphate excretion.

Urinary phosphate excretion falls as the plasma phosphate, and therefore glomerular filtrate, concentrations decrease in response to reduced dietary phosphate intake.

The measurement of urinary phosphate concentration may occasionally be useful to distinguish hypophosphataemia due to true depletion (low urinary phosphate) and the increased urinary phosphate excretion found in renal tubular disorders, such as X-linked hypophosphataemic rickets.

The urinary phosphate excretion threshold can be derived from nomograms and a low value implies renal phosphate loss. Another way to assess renal phosphate loss is to calculate the fractional phosphate excretion (FEPi%):

$$\text{FEPi\%} = \frac{\text{urinary[phosphate]} \times \text{plasma[creatinine]}}{\text{plasma[phosphate]} \times \text{urinary[creatinine]}} \quad (6.4)$$

An FEPi% of more than 10 per cent implies a renal phosphate loss.

> **Box 6.3 Some causes of hyperphosphataemia**
>
> Artefact due to in-vitro haemolysis or old blood sample
> Inappropriately high phosphate intake, usually intravenously
> Increased tissue breakdown
> Tumour lysis syndrome
> Malignant hyperpyrexia
> Crush injuries
> Acute or chronic renal failure
> Acidaemia (metabolic or respiratory acidosis)
> Diabetic ketoacidosis
> Hypoparathyroidism
> Acromegaly
> Excess vitamin D intake

THE FUNCTION OF PHOSPHATE IN VIVO

Phosphate is an important intracellular buffer as well as being essential for buffering hydrogen ions in urine. In addition, it has a structural role as a component of phospholipids, nucleoproteins and nucleic acids.

Phosphate plays a central role in cellular metabolic pathways, including glycolysis and oxidative phosphorylation. A by-product of glycolysis is 2,3-diphosphoglycerate (2,3-DPG). This is a regulator of haemoglobin oxygen dissociation. Nucleotides such as adenosine triphosphate consist of phosphate. Other actions include excitation-stimulus response coupling and nervous system conduction. Phosphate also has a role in the optimal function of leucocytes, for example chemotaxis and phagocytosis, and for platelets in clot retraction.

ABNORMALITIES OF PLASMA PHOSPHATE CONCENTRATION

Hyperphosphataemia

The causes of hyperphosphataemia are listed in Box 6.3. The majority of the clinical effects are the result of hypocalcaemia, particularly if the plasma phosphate concentration is more than 3.0 mmol/L. The reason for this is that calcium/phosphate precipitation into the tissues can ensue when the phosphate and calcium plasma concentrations exceed their solubility product. Thus metastatic calcification is a clinical consequence of hyperphosphataemia.

The treatment for hyperphosphataemia is with oral phosphate-binding agents, for example magnesium hydroxide or calcium carbonate. These agents have been used in the management of patients with chronic renal failure (see Chapter 3). There has been recent controversy about the toxicity of aluminium-containing phosphate-binding agents in view of possible side-effects, including nausea, vomiting, constipation and, more seriously, microcytic anaemia and encephalopathy. In the face of acute or chronic renal failure and persistently severe hyperphosphataemia, haemodialysis or peritoneal dialysis may be indicated.

Hypophosphataemia

Hypophosphataemia associated with disturbances of calcium metabolism is usually due to high circulating PTH concentrations. In such conditions, and in renal tubular disorders of phosphate reabsorption, phosphate is lost from the body in urine. Hypophosphataemia may also be caused by severe and prolonged dietary deficiency; urinary phosphate excretion is then usually significantly reduced.

Phosphate, like potassium, enters cells from the ECF if the rate of glucose metabolism is increased. This may be associated with glucose infusion during, for example, the treatment of diabetic coma with insulin. The redistribution of phosphate is a common cause of hypophosphataemia in patients receiving parenteral nutrition with insulin and glucose. Long-term parenteral feeding without phosphate supplementation may cause true phosphate depletion, as may

> **Box 6.4 Some causes of hypophosphataemia**
>
> Cellular redistribution
>   Intravenous glucose
>   Alkalaemia (metabolic or respiratory alkalosis)
>   Administration of insulin
>   Re-feeding syndrome
> Poor intake, e.g. total parenteral nutrition
> Malabsorption states
> Chronic alcoholism
> Post-trauma or myocardial infarction or operation
> Renal tubular loss
>   Isolated phosphate disorder
>   Hypophosphataemic osteomalacia
>   X-linked hypophosphataemia
>   Oncogenic hypophosphataemia
>   Paracetamol poisoning
>   As part of the Fanconi syndrome
> Miscellaneous
>   Liver disease
>   Septicaemia
>   Hyperparathyroidism or parathyroid hormone-related peptide release

feeding after prolonged starvation (re-feeding syndrome; Box 6.4).

Severe hypophosphataemia, often quoted as a plasma inorganic phosphate concentration less than 0.30 mmol/L, can result in a plethora of clinical features. Rhabdomyolysis has been described, as has impaired skeletal muscle function, including weakness and myopathy. Hypophosphataemia is also reported to impair diaphragmatic contractility, which may help to explain the difficulty in weaning patients off mechanical ventilators. Cardiomyopathy is another possible complication of severe hypophosphataemia.

Hypophosphataemia can evoke seizures, perturbed mental state and paraesthesiae as well as renal tubular impairment. If prolonged, it can lead to osteomalacia. The haematological effects caused by severe hypophosphataemia include thrombocytopenia, impaired clotting processes and also reduced leucocyte function. Haemolysis can also occur, as can erythrocyte 2,3-DPG depletion, resulting in a shift in the haemoglobin/oxygen dissociation curve to the left, i.e. haemoglobin has a greater affinity for oxygen.

Treatment of hypophosphataemia is usually not necessary unless the plasma phosphate concentration is less than 0.30 mmol/L or the patient is symptomatic. Sometimes oral phosphate salts have been used, although diarrhoea can be a problem. If intravenous phosphate replacement is indicated, the following regimen can be used, namely 9 mmol of monobasic potassium phosphate in half-normal saline by continuous intravenous infusion over 12 hours. This should not be given to patients with hypercalcaemia, because of the risk of metastatic calcification, or to patients with hyperkalaemia.

MAGNESIUM METABOLISM

PLASMA MAGNESIUM AND ITS CONTROL

Magnesium is predominately an intracellular divalent cation and is important for optimal cell function. It is an essential cofactor to many enzymes as well as being important for membrane function. Furthermore, it can act as an antagonist to calcium in cellular responses and has a structural role within the cell.

The body contains about 1 mol (approximately 25 g) of magnesium, mostly in the bone and muscle. The recommended daily allowance of magnesium for adults is about 4.5 mg/kg; rich dietary sources include cereal, nuts and vegetables.

Magnesium is largely absorbed in the upper small intestine but the large intestine may also be important; unlike calcium, its absorption is not vitamin D dependent. As much as 70 per cent of dietary-intake magnesium is not absorbed but eliminated in the faeces. The major excretory route is via the kidneys and about 65 per cent of glomerular-filtered magnesium is reabsorbed in the loop of Henle. The exact mechanisms of magnesium homeostatic control are unclear, although PTH, insulin and calcitonin are important. Parathyroid hormone can increase magnesium reabsorption, although hypercalcaemia can increase the renal excretion of magnesium. About 35 per cent of plasma magnesium is protein bound, and the plasma concentration is normally 0.7–1.2 mmol/L.

CLINICAL EFFECTS OF ABNORMAL PLASMA MAGNESIUM CONCENTRATIONS

Hypermagnesaemia

Some causes of hypermagnesaemia are shown in Box 6.5.

> **Box 6.5 Some causes of hypermagnesaemia**
>
> *Increased intake of magnesium*
> Antacids, milk-alkali syndrome
> Purgatives
> Parenteral nutrition
>
> *Impaired renal excretion of magnesium*
> Acute and chronic renal failure
> Familial hypocalciuric hypercalcaemia
> Lithium treatment
>
> *Miscellaneous causes*
> Hypothyroidism
> Adrenal insufficiency

> **Box 6.6 Some causes of hypomagnesaemia**
>
> *Redistribution of magnesium between cells*
> Excess of catecholamines
> Re-feeding syndrome
> Hungry bone syndrome
>
> *Reduced intake of magnesium*
> Parenteral nutrition
> Starvation/malnutrition
>
> *Poor magnesium absorption*
> Intestinal resection
> Gastrointestinal fistulae
> Malabsorption states
>
> *Increased renal loss of magnesium*
> Post-renal transplantation
> Dialysis
> Bartter's and Gitelman's syndromes
>
> *Drugs*
> Diuretics
> Cytotoxics
> Aminoglycosides
> Beta-2-adrenergic agonists
> Cyclosporin and tacrolimus
> Pamidronate, pentamidine, amphotericin B, foscarnet
>
> *Miscellaneous causes*
> Alcoholism
> Hypercalcaemia
> Hyperthyroidism
> Hyperaldosteronism
> Diabetes mellitus

Clinical consequences of hypermagnesaemia

Hypermagnesaemia can result in cardiac arrhythmias, such as heart block and inhibition of AV conduction leading to cardiac arrest, seizures, altered nerve conduction, reduced tendon reflexes, paralytic ileus, nausea, respiratory depression and hypotension. Clinical features do not usually become manifest until the plasma magnesium concentration exceeds 2 mmol/L.

Clinical management of severe hypermagnesaemia

If there is severe hypermagnesaemia, 10 mL of 10 per cent calcium gluconate given slowly intravenously may relieve symptoms. Analogous to the treatment of hyperkalaemia, insulin and glucose infusion can be used in severe hypermagnesaemia (see Chapter 5). Failing this, and if there is impaired renal function, dialysis may be indicated (see Chapter 3).

Hypomagnesaemia

Some causes of hypomagnesaemia are shown in Box 6.6. The symptoms of hypomagnesaemia are very similar to those of hypocalcaemia. If the plasma calcium concentrations (allowing for that of albumin) and blood pH are normal in a patient with tetany, the plasma magnesium concentration should be assayed.

Hypomagnesaemia can result in cardiac arrhythmias, including torsade de pointes, and digoxin sensitivity. In addition, abdominal discomfort and anorexia have been described, as well as neuromuscular sequelae including tremor, paraesthesiae, vertigo, tetany, seizures, irritability, confusion, weakness and ataxia. Severe hypomagnesaemia can lead to hypocalcaemia due to decreased PTH release and activity.

Long-term magnesium deficiency may be a risk factor for coronary artery disease, perhaps increasing atherosclerosis and platelet aggregation. There are data suggesting that reduced magnesium intake is associated with hypertension and insulin resistance.

Treatment of hypomagnesaemia

Sometimes the symptoms and signs of magnesium deficiency occur in the face of borderline magnesium plasma concentrations as plasma levels poorly reflect intracellular magnesium stores. In such circumstances the intravenous magnesium-loading test may be useful: 30 mmol of magnesium (usually as sulphate) is infused intravenously in 500 mL 5 per cent dextrose and urine is collected over 24 hours for magnesium determination. Magnesium depletion is unlikely if more than 24 mmol of magnesium is excreted in 24 hours.

Severe hypomagnesaemia, less than 0.5 mmol/L or if symptomatic, can be corrected by oral magnesium salts but these may be poorly absorbed and lead to gastrointestinal upset. A possible regimen would be oral magnesium gluconate 12 mmol/day to a maximum of 48 mmol/L, if required, in three or four divided doses. Intravenous replacement is often given as magnesium sulphate. Generally, 0.5 mmol/kg per day can be given by intravenous infusion. Close monitoring of plasma magnesium is necessary.

The treatment of hypomagnesaemia may facilitate the treatment of refractory hypokalaemia and hypocalcaemia.

CONCLUSIONS

- Calcium, phosphate and magnesium metabolism are closely related and abnormalities are clinically relatively common.
- Plasma calcium levels are controlled by PTH (raises plasma calcium), vitamin D activity and optimal renal and intestinal function.
- Hypercalcaemia can result in various symptoms: 'bones, stones, moans and groans'. The causes include malignant disease, primary or tertiary hyperparathyroidism, certain drugs such as thiazides, granulomatous disease such as sarcoidosis, milk-alkali syndrome, thyrotoxicosis, Addison's disease, hypocalciuric hypercalcaemia and acromegaly.
- Hypocalcaemia can present with paraesthesiae, tetany, osteomalacia and seizures. The causes may be due to poor diet, including vitamin D deficiency, chronic renal failure, malabsorption, certain drugs, such as loop diuretics, and hypoparathyroidism.

7 THE HYPOTHALAMUS AND PITUITARY GLAND

General principles of endocrine diagnosis	115	Disorders of anterior pituitary hormone secretion	118
Hypothalamus and pituitary gland	116	Disorders of the posterior pituitary	123

GENERAL PRINCIPLES OF ENDOCRINE DIAGNOSIS

A hormone can be defined as a substance secreted by an endocrine gland that is transported in the blood, thereby regulating the function of another tissue(s). Certain hormones, such as growth hormone (GH, secreted from the anterior pituitary gland), thyroxine (T_4, from the thyroid gland) and insulin (from the pancreatic islet cells), influence tissue metabolism directly. Conversely, trophic hormones from the pituitary gland stimulate target endocrine glands to synthesize and secrete further hormones, which in turn partly control trophic hormone release, usually by negative feedback inhibition. For example, hypercalcaemia inhibits the secretion of parathyroid hormone (PTH) and elevation of plasma T_4 concentration inhibits the secretion of thyroid-stimulating hormone (TSH).

Endocrine glands may secrete excessive or deficient amounts of hormone. Abnormalities of target glands may be primary, or secondary to dysfunction of the controlling mechanism, usually located in the hypothalamus or anterior pituitary gland.

Hormone secretion may vary predictably over a 24-hour (circadian) or longer period. It may be episodic or may respond predictably to physiological stimuli such as stress. Simultaneous measurement of both the trophic hormones and their controlling factors, whether hormones or metabolic products, may be more informative than the measurement of either alone. An important endocrine principle is that an apparently 'normal' hormone result should be interpreted in the context of the associated hormone axis, for example a plasma PTH concentration within the reference range may be abnormal if the plasma calcium concentration is elevated.

It is also important to know about the assay's performance, as sometimes heterophilic interfering antibodies may cross-react with various hormones, as can certain immunoglobulins, for example macroprolactin (see later).

If the results of preliminary tests are definitely abnormal, this may be primary, or secondary to a disorder of one of the controlling mechanisms. Should the results be equivocal when considered together with the clinical findings, so-called 'dynamic' tests should be carried out. In such tests the response of the gland or the feedback mechanism is assessed after stimulation or suppression by the administration of exogenous hormone.

Suppression tests are used mainly for the differential diagnosis of excessive hormone secretion. The substance (or an analogue) that normally suppresses secretion by negative feedback is administered and the response is measured. Failure to suppress implies that secretion is not under normal feedback control (autonomous secretion).

Stimulation tests are used mainly for the differential diagnosis of deficient hormone secretion. The trophic hormone that normally stimulates secretion is administered and the response is measured. A normal response excludes an abnormality of the target gland, whereas failure to respond confirms it.

Disorders of the pituitary gland and hypothalamus are discussed in this chapter. Diseases of the target endocrine organs, the adrenal cortex, gonads and thyroid gland are considered in Chapters 8, 9 and 11 respectively. The parathyroid glands and endocrine pancreas are discussed in Chapters 6 and 12.

HYPOTHALAMUS AND PITUITARY GLAND

The anterior and posterior lobes of the pituitary gland are developmentally and functionally distinct; both depend on hormones synthesized in the hypothalamus for normal function. The hypothalamus also has extensive neural connections with the rest of the brain, and stress and some psychological disorders affect the secretion of pituitary hormones and of the hormones from other endocrine glands.

Control of posterior pituitary hormones

Two structurally similar peptide hormones, antidiuretic hormone (ADH) and oxytocin, are synthesized in the hypothalamus and transported down the nerve fibres of the pituitary stalk attached to specific carrier proteins – neurophysins. The hormones are stored in the posterior pituitary gland and are released independently of each other into the bloodstream under hypothalamic control together with neurophysin. Neurophysin has no apparent biological function and is rapidly cleared from plasma.

Antidiuretic hormone (arginine vasopressin) is mainly synthesized in the supraoptic nuclei of the hypothalamus and enhances water reabsorption from the collecting ducts in the kidneys (see Chapters 2 and 3).

Oxytocin is synthesized in the paraventricular nuclei of the hypothalamus. It controls the ejection of milk from the lactating breast and may have a role in initiating uterine contractions, although normal labour can proceed in its absence. It may be used therapeutically to induce labour.

Anterior pituitary hormones

There is no direct neural connection between the hypothalamus and the anterior pituitary gland. The hypothalamus synthesizes small molecules (regulating hormones or factors) that are carried to the cells of the anterior pituitary lobe by the hypothalamic portal system. This network of capillary loops in the median eminence forms veins, which, after passing down the pituitary stalk, divide into a second capillary network in the anterior pituitary gland, from where hypothalamic hormones stimulate or inhibit pituitary hormone secretion into the systemic circulation.

The cells of the anterior pituitary lobe can be classified simply by their staining reactions as acidophils, basophils or chromophobes. More sophisticated immunological techniques can identify specific hormone-secreting cells.

Acidophils are of two cell types:

- lactotrophs, which secrete prolactin,
- somatotrophs, which secrete GH (somatotrophin).

These hormones, which are simple polypeptides with similar amino acid sequences, mainly affect peripheral tissues directly. Stimulation and inhibition of secretion via the hypothalamus is influenced by neural stimuli.

Basophils secrete hormones that affect other endocrine glands. The hypothalamic control is mainly stimulatory. There are three cell types.

- Corticotrophs synthesize a large polypeptide (pro-opiomelanocortin), which is a precursor of both adrenocorticotrophic hormone (ACTH; corticotrophin) and β-lipotrophin (Fig. 7.1). Secretion of these hormones occurs in parallel.

    Adrenocorticotrophic hormone stimulates the synthesis and secretion of steroids, other than aldosterone, from the adrenal cortex and maintains adrenal cortical growth. Part of the molecule has melanocyte-stimulating activity, and high circulating concentrations of ACTH are often associated with pigmentation.

    Beta-lipotrophin is inactive until rapidly converted to endorphins. These are neurotransmitters which, because they have opiate-like effects, help control pain.
- Gonadotrophs secrete the gonadotrophins, follicle-stimulating hormone (FSH) and luteinizing hormone (LH), which act on the gonads.
- Thyrotrophs secrete TSH (thyrotrophin), which acts on the thyroid gland.

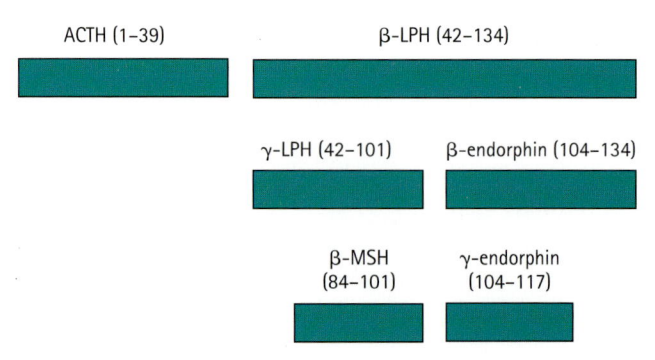

Fig. 7.1 The products of pro-opiomelanocortin (POMC), adrenocorticotrophic hormone (ACTH), β-lipotrophin (LPH), melanocyte-stimulating hormone (MSH) and endorphin. The numbers indicate the amino acid sequence in POMC.

These hormones are structurally similar glycoproteins consisting of two subunits, alpha and beta. The α-subunit is common to all three hormones; the β-subunit is important for receptor recognition and therefore in specific biological activity.

Chromophobes, once thought to be inactive, do contain secretory granules. Chromophobe adenomas often secrete hormones, particularly prolactin.

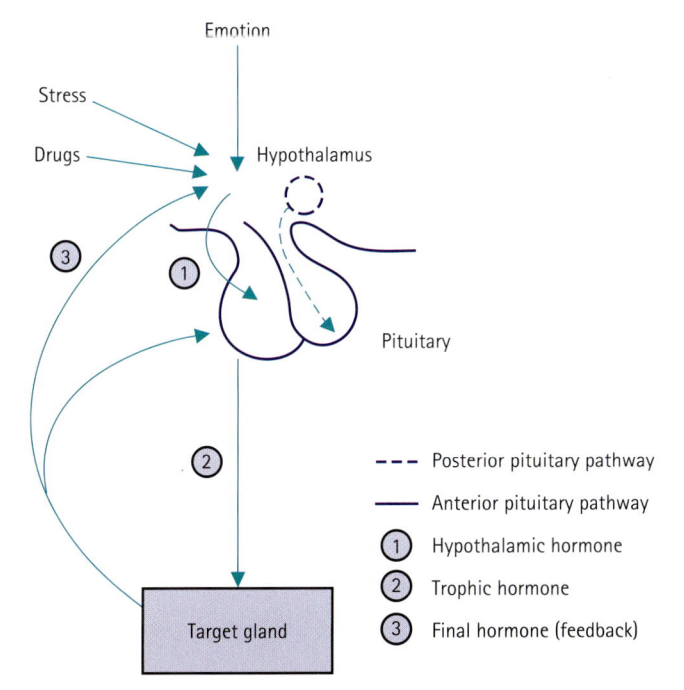

Control of anterior pituitary hormone secretion

Neural and feedback controls are the two most important physiological factors influencing the secretion of the anterior pituitary hormones (Fig. 7.2).

Extrahypothalamic neural stimuli modify, and at times override, other control mechanisms. Physical or emotional stress and mental illness may give similar findings to, and even precipitate, endocrine disease. The stress caused by insulin-induced hypoglycaemia is used to test anterior pituitary function. Stress may also stimulate the secretion of ADH from the posterior pituitary.

Feedback control is mediated by the concentrations of circulating target-cell hormones; a rising concentration usually suppresses trophic hormone secretion. This negative feedback may directly suppress hypothalamic hormone secretion or may modify its effect on pituitary cells (long feedback loop). The secretion of hypothalamic hormones may also be suppressed by rising concentrations of pituitary hormone in a short feedback loop.

Inherent rhythms: hypothalamic, and consequently pituitary, hormones are released intermittently, either in pulses or in a regular circadian rhythm. Disturbances of such rhythms may be of diagnostic value. This subject is considered further in the relevant sections.

Drugs may also stimulate or block the action of neurotransmitters, such as catecholamines, acetylcholine and serotonin, and influence the secretion of hypothalamic, and consequently pituitary, hormones. The following are some examples.

- Certain neuroleptic drugs, such as chlorpromazine and haloperidol, interfere with the action of dopamine. This results in reduced GH secretion (reduced effect of releasing factor) and increased prolactin secretion (reduced inhibition).
- Bromocriptine, which has a dopamine-like action, and L-dopa, which is converted to dopamine, have the opposite effect in normal subjects. Bromocriptine causes a paradoxical suppression of excessive GH secretion in acromegalics; the reason for this anomalous response is unknown.

All these effects have been used in both the diagnosis and treatment of hypothalamic–pituitary disorders; they are discussed in later sections.

Evaluation of anterior pituitary function

The interpretation of the results of basal pituitary hormone assays is often difficult. Low plasma concentrations are not necessarily abnormal, and plasma concentrations within the reference range do not exclude pituitary disease. The diagnosis of suspected hypopituitarism is best excluded by the direct measurement of pituitary hormones after stimulation or by demonstrating target-gland hyposecretion after the administration of the relevant trophic hormone. However, prolonged hypopituitarism may result in secondary failure of the target gland with diminished response to stimulation.

Laboratory tests only establish the presence or absence of hypopituitarism and the cause must be sought by other clinical means such as radiological imaging.

Hypothalamus or pituitary dysfunction?

It may be difficult to distinguish between hypothalamic and pituitary causes of pituitary hormone deficiency or, more correctly, between deficient releasing factor and a primary deficiency of pituitary hormone secretion. Isolated hormone deficiencies are more likely to be of hypothalamic

Fig. 7.2 Control of pituitary hormone secretion.

than of pituitary origin. The coexistence of diabetes insipidus suggests a hypothalamic disorder, but symptoms of water loss may not occur at first because of ACTH, and therefore cortisol, deficiency causing water retention.

Some biochemical investigations evaluate both hypothalamic and pituitary function and some only the latter, although it may be possible to distinguish the anatomical site of the lesion. For example, the TSH response to thyrotrophin-releasing hormone (TRH) may differ in hypothalamic and pituitary causes of secondary hypothyroidism (see Chapter 11). In cases of hypogonadism due to gonadotrophin deficiency, differentiation on the basis of the response to gonadotrophin-releasing hormone (GnRH) is less clear cut (see Chapter 9).

DISORDERS OF ANTERIOR PITUITARY HORMONE SECRETION

The main clinical syndromes associated with excessive or deficient anterior pituitary hormone secretion are shown in Table 7.1. Excessive secretion usually involves a single hormone, but deficiencies are often multiple. However, many pituitary tumours are non-secretory and may present clinically with eye signs or headaches.

Growth hormone

Growth hormone secretion from the anterior pituitary gland is mainly controlled by hypothalamic GH-releasing hormone (GHRH). After synthesis by the hypothalamus, this is transported via the hypothalamic portal system to the somatotrophs of the anterior pituitary. Secretion of GHRH, and therefore of GH, is pulsatile, occurring about seven or eight times a day, usually associated with:

- exercise,
- onset of deep sleep,
- in response to the falling plasma glucose concentration about an hour after meals.

At other times, plasma concentrations are usually very low or undetectable, especially in children.

Growth hormone release is inhibited in a negative feedback pathway by another hypothalamic hormone, somatostatin (GH-release inhibiting hormone). Somatostatin is found not only in the hypothalamus and elsewhere in the brain, but also in the gastrointestinal tract and pancreatic islet cells, where it inhibits the secretion of many gastrointestinal hormones. Insulin-like growth factor 1 (IGF-1) acts by feedback to inhibit GHRH action.

Growth hormone secretion may be stimulated by:

- stress, one cause of which is hypoglycaemia,
- glucagon,
- some amino acids, for example arginine,
- drugs such as L-dopa and clonidine.

All these stimuli have been used to assess GH secretory capacity, which may also be impaired in obese patients, in hypothyroidism and hypogonadism, in some cases of Cushing's syndrome and in patients receiving large doses of steroids.

Growth hormone secretion is inhibited by hyperglycaemia in the normal subject.

Table 7.1 Disorders associated with primary abnormalities of anterior pituitary hormone secretion

Hormone	Excess	Deficiency
Growth hormone	Acromegaly or Gigantism	Short stature
Prolactin	Amenorrhoea Infertility Galactorrhoea	Lactation failure
Adrenocorticotrophic hormone (corticotrophin)	Cushing's disease	Secondary adrenal hypofunction
Thyroid-stimulating hormone	Hyperthyroidism (very rare)	Secondary hypothyroidism
Luteinizing hormone/ follicle-stimulating hormone	Precocious puberty	Secondary hypogonadism Infertility

Actions of growth hormone

The main function of GH is to promote growth. Its action is primarily mediated by IGFs, polypeptides that are synthesized in many tissues, where they act locally. Plasma concentrations of one of these, IGF-1 (also known as somatomedin C), correlate with GH secretion.

Carbohydrate metabolism is affected by GH: GH antagonizes the insulin-mediated cell uptake of glucose, and excess secretion may produce glucose intolerance.

Fat metabolism is stimulated by GH: lipolysis is stimulated, with a consequent increase in the concentration of circulating free fatty acids. Free fatty acid antagonizes insulin release and action.

Growth hormone (the action of which is mediated by IGF-1) enhances protein synthesis in conjunction with insulin, to stimulate amino acid uptake by cells.

The production of IGF-1 is also influenced by other factors, the most important of which is nutritional status. In malnutrition, plasma concentrations are low, whereas GH concentrations are elevated, suggesting that plasma IGF-1 may influence GH secretion by negative feedback. Other factors, such as adequate nutrition and T_4, are also needed for normal growth. The growth spurt during puberty may be enhanced by androgens.

Growth hormone excess: gigantism and acromegaly

Growth hormone excess causes gigantism during childhood and acromegaly in adults.

Most patients with GH excess have acidophil adenomas of the anterior pituitary gland, which may be secondary to excessive hypothalamic stimulation. Rarely, malignant tumours may release GH or GHRH.

Acromegaly is sometimes one of the manifestations of multiple endocrine neoplasia (MEN).

The clinical manifestations of GH excess depend on whether the condition develops before or after fusion of the bony epiphyses. Gigantism is caused by excess GH secretion in childhood before fusion of the epiphyseal plates, which may be delayed by accompanying hypogonadism. Heights of up to about 2 metres may be reached. Acromegalic features may develop after bony fusion, but these patients may die in early adult life from infection or cardiac failure or as a consequence of progressive pituitary tumour growth.

The features of acromegaly may include the following.

- An increase in the bulk of bone and soft tissues with enlargement of, for example, the hands, tongue, jaw and heart. Changes in facial appearance are often marked, due to the increasing size of the jaw and sinuses; the gradual coarsening of the features may pass unnoticed for many years. Thyroid gland enlargement may be clinically detectable, but the patient is usually euthyroid.
- Excessive hair growth, hyperhidrosis and sebaceous gland secretion.
- Menstrual disturbances, which are common in females.
- Impaired glucose tolerance is present in about 25 per cent of cases, about half of whom develop symptomatic diabetes mellitus. In most cases the pancreas can secrete enough insulin to overcome the antagonistic effect of GH.
- Predisposition to multiple pre-malignant colon polyposis and hypertension.
- Hyperphosphataemia, hypercalcaemia and hypertriglyceridaemia may also be present.

Many of these features are due to the action of IGF-1, which acts as a general growth factor.

A different group of symptoms may occur due to the encroachment of a pituitary tumour on surrounding structures.

- Compression of the optic chiasma may cause visual field defects such as bitemporal hemianopsia.
- If destruction of the gland progresses, other anterior pituitary hormones such as ACTH, LH, FSH and TSH may become deficient (see above). Plasma prolactin concentrations may, however, be raised.

Diagnosis

The diagnosis of GH excess is suggested by the clinical presentation, biochemical tests and radiological findings of the pituitary. Magnetic resonance imaging (MRI) is more sensitive than computerized tomography (CT) scanning. Plasma GH concentrations are usually higher than normal and may reach several hundred milli-units per litre (mU/L), but, because of the wide reference range, the results from ambulant patients may fail to distinguish those with only moderately raised plasma concentrations from normal subjects. Random GH measurements are often not diagnostic due to episodic secretion and a short half-life.

The diagnosis is confirmed by demonstrating a raised plasma GH concentration that is not suppressed by a rise in plasma glucose concentration. In normal subjects, plasma GH concentrations fall to very low levels – to below 1 mU/L after a 75 g oral glucose load. In acromegaly, the secretion of GH is autonomous and this fall may not occur or be only slight, or there may even be a paradoxical rise.

Glucose suppression test for suspected acromegaly

Procedure
After an overnight fast, insert an indwelling intravenous cannula. After at least 30 minutes, take basal samples for plasma glucose and GH estimation. The patient should drink 75 g of glucose dissolved in about 300 mL of water, or an equivalent glucose load. Take samples for glucose and GH assays at 30, 60, 90 and 120 minutes after the glucose load has been taken.

Interpretation
In normal subjects, plasma GH concentrations fall to undetectable levels. Although failure to suppress suggests acromegaly or gigantism, it may be found in some patients with severe liver or renal disease, in heroin addicts or in those taking L-dopa. Fasting plasma GH can be normal in 8 per cent of acromegalic patients. The plasma glucose concentrations may demonstrate impaired glucose tolerance or diabetes mellitus in acromegaly. Note that the test is usually unnecessary in patients who are diabetic, as GH should already be suppressed.

If acromegaly is confirmed, it is wise to investigate for other pituitary hormone defects, for example TSH, LH, FSH and ACTH. Acromegaly can also be associated with the MEN syndrome (see Chapter 24).

Plasma IGF-1 has a long half-life and may be used in screening for acromegaly. Plasma concentrations correlate with the activity of the disease. Measurement of the plasma concentrations of GH, or of IGF-1, may be used to monitor the efficacy of treatment. Remember that pregnancy increases IGF-1 concentration, and starvation, obesity and diabetes mellitus decrease it. Insulin-like growth-factor-binding protein-3 is the main binding protein for IGF-1 and its concentration is also increased in acromegaly.

Sometimes plasma GHRH concentrations are useful and can be raised where there is an ectopic source or may be suppressed in pituitary disease. Computerized tomography or MRI body scanning may help to find an ectopic source of GH or GHRH.

Treatment
There are various approaches to treatment, often with surgery to remove the adenoma, usually by trans-sphenoidal hypophysectomy. Residual disease requires medical therapy, usually with either bromocriptine (a dopamine receptor agonist that may have limited effectiveness) or somatostatin analogues (somatostatin itself has too short a half-life for effective therapeutic use). Octreotide can be used and binds to somatostatin receptors. Radiation therapy is sometimes used as an adjuvant for large invasive tumours or when surgery is contraindicated.

The aim of treatment is to ameliorate symptoms and to obtain an oral glucose suppressed GH concentration of less than 1 mU/L (this cut-off can be GH assay dependent) and normalization of plasma IGF-1 concentrations.

Growth hormone deficiency

In adults, GH deficiency rarely causes clinical symptoms, although it may be associated with tiredness, dyslipidaemia and increased cardiovascular disease.

CASE 1

A 48-year-old man noticed that his hat size had increased and his wife thought that his appearance had changed since their marriage, his features becoming coarser and his hands larger. Plasma IGF-1 concentration was raised and an oral glucose suppression test was performed. The results were as follows.

Plasma
0 minutes: GH 24.5 mU/L
30 minutes: GH 24.6 mU/L
60 minutes: GH 23.7 mU/L
90 minutes: GH 20.5 mU/L
120 minutes: GH 25.8 mU/L

DISCUSSION
The plasma GH concentration was not suppressed during the test in any of the samples. These findings are indicative of acromegaly; the clinical features are typical of acromegaly. This case illustrates the principle of using a suppression test when considering a condition involving a hormone excess. In normal individuals, plasma GH concentration would be suppressed to less than 1 mU/L by the glucose intake.

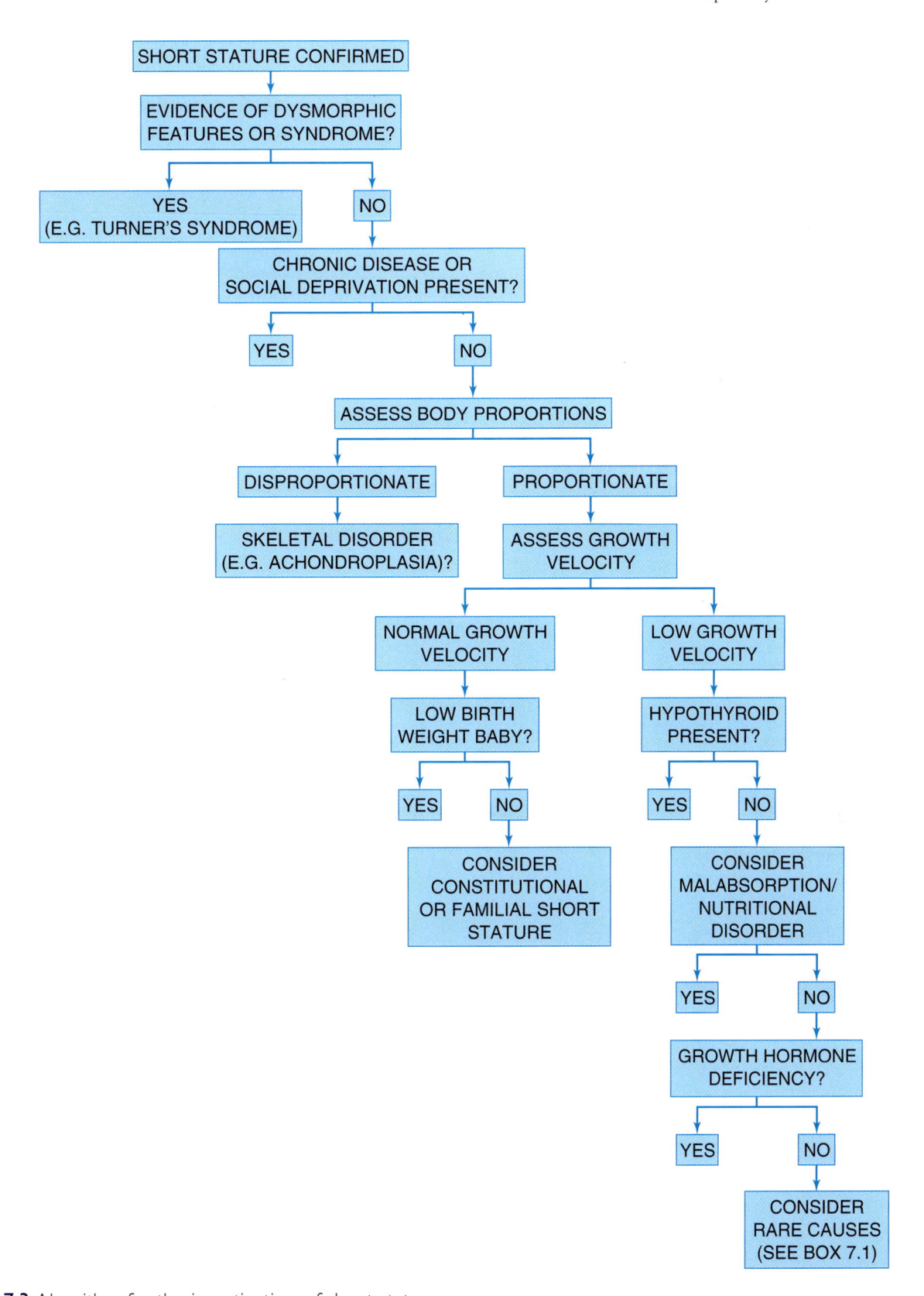

Fig. 7.3 Algorithm for the investigation of short stature

Growth hormone deficiency can cause short stature in children. It is present in a small percentage of normally proportioned small children; the birth weight may be normal but the rate of growth is subnormal. Other causes of growth retardation and short stature must be excluded before a diagnosis of GH deficiency is made (Box 7.1).

Emotional deprivation may be associated with GH deficiency that is indistinguishable by laboratory tests from that due to organic causes. Laron dwarfs have a GH receptor defect and pygmies have a GH receptor defect and low IGF-1 concentrations.

It is important to investigate children with reduced growth rate to identify those who may benefit from recombinant human GH replacement treatment.

Isolated GH deficiency is most commonly secondary to idiopathic deficiency of hypothalamic GHRH. In some cases, the secretion of other hormones is also impaired. Sometimes there may be an organic disorder of the anterior pituitary gland or hypothalamus; rare inherited forms have been described.

Diagnosis

The clinical history should include information about birth weight and whether intrauterine growth retardation was an issue. The sex-adjusted mid-parental height or target height is useful and can be calculated by adding 6.5 cm to the mean of the parents' heights for boys and subtracting 6.5 cm from the mean of the parents' heights for girls. Normal growth may be defined as more than 5 cm per year in mid-childhood. It is, of course, important to exclude hypothyroidism, chronic diseases and malabsorption states, poor nutritional state and failure to thrive. Clinical examination should assess for obvious syndromes, pubertal status, bone age, growth or growth velocity, for example Tanner Whitehouse charts and proportionality of limbs. Karyotyping may be indicated if a chromosomal disorder such as Turner's syndrome (45,X0) is suspected.

There is a physiological reduction in GH secretion at the end of pre-puberty. Thus, in children with bone age more than 10 years, priming with sex hormones before investigation may be necessary. For example, ethinyloestradiol may be given to girls and testosterone to boys prior to testing.

There is no general agreement about the best way to investigate such children biochemically. This is partly because GH secretion is episodic, GH assays vary between laboratories and there is a variable response of GH to provocative stimuli. Plasma GH concentrations in normal children are often low and assays under basal conditions rarely exclude the diagnosis. A low plasma IGF-1 concentration may be a useful screening test. Urinary GH

> **Box 7.1 Some causes of growth retardation and short stature**
>
> Familial short stature
> Social/emotional deprivation
> Malnutrition and chronic disease, e.g.
>   Coeliac disease
>   Rickets
>   Chronic renal failure
> Endocrine disorders
>   Growth hormone deficiency, congenital or acquired
>   Hypothyroidism
>   Cushing's syndrome
>   Congenital adrenal hyperplasia
> Chromosomal abnormalities
>   Turner's syndrome (45,X0)
> Skeletal disorders
>   Achondroplasia
> Laron dwarfs and pygmies

CASE 2

A 10-year-old boy was referred to paediatric out-patients because of short stature. His height was 1.08 m and he had normal body proportions. Physical examination and preliminary biochemical tests showed no obvious explanation for his small stature. A random plasma GH was less than 2 mU/L. After a glucagon stimulation test, the plasma GH concentration failed to increase above 4 mU/L. However, other pituitary hormone concentrations were normal on biochemical testing.

DISCUSSION

A diagnosis of isolated GH deficiency was made. Note the failure of GH concentration to increase after stimulation by glucagon. This illustrates well the concept of using stimulation dynamic tests when considering a hormone deficiency state.

excretion, either in 24-hour collections or timed overnight, may offer relatively safe screening tests. If blood is taken at a time when physiologically high concentrations are expected, the need for the more unpleasant stimulation tests may be avoided, for example 60–90 minutes after the onset of sleep and about 20 minutes after vigorous exercise. A plasma GH more than 40 mU/L (20–40 equivocal) makes GH deficiency unlikely.

If GH deficiency is not excluded by the above measurements, it is necessary to perform one or more stimulation tests. The response of GH to insulin may be the most reliable to detect GH deficiency, but it is not without the risk of fatal hypoglycaemia. Glucagon could also be used as an alternative (see later). A GH response more than 40 mU/L (20–40 equivocal) tends to exclude GH deficiency after the presentation of provocative stimuli on two occasions. Other such stimuli include arginine, clonidine or the GHRH test. (See below for a brief summary of some of these tests.) An unequivocally normal response to a stimulation test excludes the diagnosis and a clearly impaired one confirms it. Once GH deficiency has been established, a cause should be sought by appropriate clinical and imaging means.

The following are second-line dynamic tests sometimes used for suspected GH deficiency. Clonidine at 0.15 mg/m^2 body surface area is given orally after an overnight fast. Blood samples for plasma GH are collected at 0, 30, 60, 90, 120 and 150 minutes. The patient should be closely monitored for hypotension. Arginine hydrochloride, like clonidine, is another agent used in provocative dynamic tests for suspected GH deficiency. Arginine should not be given to patients with renal, hepatic or acid–base disorders or diabetes mellitus. After an overnight fast, 0.5 g/kg body weight to a maximum of 30 g is intravenously infused. Blood samples for plasma GH are collected at 0, 30, 60, 90 and 120 minutes. Arginine may evoke allergic reactions and the necessary precautions should be in place in case of this.

Figure 7.3 shows an algorithm for the investigation of short stature.

DISORDERS OF THE POSTERIOR PITUITARY

Disorders of the posterior pituitary are rare compared with those of the anterior pituitary. Deficiency of ADH in diabetes insipidus may present as polyuria. In the syndrome of inappropriate ADH, hyponatraemia due to water excess occurs. (These are discussed in Chapters 2 and 3.)

Hypopituitarism

Hypopituitarism is a syndrome of deficiency of pituitary hormone production which may result from disorders of the hypothalamus, pituitary or surrounding structures. The anterior pituitary gland has considerable functional reserve. Clinical features of deficiency are usually absent until about 70 per cent of the gland has been destroyed, unless there is associated hyperprolactinaemia, when amenorrhoea and infertility may be early symptoms. Panhypopituitarism alludes to the involvement of all pituitary hormones; alternatively, only one or more may be involved, as in partial hypopituitarism.

Some of the causes of hypopituitarism are shown in Box 7.2

Panhypopituitarism with the full clinical picture described below is uncommon. Suspicion of anterior pituitary hypofunction usually arises in patients presenting with various features such as clinical and radiological evidence of a pituitary or localized brain tumour, hypogonadism, adrenocortical insufficiency, short stature caused by GH deficiency, and hypothyroidism.

Although isolated hormone deficiency, particularly of GH, may occur, several hormones are usually involved. If a deficiency of one hormone is demonstrated, it is important to establish whether the secretion of others is also abnormal. Gonadotrophins are often the first to decrease in

> **Box 7.2 Some causes of hypopituitarism**
>
> Tumours
>   Craniopharyngiomas
>   Pituitary adenomas (microadenoma <10 mm, macroadenoma >10 mm)
>   Secondary tumour deposits
> Infections
>   Tuberculosis
>   Meningitis
>   Syphilis
> Infiltrations
>   Sarcoidosis
>   Haemochromatosis
>   Histiocytosis X
> Vascular
>   Sheehan's syndrome
>   Apoplexy
> Empty sella syndrome
> Autoimmune – lymphocytic hypophysitis
> Iatrogenic – radiation, surgery

hypopituitarism and it is unusual for the post-pituitary hormones such as ADH and oxytocin to be affected.

Consequences of pituitary hormone deficiencies

Progressive pituitary damage usually presents with evidence of deficiencies of gonadotrophins and GH. Plasma ACTH and/or TSH concentrations may remain normal, or become deficient months or even years later. The clinical and biochemical consequences of the target-gland failure include the following.

- *Growth retardation in children*: this may be due to deficiency of GH; deficiency of TSH, and therefore of thyroid hormone, may contribute.
- *Secondary hypogonadism*: this is due to gonadotrophin deficiency, presenting as amenorrhoea, infertility and atrophy of secondary sexual characteristics with loss of axillary and pubic hair and impotence or loss of libido. Puberty is delayed in children.
- *Secondary adrenocortical hypofunction* (ACTH deficiency): in contrast to the primary form (Addison's disease), patients are not hyperpigmented because ACTH secretion is not raised. The sodium and water deficiency and hyperkalaemia characteristic of Addison's disease do not usually occur because aldosterone secretion (which is controlled by angiotensin and not by ACTH) is normal. However, cortisol is needed for normal free water excretion, and consequently there may be a dilutional hyponatraemia due to cortisol deficiency. Cortisol is also necessary for the maintenance of normal blood pressure. Hypotension may be associated with ACTH deficiency. Cortisol and/or GH deficiency may cause increased insulin sensitivity with fasting hypoglycaemia.
- *Secondary hypothyroidism* (TSH deficiency): this may sometimes be clinically indistinguishable from primary hypothyroidism.
- *Prolactin deficiency* with failure to lactate may occur after postpartum pituitary infarction (Sheehan's syndrome). However, in hypopituitarism due to a tumour, plasma prolactin concentrations are often raised and may cause galactorrhoea (secretion of breast fluid).

Patients with hypopituitarism, like those with Addison's disease, may die because of an inability to secrete an adequate amount of cortisol in response to stress caused by, for example, infection or surgery. Other life-threatening complications are hypoglycaemia and hypothermia.

Pituitary tumours

The clinical presentation of pituitary tumours depends on the type of cells involved and on the size of the tumour (microadenomas less than 10 mm and macroadenomas more than 10 mm).

Tumours of secretory cells may produce the clinical effects of excess hormone secretion:

- excess prolactin causes infertility, amenorrhoea and varying degrees of galactorrhoea (see Chapter 9),
- excess GH causes acromegaly or gigantism,
- excess ACTH causes Cushing's syndrome (see Chapter 8).

CASE 3

A 17-year-old female presented to the endocrine clinic because of headaches, weakness and amenorrhoea. The following baseline biochemical endocrine test results were obtained.

Plasma
Luteinizing hormone 0.46 mU/L (1–25)
Follicle-stimulating hormone 0.87 mU/L (1–15)
09.00 hours cortisol 56 nmol/L (180–720)
Prolactin 460 mU/L (<470)
Thyroid-stimulating hormone 0.21 mU/L (0.20–5.0)
Free T_4 10.4 pmol/L (12–25)
Oestradiol 60 pmol/L (70–880)

DISCUSSION
The patient has panhypopituitarism. Note the low concentrations of plasma gonadotrophins and secondary hypogonadism. A low 09.00 hours plasma cortisol concentration implies also low ACTH concentration. The panhypopituitarism was subsequently found to be due to a craniopharyngioma that had infiltrated the pituitary gland.

Note that this case illustrates another important principle of endocrine testing: that the plasma free T_4 concentration is low but the TSH concentration is within the reference range, which is abnormal given the hypothyroxinaemia.

Large pituitary tumours may present with:

- visual disturbances caused by pressure on the optic chiasma or headache due to raised intracranial pressure,
- deficiency of some or all of the pituitary hormones due to destruction of secretory cells in the gland.

Non-secreting tumours are difficult to diagnose using biochemical tests, although the combined pituitary stimulation test (see later) may indicate subclinical impairment of function. Hyperprolactinaemia, which may be asymptomatic, is a valuable biochemical marker of the presence of a pituitary tumour. Prolactin may be secreted by the tumour cells or by unaffected lactotrophs if tumour growth interferes with the normal inhibition of prolactin secretion (see Chapter 9).

Investigation of suspected hypopituitarism

The laboratory should always be consulted before any complex investigation or uncommon test is performed, in order to check the details of specimen collection and handling.

Deficiency of pituitary hormones causes hypofunction of the target endocrine glands. Investigation aims to confirm such deficiency, to exclude disease of the target gland and then to test pituitary hormone secretion after maximal stimulation of the gland.

Measurement should be made of the plasma concentrations of:

- LH, FSH and oestradiol (female) or testosterone (male),
- total or free T_4 and TSH,
- prolactin, to test for hypothalamic or pituitary stalk involvement,
- cortisol at 09.00 hours, to assess the risk of adrenocortical insufficiency during later testing.

If the plasma concentration of the target-gland hormone is low and the concentration of trophic hormone is raised, the affected target gland should be investigated. Conversely, if the plasma concentrations of both the target gland and trophic hormones are low or low-normal, consider a pituitary stimulation test (see below).

Investigation of the pituitary region using radiological techniques such as CT or MRI scanning may help elucidate a cause of the hypopituitarism.

Although some textbooks talk about the combined pituitary stimulation test (insulin or glucagon plus TRH and GnRH given as one test), this is rarely required, as useful information can be obtained from the basal pituitary hormones and, if indicated, an insulin stimulation/hypoglycaemia test, although this is not without risk.

Insulin tolerance or insulin stimulation test

This test is potentially dangerous and must be done under direct medical supervision. Fatalities have been reported due to severe hypoglycaemia and the test should only be carried out in specialist units by experienced staff. It is contraindicated in the following patient groups: the elderly, patients with ischaemic heart disease, epilepsy or severe panhypopituitarism, and patients in whom 09.00 hours plasma cortisol is less than 100 nmol/L. A resting electrocardiogram should be normal. Hypothyroidism should be treated beforehand as this can impair the cortisol and GH responses. However, note that treatment with thyroxine can precipitate an adrenal crisis in such patients and thus corticosteroid replacement is also necessary.

Indications of the insulin stimulation test may include:

- assessment of GH in growth deficiency,
- assessment of ACTH/cortisol reserve (although the development of plasma ACTH assays has made such testing less necessary),
- differentiation of Cushing's syndrome from pseudo-Cushing's syndrome, for example depression or alcohol excess.

Both ACTH and GH are released in response to the stress of hypoglycaemia.

Fifty millilitres of 20 per cent glucose for intravenous administration must be immediately available in case severe symptomatic hypoglycaemia develops. Care should be taken not to induce severe hyperglycaemia during infusion, as it may cause hyperosmolality, which can be dangerous. Plasma cortisol is usually measured as an index of ACTH secretion. If glucose needs to be given, continue with the sampling.

Procedure

After an overnight fast, insert an indwelling intravenous cannula, for example 19 gauge. After at least 30 minutes, take basal samples at time 0 minutes for cortisol, GH and glucose.

Inject soluble insulin in a dose sufficient to lower plasma glucose concentrations to less than 2.5 mmol/L and evoke symptomatic hypoglycaemia. The recommended dose of insulin must be adjusted for the patient's body weight and for the suspected clinical condition under investigation. The usual dose is 0.15 U/kg body weight. If either pituitary or adrenocortical hypofunction is suspected, or if a low fasting glucose concentration has been found, reduce the dose to 0.1 or 0.05 U/kg. If there is likely to be resistance to the action of insulin because of Cushing's syndrome, acromegaly or obesity, 0.2 or 0.3 U/kg may be needed.

Take blood samples at 30, 45, 60, 90 and 120 minutes after the injections for cortisol, GH and glucose assays.

Interpretation

Methods of hormone assay vary and results should not be compared with reference values issued by other laboratories. Interpretation is not possible if hypoglycaemia is not attained, and the dose of insulin can cautiously be repeated if this is not attained in the 45-minute blood sample.

If hypoglycaemia has been adequate, plasma cortisol concentrations should rise by more than 200 nmol/L and exceed 580 nmol/L, whilst plasma GH concentrations should exceed 40 mU/L (20–40 mU/L are equivocal). In Cushing's syndrome, neither plasma cortisol nor GH concentrations rise significantly, although they usually do in cases of pseudo-Cushing's syndrome (Chapter 8). See Chapters 9 and 11 for details of GnRH and TRH tests if the combined pituitary test is used.

After the test, a supervised meal should be given and the patient should not drive for at least 2 hours.

Glucagon stimulation test of the hypothalamus–pituitary axis

This test is useful if the insulin hypoglycaemic test is contraindicated. However, fatalities have been described and it is essential that the test is carried out in a specialist unit by experienced staff.

The basic principle is that glucagon stimulates GH and ACTH release probably via a hypothalamic route.

The test is contraindicated if there is severe adrenal failure, for example if 09.00 hours cortisol is less than 100 nmol/L or in hypothyroidism. It is also unreliable in the presence of diabetes mellitus. Hypoglycaemia is not normally provoked by the test.

Procedure

Patients should fast overnight, although they can drink water. An indwelling intravenous cannula, for example gauge 19, is inserted. For adults, 1 mg of glucagon is injected subcutaneously at 09.00 hours.

Blood samples are taken at 0, 90, 120, 150, 180, 210 and 240 minutes for cortisol and GH.

Interpretation

Plasma cortisol should normally rise by at least 200 nmol/L to more than 580 nmol/L, and plasma GH should rise to more than 40 mU/L (20–40 mU/L are equivocal).

Treatment of hypopituitarism

This consists of specific therapy depending on its cause and may include surgical removal of a large adenoma. If the ACTH axis is impaired, it is essential to prescribe a glucocorticoid, for example hydrocortisone in the acute situation or prednisolone for maintenance. Secondary hypothyroidism will need thyroid replacement.

Adrenal replacement should precede T_4 therapy to avoid an Addisonian crisis (see Chapter 8). Gonadotrophin deficiency may require testosterone in males and oestrogen replacement in women, with or without progesterone as appropriate. In children and sometimes in adults, GH may be indicated.

CONCLUSIONS

- The anterior pituitary gland releases a number of peptide hormones, which are themselves regulated by hypothalamus hormones that reach the pituitary via the portal blood system. The anterior pituitary hormones include ACTH, TSH, LH and FSH; their respective target organs are the adrenal, thyroid and ovaries/testes. Growth hormone is also an anterior pituitary hormone but does not have a specific target organ, instead it influences most tissues.
- Hypopituitarism can be due to many conditions, such as pituitary infiltration or destruction, and results in a deficiency of all (panhypopituitarism) or some of the pituitary hormones.
- Conversely, excess release of certain anterior pituitary hormones can occur because of pituitary tumours. For example, acromegaly is due to excess GH, and Cushing's disease to excess ACTH release.
- The posterior pituitary releases oxytocin and ADH. The former is involved in uterine contraction during labour. Antidiuretic hormone controls water elimination by changing the renal collecting ducts' permeability. Deficiency of ADH results in diabetes insipidus (discussed in Chapter 2).

8 THE ADRENAL CORTEX

Chemistry and biosynthesis of steroids	127	Primary adrenocortical hypofunction (Addison's disease)	134
Physiology	128	Investigation of suspected adrenal hypofunction	136
The hypothalamic–pituitary–adrenal axis	129	Corticosteroid therapy	137
Factors affecting plasma cortisol concentrations	129	Congenital adrenal hyperplasia	138
Disorders of the adrenal cortex	130	Primary hyperaldosteronism (Conn's syndrome)	140
Adrenocortical hyperfunction	130		

A number of endocrine abnormalities involve the adrenal glands, and some of the more common conditions are discussed in this chapter, which should perhaps be read in conjunction with Chapter 7 (on pituitary function) and Chapter 9 (which deals with reproductive endocrinology).

The adrenal glands are divided into two embryologically and functionally distinct parts. The *adrenal cortex* is part of the hypothalamic–pituitary–adrenal endocrine system. Morphologically, the adult adrenal cortex consists of three layers. The outer thin layer (zona glomerulosa) secretes only aldosterone. The inner two layers (zona fasciculata and zona reticularis) form a functional unit and secrete most of the adrenocortical hormones. In the fetus there is a wider fourth layer, which disappears soon after birth. One of its most important functions during fetal life is, together with the adrenal cortex, to synthesize oestriol, in association with the placenta. The *adrenal medulla* is part of the sympathetic nervous system. Glucocorticoids are involved in the synthesis of adrenaline (epinephrine).

CHEMISTRY AND BIOSYNTHESIS OF STEROIDS

Steroid hormones are derived from the lipid cholesterol. Figure 8.1 shows the internationally agreed numbering of the 27 carbon atoms of steroid molecules and the lettering of the four rings. The products of cholesterol are also indicated. If the molecule contains 21 carbon atoms, it is referred to as a C21 steroid. The carbon atom at position 21 of the molecule is written as C-21. The side chain on C-17 is the main determinant of the type of hormonal activity (Fig. 8.1), but substitutions in other positions modify activity within a particular group.

The first hormonal product of cholesterol is pregnenolone. Several important synthetic pathways diverge from it (Fig. 8.1). The final product is dependent upon the tissue and its enzymes.

The zona glomerulosa secretes aldosterone, produced by 18-hydroxylation. Synthesis of this steroid is controlled by the renin–angiotensin system and not normally by adrenocorticotrophic hormone (ACTH). Although ACTH is important for maintaining growth of the zona glomerulosa, deficiency does not significantly reduce output.

The zonae fasciculata and reticularis synthesize and secrete two groups of steroid:

- *cortisol*, a glucocorticoid (the most important C21 steroid), is formed by progressive addition of hydroxyl groups at C-17, C-21 and C-11,
- *androgens* (for example androstenedione) are formed after the removal of the side chain to produce C19 steroids.

Adrenocorticotrophic hormone secreted by the anterior pituitary gland stimulates synthesis of these two steroid groups. Its secretion is influenced by negative feedback from changes in plasma cortisol concentrations. Impaired cortisol synthesis due, for example, to an inherited

128 THE ADRENAL CORTEX

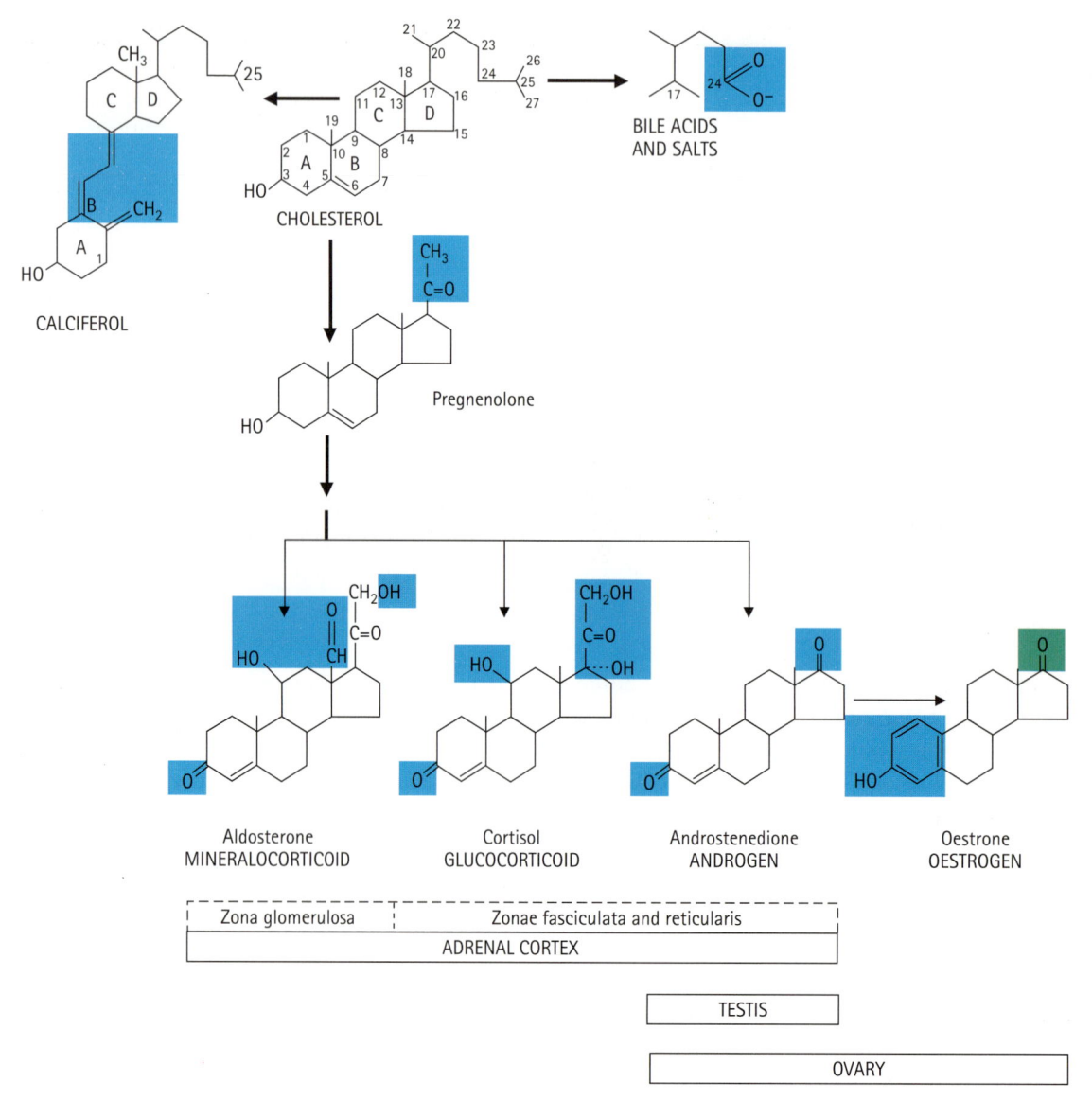

Fig. 8.1 Numbering of the steroid carbon atoms of cholesterol and the synthetic pathway of steroid hormones; the chemical groups highlighted determine the biological activity of the steroid.

21-α-hydroxylase or 11-β-hydroxylase deficiency (congenital adrenal hyperplasia) results in increased ACTH stimulation with increased activity of both pathways. The resultant excessive androgen production may cause hirsutism or virilization.

PHYSIOLOGY

The adrenocortical hormones can be classified into groups depending on their predominant physiological effects.

Glucocorticoids

Cortisol and corticosterone are naturally occurring glucocorticoids. They stimulate gluconeogenesis and the breakdown of protein and fat, i.e. they antagonize some of insulin's action. Glucocorticoids in excess may impair glucose tolerance and alter the distribution of adipose tissue. Cortisol helps maintain the extracellular fluid volume and normal blood pressure.

Circulating cortisol is bound to cortisol-binding globulin (CBG; transcortin) and to albumin. At normal concentrations, only about 5 per cent of the total is unbound and physiologically active. Plasma CBG is almost fully saturated, so that increased cortisol secretion causes a disproportionate rise in the free active fraction. Cortisone is not secreted in significant amounts by the adrenal cortex. It is biologically inactive until it has been converted in vivo to cortisol (hydrocortisone).

Glucocorticoids are conjugated with glucuronate and sulphate in the liver to form inactive metabolites, which, because they are more water soluble than the mainly protein-bound parent hormones, can be excreted in the urine.

Mineralocorticoids

In contrast to other steroids, aldosterone is not transported in plasma bound to specific proteins. It stimulates the exchange of sodium for potassium and hydrogen ions across cell membranes and its renal action is especially important for sodium and water homeostasis. It is discussed more fully in Chapters 2, 3 and 4. Like the glucocorticoids, it is inactivated by hepatic conjugation and is excreted in the urine.

There is overlap in the actions of C21 steroids. Cortisol, in particular, may have a significant mineralocorticoid effect at high plasma concentrations when the free fraction is significantly increased.

Adrenal androgens

The main adrenal androgens are dehydroepiandrosterone (DHEA), its sulphate (DHEAS) and androstenedione. They promote protein synthesis and are only weakly androgenic at physiological concentrations. Testosterone, the most powerful androgen, is synthesized in the testes or ovaries but not in the adrenal cortex. Most circulating androgens, like cortisol, are protein bound, mainly to sex-hormone-binding globulin and albumin.

There is extensive peripheral interconversion of adrenal and gonadal androgens. The end products, androsterone and aetiocholanolone, together with DHEA, are conjugated in the liver and excreted as glucuronides and sulphates in the urine.

THE HYPOTHALAMIC–PITUITARY–ADRENAL AXIS

The hypothalamus, anterior pituitary gland and adrenal cortex form a functional unit – the hypothalamic–pituitary–adrenal axis (see Chapter 7).

Cortisol is synthesized and secreted in response to ACTH from the anterior pituitary gland. The secretion of ACTH is dependent on corticotrophin-releasing hormone (CRH), released from the hypothalamus. High plasma free-cortisol concentrations suppress CRH secretion (negative feedback) and alter the ACTH response to CRH, thus acting on both the hypothalamus and the anterior pituitary gland (Fig. 8.2).

The melanocyte-stimulating effect of high plasma concentrations of ACTH, or related peptides, causes skin pigmentation in two conditions associated with low plasma cortisol concentrations:

- *Addison's disease*,
- *Nelson's syndrome*: after bilateral adrenalectomy for Cushing's disease (see later), removal of the cortisol feedback causes a further rise in plasma ACTH concentrations from already high levels.

Inherent rhythms and stress

Adrenocorticotrophic hormone is secreted episodically, each pulse being followed 5–10 minutes later by cortisol secretion. These episodes are most frequent in the early morning (between the fifth and eighth hour of sleep) and least frequent in the few hours before sleep. Plasma cortisol concentrations are usually highest between about 07.00 and 09.00 hours and lowest between 23.00 and 04.00 hours.

The secretion of ACTH and cortisol usually varies inversely and the almost parallel circadian rhythm of the two hormones may be due to cyclical changes in the sensitivity of the hypothalamic feedback centre to cortisol levels. Inappropriately high plasma cortisol concentrations at any time of day suppress ACTH secretion. This effect can be tested by the dexamethasone suppression test. Loss of circadian rhythm is one of the earliest features of Cushing's syndrome. Stress, either physical or mental, may override the first two mechanisms and cause sustained ACTH secretion. An inadequate stress response may cause acute adrenal insufficiency. Stress caused by insulin-induced hypoglycaemia can be used to test the axis.

FACTORS AFFECTING PLASMA CORTISOL CONCENTRATIONS

Plasma cortisol is usually measured by immunoassay, but the antibody may cross-react with other steroids or drugs. Factors that may affect results include hydrocortisone (cortisol), cortisone (converted to cortisol by metabolism)

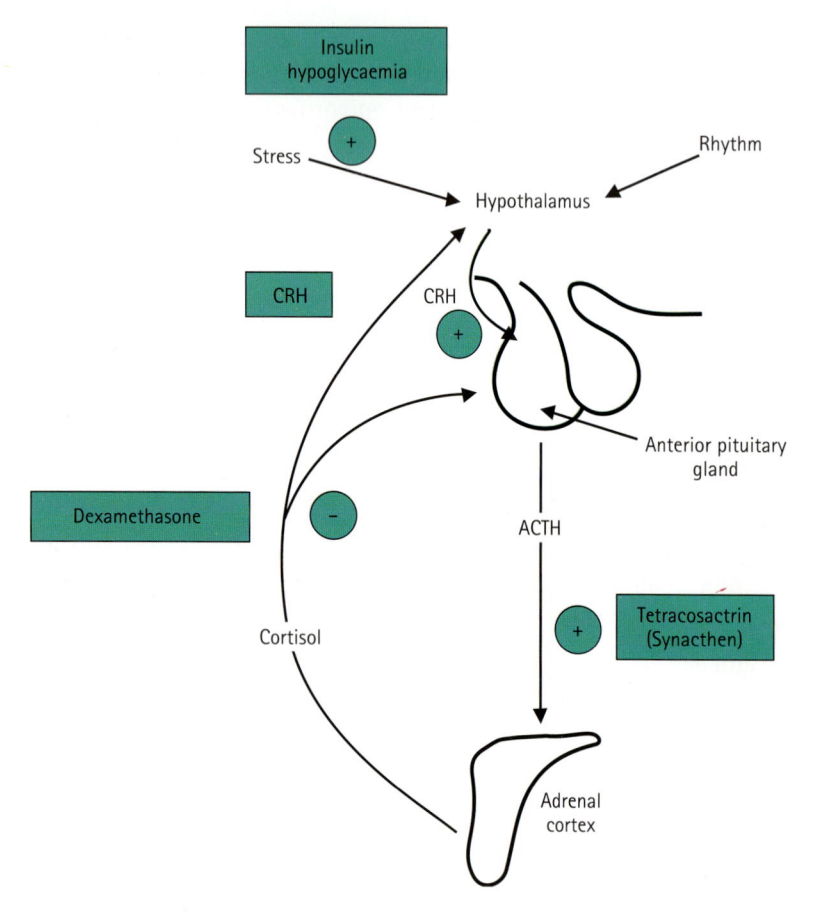

Fig. 8.2 The factors controlling the secretion of cortisol from the adrenal gland, including the site of action of dynamic function tests (shaded). (+ = stimulates; − = inhibits; CRH = corticotrophin-releasing hormone; ACTH = adrenocorticotrophic hormone.)

and prednisolone, which may contribute to the 'cortisol' concentration of some immunoassay methods. Thus, it is recommended either that the patient is prescribed dexamethasone (which is less likely to cross-react with cortisol assays) or, if possible, that the prednisolone is gradually reduced and then stopped for about 3 days before sampling. Oestrogens and some oral contraceptives increase the plasma CBG concentration, and therefore the protein-bound cortisol concentration.

Adrenocorticotrophic hormone (corticotrophin)

Adrenocorticotrophic hormone is a single-chain polypeptide made up of 39 amino acids with biological activity at the N-terminal end of the peptide. A peptide consisting of this sequence has been synthesized (tetracosactrin, Synacthen) and can be used for diagnosis and treatment in place of ACTH. The ACTH stimulates cortisol synthesis and secretion by the adrenal cortex. It has much less effect on adrenal androgen production and, at physiological concentrations, virtually no effect on aldosterone production.

DISORDERS OF THE ADRENAL CORTEX

The main disorders of adrenocortical function are shown in Table 8.1.

ADRENOCORTICAL HYPERFUNCTION

Cushing's syndrome

Cushing's syndrome is caused by an excess of circulating cortisol. Many of the clinical and metabolic disturbances can be explained by glucocorticoid excess. The clinical and metabolic features may include the following:

- Obesity, typically involving the trunk and face, and a round, red 'moon' face.
- Impaired glucose tolerance and hyperglycaemia. Cortisol has an opposite action to that of insulin, causing increased gluconeogenesis, and some patients may have diabetes mellitus.

Table 8.1 Disorders of adrenocortical function

Altered hormone secretion	Associated clinical disorder
Hypersecretion	
Cortisol	Cushing's syndrome
Aldosterone	Primary hyperaldosteronism (Conn's syndrome)
Androgens	Congenital adrenal hyperlasia
	Adrenocortical carcinoma
Hyposecretion	
Cortisol and aldosterone	Primary adrenal disorders, e.g. Addison's disease or congenital adrenal hyperplasia
Cortisol and adrenocorticotrophic hormone	Adrenal insufficiency secondary to pituitary disease

- Increased protein catabolism, which also increases urinary protein loss. Thus there is a negative nitrogen balance associated with proximal muscle wasting with weakness, thinning of the skin and osteoporosis. The tendency to bruising, and the purple striae (most obvious on the abdominal wall) are probably due to this thinning.
- Hypertension, caused by urinary retention of sodium and therefore of water, which are due to the mineralocorticoid effect of cortisol. Increased urinary potassium loss may cause hypokalaemia.
- Androgen excess, which may account for the common findings of greasy skin with acne vulgaris and hirsutism and menstrual disturbances in women.
- Psychiatric disturbances, such as depression.

Laboratory findings include a hypokalaemic alkalosis, leucocytosis and eosinophilia.

Causes of Cushing's syndrome

One of the commonest causes of Cushing's syndrome is iatrogenic and related to excessive steroid treatment. Increased endogenous cortisol production may be due to hyperstimulation of the adrenal gland by ACTH, either from the pituitary gland or from an 'ectopic' source, or due to largely autonomous secretion by an adrenal tumour such as an adenoma or carcinoma (Fig. 8.3).

The secretion of ACTH is increased in the following conditions.

- *Cushing's disease*: it is associated with bilateral adrenal hyperplasia, often secondary to a basophil adenoma of the anterior pituitary gland.
- In *ectopic ACTH secretion*, usually from a small-cell carcinoma of the bronchus, ACTH concentrations may be high enough to cause skin pigmentation. The patient may have weight loss with cachexia. One metabolic complication is a hypokalaemic alkalosis. The clinical features may be indistinguishable from those of Cushing's disease.

The secretion of ACTH is appropriately suppressed in primary cortisol-secreting tumours of the adrenal cortex. The tumours may be benign or malignant and are usually derived from the zona fasciculata/zona reticularis of the adrenal. These glucocorticoid-secreting tumours do not normally secrete aldosterone, which is produced in the zona glomerulosa layer of the adrenal cortex. Benign adenomas occur and also carcinomas. The latter secrete a variety of steroids, including androgens, and thus may cause hirsutism or virilization. In these cases plasma ACTH is suppressed by the excess glucocorticoids.

Basis of investigation of suspected Cushing's syndrome

The following questions should be asked.

- Is there abnormal cortisol secretion?
- If so, does the patient have any other condition that may cause it?
- If Cushing's syndrome is confirmed, what is the cause?

Is there abnormal cortisol secretion?

Plasma cortisol concentrations reflect ACTH activity at that moment and, because of the episodic nature of cortisol secretion, such isolated values may be misleading. Indeed, cyclical Cushing's syndrome may require repeated investigation. The level of cortisol measured in a 24-hour urine sample reflects the overall daily secretion.

One of the earliest features of Cushing's syndrome is the loss of the diurnal variation in cortisol secretion, with high concentrations in the late evening, when secretion is normally at a minimum. However, it is not a diagnostic finding because it can also be caused by, for example, stress and endogenous depression. The assessment of diurnal rhythm is not a practical out-patient procedure.

Out-patient screening tests therefore may include the following.

Estimation of 24-hour urinary free cortisol

Only the unbound fraction of cortisol in plasma is filtered at the glomeruli and excreted in the urine (urinary 'free' cortisol). In Cushing's syndrome, because of the loss of circadian rhythm, raised plasma values are present for longer than normal and daily urinary cortisol excretion is further increased (i.e. there is a disproportionately raised free fraction of cortisol).

Plasma and urinary cortisol concentrations are much higher when Cushing's syndrome is due to adrenocortical carcinoma or overt ectopic ACTH secretion.

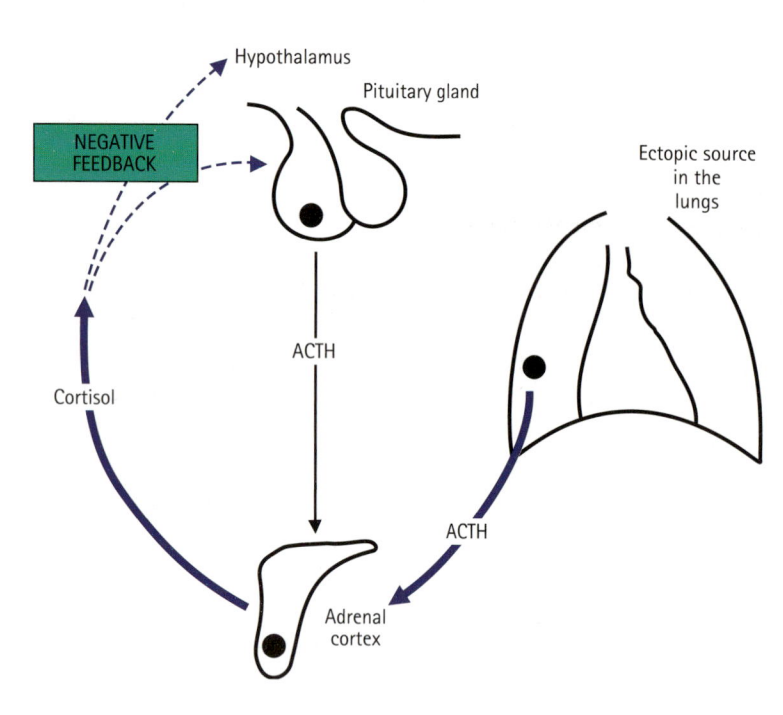

Fig. 8.3 Cushing's disease, indicating excess cortisol production caused either as a result of hyperstimulation of the adrenal gland by adrenocorticotrophic hormone (ACTH), from either the pituitary or an ectopic source, or by autonomous hormone secretion from an adrenal tumour

CASE 1

A 45-year-old female was referred to the endocrine clinic because of skin pigmentation, obesity, hypertension and muscle weakness. The following biochemical results were returned.

Plasma
Sodium 140 mmol/L (135–145)
Potassium 3.0 mmol/L (3.5–5.0)
Urea 5.5 mmol/L (2.5–7.5)
Creatinine 100 μmol/L (60–120)
Glucose 12.5 mmol/L (3.5–6.0)

Urine
24-hour free cortisol 1700 nmol (100–350)

The following were further results of an overnight dexamethasone suppression test.

Plasma
09.00 hours cortisol 969 nmol/L (180–720)
Cortisol after low-dose 1 mg dexamethasone test 990 nmol/L
Adrenocorticotrophic hormone 454 ng/L (20–80)

DISCUSSION

The raised 24-hour urinary free cortisol and 09.00 hours cortisol concentrations are suggestive of Cushing's syndrome. This is supported by the fact that there was a failure of cortisol suppression by low-dose dexamethasone. The raised plasma ACTH concentration could be indicative of either Cushing's disease or ectopic ACTH secretion. Further tests, including computerized tomography (CT) scanning and a CRH test, confirmed ectopic ACTH secretion due to a lung tumour. Note also the hypokalaemia and hyperglycaemia and the other clinical features typical of Cushing's syndrome.

Determinations of 24-hour urinary free cortisol have about a 5 per cent false-negative rate, but if three separate determinations are normal, Cushing's syndrome is most unlikely.

Low-dose overnight dexamethasone suppression test

A small dose, for example 1 mg, of this synthetic steroid inhibits ACTH, and thereby cortisol secretion by negative feedback. This is usually given at midnight and blood is taken for cortisol assay at 09.00 hours the following morning.

The overnight dexamethasone suppression test is a sensitive, but not completely specific, test in evaluating such patients. The false-positive rate is about 12 per cent and the false-negative rate about 2 per cent. A normal fall in plasma cortisol concentrations makes the diagnosis of Cushing's syndrome very unlikely, but failure to suppress plasma cortisol to less than 50 nmol/L does not confirm it with certainty.

There are some pitfalls, for example certain anticonvulsant drugs, such as phenytoin, may interfere with dexamethasone suppression tests, inducing liver enzymes that increase the rate of metabolism of the drug. Plasma concentrations may therefore be too low to suppress the feedback centre.

Additional tests

In some cases, additional tests are needed to confirm the diagnosis of excess cortisol production. The 48-hour low-dose dexamethasone suppression test may be useful: 0.5 mg dexamethasone is given orally at 6-hourly intervals from 09.00 hours on day 1 for eight doses and then plasma cortisol is measured after 48 hours at 09.00 hours. Plasma cortisol should normally suppress to less than 50 nmol/L, but not in Cushing's syndrome.

Is there another cause for the abnormal cortisol secretion?

Various conditions can mimic Cushing's syndrome (pseudo-Cushing's) and thus give false-positive results for screening tests.

The following non-Cushing's causes of abnormal cortisol secretion are important to remember.

- *Stress* overrides the other mechanisms controlling ACTH secretion, with loss of the normal circadian variation of plasma cortisol and a reduced feedback response. Urinary free-cortisol excretion may be increased even in relatively minor physical illness or mental stress.
- *Endogenous depression* may be associated with sustained high plasma cortisol and ACTH concentrations that may not be suppressed even by a high dose of dexamethasone. However, these patients often have a normal cortisol response to insulin-induced hypoglycaemia, whereas those with Cushing's syndrome do not (see Chapter 7).
- *Severe alcohol abuse* can cause hypersecretion of cortisol that mimics Cushing's syndrome clinically and biochemically. The abnormal findings revert to normal when alcohol is stopped.
- *Severe obesity* can also imitate Cushing's syndrome.

What is the cause of Cushing's syndrome?

The following biochemical investigations may help to elucidate the cause and ideally should be carried out on a metabolic ward by experienced staff (Table 8.2).

- Plasma ACTH is detectable only in ACTH-dependent Cushing's syndrome, and plasma concentrations are suppressed in patients with secreting adrenocortical

Table 8.2 Some biochemical test results in patients with Cushing's syndrome

	Pituitary dependent (Cushing's disease)	Ectopic ACTH	Adrenocortical carcinoma	Adrenocortical adenoma
Plasma cortisol				
Morning	Raised or normal	Raised	Raised	Raised or normal
Evening	Raised	Raised	Raised	Raised
After low-dose dexamethasone	No suppression	No suppression	No suppression	No suppression
After high-dose dexamethasone	Suppressed	No suppression	No suppression	No suppression
Urinary free cortisol	Raised	Raised	Raised	Raised
Plasma ACTH	Raised or normal	Raised	Low	Low

ACTH = adrenocorticotrophic hormone.

tumours. In patients with Cushing's disease, plasma ACTH concentration may be either high-normal or moderately raised but inappropriate for the high plasma cortisol concentration. Conversely, plasma ACTH concentrations are markedly raised in patients with 'ectopic' ACTH production.

- The high-dose dexamethasone suppression test may be useful. The principle of this test is the same as that of the low-dose test described above, but a higher dose (2 mg) given over 48 hours at 6-hourly intervals may suppress the relatively insensitive feedback centre of pituitary-dependent Cushing's disease (this occurs in about 90 per cent of cases). Plasma cortisol concentration suppression by about 50 per cent is usual. In the other two categories, ectopic ACTH production or adrenal tumours, when pituitary ACTH is already suppressed, even this high dose will usually have no effect, although there may be some suppression in some cases of 'ectopic' ACTH secretion.
- If there is virilization, measure the plasma androgens such as testosterone, DHEA and DHEAS. High concentrations suggest an adrenocortical carcinoma (see Chapter 9).
- In cases of Cushing's syndrome with raised plasma ACTH concentration, the intravenous CRH test (100 μg in adults or 1 μg/kg body weight in children) has gained popularity. In Cushing's disease (pituitary disorder), an increase in baseline plasma cortisol concentration of about 25 per cent occurs in 90 per cent of patients, whereas patients with ectopic ACTH, for example with lung carcinoma, usually fail to show this rise.
- The insulin tolerance test may be appropriate. Elevated plasma cortisol concentrations suppress the stress response to hypoglycaemia and this test may be of value in differentiating Cushing's syndrome from pseudo-Cushing's syndrome due to depression or obesity. This test is not without hazards due to severe hypoglycaemia.

Confirmation of Cushing's disease will require pituitary imaging techniques, for example magnetic resonance imaging (MRI) as well as pituitary hormone assessment (see Chapter 7). Specialized units may perform simultaneous petrosal sinus sampling in an attempt to localize the pituitary tumour and confirm differentiation from an ectopic ACTH source. A peripheral blood sample:petrosal blood sample ACTH ratio of more than 2 is indicative of Cushing's disease (ratio more than 3 if CRH stimulation used).

In cases of ectopic ACTH secretion, imaging techniques are important to try to locate the tumour, such as thin-slice MRI of the chest and abdomen. Seventy per cent of these tumours co-secrete other peptide hormones such as glucagon, somatostatin, calcitonin and bombesin. Ectopic ACTH-induced Cushing's syndrome is more likely to present with hypokalaemia, skin pigmentation, short clinical history and severe myopathy. Plasma ACTH concentrations are also often much higher than those found in Cushing's disease. Sometimes venous sampling of ACTH is necessary to locate the tumour. Rarely, a tumour may secrete CRH and thus mimic Cushing's disease. Abdominal imaging, for example CT scanning, may locate an adrenal tumour. Here, of course, plasma ACTH will usually be suppressed and the tumour may also secrete androgens.

The treatment of Cushing's syndrome depends upon the cause. Surgery is usually the treatment of choice. In Cushing's disease, pituitary removal by trans-sphenoidal surgery with pituitary radiation as an adjunct may be necessary. Adrenal tumours also usually require surgery, although the prognosis may be poor with carcinoma. Bilateral adrenal removal can lead to skin pigmentation due to pituitary ACTH release – Nelson's syndrome. Similarly, if the source of ectopic ACTH is found, surgery may be indicated to remove the tumour, for example lung carcinoma.

PRIMARY ADRENOCORTICAL HYPOFUNCTION (ADDISON'S DISEASE)

Addison's disease is caused by bilateral destruction of all zones of the adrenal cortex, usually as the result of an autoimmune process. The association of Addison's disease with hypoparathyroidism and mucocutaneous candidiasis is described as polyglandular autoimmune syndrome type 1 and has autosomal recessive inheritance. Polyglandular autoimmune syndrome type 2 occurs when Addison's disease is associated with type 1 diabetes mellitus and autoimmune thyroid disease, either Hashimoto's thyroiditis or Graves' disease, and is also related to HLA-B8 and DR-3 types.

Tuberculosis affecting the adrenals is an important cause in countries where this disease is common. Other causes of bilateral destruction of the adrenal glands include amyloidosis, mycotic infections, acquired immunodeficiency

> **CASE 2**
>
> A 28-year-old female attended endocrine out-patients because of weight loss, weakness, amenorrhoea, buccal pigmentation and vitiligo. Some of her biochemical tests were as follows.
>
> *Plasma*
> Sodium 118 mmol/L (135–145)
> Potassium 5.8 mmol/L (3.5–5.0)
> Urea 4.5 mmol/L (2.5–7.5)
> Creatinine 90 µmol/L (60–120)
> 09.00 hours cortisol 89 nmol/L (180–720)
> Cortisol 30 minutes later after 250 µg intramuscular Synacthen 80 nmol/L
>
> **DISCUSSION**
> These studies support the diagnosis of adrenal insufficiency (Addison's disease), with a failure of plasma cortisol to rise after Synacthen stimulation. The symptoms and signs are typical of the condition. The patient was subsequently shown to have polyendocrine syndrome with premature ovarian failure, vitiligo and auto-immune Addison's disease. The buccal mucosa pigmentation is due to increased ACTH concentration. Note the hyponatraemia and hyperkalaemia.

syndrome and secondary deposits often originating from a bronchial carcinoma.

An important cause of acute adrenal crisis is bilateral adrenal haemorrhage, which can occur on warfarin therapy or in patients with meningococcus septicaemia, as in Waterhouse–Friderichsen syndrome. Certain drugs can inhibit glucocorticoid synthesis, including ketoconazole, aminoglutethimide, methadone and etomidate.

Glucocorticoid deficiency contributes to the hypotension and causes marked sensitivity to insulin; hypoglycaemia may be a presenting feature.

The clinical presentation of Addison's disease depends on the degree of adrenal destruction. In cases of massive haemorrhagic adrenal destruction, as in Waterhouse–Friderichsen syndrome of meningococcaemia, the patient may be shocked, with volume depletion; this adrenal crisis should be treated as a matter of urgency. Conversely, sometimes the presentation can be surreptitious; a prolonged period of vague ill-health, tiredness, weight loss, mild hypotension and pigmentation of the skin and buccal mucosa may occur. The cause of these vague symptoms may only become evident if an Addisonian crisis is precipitated by the stress of some other, perhaps mild, illness or surgery.

Androgen deficiency is not clinically evident because testosterone production by the testes is unimpaired in males and because androgen deficiency does not produce obvious effects in women. The pigmentation that develops in some cases of Addison's disease is due to the high circulating levels of ACTH or related peptides resulting from the lack of cortisol suppression of the feedback mechanism. Patients with primary adrenal insufficiency, as in Addison's disease due to autoimmune disease, may also show vitiligo.

Patients with acute cortisol deficiency may present with nausea, vomiting and hypotension. Dilutional hyponatraemia may be present because cortisol is needed for sodium-free water excretion by the kidneys. The biochemical changes therefore resemble those of inappropriate ADH secretion.

Other causes of hypoadrenalism

Hypoaldosteronism hyporeninism is discussed in Chapters 4 and 5 and is associated with type 2 diabetes mellitus and type IV renal tubular acidosis.

Another, rarer, cause of hypoadrenalism is Allgrove's syndrome due to congenital adrenocortical unresponsiveness to ACTH. Abnormalities of β-oxidation of very long-chain fatty acids (VLCFAs) are X-linked recessive defects in which VLCFAs accumulate in the tissues, including the adrenals, for example adrenoleucodystrophy.

Pseudohypoadrenalism

Pseudohypoaldosteronism type 1 usually presents in infancy with failure to thrive and salt wasting associated with hypotension, hyperkalaemia and large elevations in plasma renin and aldosterone. Defects are either in the epithelial sodium channel or in the mineralocorticoid receptor. Treatment is with a high sodium diet and high-dose fludrocortisone or carbenoxolone.

Pseudohypoaldosteronism type 2, or Gordon's syndrome, is an autosomal dominant condition typified by hyperkalaemia, hypertension and a mild hyperchloraemic acidosis. There is a mutation in the distal tubule chloride channel, resulting in enhanced distal chloride reabsorption in preference to excretion of potassium. Treatment is with a low-potassium diet and a thiazide diuretic.

Secondary adrenal hypofunction (ACTH deficiency)

Adrenocorticotrophic hormone release may be impaired by disorders of the hypothalamus or the anterior pituitary gland, most commonly due to a tumour or infarction (see Chapter 7). Corticosteroids suppress ACTH release and, if such drugs have been taken for a long time, the ACTH-releasing mechanism may be slow to recover. There may be temporary adrenal atrophy after prolonged lack of stimulation.

Extensive destruction of the anterior pituitary gland may cause panhypopituitarism (see Chapter 7), but if it is only partial, ACTH secretion may be adequate for basal requirements. Adrenocortical deficiency may then only become clinically evident under conditions of stress, which may precipitate acute adrenal insufficiency. The most common causes of stress are infection and surgery.

Patients may present with non-specific symptoms such as weight loss and tiredness. Hypoglycaemia may occur because of marked insulin sensitivity. Unlike primary adrenal hypofunction, pigmentation is absent because plasma ACTH concentrations are not raised.

Basis of investigation of suspected adrenocortical hypofunction

If a diagnosis of acute adrenal insufficiency is suspected clinically, blood should be taken so that the plasma cortisol concentration can be measured later; steroid treatment must be started immediately, as the condition can be life threatening. Adrenocorticol hypofunction may not be excluded on the results of a random plasma cortisol concentration, as this gives little idea as to adrenal stress reserve. Nor will plasma cortisol estimation distinguish between primary and secondary adrenal failure.

The tetracosactrin (Synacthen) stimulation test should be performed as soon as possible. Tetracosactrin has the same biological action as ACTH but, because it lacks the antigenic part of the molecule, there is much less danger of an allergic reaction. If the patient cannot stop using steroids, a steroid such as dexamethasone, which does not normally interfere with the assay of cortisol, should be prescribed. (See later for details of the Synacthen test.)

A plasma autoantibody screen including adrenal antibodies may point to a primary adrenal autoimmune problem.

Plasma ACTH assay may be of value when inappropriately low plasma cortisol concentrations have been found; a raised plasma ACTH concentration indicates primary insufficiency, whereas a low ACTH concentration suggests secondary insufficiency.

The essential abnormality in adrenocortical hypofunction is that the adrenal gland cannot adequately increase cortisol secretion in response to stress. This may be due to adrenal (primary) or hypothalamic–pituitary (secondary) pathology. In the case of the latter, it may be necessary to test the whole axis (see Chapter 7). Insulin-induced hypoglycaemia normally causes ACTH secretion from the anterior pituitary gland. This can be assessed by demonstrating a rise in plasma cortisol concentrations. An impaired response indicates pituitary dysfunction only if the adrenal cortices have already been shown to be capable of responding to exogenous ACTH.

INVESTIGATION OF SUSPECTED ADRENAL HYPOFUNCTION

Suspected Addisonian crisis (acute)

Before starting treatment, take blood for immediate plasma urea, creatinine and electrolyte estimations as well as plasma glucose, calcium and cortisol.

Hyponatraemia, hyperkalaemia, hypoglycaemia and uraemia are compatible with an Addisonian crisis. Hypercalcaemia may also occur (see Chapter 6).

Start steroid treatment once blood has been taken, as the condition is life threatening.

If the plasma cortisol is very high, an Addisonian crisis is unlikely. Conversely, if the plasma cortisol concentration is very low or undetectable, and if there is no reason to suspect severe CBG deficiency, for example due to the nephrotic syndrome, an Addisonian crisis is likely. Plasma cortisol concentrations, which would be normal under basal conditions, may be inappropriately low for the degree of stress. To confirm this, perform a short Synacthen test (see below).

Suspected chronic adrenal hypofunction

Measure the 09.00 hours plasma cortisol concentration. If more than 580 nmol/L, Addison's disease is unlikely, but this does not provide information about the adrenal glands' reserve to a stressful stimulus.

If the plasma cortisol concentrations are equivocal, perform a short Synacthen test. A normal result makes long-standing secondary adrenal insufficiency unlikely. Prolonged ACTH deficiency causes reversible adrenal insensitivity to trophic stimulation.

Send a blood specimen for plasma ACTH. If the plasma ACTH concentration is high, this confirms primary adrenal hypofunction. A low ACTH concentration suggests secondary adrenal hypofunction, and pituitary assessment is indicated (see Chapter 7).

If the diagnosis is still unclear, admit the patient to a hospital metabolic ward and perform a prolonged Synacthen test. A normal result excludes primary adrenal hypofunction.

An increasing response over time to the short and prolonged Synacthen tests indicates gradual recovery of the adrenal cortex and suggests hypothalamic or pituitary hypofunction (see Chapter 7).

Tetracosactrin (Synacthen) test of adrenal function

Tetracosactrin is marketed as Synacthen.

Short Synacthen stimulation test

Procedure
The patient should be resting quietly but not fasting. It is recommended that the test is done in the morning. Resuscitation facilities should be available in case of an allergic reaction.

Blood is taken for basal cortisol assay.

Synacthen 250 µg is given by intramuscular injection. Blood is taken for cortisol assay at baseline, 30 and 60 minutes.

Interpretation
Normally the plasma cortisol concentration increases by at least 200 nmol/L, to a concentration of at least 580 nmol/L. The peak is usually at 30 minutes, although a steady increase at 60 minutes may imply secondary hypoadrenalism due to pituitary or hypothalamic disease.

Depot or prolonged Synacthen stimulation test

Repeated injections of depot Synacthen are painful and may cause sodium and water retention. Therefore this test is contraindicated in patients in whom sodium retention may be dangerous, such as those with congestive cardiac failure. The test is rarely indicated if a basal plasma ACTH concentration is known. Its main indication is to differentiate primary from secondary adrenal insufficiency (due either to pituitary failure or to prolonged corticosteroid therapy) when adrenal failure has previously been confirmed by the short Synacthen test as above.

Procedure
Depot Synacthen 1 mg is given at 09.00 hours by intramuscular injection. Blood samples are then taken at baseline, 1, 2, 4, 8 and 24 hours for plasma cortisol concentration.

Interpretation
Plasma cortisol values are usually between 600 nmol/L and 1600 nmol/L.

The plasma cortisol concentrations should peak at 4–8 hours. A delayed response peaking at 24 hours or later is seen in secondary adrenal insufficiency (ACTH deficiency or corticosteroid treatment). Plasma cortisol <50 nmol/L suggests primary adrenal failure.

CORTICOSTEROID THERAPY

There is a risk of adrenocortical hypofunction when long-term corticosteroid treatment is stopped suddenly. This may be due either to secondary adrenal atrophy or to impaired ACTH release. Excess corticosteroid therapy may cause side-effects, including hypertension, hyperglycaemia and osteoporosis.

It is probably best to give the replacement hydrocortisone in three or more doses during the day. Plasma cortisol day curves may also be useful to help tailor the individual's dose of replacement glucocorticoid. Blood samples for cortisol can be collected during the day, aiming for a 09.00 hours cortisol of between 100 nmol/L and 700 nmol/L and in the afternoon ideally more than 100 nmol/L.

Some patients require glucocorticoid therapy, for example for acute episodes of asthma or inflammatory conditions such as rheumatoid arthritis, but then need their therapy withdrawn as their condition improves. The main concern is that the hypothalamic–pituitary–adrenal axis has been suppressed, thereby putting the patient at risk of an adrenal crisis. There are no universally agreed protocols to investigate this, but the following may be useful.

If therapy is short term, i.e. less than 3 weeks, and the prednisolone dose equivalent is not higher than 40 mg, the steroid can be stopped with little likelihood of problems. In cases where a higher dose of steroid equivalent has been used and for a longer time period, particularly if the steroid has been given in the evening or at night, gradual withdrawal is important until 7.5 mg/day is reached. Afterwards, the steroid dose should slowly be withdrawn at about 1 mg/day per month. Patients should be observed closely and made aware that after withdrawal they are at a small risk of adrenal insufficiency if they develop an infection or undergo surgery, in which case steroid should be resumed. If doubt persists once the steroids have been totally withdrawn, a short Synacthen test may reveal persistent adrenal insufficiency.

CONGENITAL ADRENAL HYPERPLASIA

The term congenital adrenal hyperplasia (CAH) embraces various defects involving enzymes of cortisol or aldosterone synthesis. Many of the enzymes involved in cortisol and aldosterone pathways are cytochrome p450 proteins designated CYP. CYP21 refers to 21-α-hydroxylase, CYP11B1 refers to 11-β-hydroxylase and CYP17 to 17-α-hydroxylase.

All forms of CAH are rare. An inherited deficiency (usually autosomal recessive) of one of the enzymes involved in the biosynthesis of cortisol, with a low plasma concentration, causes a high rate of secretion of ACTH from the anterior pituitary gland (Fig. 8.4). This results in hyperplasia of the adrenal cortex, with increased synthesis of cortisol precursors before the enzyme block. The precursors may then be metabolized by alternative pathways, such as those of androgen synthesis.

Increased androgen production may cause:

- *female pseudohermaphroditism*, by affecting the development of the female genitalia in utero; ambiguous genitalia may show phallic enlargement, clitoromegaly and early pubic hair;
- *virilization in childhood*, with phallic enlargement in either sex, development of pubic hair and a rapid growth rate;
- *milder virilization in females* at or after puberty, with amenorrhoea.

All female infants with ambiguous genitalia should have plasma electrolytes estimated. In male infants with no obvious physical abnormalities the diagnosis of CAH may not be suspected.

The commonest form of CAH is CYP21 deficiency, which accounts for about 90 per cent of cases. Females have ambiguous genitalia at birth (classical) or later in adolescence (non-classical with milder enzyme deficiency) and become virilized. Males with CYP21 deficiency are not usually diagnosed in the neonatal period, as their genitalia are normal. However, if severe, the infant may present with salt wasting with vomiting, dehydration, failure to thrive and shock. Aldosterone synthesis may be

CASE 3

A 14-year-old female with primary amenorrhoea presented to endocrine out-patients. Physical examination revealed hirsutism and clitoromegaly. Some of her biochemistry tests were as follows.

Plasma
Sodium 132 mmol/L (135–145)
Potassium 5.6 mmol/L (3.5–5.0)
Urea 3.7 mmol/L (2.5–7.5)
Creatinine 101 μmol/L (60–120)
09.00 hours cortisol 128 nmol/L (180–720)
Thyroid-stimulating hormone 1.5 mU/L (0.20–5.0)
Free thyroxine 13.5 pmol/L (12–25)
Prolactin 244 mU/L (<470)
Luteinizing hormone 5.2 U/L (1–25)
Follicle-stimulating hormone 4.3 U/L (1–15)
Testosterone 6.2 nmol/L (1–3)
Sex-hormone-binding globulin 48 nmol/L (20–90)
Oestradiol 464 pmol/L (70–880)
17-hydroxyprogesterone 85 nmol/L (<35)

DISCUSSION

The results are suggestive of CAH. Note the raised plasma 17-hydroxyprogesterone and testosterone concentrations. The patient was eventually found to have 21-α-hydroxylase deficiency, which was confirmed with a 24-hour urinary steroid profile and genetic tests. Raised adrenal androgen concentrations help to explain her hirsutism and clitoromegaly. Note also the hyponatraemia and hyperkalaemia.

markedly reduced in more than half of the infants with 21-α-hydroxylase deficiency and may cause an Addisonian-like picture with marked renal sodium loss during the first few weeks of life. Volume depletion may be accompanied by hyponatraemia and hyperkalaemia. Even if plasma sodium concentrations are within the reference range, demonstrably increased plasma renin activity may suggest lesser degrees of sodium and water depletion.

CYP11B1 deficiency may also present with female ambiguous genitalia and salt loss. The child may, however, show hypertension and a hypokalaemic alkalosis. The enzyme CYP11B1 catalyses the conversion of 11-deoxycortisol to cortisol in the glucocorticoid pathway and the conversion of deoxycorticosterone to corticosterone in the mineralocorticoid pathway. CYP11B2 or aldosterone synthetase deficiency results in hyponatraemia and hyperkalaemia, although normal sexual differentiation occurs, as sex steroids are normal.

In CYP17 deficiency, ambiguous genitalia or female genitalia may be observed in male infants. A female with CYP17 deficiency appears phenotypically female at birth but will fail to develop breasts or menstruate due to inadequate oestradiol production. Hypertension due to raised deoxycorticosterone concentration may be present in CYP17 deficiency.

Diagnosis

Only the principles of the diagnosis of 21-α-hydroxylase deficiency are outlined here (see Fig. 8.4).

17-Hydroxyprogesterone can only be metabolized by the cortisol pathway in the presence of 21-α-hydroxylase, and plasma concentrations are raised in patients with CAH. In some cases a short Synacthen test may reveal elevated plasma 17-hydroxyprogesterone concentrations after stimulation. This test may be useful, as sometimes baseline elevation of cortisol precursors may be within the normal range. Those with abnormalities of 21-α-hydroxylase deficiency often show post-Synacthen 17-hydroxyprogesterone values more than 35 nmol/L. However, those with either 11-β-hydroxylase or other enzyme deficiencies may show a normal response.

Plasma androstenedione concentrations may be raised in those patients with excessive androgen synthesis. Some indication of which enzyme is deficient may be suggested by evaluating the pattern of steroid excretion in a random or 24-hour urine sample.

In 11-β-hydroxylase deficiency there is a raised concentration of 24-hour urinary tetrahydrocortisol, a metabolite of 11-deoxycortisol, and raised deoxycorticosterone concentration. In the salt-losing forms,

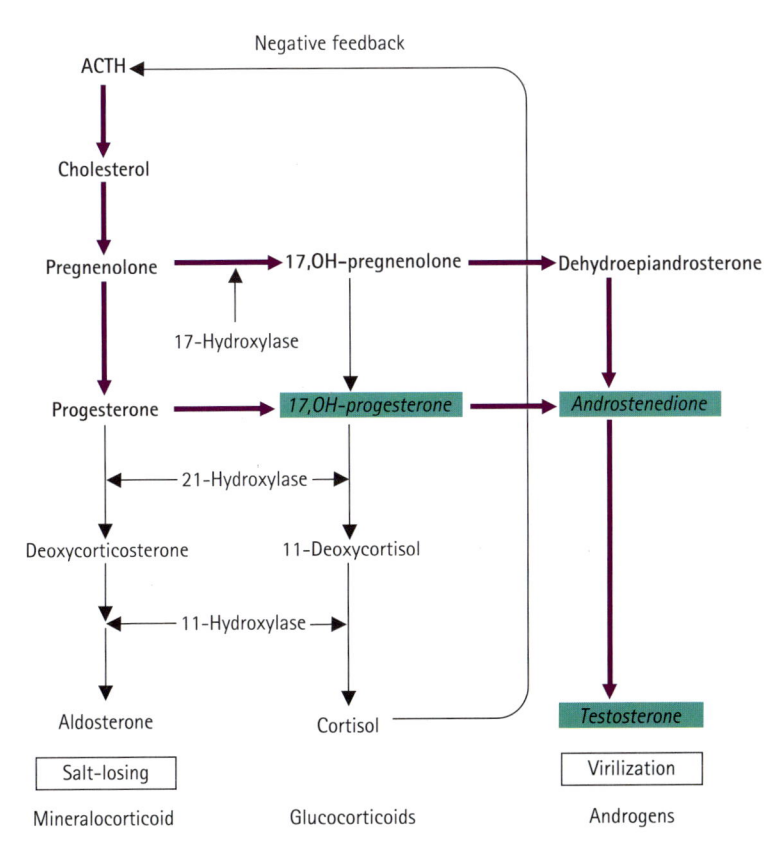

Fig. 8.4 The abnormalities occurring in congenital adrenal hyperplasia. The substances highlighted are of diagnostic importance; those shown in bold are increased in 21-α-hydoxylase deficiency. (ACTH = adrenocorticotrophic hormone.)

plasma renin and aldosterone concentrations may assist diagnosis.

If a diagnosis of CAH is confirmed, genetic counselling may be necessary, with DNA and family studies.

Treatment

Congenital adrenal hyperplasia is treated by giving a glucocorticoid, for example hydrocortisone, and, if necessary, a mineralocorticoid, for example fludrocortisone. This treatment not only replaces the deficient hormones but, by negative feedback, also suppresses ACTH secretion and therefore androgen production.

Measuring 17-hydroxyprogesterone and androstenedione concentrations in plasma or saliva enables treatment efficacy to be monitored. Salivary steroid concentrations correlate well with those in plasma, and saliva collection may be more acceptable to some patients than repeated venepuncture. Measuring the plasma renin activity may help assess mineralocorticoid replacement.

PRIMARY HYPERALDOSTERONISM (CONN'S SYNDROME)

Primary hyperaldosteronism (PH) is considered an important cause of secondary hypertension in perhaps as many as 5–15 per cent of cases, particularly in the face of hypokalaemia and kaliuria (e.g. urinary potassium more than 20 mmol/L). (See Chapter 5 for a discussion of hypokalaemia.)

The majority of cases of PH are due to adrenal aldosterone-producing adenomas (APAs), which produce 18-oxocortisol and 18-hydroxycortisol steroids in excess, although 45 per cent of cases may be due to bilateral idiopathic adrenal hyperplasia (IAH). There is also a genetic–familial variety of PH. Type 1 familial PH is glucocorticoid remediable aldosteronism (GRA), in which the associated hypertension responds to small doses of glucocorticoids in addition to antihypertensives. This condition is due to a chimeric gene product that combines the promoter of the 11-β-hydroxylase gene with the coding region of the aldosterone synthetase gene and is associated with haemorrhagic stroke.

The treatment of IAH is usually medical and the mineralocorticoid antagonist spironolactone has proved useful, sometimes in conjunction with a thiazide diuretic. The treatment of choice for unilateral variants of PH such as APA is usually surgical by adrenalectomy.

Investigation of a patient with suspected primary hyperaldosteronism

Screening tests

Hypertension and a hypokalaemic metabolic alkalosis in the face of kaliuria (urinary potassium more than 20 mmol/L) are suggestive of mineralocorticoid excess such as Conn's syndrome. A urinary potassium is thus a useful screening test. Ideally, the patient should not have taken diuretics or antihypertensive drugs for a few weeks (although this may not be safe in patients with uncontrolled severe hypertension), as they can interfere with aldosterone and renin concentrations.

In PH, plasma aldosterone concentration will be raised, with suppressed renin levels. Remember that in renal artery stenosis, Bartter's or Gitelman's syndromes, renin-secreting tumours and pseudohypoaldosteronism, both plasma

CASE 4

A 35-year-old male attended the hospital hypertension clinic (presenting blood pressure 184/100 mmHg) with the following results (off antihypertensive medication).

Plasma
Sodium 144 mmol/L (135–145)
Potassium 2.9 mmol/L (3.5–5.0)
Urea 3.4 mmol/L (2.5–7.5)
Creatinine 102 μmol/L (60–120)
Bicarbonate 40 mmol/L (24–32)

A spot urinary potassium was 63 mmol/L.

A random plasma aldosterone:renin activity ratio was 984 min/L (more than 750 min/L is suggestive of Conn's syndrome).

DISCUSSION
The results suggest Conn's syndrome (primary hyperaldosteronism). Note the hypertension, hypokalaemia and urinary potassium greater than 20 mmol/L. The patient also had a metabolic alkalosis. Further investigations, including adrenal imaging, showed an adrenal adenoma.

aldosterone and renin concentrations may be raised. Antihypertensive drugs may interfere with renin and aldosterone levels but in some cases it may not be safe to stop them, although if there is severe hypertension, α-adrenergic blockers may interfere less than other antihypertensives.

A random plasma aldosterone:renin ratio more than 750, where aldosterone is expressed in pmol/L and renin activity in μg/L per hour, is suggestive of PH and may be used as a screening test. A raised 24-hour urinary aldosterone excretion may also be a useful screening tool.

Further tests for the diagnosis of hyperaldosteronism

Sometimes dynamic tests are needed to confirm the diagnosis of PH, although in many cases the diagnosis may be obvious. The basis of these additional tests is that in PH aldosterone secretion is autonomous and thus not suppressed by physiological or pharmaceutical stimuli.

One test is the captopril test (a single oral dose of 25–50 mg), which normally suppresses plasma aldosterone levels in healthy individuals after about 2 hours, but which does not do so in PH. Captopril is an angiotensin-converting enzyme inhibitor.

Alternatively, other dynamic tests that have been used are saline-infusion, or salt-loading, tests, including the fludrocortisone suppression test. However, these tests are not without risk, as blood pressure can rise during them. Patients may need to be hospitalized during these tests as they may evoke severe hypertension.

Saline infusion test

Patients are given intravenous 0.90 per cent isotonic saline, infused over a 4-hour period. They are usually in the supine position. Plasma aldosterone is measured at baseline and 4 hours afterwards. In PH there is a failure to suppress the plasma aldosterone.

Fludrocortisone suppression test

On day 1 the plasma aldosterone is measured. Then fludrocortisone 0.1 mg is given 6-hourly for 4 days, with three tablets of 10 mmol/L slow sodium 8-hourly also for 4 days. Slow potassium tablets are also given, to maintain a normal potassium concentration during the test period.

On day 4, plasma aldosterone is measured again. Primary hyperaldosteronism is excluded if suppression of plasma aldosterone occurs.

Tests to diagnose the cause of primary hyperaldosteronism

An investigation that is sometimes useful is the postural test, which aims to distinguish between APAs and IAH. With the former there is usually a fall in plasma aldosterone on standing. Patients should be normovolaemic and have a daily sodium intake of about 100 mmol. After they have been kept recumbent for at least 8 hours, blood is taken for plasma electrolyte, renin and aldosterone assays. They then walk around for 30 minutes and a further blood sample is taken for repeat plasma renin activity and aldosterone assays.

Interpretation

The diagnosis can only be made if the plasma aldosterone concentration is high and the renin activity inappropriately low for the aldosterone concentration; the latter does not increase significantly after 30 minutes' walking around. Plasma aldosterone concentration increases after ambulation in adrenal hyperplasia (as angiotensin II responsive) and falls when there is an adrenal adenoma.

Another biochemical assay that may help distinguish adenomas from hyperplasia is based on the fact that concentrations of plasma 18-hydroxy-corticosterone are raised in adrenal adenomas compared with adrenal hyperplasia. The rare renin-responsive aldostesterone-producing adenoma, unlike APA, shows an increased plasma aldosterone concentration on ambulation.

If familial type 1 PH (GRA) is suspected from the family history, a dexamethasone suppression test (1–2 mg/day) may show improvement in blood pressure as well as suppression of plasma aldosterone concentration.

Diagnostic imaging of the adrenals by MRI or CT scanning may demonstrate adrenal adenoma or bilateral hyperplasia but gives no functional information. However, remember that 10 per cent of normal individuals may have false-positive results due to non-functioning adrenal lesions. Adrenal scintigraphy using radiolabelled iodomethyl-19 norcholesterol may also be useful to locate the adrenals. Sometimes, measuring aldosterone and renin concentrations in adrenal vein sampling may help localize the adrenal pathology, although this carries a risk of adrenal infarction. Lateralized aldosterone over-production is confirmed if the aldosterone:cortisol ratio in one adrenal vein when divided by that in the contralateral vein is more than about 4.

Treatment

Adrenal adenomas producing aldosterone are usually surgically removed, sometimes by laparoscopic adrenalectomy.

Hyperplasia of the adrenals can be treated with amiloride or spironolactone. Eplerenone is a selective aldosterone receptor antagonist, which may prove useful in preference to spironolactone. The glucocorticoid-remediable form of aldosteronism may respond to dexamethasone.

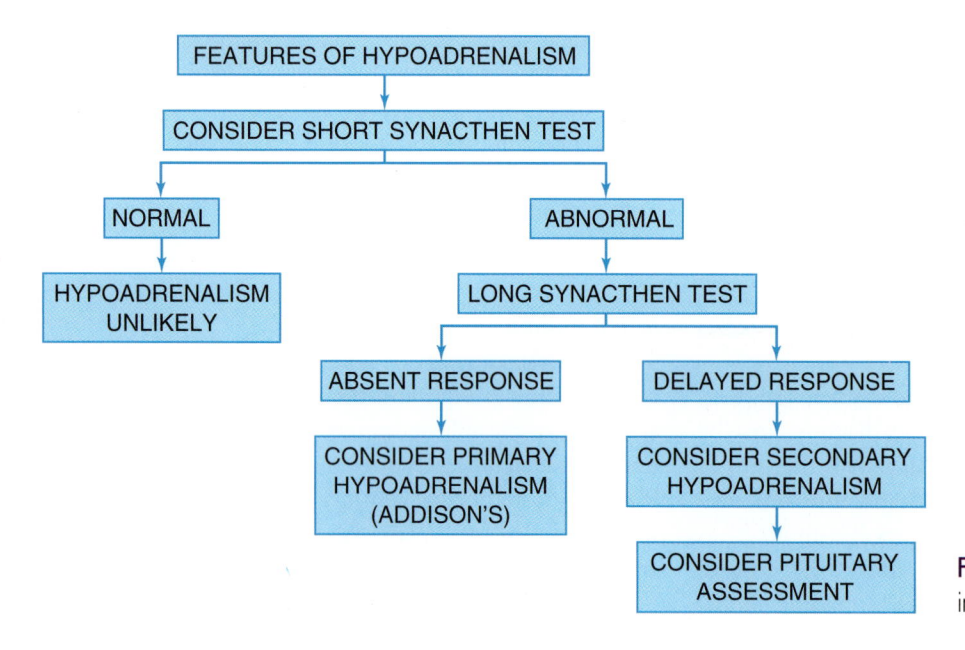

Fig. 8.5 Algorithm for the investigation of hypoadrenalism.

CONCLUSIONS

This chapter discusses adrenal cortex steroid biochemistry and abnormalities of adrenal cortical function and how clinical biochemistry tests can be used in their diagnosis and management. Disorders of the adrenal medulla are discussed in Chapter 24. The algorithms in Figs 8.5–8.7 summarize the investigation of adrenal insufficiency, Cushing's syndrome and hyperaldosteronism.

- The adrenal cortex produces three major groups of hormones: glucocorticoids, mineralocorticoids and androgens.
- Cortisol, a glucocorticoid, is a stress hormone involved in metabolism. It is controlled by pituitary ACTH.
- Aldosterone is a mineralocorticoid involved in sodium retention and potassium excretion via the kidneys. Aldosterone is controlled by the renin–angiotensin axis.
- Cushing's syndrome is due to the over-production of adrenal cortex hormones and can be due to excess ACTH from the pituitary (Cushing's disease) or ectopic ACTH release from certain tumours. Other causes include adrenal tumours, hyperplasia and excess glucocorticoid intake. Cushing's syndrome may result in hypertension, glucose intolerance, hypokalaemia, weight increase and mood changes.
- Adrenal insufficiency is due to reduced adrenal cortex hormone production; this can be due to autoimmune disease or to adrenal gland infiltration. Adrenal failure may be associated with weakness, hypotension, hyponatraemia and hyperkalaemia and is life threatening.
- Congenital adrenal hyperplasia, most commonly due to 21-α-hydroxylase deficiency, results in glucocorticoid and mineralocorticoid under-production but an excess of adrenal androgens.
- Excess adrenal mineralocorticoid production can result in hypertension, metabolic alkalosis and hypokalaemia such as Conn's syndrome.

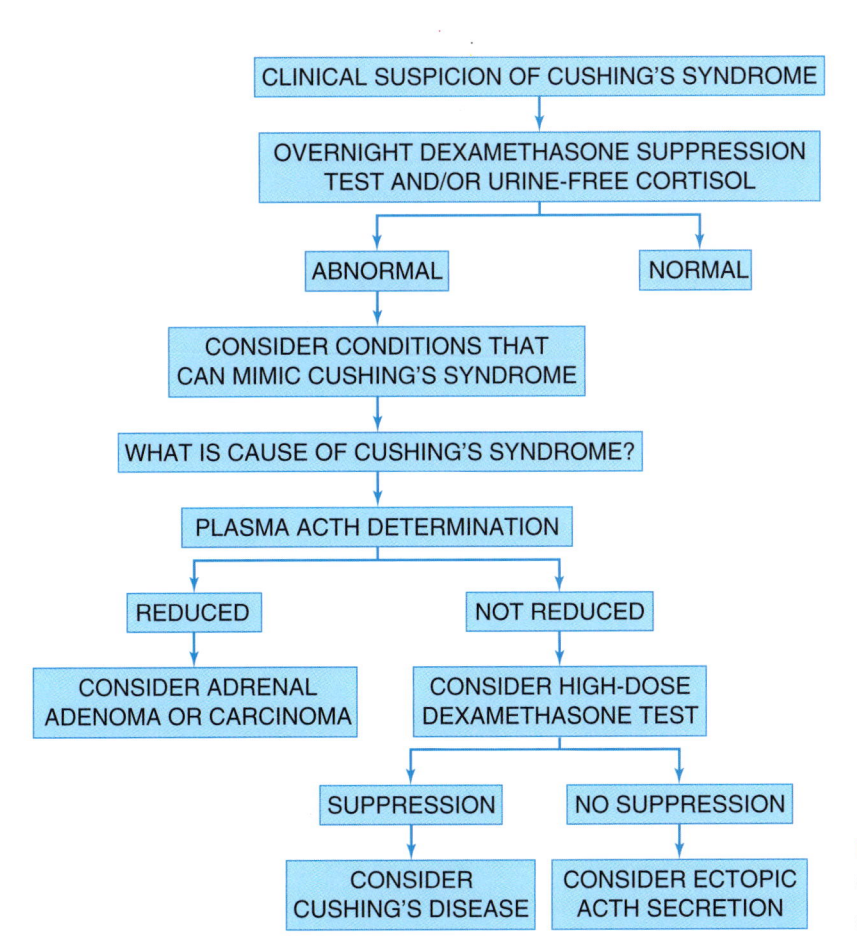

Fig. 8.6 Algorithm for the investigation of Cushing's syndrome. (ACTH = adrenocorticotrophic hormone.)

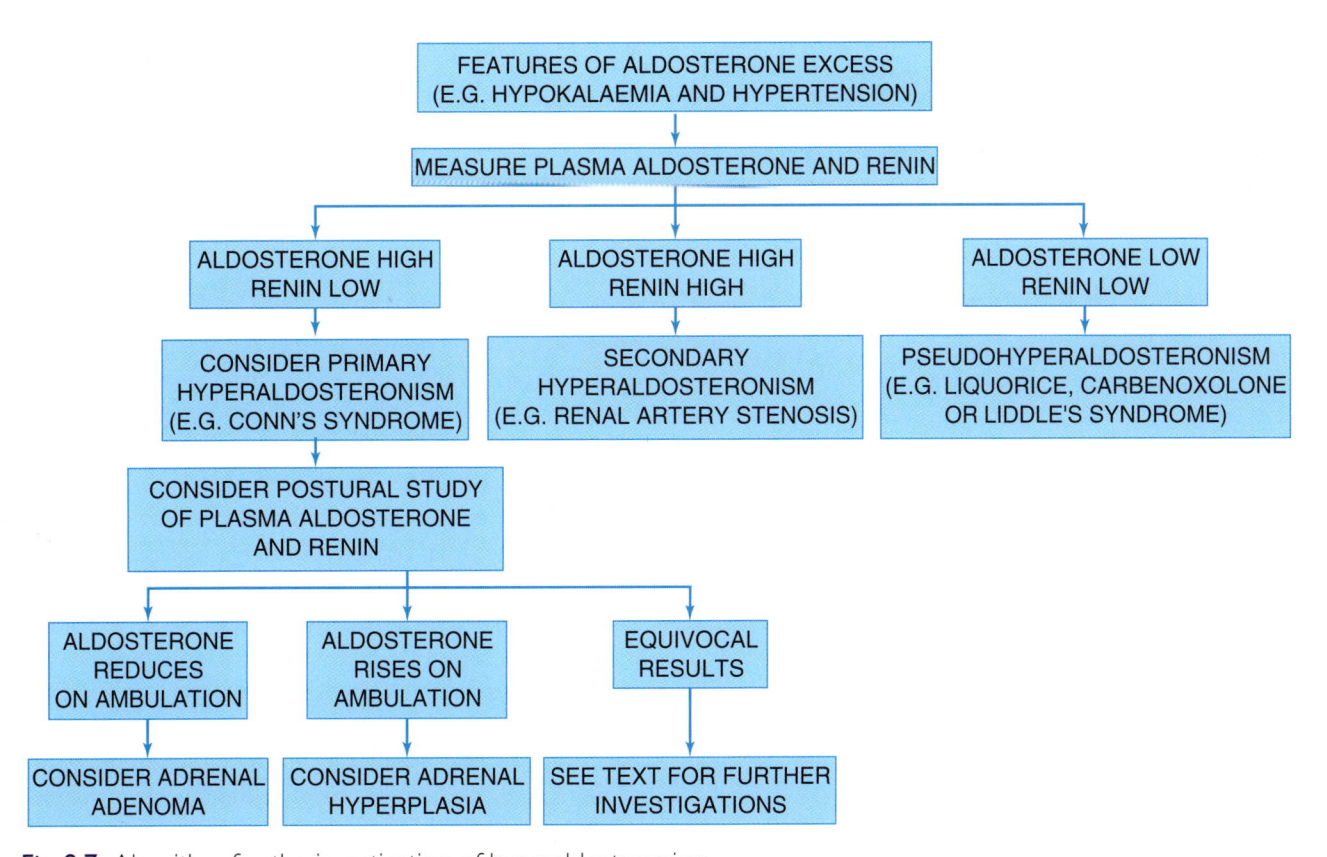

Fig. 8.7 Algorithm for the investigation of hyperaldosteronism.

9 THE REPRODUCTIVE SYSTEM

Hypothalamic–pituitary–gonadal axis	144	Other disorders of reproductive organs	153
Hyperprolactinaemia	146	Biochemical investigation of gonadal disorders	153
Sexual development from conception in females and males	147		

The study of the endocrinology of the male and female reproductive systems is a specialized field and overlaps with urology, obstetrics and gynaecology. This chapter looks at some of the commoner conditions that you are likely to encounter clinically and that have particular relevance to clinical biochemistry. Pregnancy and infertility are discussed in Chapter 10.

HYPOTHALAMIC–PITUITARY–GONADAL AXIS

The reproductive system is responsible not only for the production of hormones, but also for maturation of the germ cells in the gonads. It is important to understand the relationship between hormones with respect to these two functions if the results of reproductive endocrinology tests are to be interpreted correctly.

Hypothalamic hormones

The hypothalamus secretes two hormones concerned with the reproductive system: gonadotrophin-releasing hormone (GnRH), which regulates the secretion of the pituitary gonadotrophins, luteinizing hormone (LH) and follicle-stimulating hormone (FSH); and dopamine, a neurotransmitter, which also controls prolactin secretion (see Chapter 7).

Anterior pituitary hormones

The gonadotrophins (LH and FSH), secreted by pituitary basophil cells, control the function and secretion of hormones by the testes and ovaries. The secretion of GnRH is pulsatile and thus so, in turn, is that of LH and FSH. Although there is only one releasing hormone, secretion of LH and FSH does not always occur in parallel and may be modified by feedback from the circulating concentrations of gonadal androgens or oestrogens. The actions of the gonadotrophins are:

- LH primarily stimulates the production of hormones by the gonads,
- FSH stimulates the development of the germ cells.

Gonadotrophin analogues, for example goserelin, after an initial stimulation phase, down-regulate gonadotrophin secretion and have been used therapeutically for prostate carcinoma and endometriosis.

Prolactin, secreted by acidophil cells, is important during pregnancy and the postpartum period. It stimulates breast epithelial cell proliferation and induces milk production. Prolactin differs from all other pituitary hormones in its method of control. Secretion is inhibited, not stimulated, by dopamine; therefore, impairment of hypothalamic control causes hyperprolactinaemia. Its secretion is regulated by a short feedback loop between pituitary prolactin and hypothalamic dopamine via dopamine-2-type receptors.

Oestrogens stimulate the proliferation of pituitary lactotroph cells, although high oestrogen and progesterone concentrations inhibit secretion, as in pregnancy. Circulating prolactin concentrations are normally higher in pregnancy and increase during suckling as a result of the action of vasoactive intestinal peptide. Although thyrotrophin-releasing hormone (TRH) stimulates the secretion of prolactin, as well as of thyroid-stimulating hormone (TSH), this action does not seem to be of physiological importance; it may, however, be important in pathological conditions. Similar factors affect prolactin and growth hormone secretion. Secretion of both is pulsatile and increases during sleep and in response to physical and psychological stress.

Ovarian hormones

Oestrogens, progesterone and androgens are secreted by the ovarian follicles of the ovaries, which consist of germ cells (ova) surrounded by granulosa and theca cells. Androgens (C19 steroids), synthesized by theca cells, are converted into oestrogens (C18 steroids) in the granulosa cells, a process that involves aromatization of the A ring and the loss of the C-19 methyl group (Fig. 9.1). Oestradiol is the most important ovarian oestrogen. The liver and subcutaneous fat convert ovarian and adrenal androgens to oestrone. Both oestradiol and oestrone are metabolized to the relatively inactive oestriol. Oestrogens are essential for the development of female secondary sex characteristics and for normal menstruation, and their concentration in plasma in children is very low. Androstenedione is the main androgen secreted by the ovaries. It is converted to oestrone and to the more active testosterone in extra-ovarian tissue. A small amount of testosterone is secreted directly by the ovaries. Plasma concentrations in women are about a tenth of those in men.

Progesterone is secreted by the corpus luteum during the luteal phase of the menstrual cycle and by the placenta. It prepares the endometrium of the uterus to receive a fertilized ovum and is necessary for the maintenance of early pregnancy. It also is pyrogenic and increases the basal body temperature. In plasma, only about 2 per cent of progesterone is unbound or free, the majority being bound to albumin and transcortin.

Testicular hormones

Testosterone is secreted by the Leydig cells, which lie in the interstitial tissue of the testes between the seminiferous tubules. The production of testosterone is stimulated by LH and it, in turn, inhibits LH secretion by negative feedback. Inhibin is a hormone produced by the Sertoli cells, part of the basement membrane of the seminiferous tubules, during germ cell differentiation and spermatogenesis. These processes require testosterone and are stimulated by FSH. Inhibin controls FSH secretion by negative feedback (Fig. 9.2). Testosterone is involved in sexual differentiation, the development of secondary sexual characteristics,

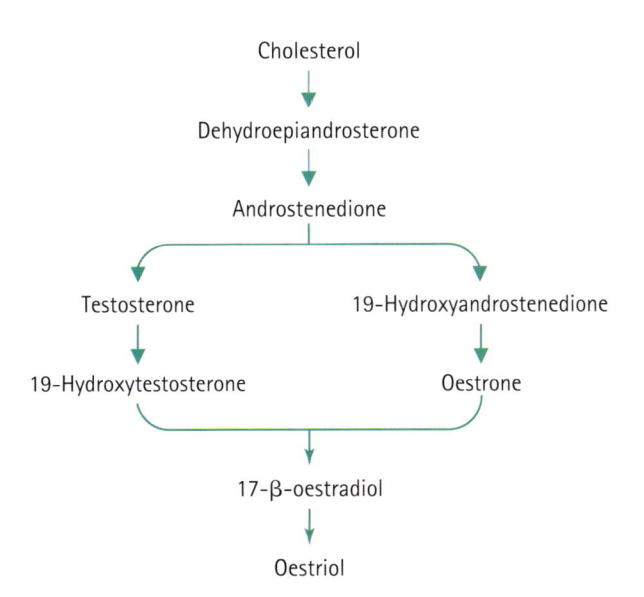

Cholesterol
↓
Dehydroepiandrosterone
↓
Androstenedione
↓
Testosterone   19-Hydroxyandrostenedione
↓   ↓
19-Hydroxytestosterone   Oestrone
↓
17-β-oestradiol
↓
Oestriol

Fig. 9.1 Pathways of sex hormone synthesis. (In this summary an arrow does not necessarily represent a single reaction.) (Reproduced with kind permission from Candlish JK and Crook M, *Notes on Clinical Biochemistry*, Singapore: World Scientific Publishing, 1993.)

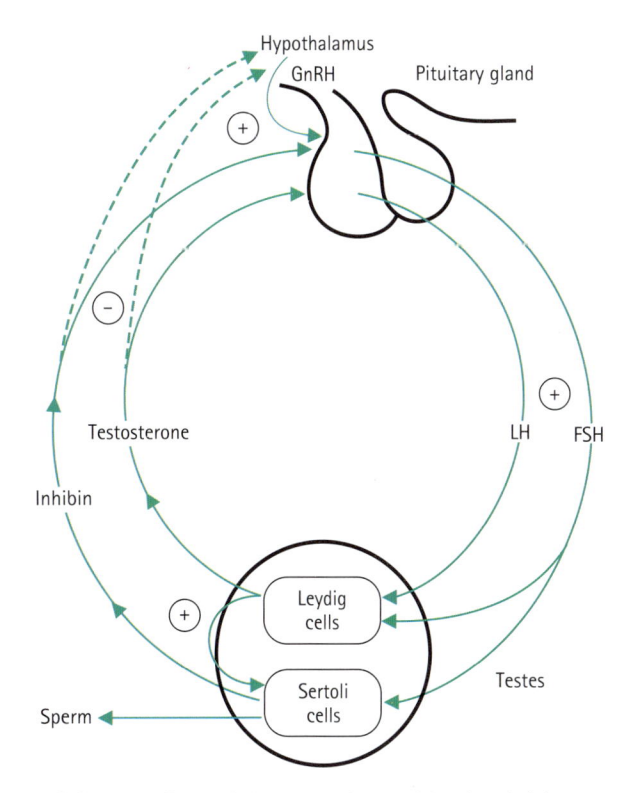

Fig. 9.2 The effect of the gonadotrophins luteinizing hormone (LH) and follicle-stimulating hormone (FSH) on testicular function. (GnRH = gonadotrophin-releasing hormone.)

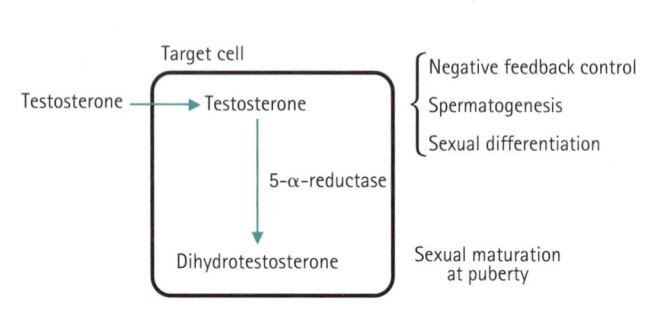

Fig. 9.3 The relationship between the biological actions of testosterone and dihydrotestosterone.

spermatogenesis and anabolism. In the male, the effects of testosterone depend on intracellular conversion to the even more potent androgen dihydrotestosterone by the enzyme 5-α-reductase in target cells (Fig. 9.3).

Luteinizing hormone stimulates testosterone production from the Leydig cells. The Sertoli cells are involved in germ cell differentiation and spermatogenesis. These functions depend on testosterone and are stimulated by FSH.

Sex-hormone-binding globulin

Testosterone and, to a lesser extent, oestradiol circulate bound to a carrier protein, sex-hormone-binding globulin (SHBG), as well as to albumin. As with other hormones, only the free or unbound fraction (about 3 per cent of the total hormone concentration) is metabolically active. Plasma SHBG levels in females are about twice those in males. Changes in SHBG concentrations change the ratio of free testosterone to free oestrogen (see Table 9.1, p. 151).

HYPERPROLACTINAEMIA

This is an important cause of amenorrhoea, sexual dysfunction and infertility. High plasma prolactin concentrations inhibit the normal pulsatile release of GnRH and inhibit gonadal steroid hormone synthesis directly. Plasma gonadotrophin and oestrogen concentrations are therefore low and the symptoms of oestrogen deficiency may occur. About a third of patients with hyperprolactinaemia have galactorrhoea.

The finding of hyperprolactinaemia should be interpreted with caution. As mentioned above, plasma prolactin concentration is raised during pregnancy and lactation. Samples for prolactin estimations should be taken at least 2–3 hours after waking in order to eliminate the misleading elevated plasma concentrations found during sleep; the stress of venepuncture may also cause prolactin secretion. A sustained increase of more than about 700 mU/L should be investigated. Macroprolactinaemia, in which the raised plasma prolactin concentration is due to a complex with immunoglobulins, should be excluded, usually by being precipitated in the plasma sample by polyethylene glycol, before extensive investigation is undertaken for true hyperprolactinaemia.

Hypothyroidism, polycystic ovary syndrome and chronic renal failure can also evoke hyperprolactinaemia. The pathological causes of hyperprolactinaemia include a prolactin-secreting tumour of the pituitary gland. If a

CASE 1

A 34-year-old female was seen in the endocrine clinic because of galactorrhoea and oligomennorhoea. She was not taking any medication, and her renal function, liver function and blood glucose were normal. Her plasma biochemical results were as follows.

Thyroid-stimulating hormone 1.6 mU/L (0.20–5.0)
Free thyroxine 13.1 pmol/L (12–25)
Prolactin 2264 mU/L (<470)
Luteinizing hormone 7.2 U/L (1–25)
Follicle-stimulating hormone 4.4 U/L (1–15)
Testosterone 2.2 nmol/L (1–3)
Sex-hormone-binding globulin 58 nmol/L (20–90)
Oestradiol 544 pmol/L (70–880)

DISCUSSION
The patient has hyperprolactinaemia, with a common presentation. A pituitary magnetic resonance imaging scan was suggestive of a microprolactinoma (microadenoma). The other pituitary hormones are normal, presumably because the microprolactinoma had not encroached on the pituitary gland. Dopamine receptor agonists such as bromocriptine or cabergoline have been used to lower prolactin concentration under these circumstances.

pituitary tumour is found, it is usually either a microadenoma (less than 10 mm) or a macroadenoma (more than 10 mm). The higher the plasma prolactin concentration, the greater the likelihood that a tumour is present, with concentrations more than 2000 mU/L suggestive of hypothalamic or microadenoma, whereas concentrations more than 6000 mU/L are more likely to indicate a macroadenoma. The latter are sometimes associated with multiple endocrine neoplasia (MEN1) syndrome (see Chapter 24).

If hyperprolactinaemia is confirmed, pregnancy must be excluded, and also renal impairment, hypothyroidism and polycystic ovary syndrome. Pituitary imaging with computerized tomography or magnetic resonance imaging may show a tumour. Dopamine receptor agonists such as bromocriptine or cabergoline are used to lower prolactin concentrations. Sometimes pituitary surgery is needed to remove a pituitary tumour.

The causes of hyperprolactinaemia are shown in Box 9.1 and a diagnostic algorithm in Fig. 9.4.

Box 9.1 Some causes of hyperprolactinaemia

Physiological, e.g. stress or pregnancy
Failure of hypothalamic inhibitory factors to reach the anterior pituitary gland:
　damage to the pituitary stalk by non-prolactin-secreting tumours of the pituitary gland or hypothalamus
　surgical section of the pituitary stalk
Other pituitary tumours, e.g.:
　microadenomas
　macroadenomas
Drugs, e.g.:
　oestrogens
　dopaminergic antagonists, e.g.:
　phenothiazines
　haloperidol
　metoclopramide
　methyldopa
　reserpine
Polycystic ovary syndrome
Chronic renal failure (due to reduced plasma clearance)
Severe primary hypothyroidism (due to anterior pituitary stimulation by high thyrotrophin-releasing hormone concentrations).
Macroprolactinaemia

SEXUAL DEVELOPMENT FROM CONCEPTION IN FEMALES AND MALES

The complex series of events leading to the development of sexual competence depends on many steps occurring at the correct time. The following simplified account aims to provide a background for the discussion of abnormalities of the system.

Chromosomal sex is determined at fertilization by the chromosomes present in the ovum and sperm, each of which contributes 22 autosomes and one sex chromosome, X or Y. Normal males have a 46,XY karyotype, and normal females 46,XX. Abnormalities occurring at this stage may result in defective gonadal development, as occurs in Klinefelter's syndrome in males (47,XXY) or Turner's syndrome in females (45,XO).

The sex chromosomes determine whether the primitive gonads become testes or ovaries. The development and disorders of gonadal function in the male and female are considered separately below.

The female

Development of female characteristics

In the absence of a Y chromosome, the fetus starts to develop female characteristics at about 12 weeks of gestation. If androgens are produced at this stage, as, for example, in congenital adrenal hyperplasia (CAH), masculinization of the external genitalia may occur, causing female pseudohermaphroditism (see Chapter 8). Proliferation of fetal germ cells produces several million oocytes. By late fetal life, all the germ cells have degenerated and no more oocytes can be produced. Those oocytes that are present enter the first stage of meiosis and their numbers decline throughout the rest of the intrauterine period and childhood; the inability to replenish them explains the limit to the span of reproductive life in women, in contrast to the continuous ability of men to produce sperm. An abnormally high rate of decline leads to premature menopause.

Female puberty

At the onset of puberty, gonadotrophin secretion increases, as it does in the male. Ovarian oestrogen secretion rises and

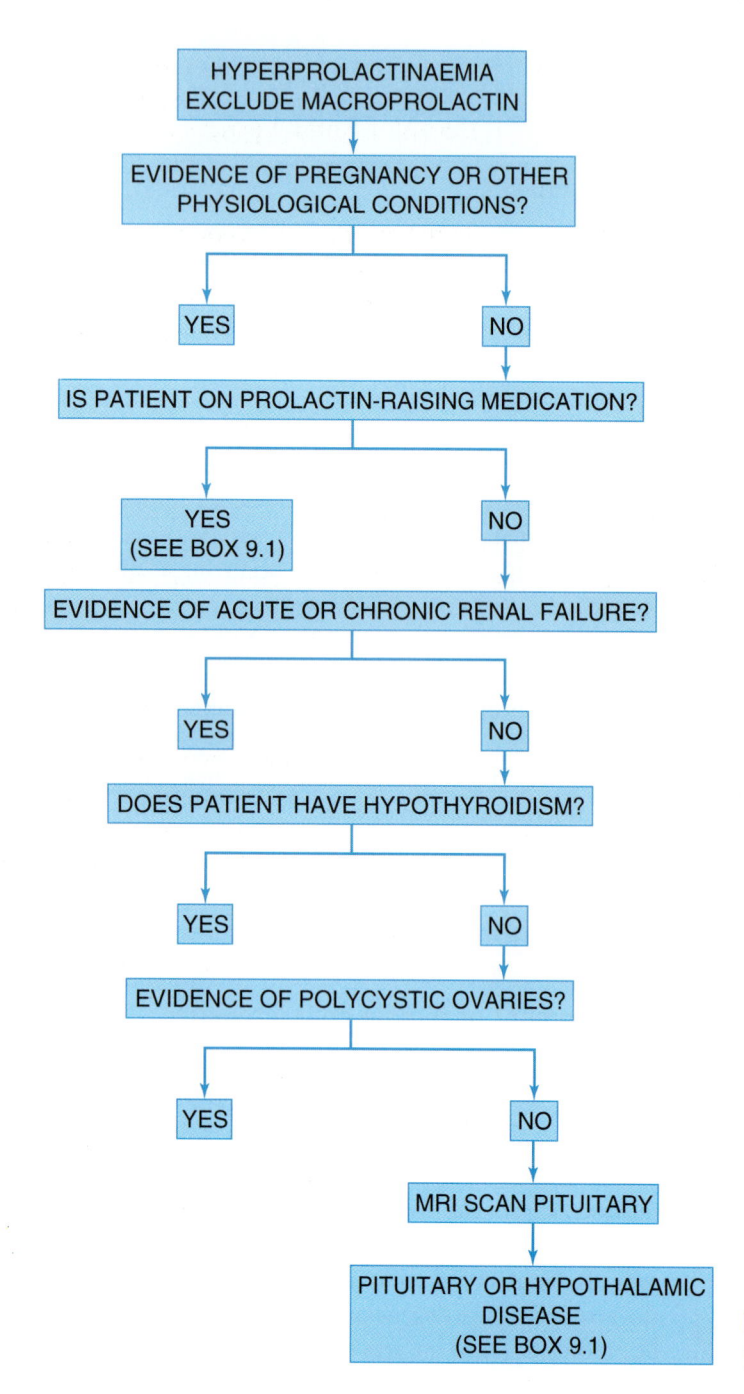

Fig. 9.4 An algorithm for the investigation of hyperprolactinaemia.

stimulates the development of female secondary sex characteristics and the onset of menstruation (menarche).

Normal gonadal function

At puberty the ovaries contain between 100 000 and 200 000 primordial follicles. During each menstrual cycle a small number develop, but usually only one reaches maturation, with extrusion of the ovum from the ovary (ovulation), and is ready for fertilization. The menstrual cycle is regulated by changing hormone concentrations (Fig. 9.5) and by changing sensitivity of ovarian tissue.

Follicular (preovulatory) phase

At the beginning of the menstrual cycle, ovarian follicles are undeveloped and plasma oestradiol concentrations are low. The secretion of LH and FSH increases because of diminished negative feedback by oestrogens. Together, LH and FSH cause the growth of a group of follicles. By about the seventh day of the cycle, one follicle becomes especially sensitive to FSH and matures, while the rest atrophy. Luteinizing hormone also stimulates oestradiol secretion, the plasma concentrations of which rise steadily. This stimulates the regeneration of the endometrium.

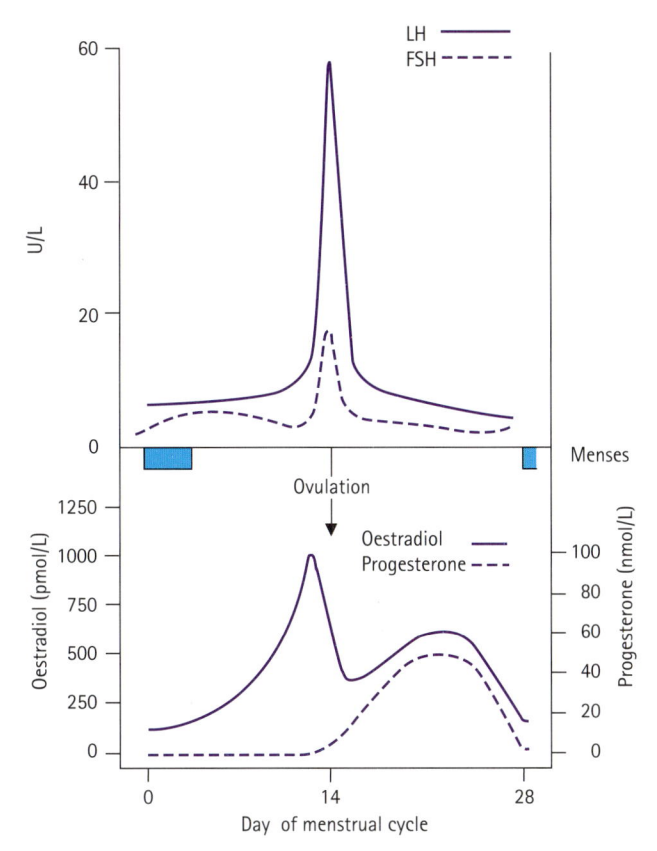

Fig. 9.5 An example of plasma hormone concentrations during the menstrual cycle. (LH = luteinizing hormone; FSH = follicle-stimulating hormone.)

Ovulation

The rapid development of the dominant follicle and the rise in plasma oestradiol concentration trigger a surge of LH release from the anterior pituitary gland by positive feedback. Ovulation occurs about 16 hours later.

Luteal (postovulatory or secretory) phase

After ovulation, the high LH concentration stimulates the granulosa cells of the ruptured follicle to luteinize and to form the corpus luteum, which synthesizes and secretes progesterone and oestradiol. Progesterone is the principal hormone of the luteal phase and prepares the endometrium for the implantation of the fertilized ovum. If the ovum is not fertilized, the corpus luteum regresses and plasma ovarian hormone concentrations fall; the menstrual cycle takes its course, with sloughing of the endometrium and menstrual bleeding. As the plasma ovarian hormone concentrations fall, the concentrations of LH and FSH in plasma begin to rise and the cycle recommences. If fertilization does occur, pregnancy may supervene (see Chapter 10).

Interpretation of plasma sex hormone concentrations must be made in relation to the stage of the cycle. It may be important to establish whether a patient who is complaining of infertility has ovulated, either spontaneously or as a result of treatment to induce ovulation. The plasma progesterone concentration should be measured in a blood sample taken during the second half of the menstrual cycle. A value within the reference range for the time of the cycle is good presumptive evidence of ovulation (see Fig. 9.5), whereas a value in the range expected in the follicular phase indicates the absence of a corpus luteum, and therefore of ovulation. Ovulation may also be detected by ultrasound examination of the ovaries. Progesterone secretion is associated with a rise in body temperature, which may be monitored serially to determine the time of ovulation. Plasma prolactin concentrations do not change cyclically during the menstrual cycle.

The menopause

The menopause is defined as the time of permanent cessation of menstruation, the average age being about 50 years. The menopause occurs when all the follicles have atrophied. Plasma concentrations of oestrogens fall and those of FSH and, to a lesser extent, LH increase after removal of the negative feedback to the pituitary. These findings are therefore similar to those of primary gonadal failure.

It may sometimes be useful to measure plasma oestradiol concentrations in women with oestradiol hormone replacement therapy (HRT) implants, as very high levels may be associated with tachyphylaxis, i.e. tolerance to dose. There may also be a place for its measurement in women on transdermal oestradiol HRT to ensure adequate absorption. Otherwise, measuring plasma oestradiol is not generally useful, as the results depend upon the type of oestrogen used in the HRT preparation.

Disorders of gonadal function in females

Gonadal dysfunction in women usually presents with any or all of the following:

- amenorrhoea,
- hirsutism,
- virilism,
- infertility (see Chapter 10).

Amenorrhoea

Amenorrhoea is defined as the absence of menstruation; it may be due to hormonal abnormalities. If there is ovarian failure, pituitary gonadotrophin concentrations in plasma are high (hypergonadotrophic hypogonadism); if the cause is in the hypothalamus or anterior pituitary gland, gonadotrophin secretion is reduced (hypogonadotrophic hypogonadism). Amenorrhoea may be classified as either primary or secondary (Box 9.2).

> **Box 9.2 Some causes of hypogonadism**
>
> *Hypogonadotrophic hypogonadism (low FSH/LH and low testosterone or oestrogen)*
> Genetic causes:
>   Kallmann's syndrome (anosmia and GnRH deficiency)
>   GnRH receptor mutations
>   isolated LH or FSH deficiency
>   *PROP1* gene mutations that lead to absence of some pituitary hormones
> Secondary causes:
>   cerebral tumours, e.g. craniopharyngioma, pituitary tumour, astrocytoma
>   head trauma
>   cerebral infections, vascular abnormalities, cerebral radiation
>   chronic systemic disease and malnutrition
>   exercise-induced amenorrhoea (females)
>   hyperprolactinaemia
>   miscellaneous causes – diabetes mellitus, marijuana use, Prader–Willi and Laurence–Moon (Bardet–Biedl) syndromes
>
> *Hypergonadotrophic hypogonadism*
> Females (raised FSH/LH and low oestrogen):
>   Turner's syndrome (45,XO)
>   LH and FSH receptor mutations
>   XX and XY gonadal dysgenesis
>   other causes of primary ovarian failure, e.g. chemotherapy, radiation, autoimmune, ovary resistance
> Males (raised FSH/LH and low testosterone):
>   Klinefelter's syndrome (47,XXY)
>   LH or FSH receptor mutations
>   primary testicular failure, e.g. chemotherapy, radiation, LH resistance, anorchism/cryptorchidism, testicular biosynthetic defects
>
> FSH = follicle-stimulating hormone, LH = luteinizing hormone, GnRH = gonadotrophin-releasing hormone.

Primary amenorrhoea occurs when the patient has never menstruated and is most commonly associated with delayed puberty. The age of the menarche is very variable. Extensive investigation should probably be postponed until around the age of 16 unless there are other clinical features of either endocrine disturbances, such as hirsutism and virilism, or chromosomal abnormalities. Turner's syndrome (45,XO) and testicular feminization syndrome may present with primary amenorrhoea.

Secondary amenorrhoea occurs when previously established menstrual cycles have stopped and is most commonly due to physiological factors such as pregnancy or the menopause. Other causes include severe illness, excess or rapid weight loss for any reason, including anorexia, or stopping oral contraceptives. These should be considered before extensive and potentially dangerous investigations are started. A number of endocrine disorders, such as hyperprolactinaemia, hyperthyroidism, Cushing's syndrome and acromegaly, may present with amenorrhoea.

Hirsutism and virilism

Increased plasma free-androgen concentrations, or increased tissue sensitivity to androgens, produce effects ranging from increased hair growth (hirsutism) to marked masculinization, with virilism. Testosterone is the most important androgen. In normal women about half the plasma testosterone comes from the ovaries, both by direct secretion and by peripheral conversion of androstenedione. The rest is derived from peripheral conversion of adrenal androgens, androstenedione and dehydroepiandrosterone (DHEA). Because of the extensive interconversion of androgens, the source of a slightly raised plasma testosterone concentration may be difficult to establish. In general, markedly raised plasma concentrations of DHEA or its sulphate (DHEAS) indicate an adrenocortical origin.

The biological activity of testosterone depends on the plasma free-hormone concentration. The plasma total concentration is also influenced by the concentration of the binding protein SHBG. Some laboratories report a free testosterone concentration or free androgen index. Conditions associated with altered plasma concentrations of SHBG are shown in Table 9.1.

Hirsutism is defined as an excessive growth of hair in a male distribution and is common, possibly occurring in 10 per cent of women. The Ferriman and Gallway score can assess its severity. A common cause is familial or racial hirsutism. For example, some Mediterranean women have more terminal hair and fair-skinned Europeans have the least. This difference may be due to racial differences in

5-α-reductase activity in skin. Plasma testosterone concentrations may be slightly raised, but are often within the female reference range. A raised testosterone concentration, particularly above 5 nmol/L, may indicate a tumour of the adrenal or ovary, which must be excluded. However, the plasma concentration of free hormone may be significantly increased if that of SHBG is low. A raised plasma 17-hydroxyprogesterone concentration may indicate CAH (see Chapter 8). Some causes of hirsutism are shown in Box 9.3.

Virilism is characterized by additional evidence of excessive androgen secretion such as an enlarged clitoris (clitoromegaly), increased hair growth of male distribution, receding temporal hair, deepening of the voice and breast atrophy. It is always associated with increased plasma androgen concentrations. Plasma DHEA and DHEAS concentrations may also be increased. Virilism usually implies an adrenal or ovarian androgen source and can be a cause of female pseudohermaphroditism (Box 9.4).

Table 9.1 Conditions associated with altered sex-hormone-binding globulin (SHBG) concentration

Increased SHBG	Decreased SHBG
Oestrogens	Androgens
Hyperthyroidism	Hypothyroidism
Liver disease	Obesity
	Protein-losing disorders
	Malnutrition

Polycystic ovary syndrome (sometimes called Leventhal–Stein syndrome)

This is a condition showing features of hyperandrogenism with anovulation and abnormal ovarian morphology and is the commonest cause of anovulatory infertility. Presenting clinical symptoms may also include hirsutism, menstrual disturbances, enlarged polycystic ovaries and infertility.

Box 9.3 Some causes of hirsutism

Idiopathic
Racial
Polycystic ovary syndrome
Cushing's syndrome
Congenital adrenal hyperplasia, e.g. 21-hydroxylase, 11β-hydroxylase
Ovarian tumours:
　arrhenoblastomas
　gonadoblastomas
Adrenal tumours:
　adenomas
　carcinomas
Exogenous androgens and drugs with androgenic activity

Box 9.4 Some causes of virilism

Idiopathic
Ovarian tumours (such as arrhenoblastomas and hilus-cell tumours) that secrete androgens, mainly testosterone
Adrenocortical disorders, e.g. carcinoma or congenital adrenal hyperplasia
Cushing's syndrome
Exogenous androgens or progestogens

CASE 2

A 28-year-old female attended the endocrine clinic because of excessive facial hair. Her periods were irregular and she was obese, with a body mass index of 32.8 kg/m². She was not taking any medication, and her renal function, liver function and blood glucose were all normal. Her plasma biochemical results were as follows.

Thyroid-stimulating hormone 2.6 mU/L (0.20–5.0)
Free thyroxine 17.1 pmol/L (12–25)
Prolactin 254 mU/L (<470)
Luteinizing hormone 27.2 U/L (1–25)
Follicle-stimulating hormone 6.4 U/L (1–15)
Testosterone 2.7 nmol/L (1–3)
Sex-hormone-binding globulin 18 nmol/L (20–90)
Oestradiol 364 pmol/L (70–880)

DISCUSSION

The clinical features and results are suggestive of polycystic ovary syndrome with raised plasma LH and low plasma SHBG concentrations. Obesity is associated with low SHBG concentrations. Polycystic ovary syndrome was confirmed by ultrasound scan of the ovaries, which showed large cysts. The SHBG concentrations are reduced in obesity, allowing increased free-testosterone concentrations.

Plasma testosterone and androstenedione concentrations are often increased. The plasma LH may be elevated with normal FSH. Because plasma SHBG concentrations are reduced in obese individuals, the plasma concentration of free testosterone is often increased. The plasma prolactin concentrations may also be high. Multiple small subcapsular ovarian cysts may be demonstrated on ultrasound scanning of the ovaries.

Polycystic ovary syndrome is also associated with insulin resistance, obesity and elevated plasma insulin concentrations, which may stimulate androgen production from the ovarian theca interna cells. Individuals may also have hyperlipidaemia, glucose intolerance and hypertension.

The male

Development of male characteristics

In the presence of the Y chromosome the fetal gonads develop into testes at about 7 weeks' gestation. The testes secrete a factor that causes degeneration of the potential female genitalia and testosterone, which stimulates the development of the potential male internal genitalia. The intracellular conversion of testosterone to dihydrotestosterone by the enzyme 5-α-reductase is essential for the development of male external genitalia. If this enzyme is deficient, varying degrees of feminization may occur, causing male pseudohermaphroditism (see later). Male penis formation is dependent upon testosterone.

Male puberty

During childhood, the rate of secretion of gonadotrophins from the anterior pituitary gland is low. As puberty approaches, the pulse amplitude and frequency of LH secretion increase. Initially, this occurs during sleep, but later continues throughout the day. Leydig cell function and testosterone secretion increase and stimulate the development of secondary male characteristics. Gonadotrophin secretion also stimulates meiosis of previously dormant germ cells in the seminiferous tubules, and thus the production of sperm.

Deficient secretion of either pituitary or gonadal hormones may cause delayed puberty.

The male germ cells produce spermatozoa continuously after puberty. Spermatogenesis is dependent on both normal Sertoli cell function and on testosterone secretion by Leydig cells. Therefore both LH and FSH are needed for normal spermatogenesis, but testosterone secretion can occur in the absence of normal seminiferous tubules.

Disorders of gonadal function in males

Gonadal dysfunction in men may present with the symptoms of androgen deficiency or of infertility, or both. Androgen deficiency is the result of impaired testosterone secretion by Leydig cells. The patient may present with delayed puberty or with regression of previously established male characteristics that are dependent on testosterone (hair distribution, potency and libido). There may be primary testicular dysfunction, in which case the low plasma testosterone concentration is accompanied by raised plasma LH concentrations (hypergonadotrophic hypogonadism). Dysfunction secondary to pituitary or hypothalamic disease conversely results in low plasma LH concentrations (hypogonadotrophic hypogonadism) (see Box 9.2).

Infertility may be caused by androgen deficiency, but most infertile men have normal plasma androgen concentrations. Sertoli cell function is dependent on both FSH and testosterone produced locally. Semen analysis is an important investigation for male infertility. However, biochemical tests may sometimes help: if the cause is primary

---

CASE 3

A 23-year-old male presented to his general practitioner with erectile dysfunction. He was not taking any medications, and his renal function, liver function and blood glucose were normal. Some of his plasma biochemical results were as follows.

Thyroid-stimulating hormone 1.0 mU/L (0.20–5.0)
Free thyroxine 14.1 pmol/L (12–25)
Prolactin 264 mU/L (<470)
Luteinizing hormone 27.2 U/L (1–7)
Follicle-stimulating hormone 41.4 U/L (1–8)
Testosterone 2.7 nmol/L (10–30)

DISCUSSION
The diagnosis is hypergonadotrophic hypogonadism – note the high plasma gonadotrophin (LH and FSH) and low testosterone concentrations. Further investigations, including karyotyping, showed XXY chromosome complement (as opposed to the normal XY male pattern), confirming Klinefelter's syndrome.

testicular failure, the plasma testosterone concentration is low, and reduced inhibin production by Sertoli cells causes a rise in FSH concentrations. If there is evidence of a failure of spermatogenesis, the plasma FSH concentration should be measured. If the cause is secondary to anterior pituitary failure, both plasma testosterone and FSH concentrations are low.

Hyperprolactinaemia is much less common in males than in females, but its presence may indicate a pituitary tumour. Chromosomal abnormalities such as Klinefelter's syndrome (47,XXY) may also cause abnormal male gonadal function.

Gynaecomastia

This is the enlargement of male breast tissue (glandular and not adipose tissue), which can be unilateral or bilateral. Important in the aetiology is an increase in the oestrogen:androgen ratio, which can be seen physiologically at puberty or in the elderly. Certain drugs, such as digoxin, spironolactone, phenothiazines and cimetidine, may be implicated. However, other causes include hyperthyroidism, human chorionic gonadotrophin (hCG)-secreting tumours and hyperprolactinaemia, as well as increased oestrogen concentration (such as in liver disease and testicular or adrenal tumours), low testosterone concentration (in pituitary or gonadal failure) and Kallmann's or Klinefelter's syndrome.

OTHER DISORDERS OF REPRODUCTIVE ORGANS

Precocious puberty

This can be defined as the appearance of secondary sexual characteristics before the age of 8 years in either females or males. It can be:

- True (central) precocious puberty caused by cerebral tumours, infection or trauma, McCune–Albright syndrome or hypothyroidism.
- Pseudoprecocious puberty caused by adrenal or ovarian/testicular tumours.

Ambiguous genitalia and intersexuality

During the fetus' second month, its indifferent gonad is stimulated to develop into a testis, initiated by testis-determining factor derived from the sex-determining region of the Y chromosome (SRY). If this region is absent or abnormal, the indifferent gonad develops into an ovary. In the gonadal male, differentiation to male phenotype is mediated by testosterone, which is converted to dihydrotestosterone by 5-α-reductase.

Female pseudohermaphrodism

Individuals with this condition usually show XX chromosomes but male genitalia characteristics and virilism. More commonly, it can be caused by high concentrations of maternal androgens during pregnancy or increased concentrations of fetal androgens, such as in CAH, including deficiency of 21-hydroxylase or 11-hydroxylase, which result in increased endogenous testosterone production (see Chapter 8).

Male pseudohermaphrodism

Individuals with this condition usually have chromosomes XY and possess two testes but female external genitalia. Causes include CAH such as 17-α-hydroxylase deficiency or 17-β-hydroxysteroid dehydrogenase deficiency. Other causes are deficient testosterone biosynthesis and androgen receptor defects such as Reifenstein's syndrome, testicular feminization or 5-α-reductase deficiency. The last condition shows a high plasma testosterone to DHT ratio.

True hermaphrodism

This is very rare, with individuals having both testicular and ovarian tissue.

BIOCHEMICAL INVESTIGATION OF GONADAL DISORDERS

In suspected cases, a careful clinical history, including medications, and physical examination can be useful. Measurement of plasma LH, FSH, TSH, prolactin, oestradiol, testosterone and SHBG may reveal a diagnosis. If intersex conditions are sought, karyotyping may be useful. (Chapters 7 and 8 should be consulted if a pituitary or adrenal disorder, respectively, is suspected.) Sometimes the more specialized tests described below are necessary.

Gonadotrophin–releasing hormone test

Gonadotrophin-releasing hormone (a decapeptide) released by the hypothalamus stimulates the release of the gonadotrophins LH and FSH from the normal anterior pituitary gland. The test is used to diagnose hypothalamic–pituitary disease in precocious and delayed puberty with low basal gonadotrophin concentrations.

Procedure

Intravenous injection of 100 μg of GnRH is given.

Plasma LH and FSH concentrations are measured in blood drawn before and at 20 and 60 minutes after the injection.

Some patients show an allergic reaction and therefore resuscitation facilities should be at hand and the test should be performed by experienced staff. Sometimes nausea and abdominal pain are experienced.

The test can sometimes be combined with the TRH and insulin or glucagon stimulation tests as part of the triple pituitary test, although this is now rarely performed (see Chapter 7).

Interpretation

In prepubertal children, plasma LH and FSH are usually both less than 2.0 U/L. In normal subjects, the levels of plasma LH and FSH at least double from their basal levels at 20 minutes, but this rise fails to occur in patients with pituitary hypofunction. Conversely, an exaggerated response may be seen in patients with hypothalamic disease. A normal response does not exclude hypothalamic or pituitary disease.

Human chorionic gonadotrophin stimulation test

Human chorionic gonadotrophin shares a common sub-unit with LH and stimulates testicular Leydig cells to release androgens. It has a long half-life and elicits a rise in plasma testosterone after 72–120 hours.

The test may be indicated in the following situations:

- to confirm the presence of testes,
- in infants with ambiguous genitalia and palpable gonads,
- in males with delayed puberty,
- in some cases of undescended testicles.

Some patients show an allergic reaction and therefore resuscitation facilities should be at hand and experienced staff should perform the test.

Procedure

On day 0, blood is taken for testosterone. Then 2000 hCG units are given on days 0 and 2 by intramuscular injection.

On day 4, blood is again taken for testosterone, androstenedione and DHT.

Normally there is at least a two-fold increase in testosterone concentration, but in the absence of testes there is no testosterone response.

CONCLUSIONS

- The gonads secrete sex hormones, although there is also some adrenal gland production. In females, the main sex hormone is the oestrogen 17-β-oestradiol, and in males testosterone.
- The anterior pituitary gonadotrophins FSH and LH stimulate the gonads.
- Prolactin is released from the anterior pituitary gland. Hyperprolactinaemia has many causes and can result in infertility and galactorrhoea.
- Plasma SHBG carries testosterone and oestrogen, the free forms of which are biologically active.
- Gonadal dysfunction in females usually presents with any or all of the following: amenorrhoea, hirsutism, virilism, infertility and ambiguous genitalia.
- Gonadal dysfunction in males may present with delayed puberty, decreased libido, gynaecomastia, infertility or ambiguous genitalia.

10 PREGNANCY AND INFERTILITY

| Pregnancy and lactation | 155 | Some drug effects on the hypothalamic–pituitary– | |
| Infertility | 159 | gonadal axis | 161 |

This chapter discusses the biochemical changes that occur in pregnancy and how clinical biochemistry tests can be used in the investigation of infertility.

PREGNANCY AND LACTATION

If the ovum is fertilized, it may implant in the endometrium, which has been prepared by progesterone during the luteal phase. The function of luteinizing hormone (LH) is taken over by human chorionic gonadotrophin (hCG), produced by the chorion and developing placenta. Human chorionic gonadotrophin is similar in structure and action to LH and prevents the involution of the corpus luteum as circulating pituitary gonadotrophin concentrations fall. Consequently, plasma oestrogen and progesterone concentrations continue to rise and endometrial sloughing is prevented. After the first trimester the placenta produces these hormones. During pregnancy the predominant oestrogen is oestriol. Prolactin concentration gradually increases during the first two trimesters and then rises steeply, to about 8000 mU/L, in the third trimester.

Prolactin, oestrogens, progesterone and (human) placental lactogen stimulate breast development in preparation for lactation. High plasma oestrogen concentrations inhibit milk secretion; lactation can only start when plasma concentrations fall after delivery of the placenta. Initially lactation depends on prolactin. Suckling stimulates secretion of the hormone, but even during lactation, plasma prolactin concentrations fall progressively postpartum and reach non-pregnant levels after 2 or 3 months. Apart from the effects on the breast, the high plasma concentration of prolactin interferes with gonadotrophin and ovarian function and produces a period of relative infertility.

Monitoring pregnancy (placental function)

Substances produced by the fetus or placenta (fetoplacental unit) may be measured in maternal plasma or urine to detect fetal abnormalities or to monitor the progress of the pregnancy. Such sampling is relatively safe and simple, but occasionally more invasive testing, such as of amniotic fluid obtained by amniocentesis, may be needed. However, the ability to visualize the fetus using ultrasound and the use of cardiotocography detecting fetal heart rate have reduced the need for such tests.

Human chorionic gonadotrophin

The secretion of hCG by the placenta reaches a peak (rising to about 500 000 U/L) at about 13 weeks of pregnancy and then falls. The fetoplacental unit then takes over hormone production, and the secretion of both oestrogen and progesterone rises rapidly. Plasma or urinary hCG concentrations, which give positive results at 1 or 2 weeks after the first missed menstrual period, are most commonly used to diagnose pregnancy. However, by using more sensitive immunoassay techniques, plasma hCG may be detected soon after implantation of the ovum and before the first missed period. Such early diagnosis may be of value if an ectopic pregnancy is suspected, in conjunction with ultrasonography, or if the patient is being treated for infertility.

Serial hCG measurements may be used to assess the progress of early pregnancy; single values are difficult to interpret because of the wide reference range. As a rough guide, plasma concentrations should double every 2 days in a normal pregnancy.

Human placental lactogen

This is a peptide hormone synthesized by the placenta. It is detectable in maternal plasma after about the eighth week of gestation and has been used to assess the likelihood of threatened miscarriage and to monitor late pregnancy, but now is rarely used.

Detection of fetal abnormalities

Some fetal abnormalities may be diagnosed by tests carried out on maternal plasma or amniotic fluid. Amniocentesis is a procedure by which amniotic fluid is obtained through a needle inserted through the maternal abdominal wall into the uterus and is usually carried out after about 14 weeks' gestation. The procedure carries a small risk to the fetus. Both the safety and the reliability of the procedure can be improved if combined with ultrasound examination in order to locate the position of the fetus, placenta and maternal bladder.

Analytical results may be misleading if, for example, the specimen is contaminated with maternal or fetal blood or maternal urine, is not fresh or is not properly preserved. Close liaison between the clinician and the laboratory staff helps to ensure the suitability of the specimen and the speed of the assay. Amniotic fluid is probably derived from both maternal and fetal sources, but its value in reflecting abnormalities arises from its intimate contact with the fetus and from the increasing contribution of fetal urine in later pregnancy.

Detection of neural tube defects

Alpha-fetoprotein (AFP) is a low-molecular-weight glycoprotein synthesized mainly in the fetal yolk sac and liver. Its production is almost completely repressed in the normal adult. It can diffuse slowly through capillary membranes and appears in the fetal urine, and hence in the amniotic fluid, and in maternal plasma. Severe fetal neural tube defects, such as open spina bifida and anencephaly, are associated with abnormally high concentrations in these fluids. The reason for this is not clear, but the protein may leak from the exposed neural tube vessels.

As well as neural tube defects, the causes of raised AFP concentration in amniotic fluid and maternal plasma include:

- multiple pregnancy,
- serious fetal abnormalities,
- exomphalos.

In some countries, pregnant women attending for antenatal care are offered plasma AFP assay at between 16 and 18 weeks of gestation to screen for the presence of a fetus with a neural tube defect (although high resolution ultrasound is beginning to replace this test). The gestational age should be confirmed by ultrasound, which should also exclude a multiple pregnancy as a cause of high concentrations.

Positive results should be confirmed on a fresh sample, which, if still high and if the diagnosis has not been confirmed by ultrasound, may be followed by AFP estimation on amniotic fluid. This is a more precise diagnostic test and yields fewer false-positive results than plasma assays if sampling is properly performed. It should be reserved for subjects known to be at risk, either because of a family history of neural tube defects or because of the finding of a high concentration in maternal plasma with a normal or equivocal ultrasound scan.

Amniotic fluid acetylcholinesterase assay is now rarely used to detect certain fetal malformations, including neural tube defects and exomphalos. It gives reliable results up to about 23 weeks of gestation. The interpretation of the result is less dependent on fetal age than AFP, but is equally invalidated by contamination with fetal or maternal blood. The assay is less widely available than that for AFP.

Detection of Down's syndrome

Low maternal plasma AFP and unconjugated oestriol, and raised hCG and inhibin-A concentrations, measured

CASE 1

A 20-year-old female attended the antenatal clinic in the 17th week of pregnancy for a Down's syndrome screen test. A plasma AFP was 67 kU/L (reference median being 38 kU/L for 17 weeks). Her other blood tests were normal.

DISCUSSION

It was feared that the fetus had a neural tube defect because of the raised plasma AFP concentration. However, an ultrasound scan showed a twin pregnancy and no evidence of a neural tube defect. Other causes of a raised plasma AFP concentration include incorrect gestational dating, fetal renal disease, duodenal/oesophageal atresia and ventral wall defects or exomphalos.

between the 16 and 18 weeks of gestation, are associated with an increased risk of the fetus having Down's syndrome (trisomy 21). This combination of tests (quadruple test) to screen for the congenital disorder is available in specialized laboratories. Fetal nuchal translucency determined by high-resolution ultrasound may also have a role as a screening test; increased thickness is associated with chromosomal abnormalities and may be used in conjunction with the biochemical tests. A definitive test is amniocentesis, which allows the collection of fetal cells for karyotyping.

Detection of other fetal abnormalities

Chromosomal abnormalities and some inborn errors of metabolism may be detected by cytogenetic, biochemical or enzymatic assays on cells cultured from amniotic fluid or after biopsy of chorionic villi. These tests are performed only in special centres and usually on individuals with a family history of a genetic condition.

Assessment of fetomaternal blood group incompatibility

Rhesus or other blood group incompatibility has effects on the fetus, which may be assessed by measuring amniotic fluid concentrations of bilirubin in conjunction with maternal antibody titres. Normally bilirubin concentrations in amniotic fluid decrease during the last half of pregnancy. The concentrations at any stage correlate with the severity of haemolysis. The result is read off a Liley chart relating optical density of amniotic fluid at 450 nm (an indirect measure of bilirubin) against gestational time. Such tests may allow the optimum time for induction of labour or the need for intrauterine transfusion to be assessed.

Assessment of fetal lung maturity

The examination of amniotic fluid has also been used to assess pulmonary maturity. Immature lungs do not expand normally at birth and may cause neonatal respiratory distress syndrome (hyaline membrane disease), with the need for respiratory support. It is therefore important to have evidence of pulmonary maturity before labour is induced. At about 32 weeks of gestation, the cells lining the fetal alveolar walls start to synthesize a surface-tension-lowering complex (surfactant), 90 per cent of which is the phospholipid lecithin, which contains palmitic acid. Surfactant is probably washed from, or secreted by, the alveolar walls into the surrounding amniotic fluid, in which both lecithin and palmitic acid concentrations steadily increase. The concentration of lecithin, relative to another lipid, sphingomyelin, which remains constant in amniotic fluid, can be measured. A rise in the lecithin:sphingomyelin (L:S) ratio may help determine pulmonary maturity and a ratio less than 2 implies immaturity. This invasive test is rarely indicated now as steroids, which induce surfactant synthesis, are sometimes given to patients who have premature rupture of the membranes.

Maternal biochemical changes in pregnancy

Weight gain of about 12 kg occurs due to increased maternal fluid retention, increased maternal fat stores and also the products of conception, including the fetus, placenta and amniotic fluid.

Many plasma constituents are influenced by sex hormones. For example, the reference ranges of plasma urate and iron differ in males and females after puberty. Therefore it is not surprising to find that during pregnancy the very high circulating concentrations of oestrogens and progesterone alter the concentrations of many substances in plasma (Table 10.1).

The plasma concentrations of many specific carrier proteins increase during pregnancy, accompanied by a proportional increase of the substance bound to them, without any change in the unbound free fraction. Because the protein-bound fraction is a transport form and because, in all cases, it is the free substance that is physiologically active, this rise in concentration is of importance in the interpretation of the results of such assays as those of plasma thyroxine.

Other changes in maternal plasma are due to progressive haemodilution by fluid retained during pregnancy. This is maximal at about the thirtieth week and the effects are most evident in reduced concentrations of albumin, and of calcium, which is bound to albumin. These changes are more marked in pre-eclamptic toxaemia, in which fluid retention may be greater than normal. The glomerular filtration rate increases and creatinine clearance can be over 140 mL/min by about 28 weeks. There is a reduced renal threshold for glucose and increased excretion of urate and some amino acids.

There is a mild increase in ventilation rate. Oxygen consumption is increased, but P_{O_2} maintains fairly constant despite a small decrease in P_{CO_2}. There is increased fasting glucose utilization, and therefore fasting glucose concentration is lower.

Renal glycosuria is common in pregnancy and sometimes in individuals taking oral contraceptives. The glomerular filtration rate increases by about 50 per cent during pregnancy,

Table 10.1 Some biochemical changes that may occur during pregnancy

Test	Effect	Comment
Plasma		
Total T$_4$[a]	Increased	Increased TBG
		Free T$_4$ usually normal
Cortisol[a]	Increased	Increased transcortin
		Free cortisol usually normal
Transferrin or TIBC[a]	Increased	
Iron[a]	Increased	
Copper[a]	Increased	Increased caeruloplasmin
Alkaline phosphatase	Increased	Placental isoenzyme
Total protein and albumin	Decreased	Dilution by fluid retention
Creatinine	Decreased due to increased GFR	
Urea	Anabolism due to fetal growth and increased GFR	
Cholesterol	Raised	
Triglyceride[a]	Raised	
Oestrogen[a]	Increased	
Progesterone	Increased	
LH and FSH	Decreased	
Pco$_2$	Decreased due to mild hyperventilation	
Glucose	Some women may develop gestational diabetes	
Urate	Decreased but may be increased if hypertension	
Urine		
Glucose	Glycosuria	Reduced renal threshold
Proteinuria	May be associated with hypertension	

[a] These changes may also occur in women taking oestrogen oral contraceptives.
T$_4$ = thyroxine; TBG = thyroxine-binding globulin; TIBC = total iron-binding capacity; GFR = glomerular filtration rate; LH = luteinizing hormone; FSH = follicle-stimulating hormone.

CASE 2

A 35-year-old female was 23 weeks' pregnant and was noted to have glycosuria. She had the following biochemical results.

Plasma
Sodium 136 mmol/L (135–145)
Potassium 3.6 mmol/L (3.5–5.0)
Urea 2.1 mmol/L (2.5–7.0)
Creatinine 60 μmol/L (70–110)
Alkaline phosphatase 344 U/L (<250)
Albumin 34 g/L (35–45)
Random plasma glucose 4.1 mmol/L (3.5–5.5)

DISCUSSION
The results are typical of pregnancy; note the low plasma urea and creatinine and albumin concentrations, in part due to increased glomerular filtration rate and plasma volume. Plasma alkaline phosphatase concentration is elevated due to placental isoenzyme release. Glycosuria was present due to a lowered renal threshold for glucose that occurs during pregnancy and not necessarily as a result of diabetes mellitus.

resulting in a reduced plasma creatinine. Glycosuria may partly be due to an increased glucose load in normal tubules. The positive protein and purine balance during the growth of the fetus and the increase in glomerular filtration rate that occurs during pregnancy result in lowered maternal plasma urea and urate concentrations. Plasma alkaline phosphatase activity rises during the last 3 months of pregnancy due to the presence of the placental isoenzyme and should not be misinterpreted (see Chapter 18). Placental alkaline phosphatase does not cross the placenta and therefore it is not present in the plasma of the newborn infant.

Delivery

During delivery, blood gases and lactate can be measured in fetal blood to monitor for hypoxia. Capillary blood samples may be collected from the fetal scalp during delivery. Transcutaneous oxygen electrodes can determine fetal Po_2.

Hypertension in pregnancy

Pregnancy-induced hypertension or pre-eclampsia is associated with convulsions, oedema, impaired renal function, proteinuria and maternal death as well as with placental insufficiency and intrauterine fetal growth retardation.

Pregnant women should thus be closely monitored for hypertension and those with pre-eclampsia should have their urinary protein excretion and creatinine clearance measured. Plasma urate may rise in pre-eclampsia.

Detection and follow-up of trophoblastic tumours

Trophoblastic tumours (hydatidiform mole, choriocarcinoma), which may follow abnormal pregnancy or a miscarriage, and some teratomas secrete hCG, which can be estimated in plasma or urine by sensitive tests allowing early detection and treatment of recurrence. However, these tests will not necessarily differentiate pregnancy from recurrence of a tumour because plasma hCG concentrations rise in both situations (see Chapter 24).

INFERTILITY

Infertility can be defined as primary when conception has never occurred despite at least 1 year of unprotected coitus, and secondary when there has been a previous pregnancy, either successful or not.

In cases of infertility, both partners should be investigated. The history should include coital frequency and success, serious illnesses, use of alcohol and drugs, and sexually transmitted diseases.

Female

Examination should include looking for anorexia, hirsutism, virilism, galactorrhoea and ambiguous genitalia. A history should also be taken for medications and drugs (see Chapter 9).

Investigations

A woman may be infertile despite having a clinically normal menstrual cycle (about 95 per cent of such cycles are ovulatory). Thus even if the cycle seems to be regular, it is important to determine whether ovulation is occurring and if luteal development is normal. Anovulatory infertility is probably the commonest form of female infertility and is associated with oligomenorrhoea or amenorrhoea. (Discussion of the complete investigation of female infertility, including tests such as that for tubal patency, is beyond the scope of this book.)

- If the patient is menstruating regularly, measure plasma progesterone concentration during the luteal phase on day 21 of the cycle. A normal plasma concentration is strong evidence that the patient has ovulated. A low plasma concentration of <30 nmol/L suggests either ovulatory failure or impaired luteal function. This investigation should be repeated on more than one occasion. The commonest cause of a low progesterone concentration (less than 30 nmol/L) is inaccurate sample timing, although, if authentic, it suggests lack of ovulation. However, a plasma progesterone concentration of more than 100 nmol/L suggests pregnancy.
- Follicular development and ovulation may be monitored by ovarian ultrasound examination. Polycystic ovary syndrome should be excluded (see Chapter 9). Plasma follicle-stimulating hormone (FSH), LH, oestrogen and testosterone concentrations are useful, as is the exclusion of thyroid disease.
- If there is primary amenorrhoea, consider karyotyping the patient, for example Turner's syndrome (45,XO).
- Sometimes histological examination of an endometrial biopsy specimen or the appearance of cervical mucus

> **CASE 3**
>
> A 28-year-old female attended the gynaecology outpatient clinic because of infertility. Her periods were noted to be irregular. She was on no medication, and her renal function, liver function and blood glucose concentration were normal. Her plasma results were as follows.
>
> Thyroid-stimulating hormone 2.1 mU/L (0.20–5.0)
> Free thyroxine 14.3 pmol/L (12–25)
> Prolactin 414 mU/L (<470)
> Luteinizing hormone 7.2 U/L (1–25)
> Follicle-stimulating hormone 5.4 U/L (1–15)
> Testosterone 1.7 nmol/L (1–3)
> Sex-hormone-binding globulin 33 nmol/L (20–90)
> Oestradiol 564 pmol/L (70–880)
> 21-day plasma progesterone 6.6 nmol/L (>30 suggests ovulation)
>
> **DISCUSSION**
> The low 21-day plasma progesterone concentration suggests a poor luteal phase and possible anovulation. The patient was having anovulatory menstrual cycles, which explained her infertility.

can indicate whether luteal function is normal. An oral progestogen challenge can be used: a withdrawal bleed 5–7 days later implies adequate endometrial oestrogen, whereas failure to bleed despite oestrogen treatment implies uterine disease.
- Hyperprolactinaemia should be excluded by checking the plasma prolactin concentration (see Chapter 9).
- Do the plasma FSH, LH and oestrogen results suggest hypergonadotrophic hypogonadism or hypogonadotrophic hypogonadism? In the presence of amenorrhoea, a plasma FSH of more than 50 U/L is suggestive of ovarian failure. (See Chapter 9 for the causes of hypergonadotrophic hypogonadism and hypogonadotrophic hypogonadism.)
- Low concentrations of plasma gonadotrophins may necessitate a gonadotrophin-releasing hormone (GnRH) test to look for pituitary or hypothalamic disease (see Chapter 9).

Male

Systemic illness, for example cystic fibrosis, thyroid disease, gynaecomastia, eunuchoid appearance and ambiguous genitalia, should be excluded and any history of mumps, drugs and medications should be obtained.

Investigations

- Semen analysis. The volume should be at least 2 ml. There should be more than 20×10^9/L spermatozoa, more than 50 per cent being motile at 4 hours post-ejaculation and more than 30 per cent normal morphology. A post-coital test is useful so that cervical mucus can be examined for the presence of spermatozoa and their activity. Sperm antibodies may exist.
- Plasma testosterone, LH and FSH concentrations should be measured.

  Raised plasma FSH and LH concentrations with a low testosterone concentration (hypergonadotrophic hypogonadism) indicate a testicular problem such as Leydig cell failure. Low plasma FSH and LH and testosterone concentrations suggest pituitary or hypothalamic disease (hypogonadotrophic hypogonadism). In the case of the latter, a GnRH test may be required (see Chapter 9).

  A raised plasma FSH concentration in comparison with LH may indicate seminiferous tubular failure, irrespective of the plasma testosterone concentration. There is usually azoospermia or oligospermia. Oligospermia with a low plasma FSH concentration suggests pituitary or hypothalamic disease.
- If there is evidence of feminization, karyotype should be considered. This should also be considered if azoospermia is present, for example Klinefelter's syndrome (47,XXY).
- Plasma prolactin should be measured and hyperprolactinaemia and thyroid disease excluded (see Chapter 9).
- Defects of the male reproductive tract may also be found and necessitate a urology opinion, but are beyond the scope of this book.
- An hCG stimulation test may be indicated if absence of testes is suspected or to assess Leydig cell reserve (see Chapter 9).

- Some tumours can release β-hCG or oestrogens and may induce features of feminization. These can be assayed in plasma if the cause of infertility is unclear.

Sometimes, despite both partners being investigated, no cause for the infertility can be found.

SOME DRUG EFFECTS ON THE HYPOTHALAMIC–PITUITARY–GONADAL AXIS

Oral contraceptives contain synthetic oestrogens and/or progestogens. They suppress pituitary gonadotrophin secretion and thus inhibit ovulation. Withdrawal mimics involution of the corpus luteum and results in menstrual bleeding. Clomiphene blocks oestrogen receptors in the hypothalamus and so prevents negative feedback. It may stimulate gonadotrophin release, even when circulating oestrogen concentrations are high. Clomiphene may be used to induce ovulation in patients with amenorrhoea or infertility.

Gonadotrophin treatment may be used if clomiphene fails to induce ovulation. This therapy may cause dangerous follicular enlargement due to hyperstimulation, or may stimulate many follicles and so cause multiple pregnancy. Treatment must therefore be monitored either by frequent plasma oestradiol estimations (which would be expected to be very high) and by ovarian ultrasound examination. Ovulation may be assessed by demonstrating rising plasma progesterone concentrations or by ultrasound. Gonadotrophins may also be used to stimulate the production of enough oocytes to enable them to be 'harvested' for in-vitro fertilization or gamete intrafallopian transfer.

Gonadotrophin-releasing hormone treatment can be used for patients with infertility secondary to hypogonadotrophic hypogonadism. It is given subcutaneously in pulses, such as every 90 minutes, using a portable syringe pump. Bromocriptine may reduce high plasma prolactin concentrations, after which menstruation may resume and fertility may be restored.

CONCLUSIONS

- A number of physiological changes may take place during pregnancy that may affect laboratory tests. In some cases this is due to increased concentrations of hormone or transport proteins, although the free-hormone concentrations are normal.
- Increased urinary (or plasma) hCG concentration can be used to diagnose pregnancy.
- Biochemical tests can be used to monitor the progression of pregnancy as well as to detect fetal abnormality.
- Infertility may be primary or secondary and can be the result of problems with the man or woman, or both. Biochemical tests can also be useful in the diagnosis of infertility in conjunction with other investigations.

11 THYROID FUNCTION

Physiology	162	Disorders of the thyroid gland	166
Thyroid function tests	164	Strategy for thyroid function testing and interpretation	172

It is important to understand thyroid biochemistry, as it helps to interpret thyroid function tests, which are amongst the most common endocrine requests in clinical practice. Thyroid disease is relatively common and therefore is likely to be encountered clinically.

Briefly, thyroxine (T_4), tri-iodothyronine (T_3) and calcitonin are secreted by the thyroid gland. Both T_4 and T_3 are products of the follicular cells and influence the rate of all metabolic processes. Calcitonin is produced by the specialized C-cells and influences calcium metabolism (see Chapter 6).

PHYSIOLOGY

Thyroid hormones are synthesized in the thyroid gland by the iodination and coupling of two molecules of the amino acid tyrosine, a process that is dependent on an adequate supply of iodide. Iodide in the diet is absorbed rapidly from the small intestine. In areas where the iodide content of the soil is very low, there used to be a high incidence of enlargement of the thyroid gland (goitre), but the general use of artificially iodized salt has made this a less common occurrence. Seafoods generally have a high iodide content. Therefore fish and iodized salt are the main dietary sources of the element. Normally about a third of dietary iodide is taken up by the thyroid gland and is renally excreted.

Synthesis of thyroid hormones

Iodide is actively taken up by the thyroid gland under the control of thyroid-stimulating hormone (TSH) via a sodium/iodide symporter. Uptake is blocked by thiocyanate and perchlorate. The concentration of iodide in the gland is at least 20 times that in plasma and may exceed it by 100 times or more.

Iodide is rapidly converted to iodine within the thyroid gland, catalysed by thyroperoxidase (TPO).

Iodination of tyrosine residues in a large 660 kDa glycoprotein, thyroglobulin, takes place to form mono-iodotyrosine (MIT) and di-iodotyrosine (DIT) mediated by the enzyme TPO. This step is inhibited by carbimazole and propylthiouracil.

Iodotyrosines are coupled to form T_4 (DIT and DIT) and T_3 (DIT and MIT) (Fig. 11.1), which are stored in the lumen of the thyroid follicular cells. Normally much more T_4 than T_3 is synthesized, but if there is an inadequate supply of iodide, the ratio of T_3 to T_4 in the gland increases. The thyroid hormones, still incorporated in thyroglobulin, are stored in the colloid of the thyroid follicle.

Prior to the secretion of thyroid hormones, thyroglobulin is taken up by the follicular cells, by a process involving endocytosis and then phagocytosis, and T_4 and T_3 are released by proteolytic enzymes into the bloodstream. This process is stimulated by TSH and inhibited by iodide. The thyroid hormones are immediately bound to plasma proteins. Mono-iodotyrosine and DIT, released at the same time, are de-iodinated and the iodine is re-used.

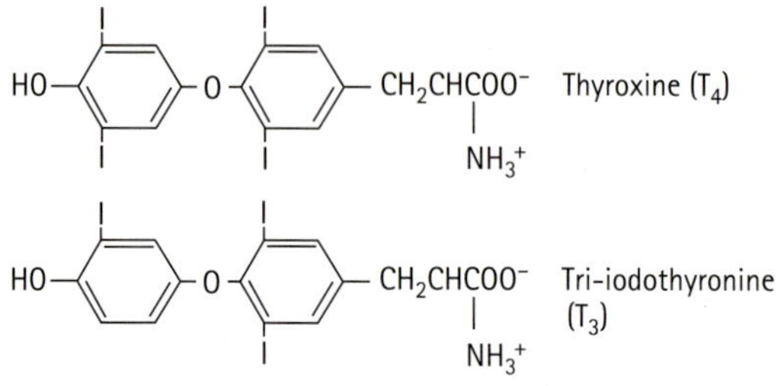

Fig 11.1 Chemical structure of the thyroid hormones.

Each step is controlled by specific enzymes, and congenital deficiency of any of these enzymes can lead to goitre and, if severe, hypothyroidism. The uptake of iodide, as well as the synthesis and secretion of thyroid hormones, is regulated by TSH, secreted from the anterior pituitary gland. About ten times more T_4 than T_3 is formed, with most of the latter being formed by de-iodination in the liver, kidneys and muscle.

Protein binding of thyroid hormones in plasma

Most of the plasma T_4 and T_3 is protein bound, mainly (70 per cent) to an α-globulin, thyroxine-binding globulin (TBG), and, to a lesser extent (15 per cent), transthyretin, with about 10–15 per cent bound to albumin and thyroxine-binding pre-albumin (TBPA). In keeping with many other hormones, the free unbound fraction is the physiologically active form, which also regulates TSH secretion from the anterior pituitary. Modern laboratory assays tend to measure the free hormones. Changes in the plasma concentrations of the binding proteins, particularly TBG, alter plasma total T_4 and T_3 concentrations, but not the concentrations of free hormones.

Peripheral conversion of thyroid hormone

Some of the circulating T_4 is de-iodinated by enzymes in peripheral tissues, especially in the liver and kidneys. About 80 per cent of the plasma T_3 is produced by the removal of an iodine atom from the outer (β) ring; the remaining 20 per cent is secreted by the thyroid gland. De-iodination of the inner (α) ring produces reverse T_3, which is probably inactive. The T_3 binds more avidly to thyroid receptors than T_4 and is the main active form. The conversion of T_4 to T_3 may be:

- *reduced* by many factors, of which the most important are:
  - systemic illness,
  - prolonged fasting,
  - drugs such as β-blockers, for example propranolol or amiodarone (200 mg of this anti-arrhythmic drug contains about 75 mg of iodine);
- *increased* by drugs that induce hepatic enzyme activity, such as phenytoin.

The plasma T_3 concentration is therefore a poor indicator of thyroid hormone secretion because it is influenced by many non-thyroidal factors and its measurement is rarely indicated, except if thyrotoxicosis is suspected.

Action of thyroid hormones

Thyroid hormones affect many metabolic processes, increasing oxygen consumption. They bind to specific receptors in cell nuclei and change the expression of certain genes. Thyroid hormones are essential for normal growth, mental development and sexual maturation and also increase the sensitivity of the cardiovascular and central nervous systems to catecholamines, thereby influencing cardiac output and heart rate.

Control of thyroid-stimulating hormone secretion

Thyroid-stimulating hormone stimulates the synthesis and release of thyroid hormones from the thyroid gland. Its secretion from the anterior pituitary gland is controlled by thyrotrophin-releasing hormone (TRH) and circulating concentrations of thyroid hormones.

Effect of thyrotrophin-releasing hormone

Pituitary TSH synthesis and release are stimulated by TRH, a tripeptide produced in the hypothalamus and released into the portal capillary plexus. The action of TRH can be

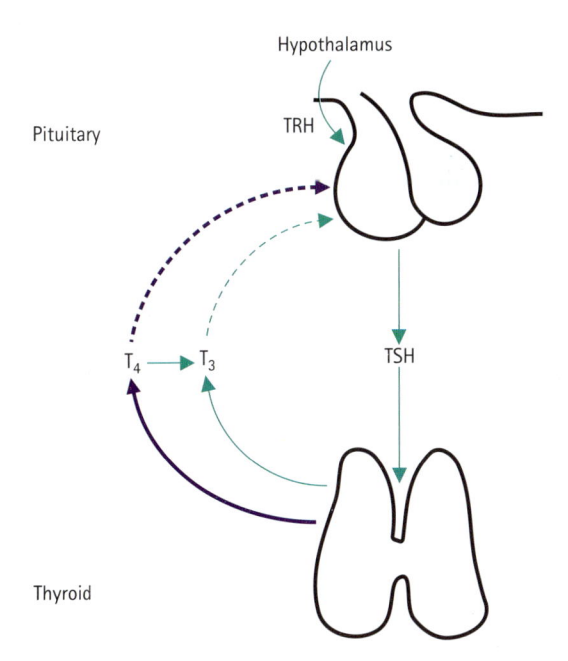

Fig. 11.2 Secretion and control of thyroid hormones. (Solid lines indicate secretion and interconversion of hormones; dotted lines indicate negative feedback. TRH = thyrotrophin-releasing hormone; TSH = thyroid-stimulating hormone; T_4 = thyroxine; T_3 = tri-iodothyronine.)

overridden by high circulating free T_4 (fT_4) concentrations, and therefore exogenous TRH has little effect on TSH secretion in hyperthyroidism (see later for TRH test). Once TRH reaches the pituitary, it binds to TRH receptors, members of the seven-transmembrane-spanning receptor family, which are coupled to G proteins.

Effects of thyroid hormones in the control of thyroid-stimulating hormone secretion

Thyroid hormones reduce TSH secretion by negative feedback. Tri-iodothyronine binds to anterior pituitary nuclear receptors. In the anterior pituitary gland, most of the intracellular T_3 is derived from circulating fT_4. Therefore this gland is more sensitive to changes in plasma T_4 than to T_3 concentrations.

The metabolism and control of thyroid hormones are summarized in Fig. 11.2.

THYROID FUNCTION TESTS

Assessment of thyroid hormone secretion can be made by measuring plasma TSH as well as either fT_4 or total T_4 (sometimes also fT_3 or total T_3). Each test has its advantages and disadvantages, although probably most laboratories now offer fT_4 and fT_3 assays rather than total hormone concentrations.

Plasma thyroid-stimulating hormone

Concentrations of TSH are high in primary hypothyroidism and low in secondary or pituitary hypothyroidism. In hyperthyroidism, high plasma T_4 and T_3 concentrations suppress TSH release from the pituitary, resulting in very low or undetectable plasma TSH concentrations. Plasma TSH assays are used as first-line assays for thyroid function assessment. New generation assays have high sensitivity and have a detection limit for plasma TSH of less than 0.1 mU/L. In normal individuals there is a log-linear relationship between plasma fT_4 and TSH concentrations; that is to say, exponential increases in TSH concentration occur with small incremental changes in fT_4 concentration.

Plasma total thyroxine or free thyroxine assays

Plasma T_4 is more than 99 per cent protein bound; therefore, plasma total T_4 assays reflect the protein-bound rather than the free hormone fraction. Total T_4 reflects fT_4 concentrations unless there are abnormalities of binding proteins.

- In the *euthyroid* state, about a third of the binding sites on TBG are occupied by T_4 and the remainder are unoccupied, irrespective of the concentration of the binding protein.
- In *hyperthyroidism*, both plasma total and fT_4 concentrations are increased and the number of unoccupied binding sites on TBG is decreased.
- In *hypothyroidism*, the opposite to the above occurs.

An increase in plasma TBG concentration causes an increase in both bound T_4 and unoccupied binding sites but no change in plasma fT_4 concentrations. Such an increase may occur because of:

- a high oestrogen concentration during pregnancy or in the newborn infant,
- oestrogen therapy, for example certain oral contraceptives or hormone replacement therapy,
- inherited TBG excess (rare).

A decrease in plasma TBG concentration decreases both bound T_4 concentrations and unoccupied binding sites but does not alter the plasma fT_4 concentration. Such changes may occur because of:

- severe illness, but this is usually temporary,
- loss of low-molecular-weight proteins, usually in the urine, for example nephrotic syndrome,
- androgens or danazol treatment,
- inherited TBG deficiency (rare).

These changes might be misinterpreted as being diagnostic of hyperthyroidism or hypothyroidism respectively if only plasma total T_4 was assayed and it is for this reason that fT_4 concentrations are now generally preferred.

Some drugs, such as salicylates and danazol, bind to TBG and displace T_4. The change in unoccupied binding sites is variable and TBG concentrations are unaffected. Measurement of plasma TBG concentrations may occasionally be indicated to confirm either congenital TBG excess or deficiency.

Plasma total or free tri-iodothyronine

Total T_3 or free T_3 (fT_3) concentrations may help in the diagnosis of hyperthyroidism but are not usually used routinely to diagnose hypothyroidism because normal plasma concentrations are very low. In hyperthyroidism, the increase in plasma T_3 or fT_3 concentrations is greater, and usually occurs earlier than that of T_4 or fT_4.

Occasionally in hyperthyroidism the plasma T_3 or fT_3 concentrations are elevated but not those of T_4 or fT_4 (T_3 toxicosis). Like T_4, T_3 is bound to protein. It is usually preferable to measure the plasma concentration of fT_3 rather than total T_3, as the latter may be altered by changes in the plasma concentrations of TBG.

Thyrotrophin-releasing hormone test

The TRH test is used to confirm the diagnosis of secondary hypothyroidism, or occasionally to diagnose early primary hypothyroidism. Since the development of sensitive TSH assays, it is rarely used to diagnose hyperthyroidism, although it may have a place in the differential diagnosis of thyroid resistance syndrome or TSH-secreting pituitary tumours (TSHomas). It is sometimes used as part of the combined pituitary stimulation test (see Chapter 7).

Allergic reactions may occur and therefore resuscitation facilities should be available and the test should be carried out by experienced staff.

Procedure
- A basal blood sample is taken.
- 200 μg of TRH is injected intravenously over about a minute.
- Further blood samples are taken 20 and 60 minutes after the TRH injection and TSH is measured in all samples.

Note that certain drugs, such as dopamine agonists and glucocorticoids, reduce the response, and oestrogens, metoclopramide and theophylline enhance it.

Interpretation
In normal subjects, plasma TSH concentration increases at 20 minutes by at least 2 mU/L and exceeds the upper limit of the reference range, with a small decline at 60 minutes.

- An exaggerated response at 20 minutes and a slight fall at 60 minutes are suggestive of primary hypothyroidism.
- A normal or exaggerated increment but delayed response, with plasma TSH concentrations higher at 60 minutes than at 20 minutes, suggests secondary hypothyroidism due to hypothalamic dysfunction. If clinically indicated, pituitary and hypothalamic function should be investigated.
- A flat response of TSH of less than 5 mU/L is compatible with primary hyperthyroidism, although this may also occur in some euthyroid patients with multinodular goitre.

Drug effects on thyroid function tests

Drugs may alter plasma T_4 and T_3 concentrations. The more common effects are summarized in Table 11.1. If the primary change is in binding protein concentrations, plasma free hormone concentrations are usually normal.

TABLE 11.1 Drug effects on thyroid function tests

Drug	T_4	fT_4	T_3	fT_3	Remarks
Amiodarone	↑	Normal or ↑	Normal	Normal	Blocking T_4 to T_3 conversion
Androgens	↓	Normal	↓	Normal	Reduced TBG
Carbamazepine	↓	↓	Normal	Normal	Increased T_4 to T_3 conversion
Carbimazole	↓	↓	↓	↓	Therapeutic
Lithium	↓	↓	↓	↓	Lithium may inhibit iodination
Oestrogens	↑	Normal	↑	Normal	Increased TBG
Phenytoin	↓	↓	Normal	Normal	Increased T_4 to T_3 conversion
Propranolol	Normal	Normal	↓	↓	Blocking T_4 to T_3 conversion
Propylthiouracil	↓	↓	↓	↓	Therapeutic
Salicylate	↓	Normal	↓	Normal	Reduced TBG binding
Some radiocontrast media	↑	Normal	↓	Normal or ↓	Blocking T_4 to T_3 conversion (transient effect)

T_4 = thyroxine; T_3 = tri-iodothyronine; fT_4 = free thyroxine; fT_3 = free tri-iodothyronine; TBG = thyroxine-binding globulin.

Interference of assays by immunoglobulins

Anti-T_4 or anti-T_3 immunoglobulins such as heterophilic antibodies can cause a spurious elevation of T_4 or T_3 (or free hormones), respectively, when assayed by immunoassay. This needs to be remembered when interpreting thyroid function test results.

DISORDERS OF THE THYROID GLAND

The most common presenting clinical features of thyroid disease are the result of:

- *hypothyroidism*, due to deficient thyroid hormone secretion,
- *hyperthyroidism*, due to excessive thyroid hormone secretion,
- *goitre*, either diffuse or due to one or more nodules within the gland. There may or may not be abnormal thyroid hormone secretion and thus the patient may be euthyroid.

Hypothyroidism

Hypothyroidism is caused by suboptimal circulating concentrations of thyroid hormones. It becomes more prevalent with age, affecting about 6 per cent of people over 60 years, and is more common in women.

The condition may develop insidiously and in its early stages may cause only vague symptoms. There is a generalized slowing down of metabolism, with lethargy, bradycardia, depression and weakness.

If the hormone deficiency is caused by a primary disorder of the thyroid gland, the patient may present with weight gain, myopathy, menstrual disturbances, such as menorrhagia, and constipation. The skin may be dry, the hair may fall out and the voice may be hoarse. Subcutaneous tissues are thickened; this pseudo-oedema, with a histological myxoid appearance, accounts for the term myxoedema, which is sometimes used to describe advanced hypothyroidism. In severe cases, coma with profound hypothermia may develop.

The following laboratory changes may be associated with hypothyroidism, particularly if severe.

- Plasma cholesterol concentration. In hypothyroidism the clearance of plasma low-density lipoprotein (LDL)-cholesterol is impaired and plasma cholesterol concentrations may be moderately high.
- Plasma creatine kinase activity is often raised in hypothyroidism, due to possible myopathy.
- Hyponatraemia may occasionally be present in patients with profound hypothyroidism or myxoedema coma. It is caused by increased antidiuretic hormone release with excessive water retention, occasionally precipitated by a constrictive pericardial effusion that some patients develop.
- Hypothyroidism may be associated with hyperprolactinaemia.
- Plasma sex-hormone-binding globulin (SHBG) concentration is reduced in hypothyroidism.
- A macrocytic anaemia may be observed, with raised mean corpuscular volume.
- Sometimes the results of liver and renal function tests are abnormal.

The commonest cause of hypothyroidism worldwide is iodine deficiency. In areas of adequate iodine intake, acquired hypothyroidism is mainly due to autoimmune thyroiditis or Hashimoto's thyroiditis, which is more frequently seen in women and the elderly. About 90 per cent of patients have positive thyroid antibodies, for example anti-thyroid peroxidase (anti-TPO), anti-thyroglobulin (anti-Tg) or TSH receptor blocking antibodies. There may

---

CASE 1

A 57-year-old female consulted her general practitioner because of weight gain, constipation and weakness. The following thyroid function test results were returned.

Plasma TSH 54.6 mU/L (0.20–5.0)
Free T_4 5.7 pmol/L (12–25)

DISCUSSION

The results show primary hypothyroidism with high plasma TSH and low fT_4 concentrations. The symptoms are typical of hypothyroidism. The patient was also shown to have positive thyroid antibodies (anti-TPO). The thyroid function tests normalized on treatment with 100 μg/day of T_4.

also be a goitre. Hypothyroidism may also be associated with other autoimmune diseases such as type 1 diabetes mellitus, adrenal insufficiency and pernicious anaemia.

Rare causes of primary hypothyroidism are exogenous goitrogens and dyshormonogenesis, a term that includes inherited deficiencies of any of the enzymes involved in thyroid hormone synthesis, which may present in childhood. Although the biochemical and clinical features differ, the end result is hypothyroidism. In most cases prolonged TSH stimulation, due to reduced negative feedback, causes goitre. The commonest form is due to failure to incorporate iodine into tyrosine. The perchlorate discharge test may be useful to diagnose iodination and trapping defects, although it is rarely used.

Secondary hypothyroidism is due to low concentrations of TSH from the anterior pituitary or to hypothalamic TRH deficiency; this is much less common than primary hypothyroidism. In longstanding secondary hypothyroidism, the thyroid gland may atrophy irreversibly. The essential biochemical difference between primary and secondary hypothyroidism is in the plasma TSH concentration, which is high in the former and inappropriately low in the latter.

Pathophysiology

As primary hypothyroidism develops, TSH secretion from the anterior pituitary gland increases as the negative feedback (associated with the falling plasma T_4 or fT_4 concentration) decreases. Plasma T_3 or fT_3 concentrations are often normal and thus not usually useful in making the diagnosis.

Generally in primary hypothyroidism the plasma TSH concentration is high, but it is low in secondary hypothyroidism due to pituitary or hypothalamic disease. Initially, the plasma T_4 or fT_4 concentration may be within the population reference range, although abnormally low for the individual. For this reason the plasma TSH concentration is the most sensitive index of early hypothyroidism. If the patient is very ill, investigations should be deferred (see 'Sick euthyroid' below).

Neonatal hypothyroidism

Routine screening for congenital hypothyroidism is discussed in Chapters 26 and 27.

Treatment of hypothyroidism

This is usually with T_4, which can be titrated until the plasma TSH is within the reference range. However, this has recently been challenged, as plasma TSH concentrations may not adequately reflect tissue hypothyroidism and it may be better to be guided by plasma fT_4 concentrations and clinical features. On rare occasions, such as in hypothyroid comas, T_3 is given instead, as its action is more immediate. The response to T_4 therapy can be checked 2–3 monthly until the patient is stable, when 6–12-monthly blood checks may be useful.

Thyroxine should be used with caution in patients with ischaemic heart disease for fear of worsening angina pectoris, and low doses initially plus β-blockers may be indicated. Thyroid-stimulating hormone assays are of no value in monitoring secondary hypothyroidism; fT_4 is better. Thyroxine therapy may precipitate an Addisonian crisis in patients with concomitant adrenal insufficiency. Overtreatment with T_4 can evoke atrial fibrillation and osteoporosis; in such cases, plasma TSH concentrations are often low or suppressed.

If a patient is non-compliant with treatment and only takes T_4 near to the time of thyroid function testing, a high plasma TSH may be observed with high plasma fT_4 concentrations. This is because there is insufficient T_4 to normalize plasma TSH and yet the high plasma fT_4 reflects the recent taking of T_4.

Compensated hypothyroidism

Compensated or subclinical hypothyroidism is the state in which plasma TSH concentration is raised but the total or fT_4 concentration still falls within the reference range. In individuals over the age of 60 years, the prevalence may be as high as 10 per cent. Some of these patients have positive thyroid antibodies, for example anti-TPO or anti-Tg, and each year about 2–5 per cent of thyroid-antibody-positive patients go on to develop hypothyroidism.

Some patients may be asymptomatic, whereas others have symptoms suggestive of hypothyroidism. Thyroxine therapy may be indicated particularly in pregnancy, when the patient is symptomatic, or with positive thyroid antibodies and plasma TSH more than 10 mU/L.

Thyroid hormone resistance

In generalized thyroid hormone resistance, the plasma total and T_4 and fT_4 concentrations are elevated, with normal or slightly raised TSH concentration. Some patients appear euthyroid, but others may present with hypothyroid symptoms, and the defect may be inherited as an autosomal dominant trait in some patients. The defect is thought to be due to a defect in T_4 and/or T_3 receptors and may be associated with other end-organ resistance states.

> **CASE 2**
>
> A 49-year-old female was investigated in the medical out-patients department for tiredness. The following test results were returned.
>
> Plasma TSH 10.6 mU/L (0.20–5.0)
> Free T_4 13.9 pmol/L (12–25)
>
> **DISCUSSION**
> These results are suggestive of compensated hypothyroidism, in which the plasma TSH concentration is raised and the fT_4 concentration still remains within the reference range. The patient also had positive thyroid antibodies (anti-TPO). A trial of T_4 50 μg/day brought her plasma TSH concentration to within the reference range and improved her symptoms.

Laboratory investigation of suspected hypothyroidism

A careful history (including drugs) should be taken and an examination performed, checking for a goitre.

- The plasma TSH and total T_4 or fT_4 concentrations should be measured.
- Slightly elevated plasma TSH and normal fT_4 concentrations suggest compensated hypothyroidism. Measuring circulating thyroid antibodies may be useful, i.e. anti-TPO and anti-Tg. Tests should be repeated after 3–6 months as some patients may develop full-blown hypothyroidism.
- Raised plasma TSH and low fT_4 concentrations suggest primary hypothyroidism. The thyroid antibodies should be measured and, if positive, other autoimmune diseases excluded.
- Low plasma TSH and low fT_4 concentrations may indicate that the hypothyroidism is caused by a hypothalamic or pituitary disorder. A TRH test should be done, if indicated, and the pituitary gland assessed (see Chapter 7).
- Raised plasma TSH and raised/normal plasma fT_4 concentrations in the presence of hypothyroid symptoms may indicate thyroid hormone resistance.

Some causes of hypothyroidism are shown in Box 11.1.

Hyperthyroidism (thyrotoxicosis)

Hyperthyroidism causes sustained high plasma concentrations of T_4 and T_3. There is often generalized increase in the metabolic rate, evidenced clinically by, for example, heat intolerance, a fine tremor, tachycardia including atrial fibrillation, weight loss, tiredness, anxiety, sweating and diarrhoea.

The following biochemical features may be associated with hyperthyroidism.

- Hypercalcaemia is occasionally found in patients with severe thyrotoxicosis. There is an increased turnover of bone cells, probably due to a direct action of thyroid hormone.

> **Box 11.1 Some causes of hypothyroidism**
>
> *Primary hypothyroidism*
> Iodine deficiency
> Autoimmune thyroid disease:
>   Hashimoto's disease
>   subacute thyroiditis
>   transient subacute thyroiditis (de Quervain's)
> Following treatment of hyperthyroidism:
>   post-thyroidectomy
>   post-radio-iodine treatment
> External irradiation to neck region
> Surgery or trauma to neck
> Defects of thyroid hormone synthesis
> Congenital absence of thyroid gland
> Infiltrative disease of the thyroid, e.g. sarcoid, haemochromatosis, fibrosis (Riedel's struma)
> Drugs:
>   carbimazole
>   propylthiouracil
>   amiodarone
>   lithium
>   interferon-alpha
>
> *Secondary hypothyroidism*
> Pituitary or hypothalamic disease
>
> *Thyroid hormone resistance*
> Generalized thyroid resistance

- Hypocholesterolaemia can occur, due to increased LDL clearance.
- Hypokalaemia may also occur, associated with hyperthyrotoxic periodic paralysis.
- Plasma SHBG is increased.
- Plasma creatine kinase may be increased with thyrotoxic myopathy.

Some causes of hyperthyroidism are shown in Box 11.2.

Graves' disease

This is the most common form of thyrotoxicosis and occurs more often in females than in males. It may be caused by relatively autonomous secretion from a diffuse goitre and is characterized by:

- exophthalmos, due to lymphocytic infiltration and swelling of retro-orbital tissues of the eyes,
- sometimes localized thickening of the subcutaneous tissue over the shin (pretibial myxoedema).

Graves' disease is an autoimmune thyroid disease characterized by a variety of circulating antibodies, including anti-TPO, as well as being associated with other autoimmune diseases such as type 1 diabetes mellitus, adrenal insufficiency and pernicious anaemia. Thyroid antibodies are detectable in some cases, such as thyroid-stimulating immunoglobulin (TSI), which is directed towards epitopes of the TSH receptor and thus acts as a TSH receptor agonist. Nuclear medicine tests may show a high radioactive uptake of iodine by the thyroid gland.

Subacute thyroiditis

This is a destructive thyroiditis resulting in the release of preformed thyroid hormones. There are three subtypes: granulomatous or painful, lymphocytic or silent and painless,

---

Box 11.2 Some causes of hyperthyroidism

Autonomous secretion
Graves' disease
Toxic multinodular goitre (Plummer's disease) or a single functioning nodule (occasionally an adenoma)
Subacute thyroiditis
Some metastatic thyroid carcinomas

Excessive ingestion of thyroid hormones or iodine
Amiodarone
Thyrotoxicosis factitia (self-administration of thyroid hormones)
Administration of iodine to a subject with iodine-deficiency goitre
Jod–Basedow syndrome

Rare causes
Thyroid-stimulating hormone (TSH) secretion by tumours, including pituitary tumours or those of trophoblastic origin
Struma ovarii (thyroid tissue in an ovarian teratoma)
Excess human chorionic gonadotrophin, e.g molar pregnancy or choriocarcinoma
Pituitary resistance to thyroid hormone

CASE 3

A 29-year-old female was seen in the thyroid clinic because of exophthalmos and a goitre. She had the following thyroid function test results.

Plasma TSH <0.05 mU/L (0.20–5.0)
Free T_4 68.8 pmol/L (12–25)
Free T_3 18.7 pmol/L (3–7)

DISCUSSION

The patient had biochemical results typical of hyperthyroidism. In fact she had Graves' disease and was shown to have positive TSIs and increased diffuse radiolabelled iodine uptake by the thyroid gland.

Compare these results with those of another patient (a 54-year-old female) in the same clinic.

Plasma TSH <0.05 mU/L (0.20–5.0)
Free T_4 18.1 pmol/L (12–25)
Free T_3 14.4 pmol/L (3–7)

Here, the plasma fT_4 concentration is within the reference range, but the plasma fT_3 concentration is raised, with suppressed plasma TSH concentration, suggesting T_3 thyrotoxicosis.

and postpartum. This condition is associated with extremely elevated thyroid hormones and no radioactive iodine uptake by the thyroid gland. The clinical course progresses through 6–8 weeks of thyrotoxicosis, 2–4 months of hypothyroidism and a return to euthyroidism in about 90 per cent of patients.

The painful or granulomatous variety is thought to be a viral disease and is associated with HLA-Bw35. The lymphocytic variety is autoimmune, as is postpartum thyroiditis. The postpartum form occurs in about 5–8 per cent of pregnant women in Europe and the USA, but in 20 per cent in Japan. Treatment is supportive, as in many cases the condition is self-limiting.

Toxic nodules

Toxic nodules, either single or multiple, in a nodular goitre may secrete thyroid hormones autonomously. The secretion of TSH is suppressed by negative feedback, as in Graves' disease. The nodules may be detected by their uptake of radioactive iodine or technetium, with suppression of uptake in the rest of the thyroid tissue ('hot nodules'). Toxic nodules are found most commonly in older patients, who may present with only one of the features of hyperactivity, usually cardiovascular symptoms such as atrial fibrillation. Toxic multinodular goitre is also called Plummer's disease.

Rare hyperthyroid states

Jod–Basedow syndrome occurs in patients with excess iodide intake and in those with regions of thyroid autonomy, as in single or multinodular goitre. High iodine intake may be assessed by urinary iodide assay. Metastatic thyroid carcinoma can produce thyroid hormones. In struma ovarii, ectopic thyroid tissue is found in dermoid tumours or ovarian teratomas. Patients with choriocarcinoma or molar hydatidiform pregnancy have extremely high concentrations of β-human chorionic gonadotrophin that can activate the TSH receptor. Rarely, the pituitary tumour releases TSH, resulting in thyrotoxicosis.

Pathophysiology

Plasma T_4 or fT_4 and T_3 and fT_3 concentrations are usually increased in hyperthyroidism. Much of the T_3 is secreted directly by the thyroid gland and the increase in plasma T_3 concentrations is greater, and usually evident earlier, than that of T_4. Rarely, only plasma T_3 and fT_3 concentrations are elevated (T_3 toxicosis). In both situations, TSH secretion is suppressed by negative feedback, and plasma TSH concentrations are either very low or undetectable.

Treatment

The aetiology of hyperthyroidism must be fully investigated and treatment started. Various forms of treatment are available, the selection of which depends on the cause, the clinical presentation and the age of the patient. Beta-blocker drugs such as propranolol, which inhibit the peripheral conversion of T_4 to T_3, may be used initially. Additional treatment includes the use of such drugs as carbimazole or propylthiouracil. Carbimazole inhibits the synthesis of T_3 and T_4; propylthiouracil additionally inhibits T_4 to T_3 conversion. Some clinicians use block-and-replace regimens: carbimazole is used to 'block' thyroid secretion and simultaneous exogenous T_4 maintains and replaces T_4 concentrations. It is important to remember that carbimazole can have the potentially lethal side-effect of bone marrow suppression, and patients should be warned about infections such as sore throats and about the need to have their full blood count monitored.

Radioactive iodine can be used in resistant or relapsing cases; surgery is rarely indicated, but may have a place if there is a large toxic goitre that is exerting pressure or if drug therapy fails but radioactive iodine is contraindicated. Thyroid function must be checked regularly, as some patients may become hypothyroid or may relapse after radio-iodine or surgery.

The progress of a patient being treated for hyperthyroidism is usually monitored by estimating plasma TSH, fT_4 and fT_3 concentrations, trying to restore these to normal (although TSH concentration may be slow to normalize). Over-treatment may induce hypothyroidism, with a rise in plasma TSH concentrations and low plasma T_4/fT_4 and T_3/fT_3 concentrations. In some patients with severe prolonged hyperthyroidism, such a rise in plasma TSH may be delayed because of the effects of prolonged feedback suppression of T_4 on the pituitary.

Subclinical hyperthyroidism

Subclinical hyperthyroidism may occur with a low or suppressed TSH concentration but normal (usually high-normal) plasma fT_4 and fT_3 concentrations. The condition may progress to full-blown hyperthyroidism with suppressed plasma TSH and raised plasma fT_4 and fT_3 concentrations. Subclinical hyperthyroidism may be associated with atrial fibrillation, decreased bone mineral density and other features of hyperthyroidism. Plasma TSI may be raised.

Laboratory investigation of suspected hyperthyroidism

A careful history (including drugs) should be taken and examination performed, checking for a goitre. The plasma TSH, fT_3 and fT_4 concentrations should be measured.

- The plasma fT_4 and fT_3 concentrations are clearly high and the TSH concentration is suppressed in clinically thyrotoxic patients.
- In the face of suppressed plasma TSH, a clearly elevated plasma fT_3 concentration confirms the diagnosis of hyperthyroidism. Remember that in T_3 thyrotoxicosis the plasma fT_4 may be normal.
- If the plasma fT_4 concentration is raised and the TSH concentration is normal, this is suggestive of biochemical euthyroid hyperthyroxaemia (see below for causes).
- Measurement of thyroid antibodies is useful, particularly if the concentration of TSIs is raised, which supports a diagnosis of Graves' disease.
- The rare TSH-secreting pituitary tumours need pituitary assessment (see Chapter 7). Raised α-subunit concentrations may be useful, as they are usually raised in such circumstances.
- In difficult cases, determination of plasma SHBG concentration can help decide whether the patient is hyperthyroid, as it is lowered in hypothyroidism and raised in hyperthyroidism.
- Radio-iodine uptake studies of the thyroid can be useful to distinguish some of the causes of hyperthyroidism (see Box 11.2).
- The TRH test is sometimes useful in the diagnosis of unclear cases.

Euthyroid goitre

If plasma T_4 concentrations fall, enlargement of the thyroid gland (goitre) may be caused by TSH stimulation resulting in cellular hyperplasia. Thyroxine synthesis may be impaired by iodide deficiency, caused by drugs such as para-aminosalicylic acid, or possibly by partial deficiency of the enzymes involved in T_4 synthesis. Under the influence of prolonged stimulation by TSH, the number of thyroid cells increases and plasma thyroid hormone concentrations are maintained at the expense of the development of a goitre.

Inflammation of the thyroid gland (thyroiditis), whether acute or subacute, may produce marked but temporary aberrations of thyroid function tests (see above).

Ultrasound scanning can be useful in the diagnosis of goitre, as can radiolabelled uptake studies to see if there are hot (T_4-producing) or cold (non-producing) nodule(s).

'Sick euthyroid'

Any severe illness may be associated with low plasma total or fT_4 concentrations and may make the interpretation of thyroid function tests extremely difficult. Plasma TSH concentrations may be normal or slightly high or low. The TSH response to TRH may also be impaired. There may be impaired conversion of T_4 to T_3 with low plasma T_3 concentrations. Consequently, the assessment of thyroid function is best deferred until the patient has recovered from the illness.

Euthyroid hyperthyroxinaemia

This is defined as a condition in which either the plasma total or fT_4 concentration is abnormally raised without clinical evidence of thyroid disease. These changes may be transient or persistent, with high, normal or low total or fT_3 concentrations. Heterophilic antibodies to fT_4 and/or fT_3 should be excluded, as these can interfere with some assays.

Causes

- Physiological conditions resulting in raised plasma TBG concentration, for example pregnancy. Concentrations of total T_4 and T_3 are both elevated, but there are usually normal fT_4 and fT_3 concentrations.
- TBG concentration is raised in newborns.
- Hereditary causes:
  - hereditary TBG excess is X-linked,
  - hereditary TBPA excess,
  - familial dysalbuminaemic hyperthyroidism (FDH) due to an abnormal form of albumin.
- Drugs causing hyperthyroxinaemia:
  - oestrogens raise TBG concentration, as do 5-fluorouracil, heroin and methadone,
  - amiodarone blocks conversion of T_4 to T_3, resulting in an elevation of T_4 and reverse T_3 concentrations,
  - heparin, due to fatty acid release, inhibits fT_4 binding to TBG,
  - propranolol inhibits extrathyroidal conversion of T_4 to T_3.
- Some patients with certain illnesses, for example hyperemesis gravidarum, have low total and fT_3 concentrations due to reduced peripheral conversion of T_4 to T_3 because 5-de-iodinase is inhibited. This results in elevated total T_4 and fT_4 concentrations. Some hepatic disorders, including acute hepatitis, result in raised concentrations of TBG and T_4 and fT_4. In up to 10 per cent of cases of acute psychosis, total and fT_4 concentrations are raised. The exact

mechanism is unknown, but it may be due to central activation of the hypothalamic–pituitary axis.

Amiodarone and thyroid function

Amiodarone is sometimes used to treat certain cardiac arrhythmias. This drug can evoke hypothyroidism, partly because it interrupts the conversion of T_4 to T_3. However, it contains iodine and can also evoke thyrotoxicosis by the Jod–Basedow or type 1 phenomenon. Conversely, it may elicit disruptive thyroiditis and thyrotoxicosis with raised interleukin-6 concentration (type 2 phenomenon). The drug has a long half-life (40–100 days) and thus takes a long time to clear from the body (see Chapter 25).

STRATEGY FOR THYROID FUNCTION TESTING AND INTERPRETATION

- A first-line test for thyroid function (as stated above) is plasma TSH, which should not be interpreted in the absence of plasma fT_4. (Sometimes fT_3 is also required, particularly if hyperthyroidism is suspected – see Table 11.2.)
- If the plasma TSH concentration is *normal* and the patient is clinically euthyroid, look at plasma fT_4.
  – If fT_4 concentration is low, consider:
    sick euthyroid/non-thyroidal illness,
    certain drugs, such as carbamazepine or phenytoin (see Table 11.1).

CASE 4

A 45-year-old male was on the coronary care unit the day after an acute myocardial infarction. One of his doctors thought that he looked hypothyroid and requested thyroid function tests, the results of which were as follows.

Plasma TSH <0.05 mU/L (0.20–5.0)
Free T_4 10.1 pmol/L (12–25)
Free T_3 1.4 pmol/L (3–7)

On repeating the tests 3 months later at a follow-up appointment in medical out-patients, the following results were obtained.

Plasma TSH 2.3 mU/L (0.20–5.0)
Free T_4 18.1 pmol/L (12–25)
Free T_3 4.5 pmol/L (3–7)

DISCUSSION

The first set of results could indicate hypothyroidism due to pituitary or hypothalamic defects (secondary hypothyroidism), i.e. low TSH and 'normal' fT_4 and fT_3 concentrations. However, the normalization of the results when the patient was not acutely ill suggested sick euthyroidism or non-thyroidal illness. Beware of requesting thyroid function tests in acutely ill patients.

TABLE 11.2 Interpretation of thyroid function tests

	Total T_4	Total T_3	fT_4	fT_3	TBG	TSH
Euthyroid	Normal	Normal	Normal	Normal	Normal	Normal
Hyperthyroid	↑	↑	↑	↑	Normal	↓ if primary ↑ if secondary
T_3 toxicosis	Normal	↑	Normal	↑	Normal	↓
Hypothyroid	↓	↓	↓	↓	Normal	↑ if primary ↓ if secondary
TBG excess	↑	↑	Normal	Normal	↑	Normal
TBG deficiency	↓	↓	Normal	Normal	↓	Normal
T_4 displacement by drug	↓	Normal	Normal/↓	Normal	Normal	Normal

T_4 = thyroxine; T_3 = tri-iodothyronine; fT_4 = free thyroxine; fT_3 = free tri-iodothyronine; TBG = thyroxine-binding globulin; TSH = thyroid-stimulating hormone.

- If fT_4 concentration is also normal, thyroid function is likely to be normal.
- If fT_4 concentration is high, consider:
  euthyroid hyperthyroxinaemia,
  interfering assay autoantibodies.
- If the plasma TSH concentration is *low*, look at plasma fT_4.
  - If fT_4 concentration is low, consider:
    sick euthyroid/non-thyroid illness,
    pituitary or hypothalamic disease (?secondary hypothyroidism),
    certain drugs (see Table 11.1).
  - If fT_4 concentration is normal, consider:
    sick euthyroid/non-thyroid illness,
    subclinical hyperthyroidism, particularly if clinically hyperthyroid,
    certain drugs, such as glucocorticoids and dopamine that may affect TSH,
    fT_3 toxicosis (fT_3 concentration is raised).
  - if fT_4 concentration is high, consider:
    hyperthyroidism (see Box 11.2),
    drugs such as amiodarone (see Table 11.1),
    iodine excess,
    hyperemesis gravidarum, molar pregnancy,
    activating TSH receptor mutations.
- If the plasma TSH concentration is *high*, look at plasma fT_4.
  - If fT_4 concentration is low, consider:
    primary hypothyroidism (see Box 11.1).
  - If fT_4 concentration is normal, consider:
    compensated hypothyroidism,
    inadequate thyroid replacement for hypothyroidism,
    drugs such as metoclopramide, domperidone.
  - If fT_4 concentration is high, consider:
    generalized thyroid hormone resistance,
    TSH-secreting tumour,
    interfering assay antibodies.

CONCLUSIONS

- Thyroid-stimulating hormone from the anterior pituitary acts upon the thyroid gland to release two iodine-containing hormones, T_4 and T_3. The latter is more active and can also be produced from T_4 peripherally. These hormones are essential for normal growth and development and increase basal metabolic rate.
- Both T_4 and T_3 are bound to proteins, including TBG, albumin and pre-albumin. Only the free or unbound form is physiologically active, although this fraction constitutes less than 1 per cent of the total hormone concentration.
- Thyroid disease is relatively common. Hypothyroidism can be primary or secondary and manifest as weight gain, tiredness and constipation – to name but a few of its clinical features. Hyperthyroidism causes thyrotoxicosis associated with weight loss, sweating and sometimes thyroid eye disease. Both can present with a goitre, although some patients with a goitre may be euthyroid (normal thyroid function tests).

12 CARBOHYDRATE METABOLISM

| Chemistry | 174 | Hyperglycaemia and diabetes mellitus | 182 |
| Physiology | 174 | Hypoglycaemia | 192 |

This chapter discusses carbohydrate metabolism and its abnormalities, with emphasis on diabetes mellitus and hypoglycaemia. In the next decade it is predicted that there will be about 250 million people worldwide with type 2 diabetes mellitus.

CHEMISTRY

The main monosaccharide hexoses are reducing sugars. Naturally occurring polysaccharides are long-chain carbohydrates composed of glucose subunits (Table 12.1):

- *starch* found in plants, is a mixture of amylose (straight chains) and amylopectin (branched chains),
- *glycogen*, found in animal tissue, is a highly branched polysaccharide.

PHYSIOLOGY

Functions of extracellular glucose

The main function of glucose is as a major tissue energy source. The basic pathways of glycolysis and the Krebs' cycle (tricarboxylic acid [TCA] cycle) are shown in Figs 12.1 and 12.2. The brain is highly dependent upon the extracellular glucose concentration for its energy supply; indeed, hypoglycaemia is likely to impair cerebral function or even lead to irreversible neuronal damage. This is because the brain cannot:

- synthesize glucose,
- store glucose in significant amounts,

Table 12.1 Common reducing and non-reducing sugars

	Reducing sugars	Non-reducing sugars
Monosaccharides	Glucose Fructose Galactose	
Disaccharides	Lactose (galactose + glucose) Maltose (glucose + glucose)	Sucrose (fructose + glucose)

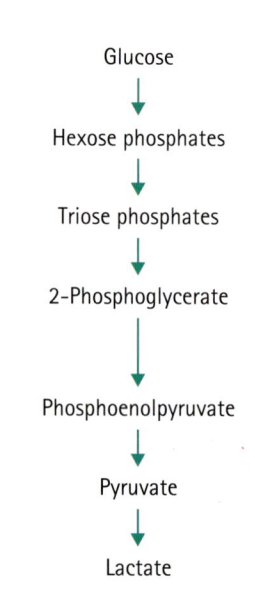

Glucose
↓
Hexose phosphates
↓
Triose phosphates
↓
2-Phosphoglycerate
↓
Phosphoenolpyruvate
↓
Pyruvate
↓
Lactate

Fig. 12.1 Simplification of glycolysis pathways. (Reproduced with kind permission from Candlish JK and Crook M, *Notes on Clinical Biochemistry*, Singapore: World Scientific Publishing, 1993.)

- metabolize substrates other than glucose and ketones – plasma ketone concentrations are usually very low and ketones are of little importance as an energy source under physiological conditions,
- extract enough glucose from the extracellular fluid at low concentrations for its metabolic needs, because entry into brain cells is not facilitated by insulin.

Normally the plasma glucose concentration remains between about 4 mmol/L and 10 mmol/L, despite the intermittent load entering the body from the diet. The maintenance of plasma glucose concentrations below about 10 mmol/L minimizes loss from the body as well as providing the optimal supply to the tissues. Renal tubular cells reabsorb almost all the glucose filtered by the glomeruli, and urinary glucose concentration is normally too low to be detected by the usual tests, even after a carbohydrate meal.

Significant glycosuria only usually occurs if the plasma glucose concentration exceeds about 10 mmol/L – the renal threshold.

How the body maintains extracellular glucose concentrations

Control of plasma glucose concentration

During normal metabolism, little glucose is lost unchanged from the body. Maintenance of plasma glucose concentrations within the relatively narrow range of 4–10 mmol/L despite the widely varying input from the diet depends on the balance between the glucose entering cells from the extracellular fluid and that leaving them into this compartment.

Hormones concerned with glucose homeostasis

Some of the more important effects of hormones on glucose homeostasis are summarized in Table 12.2.

Insulin

Insulin is the most important hormone controlling plasma glucose concentrations. A plasma glucose concentration of greater than about 5 mmol/L stimulates insulin release via glucose transporter-2 of the pancreas beta-cell. These cells produce proinsulin, which consists of the 51-amino-acid polypeptide insulin and a linking peptide (C-peptide, Fig. 12.3). Splitting of the peptide bonds by prohormone convertases releases via intermediates (mostly 32–33 split proinsulin) equimolar amounts of insulin and C-peptide into the extracellular fluid.

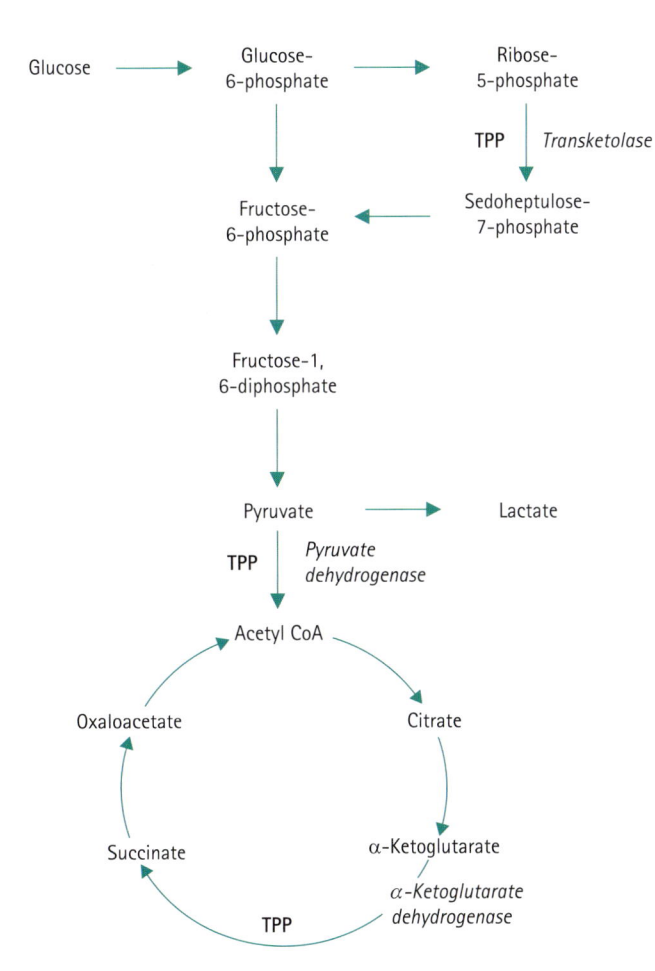

Fig. 12.2 Simplification of the tricarboxylic acid cycle. (TPP = thiamine pyrophosphate; CoA = coenzyme A). (Reproduced with kind permission from Candlish JK and Crook M, *Notes on Clinical Biochemistry*, Singapore: World Scientific Publishing, 1993.)

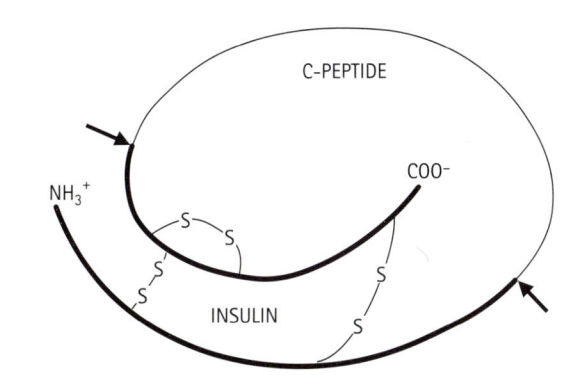

Fig. 12.3 Structure of proinsulin, indicating the cleavage sites at which insulin and C-peptide are produced.

Table 12.2 Action of hormones that affect intermediary metabolism

	Insulin	Glucagon	Growth hormone	Glucocorticoids	Adrenaline
Carbohydrate metabolism					
In liver					
glycolysis	+				
glycogenesis	+				
glycogenolysis		+			+
gluconeogenesis	−	+		+	
In muscle					
glucose uptake	+		−	−	
glycogenesis	+				
glycogenolysis					+
Protein metabolism					
synthesis	+		+		
breakdown	−			+	
Lipid metabolism					
synthesis	+				
lipolysis	−		+	+	+
Secretion					
stimulated by	Hyperglycaemia Amino acids Glucagon Gut hormones	Hypoglycaemia Amino acids Fasting	Hypoglycaemia Stress Sleep	Hypoglycaemia Stress	Hypoglycaemia Stress
inhibited by	Adrenaline Fasting Somatostatin	Insulin	Somatostatin IGF-1	Glucocorticoids	Beta blockers
Plasma NEFA concentrations	Fall	Rise	Rise	Rise	Rise
Plasma glucose concentrations	Fall	Rise	Rise	Rise	Rise

+ = stimulates − = inhibits. NEFA = non-esterified fatty acid; IGF-1 = insulin-like growth factor 1.

Insulin binds to specific cell-surface receptors on muscle and adipose tissue, thus enhancing the rate of glucose entry into these cells. Insulin-induced activation of enzymes stimulates glucose incorporation into glycogen synthesis (glycogenesis) in liver and muscle. Insulin also inhibits the production of glucose (gluconeogenesis) from fats and amino acids, partly by reducing these substrates by inhibiting fat and protein breakdown (lipolysis and proteolysis).

The transport of glucose into liver cells is insulin independent but, by reducing the intracellular glucose concentration, insulin does indirectly promote the passive diffusion of glucose into them. Insulin also directly increases the transport of amino acids, potassium and phosphate into cells, especially muscle; these processes are independent of glucose transport. In the longer term, insulin regulates growth and development and the expression of certain genes.

Glucagon

Glucagon is a single-chain polypeptide synthesized by the alpha-cells of the pancreatic islets. Its secretion is stimulated by hypoglycaemia. Glucagon enhances hepatic glycogenolysis (glycogen breakdown) and gluconeogenesis.

Somatostatin

This peptide hormone is released from the D-cells of the pancreas and inhibits insulin and growth-hormone release.

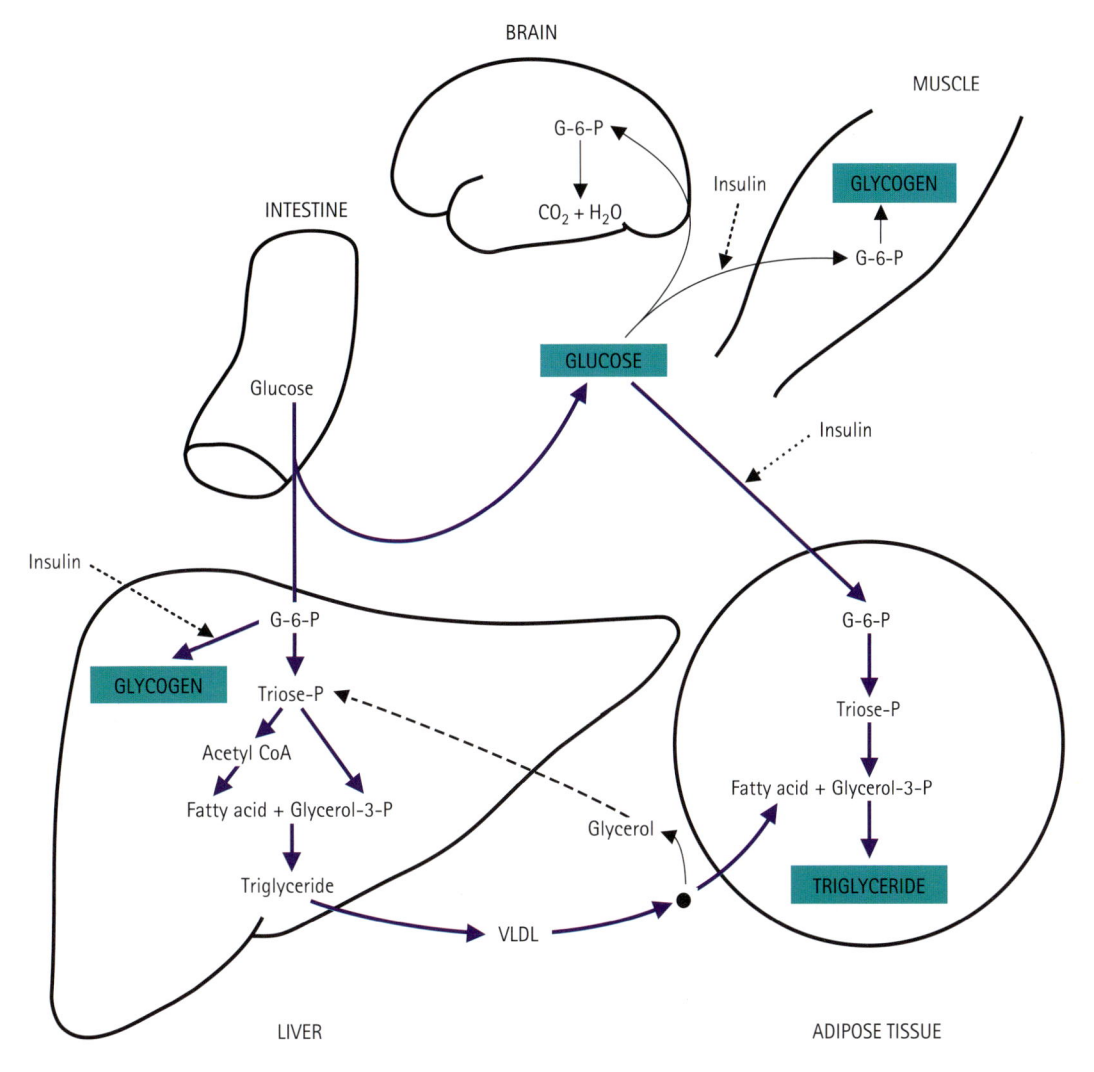

Fig. 12.4 Postprandial metabolism of glucose. (G-6-P = glucose-6-phosphate; Triose-P = triose phosphate; CoA = coenzyme A; Glycerol-3-P = glycerol-3-phosphate; VLDL = very low-density lipoprotein.)

Other hormones

When plasma insulin concentrations are low, for example during fasting, the hyperglycaemic actions of hormones, such as growth hormone (GH), glucocorticoids, adrenaline (epinephrine) and glucagon, become apparent, even if there is no increase in secretion rates. Secretion of these so-called counter-regulatory hormones may increase during stress and in patients with acromegaly (GH, see Chapter 6), Cushing's syndrome (glucocorticoids, see Chapter 8) or adrenaline and noradrenaline (norepinephrine) as in phaeochromocytoma (see Chapter 24) and thus oppose the normal action of insulin.

The liver

The liver is the most important organ maintaining a constant glucose supply for other tissues, including the brain. It is also of importance in controlling the postprandial plasma glucose concentration.

Portal venous blood leaving the absorptive area of the intestinal wall reaches the liver first, and consequently the hepatic cells are in a key position to buffer the hyperglycaemic effect of a high-carbohydrate meal (Fig. 12.4).

The entry of glucose into liver and cerebral cells is not directly affected by insulin, but depends on the extracellular glucose concentration. The conversion of glucose to glucose-6-phosphate (G-6-P), the first step in glucose metabolism in all cells, is catalysed in the liver by the enzyme glucokinase, which has a low affinity for glucose compared with that of hexokinase, which is found in most other tissues. Glucokinase activity is induced by insulin. Therefore, hepatic cells extract proportionally less glucose during fasting, when concentrations in portal venous plasma are low, than after carbohydrate ingestion. This helps to maintain a fasting supply of glucose to vulnerable tissues such as the brain.

The liver cells can store some of the excess glucose as glycogen. The rate of glycogen synthesis (glycogenesis) from G-6-P may be increased by insulin secreted by the beta-cells of the pancreas in response to systemic hyperglycaemia.

The liver can convert some of the excess glucose to fatty acids, which are ultimately transported as triglyceride in very low-density lipoprotein (VLDL) and stored in adipose tissue.

Under normal aerobic conditions, the liver can synthesize glucose by gluconeogenesis using the metabolic products from other tissues, such as glycerol, lactate or the carbon chains resulting from deamination of certain amino acids (mainly alanine) (see Table 12.3).

The liver contains the enzyme glucose-6-phosphatase, which, by hydrolysing G-6-P derived from either glycogenolysis or gluconeogenesis, releases glucose and helps to maintain extracellular fasting concentrations. Hepatic glycogenolysis is stimulated by the hormone glucagon, secreted by the alpha-cells of the pancreas in response to a fall in the plasma glucose concentration, and by catecholamines such as adrenaline or noradrenaline.

During fasting, the liver converts fatty acids, released from adipose tissue as a consequence of low insulin activity, to ketones. The carbon chains of some amino acids may also be converted to ketones (Table 12.3). Ketones can be used by other tissues, including the brain, as an energy source when plasma glucose concentrations are low.

Other organs

The renal cortex is the only other tissue capable of gluconeogenesis, and of converting G-6-P to glucose. The gluconeogenic capacity of the kidney is particularly important in hydrogen ion homeostasis and during prolonged fasting.

Other tissues, such as muscle, can store glycogen but, because they do not contain glucose-6-phosphatase, they cannot release glucose from cells and so can only use it locally; this glycogen plays no part in maintaining the plasma glucose concentration.

Table 12.3 Metabolism of the carbon skeleton of some amino acids to either carbohydrate (glycogenic) or fat (ketogenic)

Glycogenic	Glycogenic and ketogenic	Ketogenic
Alanine	Isoleucine	Leucine
Arginine	Lysine	
Glycine	Phenylalanine	
Histidine	Tyrosine	
Methionine		
Serine		
Valine		

Systemic effects of glucose intake

The liver modifies the potential hyperglycaemic effect of a high-carbohydrate meal by extracting relatively more glucose than in the fasting state from the portal plasma. However, some glucose does pass through the liver and the rise in the systemic concentration stimulates the beta-cells of the pancreas to secrete insulin. Insulin may further enhance hepatic and muscle glycogenesis. More importantly, entry of glucose into adipose tissue and muscle cells, unlike that into liver and brain, is stimulated by insulin and, under physiological conditions, the plasma glucose concentration falls to near fasting levels. Conversion of intracellular glucose to G-6-P in adipose and muscle cells is catalysed by the enzyme hexokinase, which, because its affinity for glucose is greater than that of hepatic glucokinase, ensures that glucose enters the metabolic pathways in these tissues at lower extracellular concentrations than those in the liver. The relatively high insulin activity after a meal also inhibits the breakdown of triglyceride (lipolysis) and protein (proteolysis). If there is relative or absolute insulin deficiency, as in diabetes mellitus, these actions are impaired. Both muscle and adipose tissue store the excess postprandial glucose, but the mode of storage and the function of the two types of cell are very different, as will be shown later.

Ketosis

Adipose tissue and the liver

Adipose tissue triglyceride is the most important long-term energy store in the body. Greatly increased use of fat stores, for example during prolonged fasting, is associated with ketosis. Adipose tissue cells, acting in conjunction

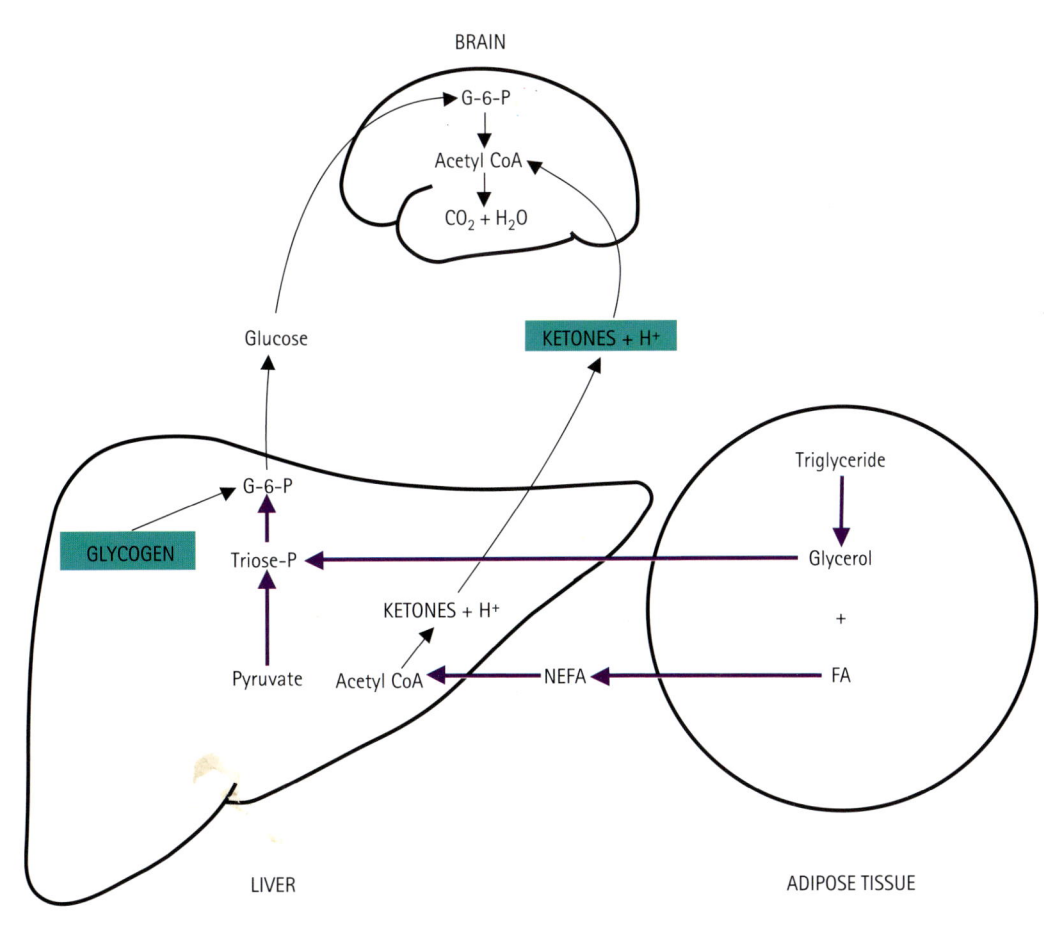

Fig. 12.5 Intermediary metabolism during fasting: ketosis. (NEFA = non-esterified fatty acid; FA = fatty acid. For other abbreviations, see Figure 12.4.)

with the liver, convert excess glucose to triglyceride and store it in this form rather than as glycogen. The components are both derived from glucose, fatty acids from the glucose entering hepatic cells and glycerol from that entering adipose tissue cells.

In the liver, triglycerides are formed from glycerol-3-phosphate (from triose phosphate) and fatty acids (from acetyl coenzyme A (CoA)).

The triglycerides are transported to adipose tissue cells incorporated in VLDL, where they are hydrolysed by lipoprotein lipase. The released fatty acids (of hepatic origin) are re-esterified within these cells with glycerol-3-phosphate, derived from glucose, which has entered this tissue under the influence of insulin. The resultant triglyceride is stored and is far more energy dense than glycogen (see Chapter 13).

During fasting, when exogenous glucose is unavailable and the plasma insulin concentration is therefore low, endogenous triglycerides are reconverted to free non-esterified fatty acids (NEFAs) and glycerol by lipolysis (Fig. 12.5). Both are transported to the liver in plasma, the NEFA being protein bound, predominantly to albumin. Glycerol enters the hepatic gluconeogenic pathway at the triose phosphate stage; the glucose synthesized can be released from these cells, thus minimizing the fall in glucose concentrations.

Most tissues, other than the brain, can oxidize fatty acids to acetyl CoA, which can then be used in the TCA cycle as an energy source. When the rate of synthesis exceeds its use, the hepatic cells produce acetoacetic acid by enzymatic condensation of two molecules of acetyl CoA; acetoacetic acid can be reduced to β-hydroxybutyric acid and decarboxylated to acetone. These ketones can be used as an energy source by brain and other tissues at a time when glucose is in relatively short supply.

Ketosis occurs when fat stores are the main energy source and may result from fasting or from reduced nutrient absorption, for example due to vomiting. Mild ketosis may occur after as little as 12 hours of fasting. After short fasts, metabolic acidosis is not usually detectable, but after longer periods, more hydrogen ions may be produced than can be dealt with by homeostatic buffering mechanisms, depleting the plasma bicarbonate concentration, which therefore falls (see Chapter 4).

The plasma glucose concentration is maintained principally by hepatic gluconeogenesis, but during prolonged starvation, such as that in anorexia nervosa or during childhood, ketotic hypoglycaemia may occur. The brain may tolerate ketotic hypoglycaemia better than the same degree of insulin-induced hypoglycaemia; in the former the brain adapts to ketone metabolism, whereas in the latter ketone concentrations are low, thus depriving the brain of its only non-glucose energy source.

During starvation, low extracellular glucose concentration reduces the supply to cells and therefore reduces adipose tissue glycolysis and fat synthesis (lipogenesis); this tendency inhibits insulin secretion and therefore the rate of lipolysis and fatty acid, and hence ketone, production is increased.

Diabetic ketoacidosis is differentiated from that of fasting by hyperglycaemia and is usually more severe. Despite the differences in plasma glucose concentrations, the ketone production in both cases is due to intracellular glucose deficiency. In diabetic ketosis this is due to low insulin activity.

Ketosis reflects the excessive use of fat as an energy source due to intracellular glucose deficiency and low insulin activity.

The low insulin activity increases the rate of production of gluconeogenic substrates by glycolysis and proteolysis, and the rate of hepatic gluconeogenesis. The resultant increased rate of glucose released into the extracellular fluid is appropriate in starvation, but aggravates the hyperglycaemia in diabetes mellitus.

Lactate production and lactic acidosis

Striated muscle and the liver

Under the influence of insulin, glucose enters muscle postprandially and is stored as glycogen. This glycogen cannot be reconverted to glucose because of the absence of glucose-6-phosphatase and can only supply local needs. Quantitatively, muscle glycogen stores are second only to those in the liver.

During muscular activity, glycogenolysis is stimulated by adrenaline (epinephrine), and the resultant G-6-P is metabolized by glycolysis and in the TCA cycle to supply energy. The rate of glycolysis may exceed the availability of oxygen needed in the TCA cycle and glycolytic products may then accumulate.

The overall reaction for anaerobic glycolysis is:

$$\text{glucose} \rightarrow 2\ \text{lactate}^- + 2\text{H}^+ \qquad (12.1)$$

The lactate is transported in the blood to the liver, where it can be used for gluconeogenesis, providing further glucose for the muscle (Cori cycle, Fig. 12.6). During gluconeogenesis, hydrogen ions are re-used. Under aerobic conditions, the liver consumes much more lactate than it produces.

The physiological accumulation of lactic acid during muscular contraction is a temporary phenomenon and rapidly disappears at rest, when slowing of glycolysis allows aerobic processes to 'catch up'.

Pathological lactic acidosis

Lactic acid, produced by anaerobic glycolysis, may either be oxidized to CO_2 and water in the TCA cycle or be reconverted to glucose by gluconeogenesis in the liver. Both the TCA cycle and gluconeogenesis need oxygen; anaerobic glycolysis is a non-oxygen-requiring pathway. Pathological accumulation of lactate may occur because:

- production is increased by an increased rate of anaerobic glycolysis,
- use is decreased by impairment of the TCA cycle or impairment of gluconeogenesis.

Tissue hypoxia (Fig. 12.7) due to the poor tissue perfusion of the 'shock' syndrome is usually the commonest cause of lactic acidosis. Hypoxia increases plasma lactate concentrations because:

- the TCA cycle cannot function anaerobically and oxidation of pyruvate and lactate to CO_2 and water is impaired,
- hepatic and renal gluconeogenesis from lactate cannot occur anaerobically,
- anaerobic glycolysis is stimulated because the falling adenosine triphosphate (ATP) levels cannot be regenerated by the TCA cycle under anaerobic conditions.

The combination of impaired gluconeogenesis and increased anaerobic glycolysis converts the liver from an organ that consumes lactate and H^+ to one that generates large amounts of lactic acid. Severe hypoxia, for example following a cardiac arrest, causes marked lactic acidosis. If diabetic ketoacidosis is associated with significant volume depletion, this hypoxic syndrome may aggravate the acidosis. (See Chapter 4 for a further discussion of lactic acidosis.)

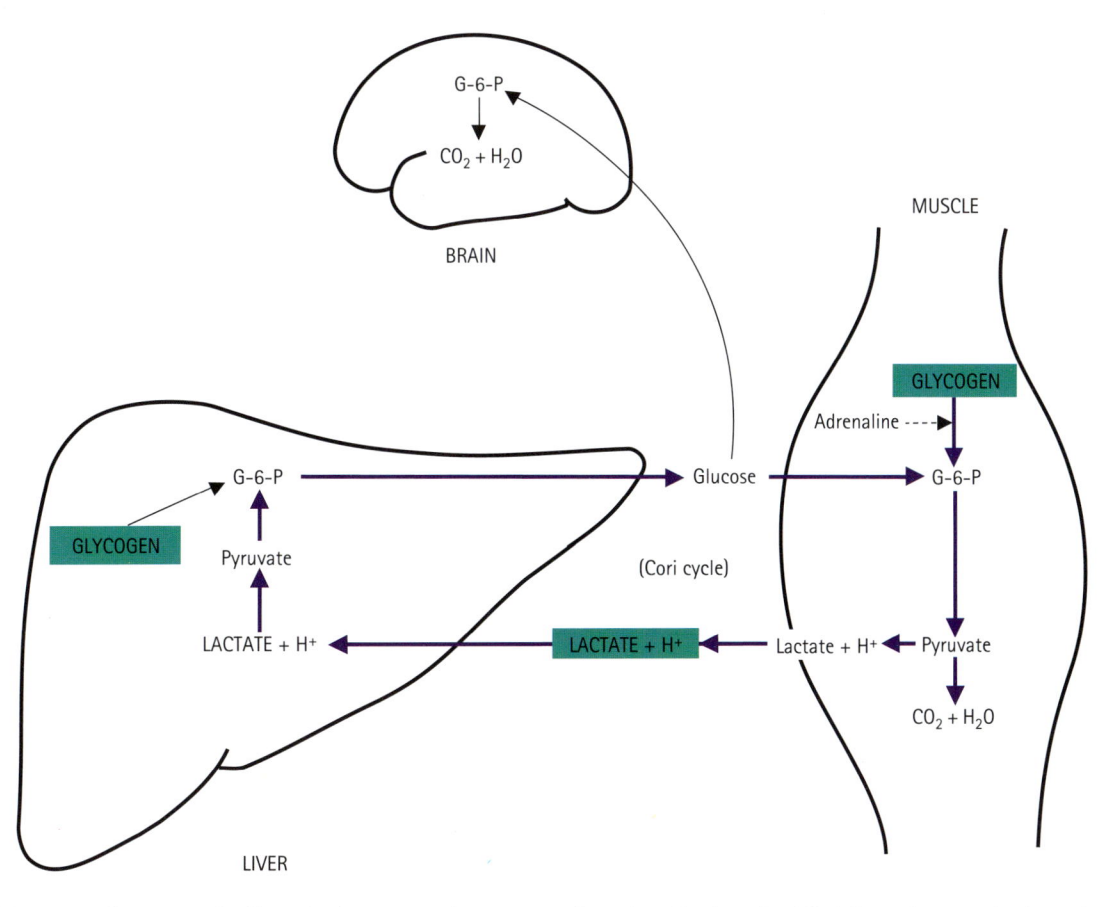

Fig. 12.6 Intermediary metabolism during muscular contraction: the Cori cycle. (G-6-P = glucose-6-phosphate.)

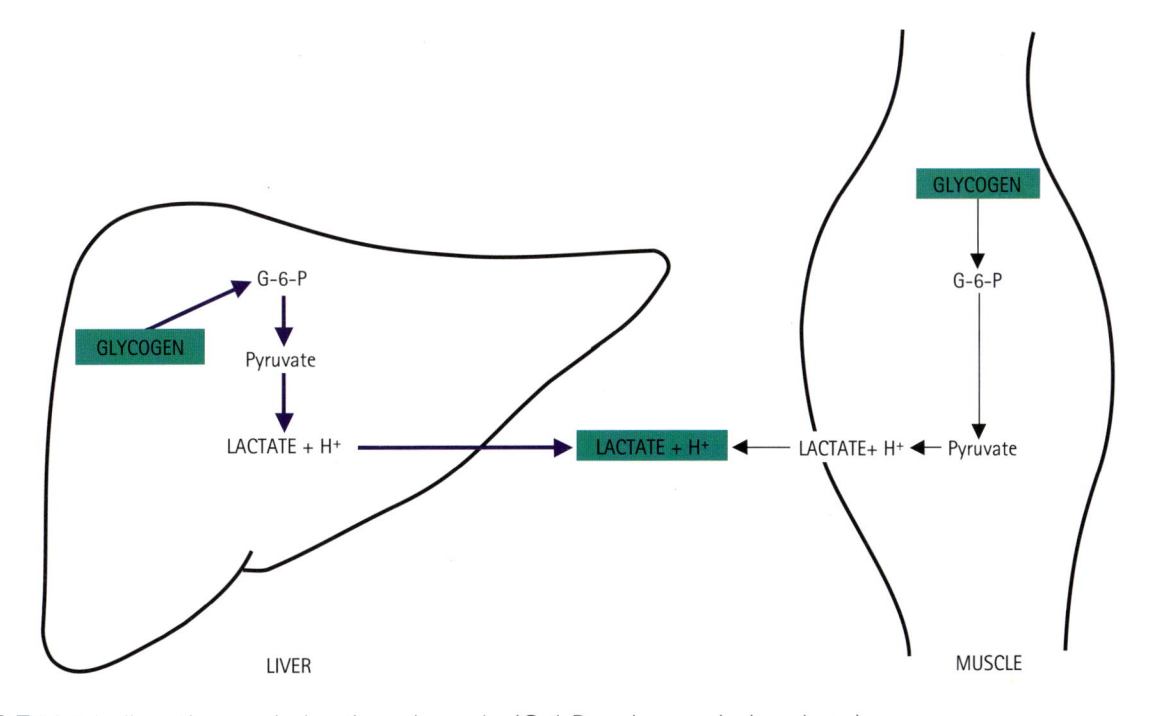

Fig. 12.7 Metabolic pathways during tissue hypoxia. (G-6-P = glucose-6-phosphate.)

The glycolytic pathway as well as the TCA cycle are summarized in Figs 12.1 and 12.2.

HYPERGLYCAEMIA AND DIABETES MELLITUS

Hyperglycaemia may be due to:

- intravenous infusion of glucose-containing fluids,
- severe stress (usually a transient effect) such as trauma, myocardial infarction or cerebrovascular accidents,
- diabetes mellitus or impaired glucose regulation.

Diabetes mellitus

Diabetes mellitus is caused by an absolute or relative insulin deficiency. It has been defined by the World Health Organization (WHO), on the basis of laboratory findings, as a fasting venous plasma glucose concentration more than or equal to 7.0 mmol/L (on more than one occasion or once in the presence of diabetes symptoms) or a random venous plasma glucose concentration more than or equal to 11.1 mmol/L. Sometimes an oral glucose tolerance test (OGTT) may be required to establish the diagnosis in equivocal cases. The interpretation of this test is shown below, but briefly, diabetes mellitus can be diagnosed if the venous plasma glucose concentration is more than or equal to 7.0 mmol/L (fasting) and/or more than or equal to 11.1 mmol/L 2 hours after the oral ingestion of the equivalent of 75 g of anhydrous glucose. Diabetes mellitus can be classified into the following categories.

Type 1 diabetes mellitus

Previously called insulin-dependent diabetes mellitus, this is the term used to describe the condition in patients for whom insulin therapy is essential because they are prone to develop ketoacidosis. It usually presents during childhood or adolescence. Most of these cases are due to immune-mediated processes and may be associated with other autoimmune disorders such as Addison's disease, vitiligo and Hashimoto's thyroiditis. It has been suggested that many cases follow a viral infection that has damaged the β-cells of the pancreatic islets. Individuals most at risk are those with HLA-types DR3 and DR4 of the major histocompatibility complex. Autoantibodies to islet cells, insulin, tyrosine phosphatases IA-2 and IA-2β and glutamic decarboxylase (GAD) are found in about 90 per cent of cases. There is a form of type 1 diabetes called idiopathic diabetes mellitus that is not autoimmune mediated but is strongly inherited and more common in Asian and African patients. The insulin requirement of affected people can fluctuate widely and the cause is unknown.

Type 2 diabetes mellitus

Previously called non-insulin-dependent diabetes mellitus, this is the commonest variety worldwide (about 90 per cent of all diabetes mellitus cases). Patients are much less likely to develop ketoacidosis than those with type 1 diabetes, although insulin may sometimes be needed. Onset is most usual during adult life; there is a familial tendency and an association with obesity. There is a spectrum of disorders ranging from mainly insulin resistance with relative insulin deficiency to a predominantly secretory defect with insulin resistance.

Other specific types of diabetes mellitus

A variety of inherited disorders may be responsible for the syndrome, either by reducing insulin secretion or by causing relative insulin deficiency because of resistance to its action or of insulin receptor defects, despite high plasma insulin concentrations.

- *Genetic defects of β-cell function:*
  - maturity-onset diabetes of the young (MODY):
    MODY 1 mutation of hepatocyte nuclear factor (HNF)-4-α gene,
    MODY 2 mutation of glucokinase gene,
    MODY 3 mutation of HNF-1-α gene.

  Some cases are thought to be point mutations in mitochondrial DNA associated with diabetes mellitus and deafness and are usually autosomal dominant.

- *Genetic defects of insulin action:*
  - type A insulin resistance (insulin receptor defect), for example leprechaunism, lipoatrophy and Rabson–Mendenhall syndrome.
- *Absolute insulin deficiency,* due to:
  - pancreatic disease,
  - chronic pancreatitis,
  - pancreatectomy,
  - haemochromatosis,
  - cystic fibrosis.
- *Endocrinopathies:*
  - relative insulin deficiency, due to excessive GH (acromegaly), phaeochromocytoma, glucocorticoid secretion (Cushing's syndrome).
- *Drugs,* such as:
  - thiazide diuretics,

- alpha-interferon,
- glucocorticoids.
- *Infections*, such as:
  - congenital rubella,
  - cytomegalovirus.
- Rare forms of *autoimmune-mediated diabetes*, such as:
  - anti-insulin receptor antibodies,
  - stiff man syndrome, with high levels of GAD autoantibodies.
- *Genetic syndromes associated with diabetes*, such as:
  - Down's syndrome,
  - Turner's syndrome,
  - Klinefelter's syndrome,
  - myotonic dystrophy.

Gestational diabetes mellitus

In the UK, about 4–5 per cent of pregnancies are complicated by gestational diabetes mellitus (GDM). It is associated with increased fetal abnormalities, for example high birth weight, cardiac defects and polyhydramnios. In addition, birth complications, maternal hypertension and the need for Caesarean section may occur. If maternal diet/lifestyle factors fail to restore glucose levels, insulin is usually required to try to reduce the risk of these complications.

Women at high risk for GDM include those who have had GDM before, have previously given birth to a high-birth-weight baby, are obese, have a family history of diabetes mellitus and/or are from high-risk ethnic groups, for example South Asian or African. These women should be screened at the earliest opportunity and, if normal, re-tested at about 24–28 weeks, as glucose tolerance progressively deteriorates throughout pregnancy. In some units 50 g oral glucose is used and the blood glucose is sampled at 1 hour – plasma glucose of more than or equal to 7.8 mmol/L being diagnostic (O'Sullivan's screening test for gestational diabetes). If fasting venous plasma glucose is more than or equal to 7.0 mmol/L and/or the random measurement gives a concentration more than or equal to 11.1 mmol/L (some doctors prefer to use a lower cut-off of about 9.0 mmol/L in pregnancy), the woman has GDM. In equivocal cases, an OGTT is indicated. Six weeks post-partum, the woman should be re-classified with repeat OGTT.

Impaired glucose tolerance

The WHO definition of impaired glucose tolerance (IGT) is a fasting venous plasma glucose concentration of less than 7.0 mmol/L and a plasma glucose concentration between 7.8 mmol/L and 11.1 mmol/L 2 hours after an OGTT. Some patients with IGT develop diabetes mellitus later and require annual OGTT to monitor for this. However, because of the increased risk of vascular complications, secondary causes of IGT should be sought, dietary advice given, if necessary, and the patient followed up. In pregnancy IGT is treated as GDM because of the risks to the fetus.

Impaired fasting glucose

A new category of impaired fasting glucose (IFG) has been defined, which, like IGT, refers to a metabolic stage intermediate between normal glucose homeostasis and diabetes mellitus. The definition is that the fasting venous plasma glucose is more than or equal to 6.1 mmol/L but less than 7.0 mmol/L, and less than 7.8 mmol/L 2 hours after an OGTT.

Subjects at risk of developing diabetes mellitus

A strong family history of diabetes mellitus may suggest that an individual is at risk of developing diabetes mellitus (particularly type 2), as may a family history of GDM, IGT or IFG. Those with predisposing HLA types and autoimmune disease may be susceptible to developing type 1 diabetes. Type 2 diabetes is commoner in certain racial groups, such as Afro-Caribbeans, South Asians and Pacific Islanders. One of the reasons why type 2 diabetes is on the increase is the increasing tendency to obesity and central adiposity in urbanized and more sedentary populations who consume high-calorie diets.

The thrifty phenotype (Barker–Hales) hypothesis proposes that nutritional deficiency in fetal and early infancy associated with low birth weight increases the risk of developing type 2 diabetes and insulin resistance.

Insulin resistance syndrome or metabolic syndrome

It has been recognized that certain coronary heart disease risk factors occur together. There is an aggregation of lipid and non-lipid risk factors of metabolic origin. A particular cluster is known as the metabolic syndrome, syndrome X or Reaven's syndrome and is closely linked to insulin resistance. One definition is the presence of three or more of the following features.

- Abdominal obesity (waist circumference):
  - male more than 102 cm (40 in)
  - female more than 88 cm (35 in).
- Fasting plasma triglycerides more than 1.7 mmol/L.

- Fasting plasma high-density lipoprotein (HDL) cholesterol:
  - male less than 1.0 mmol/L
  - female less than 1.3 mmol/L.
- Blood pressure more than or equal to 130/85 mmHg.
- Fasting blood glucose more than 5.5 mmol/L.

Plasma levels of insulin would be expected to be raised, i.e. hyperinsulinaemia. Other associated features may include polycystic ovary syndrome, fatty liver, raised fibrinogen and plasminogen activator inhibitor-1 concentrations, renal sodium retention, hyperuricaemia and dense low-density lipoprotein (LDL) particles (see Chapter 13).

Metabolic features of diabetes mellitus

Patients with type 1 diabetes tend to be diagnosed before the age of 40 years, are usually lean and have experienced weight loss at the time of presentation. They may present with diabetic ketoacidosis. Conversely, patients with type 2 diabetes often present later, usually after the age of 40 years, and are often overweight or obese. The presentation can be insidious and they may have had diabetes years before diagnosis.

Hyperglycaemia

If plasma glucose concentration exceeds about 10 mmol/L, glycosuria would be expected. High urinary glucose concentrations produce an osmotic diuresis and therefore polyuria. Cerebral cellular dehydration due to hyperosmolality, secondary to hyperglycaemia, causes thirst (polydipsia). A prolonged osmotic diuresis may cause excessive urinary electrolyte loss. These 'classical' symptoms are suggestive of diabetes mellitus.

Diabetic patients on insulin may show the following conditions. The 'dawn' phenomenon is the physiological response of the elevation of blood glucose concentration in the early morning prior to breakfast due to nocturnal spikes in GH concentration and a rise in plasma cortisol concentration that increase hepatic gluconeogenesis. Conversely, in some diabetic patients nocturnal hypoglycaemia may evoke a rebound counter-regulatory hyperglycaemia called the Somogyi phenomenon. Patient blood glucose checking at 02.00–04.00 hours may distinguish these conditions, as the Somogyi phenomenon reveals hypoglycaemia. It is sometimes possible to ameliorate these conditions by giving intermediate-acting insulin before bedtime.

Abnormalities in lipid metabolism

These may be secondary to insulin deficiency. Lipolysis is enhanced and plasma NEFA concentrations rise. In the liver, NEFAs are converted to acetyl CoA and ketones, or are re-esterified to form endogenous triglycerides and incorporated into VLDLs; the latter accumulate in plasma because lipoprotein lipase, which is necessary for VLDL catabolism, requires insulin for optimal activity. High-density lipoprotein cholesterol concentration tends to be low in type 2 diabetes. If insulin deficiency is very severe, there may also be chylomicronaemia. The rate of cholesterol synthesis is also increased, with an associated increase in plasma LDL concentrations. Consequently, patients with diabetes may show high plasma triglyceride, raised cholesterol and low HDL cholesterol concentrations.

Long-term effects of diabetes mellitus

Vascular disease is a common complication of diabetes mellitus. Macrovascular disease due to abnormalities of large vessels may present as coronary artery, cerebrovascular or peripheral vascular insufficiency. The condition is probably related to alterations in lipid metabolism and associated hypertension. The commonest cause of death is cardiovascular disease, including myocardial infarction.

Microvascular disease due to abnormalities of small blood vessels particularly affects the retina (diabetic retinopathy) and the kidney (nephropathy); both may be related to inadequate glucose control. Diabetes is one of the commonest causes of patients requiring renal dialysis. Microvascular disease of the kidney is associated with proteinuria.

Kidney disease is associated with several abnormalities, including proteinuria and progressive renal failure. Diffuse nodular glomerulosclerosis (Kimmelstiel–Wilson lesions) may cause the nephrotic syndrome. The presence of small amounts of albumin in the urine (microalbuminuria) is associated with an increased risk of developing progressive renal disease, which may sometimes be prevented by more stringent plasma glucose and blood pressure control. The renal complications may be partly due to the increased glycation of structural proteins in the arterial walls supplying the glomerular basement membrane; similar vascular changes in the retina may account for the high incidence of diabetic retinopathy. Glycation of protein in the lens may cause cataracts.

Infections are also more common in diabetic patients, for example urinary tract or chest infections, cellulitis and candida.

Diabetic neuropathy can occur, which can be peripheral symmetric sensory, peripheral painful, acute mononeuropathies or autonomic. It has been suggested that sorbitol is implicated in the aetiology of diabetic neuropathy through the action of aldolase reductase. Erectile dysfunction is also relatively common and in some cases may be partly neurologically mediated.

Diabetic ulcers, e.g of the feet, can lead to gangrene and amputation. The ulcers can be ischaemic, neuropathic or infective. The joints can also be affected, e.g Charcot's joints.

Other features of diabetes mellitus are skin disorders, such as necrobiosis lipoidica, and abscesses.

Principles of management of diabetes mellitus

The management of diabetes mellitus is considered briefly, although it is recommended to consult a specialist text if further information is required.

Insulin requirements vary in patients with type 1 diabetes. For example, the dose may need to be increased during any illness or during pregnancy and reduced if there is increased activity or meals are missed.

In patients with type 2 diabetes, plasma glucose concentrations may be controlled by diet, associated with weight reduction, and increased physical activity, but insulin may be required during periods of stress or pregnancy. In this group insulin secretion can be stimulated by the sulphonylurea drugs, such as gliclazide, glipizide, glibenclamide or glimepiride. Biguanides, usually metformin, can also be used and are particularly useful in obese patients. Metformin decreases intestinal glucose absorption and hepatic gluconeogenesis as well as increasing tissue insulin sensitivity. Metformin can inhibit oxidative phosphorylation, which can, under certain circumstances, lead to lactic acid accumulation. Acarbose delays postprandial absorption of glucose by inhibiting alpha-glucosidase. Other oral agents are the 'glitazones', for example rosiglitazone and pioglitazone, which activate γ-peroxisome proliferator-activated receptors and which can reduce insulin resistance by a number of metabolic pathways, some of which involve increasing the transcription of nuclear proteins that control free fatty acid and tissue glucose uptake. Repaglinide is a meglitinide that increases insulin release from pancreatic β-cells and enhances tissue insulin sensitivity.

It is now recognized that diabetes mellitus is not just a glucose disorder. It is important also to optimize abnormal plasma lipids (see Chapter 13) and correct hypertension, particularly if there is microalbuminuria or proteinuria (see Chapter 19).

Monitoring of diabetes mellitus

Glycosuria

Glycosuria can be defined as a concentration of urinary glucose detectable using relatively insensitive, but specific, screening tests. These tests often depend on the action of an enzyme, such as glucose oxidase, incorporated into a diagnostic strip. Usually, the proximal tubular cells reabsorb most of the glucose in the glomerular filtrate. Glycosuria, as defined above, occurs only when the plasma, and therefore glomerular filtrate, concentrations exceed the tubular reabsorptive capacity. This may be because the plasma and glomerular filtrate concentrations are more than about 10 mmol/L, and therefore the normal tubular reabsorptive capacity is significantly exceeded. Very rarely, if the glomerular filtration rate is much reduced, there may be no glycosuria despite plasma glucose concentrations more than 10 mmol/L.

A diagnosis of diabetes mellitus should *never* be made on the basis of glycosuria. However, some patients with diabetes monitor their therapy by testing for glycosuria.

Blood glucose

Blood glucose concentrations may be measured using glucose testing reagent strips. The colour change of the strip can be assessed visually or by using a portable glucose meter and the reaction often involves an enzyme determination of glucose, for example glucose oxidase. Meters should be checked regularly by laboratory staff (see Chapter 30). Although the measurement of blood glucose concentrations involves the discomfort of several skin punctures, many motivated patients are able to adjust their insulin dose more accurately based on these results than on those obtained by testing their urine. This method of testing is also useful in the detection of hypoglycaemia.

For patients who do not like blood testing, urinary glucose testing can be used, but of course cannot detect hypoglycaemia and is dependent on the renal glucose threshold.

Glycated haemoglobin

This is expressed as a percentage of total blood haemoglobin concentration and gives a retrospective assessment of the mean plasma glucose concentration during the preceding 6–8 weeks. The higher the percentage, the poorer the mean diabetic or glycaemic control. Glycated haemoglobin is formed by non-enzymatic glycation of haemoglobin and is dependent on the mean plasma glucose concentrations and on the lifespan of the red cell; falsely low values may be found in patients with haemolytic disease. Measurement of blood HbA_{1c} is an adjunct to, not a replacement for, serial plasma glucose estimations, which may be necessary to reveal potentially dangerous short-term swings. Nor does HbA_{1c} detect hypoglycaemic episodes. However, intervention trials for type 1 and type 2 diabetes have shown that trying to optimize glycaemic control, as judged by HbA_{1c}, to about 7 per cent reduces the risk of microvascular diabetic complications.

Fructosamine

The measurement of plasma fructosamine concentrations may be used to assess glucose control over a shorter time course than that of HbA_{1c} (about 2–4 weeks), but the assay has methodological limitations. Fructosamine reflects glucose bound to plasma proteins, predominantly albumin, which has a plasma half-life of about 20 days. This assay may sometimes be useful in pregnancy and also if haemoglobin variants, for example HbS or HbC, exist that may interfere with certain HbA_{1c} assays.

Urinary albumin determination and diabetic nephropathy

One of the earliest signs of diabetic renal dysfunction is the development of small amounts of albumin in the urine, called microalbuminuria. Untreated, this can progress to overt albuminuria or proteinuria (more than 300 mg/day), impaired renal function and finally end-stage renal failure.

Microalbuminuria is defined as a urinary albumin excretion of 30–300 mg/day or 20–200 μg/min. An albumin concentration less than 30 mg/day or less than 20 μg/min is defined as normoalbuminuria. A random urine sample or timed overnight collection is useful to assess urinary albumin excretion. A urinary albumin:creatinine ratio (ACR) can also be measured, which avoids a timed urine collection. This should normally be less than 2.5 g/mol in males and less than 3.5 g/mol in females. An abnormal result should be confirmed in two out of three urine samples in the absence of other causes of proteinuria (see Chapter 19). Apart from being predictive of diabetic renal complications, urinary albumin excretion is also associated with increased vascular permeability and enhanced risk of cardiovascular disease.

Optimization of glycaemic control can slow the progression of microalbuminuria, as can treating hypertension. Some recommend a target blood pressure lower than 140/80 mmHg in type 2 diabetes, or 135/75 mmHg or lower if microalbuminuria is present. The blood pressure targets are usually more aggressive in type 1 diabetes, partly as the lifetime risk of overt nephropathy is greater. Angiotensin-converting enzyme (ACE) inhibitor therapy, such as lisinopril in type 1 diabetic patients with microalbuminuria, can result in a decline in the albumin excretion rate; similar findings have been shown with enalapril in type 2 diabetes. This action of ACE inhibitors is only partially dependent on their blood pressure lowering ability, and therefore they presumably also have other important renal protective actions. Recently, the angiotensin receptor antagonists, for example irbesartan and losartan, have also been shown to have renal protective actions.

Acute metabolic complications of diabetes mellitus

Patients with diabetes mellitus may develop various metabolic complications that require emergency treatment, including coma, and these include the following.

Hypoglycaemia

This is probably the most common cause of coma seen in diabetic patients.

Hypoglycaemia is most commonly caused by accidental over-administration of insulin or sulphonylureas or meglitinides. Precipitating causes include too high a dose of insulin or hypoglycaemic drug; conversely, the patient may have missed a meal or taken excessive exercise after the usual dose of insulin or oral hypoglycaemic drugs.

Hypoglycaemia is particularly dangerous, and some patients lack awareness of this; that is to say, they lose warning signs such as sweating, dizziness and headaches. Driving is a major hazard under such circumstances. Patients should monitor their own blood glucose closely, carry glucose preparations to abort severe hypoglycaemia and avoid high-risk activities during which hypoglycaemic attacks could be dangerous.

Diabetic ketoacidosis

Diabetic ketoacidosis may be precipitated by infection, acute myocardial infarction or vomiting. The patient who reasons 'no food, therefore no insulin' could mistakenly withhold insulin. In the absence of insulin, there is increased lipid and protein breakdown, enhanced hepatic gluconeogenesis and impaired glucose entry into cells.

The clinical consequences of diabetic ketoacidosis are due to:

- hyperglycaemia causing plasma hyperosmolality,
- metabolic acidosis,
- glycosuria.

Plasma glucose concentrations are usually in the range 20–40 mmol/L, but may be considerably higher, although euglycaemic diabetic ketoacidosis has been described when plasma glucose concentrations are only slightly elevated.

Hyperglycaemia causes glycosuria and hence an osmotic diuresis. Water and electrolyte loss due to vomiting, which

CASE 1

A 34-year-old female with known type 1 diabetes mellitus was admitted to hospital following a 'black out' whilst driving. She had recently increased her insulin dose, despite having missed a couple of meals, because she felt unwell with 'flu'. The results of some of her biochemistry tests were as follows.

Plasma
Sodium 135 mmol/L (135–145)
Potassium 4.0 mmol/L (3.5–5.0)
Bicarbonate 23 mmol/L (24–32)
Urea 5.4 mmol/L (2.5–7.0)
Creatinine 100 μmol/L (70–110)
Glucose 1.5 mmol/L (5.5–11.1)
pH 7.43 (7.35–7.45)
$PaCO_2$ 5.3 kPa (4.6–6.0)
PaO_2 12.1 kPa (9.3–13.3)

DISCUSSION
The blood glucose shows hypoglycaemia, secondary to the patient having inappropriately increased her insulin. Hypoglycaemia can present with neurological impairment, including impaired memory, loss of consciousness and coma. This can be treated in the emergency situation by giving glucose intravenously to avoid irreversible neurological damage. It is important for patients on insulin to monitor their own blood glucose closely, particularly if they wish to drive.

CASE 2

A 24-year-old female was seen in casualty in a coma. The relevant biochemical results were as follows.

Urine was positive for ketones.

Plasma
Sodium 130 mmol/L (135–145)
Potassium 5.9 mmol/L (3.5–5.0)
Bicarbonate 10 mmol/L (24–32)
Chloride 92 mmol/L (95–105)
Glucose 35 mmol/L (5.5–11.1)
pH 7.10 (7.35–7.45)
$PaCO_2$ 3.1 kPa (4.6–6.0)
PaO_2 11.1 kPa (9.3–13.3)

DISCUSSION
The patient was shown to have type 1 diabetes mellitus and had presented in diabetic ketoacidosis, with hyperglycaemia, hyponatraemia, hyperkalaemia and a metabolic acidosis.

---

is common in this syndrome, increases fluid depletion. There may be haemoconcentration and reduction of the glomerular filtration rate enough to cause uraemia due to renal circulatory insufficiency. The extracellular hyperosmolality causes a shift of water out of the cellular compartment and severe cellular dehydration occurs. Loss of water from cerebral cells is probably the reason for the confusion and coma. Thus there is both cellular and extracellular volume depletion.

The rate of lipolysis is increased because of decreased insulin activity; more free fatty acids are produced than can be metabolized by peripheral tissues. The free fatty acids are either converted to ketones by the liver or, of less immediate clinical importance, incorporated as endogenous triglycerides into VLDL, sometimes causing severe hypertriglyceridaemia (see Chapter 13).

Hydrogen ions, produced with ketones other than acetone, are buffered by plasma bicarbonate. However, when their rate of production exceeds the rate of bicarbonate generation, the plasma bicarbonate falls. Hydrogen ion secretion causes a fall in urinary pH. The deep, sighing respiration (Kussmaul's respiration) and the odour of acetone on the breath are classical features of diabetic ketoacidosis.

Plasma potassium concentrations may be raised, secondarily to the metabolic acidosis, before treatment is started. This is due to failure of glucose entry into cells in the absence of insulin and because of the low glomerular filtration rate. Despite hyperkalaemia, there is a total body deficit due to increased urinary potassium loss in the presence of an osmotic diuresis. During treatment, plasma potassium concentrations may fall as potassium re-enters cells, sometimes causing severe hypokalaemia unless potassium is prescribed.

Plasma sodium concentrations may be low (hyponatraemia) or low-normal at presentation, partly because of the osmotic effect of the high extracellular glucose concentration, which draws water from the cells and dilutes the sodium. In the presence of a very high plasma glucose concentration, a normal or raised plasma sodium concentration is suggestive of significant water depletion. If there is severe hyperlipidaemia, the possibility of pseudohyponatraemia must be considered (see Chapter 2). When insulin is given, gluconeogenesis is inhibited, glucose enters cells and sodium-free water follows along the osmotic gradient. If plasma sodium concentrations rise rapidly, the patient may remain confused or even comatose as long as the plasma osmolality remains significantly raised, despite a satisfactory fall in plasma glucose concentration. This may also occur if isosmolar or stronger saline solutions are given inappropriately.

Hyperphosphataemia followed by hypophosphataemia as plasma phosphate concentrations parallel those of potassium may persist for several days after recovery from diabetic coma. Similarly, hypermagnesaemia can result, partly because of the acidosis.

Plasma and urinary amylase activities may be markedly elevated and, even in the presence of abdominal pain mimicking an 'acute abdomen', do not necessarily indicate acute pancreatitis. In some patients the amylase is of salivary rather than of pancreatic origin.

Some plasma creatinine assays cross-react with ketones, resulting in a spurious plasma creatinine elevation. Sometimes severe hypertriglyceridaemia and chylomicronaemia result due to reduced lipoprotein lipase activity in the face of insulin deficiency.

A summary of the usual clinical and biochemical findings in a patient presenting with diabetic ketoacidosis is shown in Table 12.4.

Hyperosmolal non-ketotic coma

In diabetic ketoacidosis there is always plasma hyperosmolality due to the hyperglycaemia, and many of the symptoms, including those of confusion and coma, are related to it. However, the term 'hyperosmolal' coma or 'precoma' is usually confined to a condition in which there is marked hyperglycaemia but no detectable ketoacidosis. The reason for these different presentations is not clear. It has been suggested that insulin activity is sufficient to suppress lipolysis but insufficient to suppress hepatic gluconeogenesis or to facilitate glucose transport into cells. This does

Table 12.4 Clinical and biochemical findings in a patient presenting with diabetic ketoacidosis

Findings	Underlying abnormality
Clinical	
Confusion and later coma	Hyperosmolality
Hyperventilation (Kussmaul's respiration)	Metabolic acidosis
Signs of volume depletion	Osmotic diuresis
Biochemical	
Plasma	
Hyperglycaemia	Insulin deficiency
Low plasma bicarbonate	Metabolic acidosis
Initial hyperkalaemia	Intracellular potassium moves out
Mild uraemia	Decreased glomerular filtration rate
Urine	
Glycosuria	Insulin deficiency
Ketonuria	Insulin deficiency

not explain why the plasma glucose concentration is often higher in non-ketotic coma than in ketoacidosis.

Hyperosmolal non-ketotic (HONK) coma may be of sudden onset. It is more common in older patients. Plasma glucose concentrations may exceed 50 mmol/L. The effects of glycosuria are as described above, but hypernatraemia due to predominant water loss is more commonly found than in ketoacidosis and aggravates the plasma hyperosmolality. Cerebral cellular dehydration, which contributes to the coma, may also cause hyperventilation; the consequent respiratory alkalosis may cause a slight fall in the plasma bicarbonate concentration. This should not be confused with that due to metabolic acidosis. There is also an increased risk of thrombosis.

Lactic acidosis

Lactic acidosis can cause a high anion gap metabolic acidosis and coma. It may be due to the use of metformin in certain situations, such as high doses in the very elderly, those with renal, liver or cardiac failure or those dehydrated or undergoing imaging tests with contrast media (see Chapter 4).

Other causes of coma in patients with diabetes mellitus

In addition to the comas described above, a patient with diabetes mellitus may present with other comas.

CASE 3

A 77-year-old male with known type 2 diabetes mellitus presented to the casualty department feeling drowsy. His home blood glucose monitoring had recently averaged about 20 mmol/L, and the following blood results were returned.

Urine was negative for ketones.

Plasma
Sodium 160 mmol/L (135–145)
Potassium 5.0 mmol/L (3.5–5.0)
Bicarbonate 21 mmol/L (24–32)
Urea 15 mmol/L (2.5–7.0)
Creatinine 130 μmol/L (70–110)
Glucose 65 mmol/L (5.5–11.1)
Osmolality 380 mmol/kg (285–295)
pH 7.38 (7.35–7.45)
$Pa\mathrm{CO}_2$ 5.2 kPa (4.6–6.0)
$Pa\mathrm{O}_2$ 11.8 kPa (9.3–13.3)

DISCUSSION

The patient was found to be in a HONK diabetic coma. Note the severe hyperglycaemia, hypernatraemia and high plasma osmolality and presentation in an elderly patient. HONK coma is associated with type 2 diabetes mellitus. Ketoacidosis is usually absent, as there has been no conversion to ketone metabolism. This is more common in the elderly, and severe dehydration is present and there is an increased risk of thrombotic events and focal neurological signs. Treatment is with intravenous rehydration, insulin and anticoagulation.

Table 12.5 Clinical and biochemical features of a diabetic patient presenting in coma

| | | Laboratory findings | | | | |
| | | Plasma | | | | Urine |
Diagnosis	Clinical features	Glucose	Bicarbonate	Lactate	Creatinine	Ketones
Hypoglycaemia	Sweaty, drowsy	Low	N	N	N	Neg
Ketoacidosis	Volume depletion Hyperventilating	High	Low	N	N or up	Pos
Hyperosmolar coma	Volume depletion May be hyperventilating	Very high	N or slightly low	N or up	N or up	
Lactic acidosis	Hyperventilating	Variable	Low	Up	N	Neg
Uraemia	Hyperventilating	Variable	Low	N or up	Up	Neg
Cerebrovascular accident	Neurological	May be raised	May be low	N	N	Neg

N = normal; Neg = negative; Pos = positive.

- Cerebrovascular accidents are relatively common in diabetic patients because of the increased incidence of vascular disease.
- Diabetic patients can, of course, have any other coma, for example drug overdose.
- Diabetic patients are also more at risk of diabetic nephropathy and renal failure and thus uraemic coma.

The assessment of a diabetic patient presenting in coma or precoma is outlined in Table 12.5.

Principles of treatment of diabetic coma

Only the outline of treatment will be discussed. For details of management, the reader should consult a textbook of medical emergencies.

Hypoglycaemia

Hypoglycaemic coma needs prompt glucose replacement to avoid irreversible brain damage, for example 50 mL of

20 per cent glucose intravenously. If intravenous access is not an option, glucagon 1 mg can be given intramuscularly. Once the patient is awake, glucose-containing drinks can be given.

Diabetic ketoacidosis

Repletion of fluid and electrolytes should be vigorous. A 0.9 per cent normal saline solution should be administered, usually 1 L initially and then 1 L over the next hour and then 2 hours and repeated at 4 hours. Monitoring central venous pressure may be useful to assess fluid replacement. Dextrose-saline may be used when the plasma glucose concentration is less than 15 mmol/L.

If the plasma glucose concentration is more than 20 mmol/L, 10 U soluble insulin should be given. A sliding insulin scale should be instigated. Insulin is given either by continuous intravenous infusion or by intermittent intramuscular injections, as soon as the plasma glucose and potassium concentrations are known. Once the patient is eating, subcutaneous insulin can be given instead.

If the metabolic acidosis is very severe (pH less than 7.00), bicarbonate may be infused, but only until the blood pH rises to between about 7.15 and 7.20. It is unnecessary and often dangerous to correct the plasma bicarbonate concentration completely; it rapidly returns to normal following adequate fluid and insulin therapy. Remember that 8.4 per cent sodium bicarbonate is very hyperosmolar and may cause hypernatraemia and aggravate hyperosmolality. A rapid rise in the blood pH may aggravate the hypokalaemia associated with treatment.

The plasma potassium concentration should be measured before insulin is given. It is almost always raised at presentation due to the metabolic acidosis and reduced glomerular filtration rate, although total body potassium may be decreased. The plasma potassium concentration may fall rapidly once treatment is started and therefore it should be monitored frequently and potassium given as soon as it starts to fall. Usually 20 mmol/L potassium is given to each litre bag apart from the first litre and provided there is no oliguria or hyperkalaemia.

Urinary volume should be monitored; if it fails to rise despite adequate rehydration, further fluid and potassium should only be given if clinically indicated, and then with care. The risk of deep vein thrombosis is increased, in part due to dehydration, and thus heparin 5000 U 8-hourly subcutaneously can be given.

Clinical conditions such as infection that may have precipitated the coma should be sought and treated.

Frequent monitoring of plasma glucose, potassium and sodium concentrations is essential to assess progress and to detect developing hypoglycaemia, hypokalaemia or hypernatraemia. Acid–base balance should also be assessed.

Hyperosmolal non-ketotic coma

The treatment of hyperosmolal coma is similar to that of ketoacidosis. A sudden reduction of extracellular osmolality may be harmful, and it is important to give small doses of insulin to reduce plasma glucose concentrations slowly, for example 1 U/hour. These patients are often very sensitive to the action of insulin. Hypo-osmolal solutions are often used to correct volume depletion, but these too should be given slowly. Heparin is given, as there is an increased risk of venous thrombosis.

Initial investigation of a diabetic patient presenting in coma

A diabetic patient may be in coma due to hyperglycaemia, hypoglycaemia or any of the causes shown in Tables 12.4 and 12.5. After a thorough clinical assessment, proceed as follows.

- Notify the laboratory that specimens are being taken and ensure that they are delivered promptly. This minimizes delays.
- Take blood immediately for estimation of:
  - glucose,
  - sodium and potassium,
  - urea and creatinine,
  - bicarbonate,
  - arterial blood gases.
- Do a drug screen for aspirin and paracetamol.
- Determination of plasma lactate will help diagnose a lactic acidosis (see Chapter 4).
- Test a urine sample for ketones.
- A rapid assessment of blood glucose concentration may be obtained using a reagent strip, but results may be dangerously wrong so these should always be checked against the results obtained from the laboratory.
- If severe hypoglycaemia is suspected on clinical grounds or because of the results obtained using reagent strips, glucose should be given *immediately* while waiting for the laboratory results. It is less dangerous to give glucose to a patient with hyperglycaemia than to give insulin to a patient with hypoglycaemia.
- The results of side-room tests must be interpreted with caution.
- Also look for precipitating causes such as acute myocardial infarction or infection.

Investigation of suspected diabetes mellitus

In most cases a diagnosis can be established from either fasting or random blood glucose determinations. In equivocal cases an OGTT may be required.

Initial investigations

Blood for plasma glucose estimation should be taken if a patient presents with symptoms of diabetes mellitus or glycosuria or if it is desirable to exclude the diagnosis, for example because of a strong family history.

Blood samples may be taken:

- at least 10 hours after a fast,
- at random,
- as part of an oral glucose load test.

Diabetes mellitus is confirmed if one of the following is present:

- a fasting venous plasma concentration of more than or equal to 7.0 mmol/L on two occasions or once with symptoms,
- a random venous plasma concentration of more than or equal to 11.1 mmol/L on two occasions or once with symptoms.

Diabetes mellitus is unlikely if the fasting venous plasma glucose concentration is less than 5.5 mmol/L on two occasions. Samples taken at random times after meals are less reliable for excluding than for confirming the diagnosis.

The indications for performing an OGTT to diagnose diabetes mellitus are rare. They include:

- fasting venous plasma glucose concentration between 5.5 mmol/L and less than 7.0 mmol/L,
- random venous plasma concentration between 7.0 mmol/L and less than 11.1 mmol/L,
- a high index of clinical suspicion of diabetes mellitus, such as a patient at high risk of gestational diabetes with equivocal blood glucose results.

The OGTT is sometimes also useful in the diagnosis of acromegaly (see Chapter 7).

Oral glucose tolerance test

Before starting this test, contact your laboratory: local details may vary.

Procedure

The patient should be resting and should not smoke during the test.

The patient fasts overnight (for at least 10, but not more than 16, hours). Water, but no other beverage, is allowed.

A venous sample is withdrawn for plasma glucose estimation. If the glucose concentration is measured in whole blood, the results will be approximately 1.0 mmol/L lower.

A solution containing 75 g of anhydrous glucose in 300 mL of water is hyperosmolar, and may not only cause nausea and occasionally vomiting and diarrhoea, but also, because of delayed absorption, may affect the results of the test. It is therefore more usual to give a solution of a mixture of glucose and its oligosaccharides, because fewer molecules per unit volume have less osmotic effect than the equivalent amount of monosaccharide; the oligosaccharides are all hydrolysed at the brush border, and the glucose immediately enters the cells.

A solution that contains the equivalent of 75 g of anhydrous glucose is: 113 mL of Polycal made up to approximately 300 mL with water.

This solution should be drunk slowly over a few minutes.

Further blood is taken 2 hours after the ingestion of glucose.

Note that in the investigation of acromegaly, sampling is half-hourly over the 2-hour period (see Chapter 7).

Interpretation of the OGTT is shown in Table 12.6. There is controversy as to how best to interpret the OGTT in pregnancy because of the differences in maternal glucose metabolism, as stated earlier.

Table 12.6 Interpretation of the oral glucose tolerance test (glucose mmol/L). Venous plasma preferred.

	Venous plasma		Capillary whole blood		Venous whole blood	
	Fasting	2 hours	Fasting	2 hours	Fasting	2 hours
Diabetes mellitus unlikely	<6.1	<7.8	<5.6	<7.8	<5.6	<6.7
Impaired glucose tolerance	<7.0	7.8–11.1	<6.1	7.8–11.1	<6.1	6.7–10.0
Impaired fasting glucose	6.1–6.9	<7.8	5.6–6.0	<7.8	5.6–6.0	<6.7
Diabetes mellitus	≥7.0	≥11.1	≥6.1	≥11.1	≥6.1	≥10.0

The following factors may affect the result of the test:

- *Previous diet.* No special restrictions are necessary if the patient has been on a normal diet for 3–4 days. However, if the test is performed after a period of carbohydrate restriction, for example as part of a reducing diet, this may cause abnormal glucose tolerance, probably because metabolism is adjusted to the 'fasted state' and so favours gluconeogenesis.
- *Time of day.* Most glucose tolerance tests are performed in the morning and the reference values quoted are for this time of day. There is evidence that tests performed in the afternoon yield higher plasma glucose concentrations and that the accepted 'reference values' may not be applicable. This may be due to a circadian variation in islet cell responsiveness.
- *Drugs* such as steroids, oral contraceptives and thiazide diuretics may impair glucose tolerance.

HYPOGLYCAEMIA (FIG. 12.8)

By definition, hypoglycaemia is present if the plasma glucose concentration is less than 2.5 mmol/L in a specimen collected into a tube containing an inhibitor of glycolysis. Blood cells continue to metabolize glucose in vitro and low concentrations found in a specimen collected without such an inhibitor can be dangerously misleading (pseudohypoglycaemia).

Symptoms of hypoglycaemia may develop at higher concentrations if there has been a rapid fall from a previously raised value, when adrenaline secretion is stimulated and may cause sweating, tachycardia and agitation. As discussed earlier, cerebral metabolism depends on an adequate supply of glucose from extracellular fluid, and the symptoms of hypoglycaemia may resemble those of cerebral hypoxia (neuroglycopenia). Faintness, dizziness or lethargy may progress rapidly to coma and, if untreated, permanent cerebral damage or death may occur. Existing cerebral or cerebrovascular disease may aggravate the clinical picture. Whipple's triad is defined as hypoglycaemia, neuroglycopenic symptoms, and relief of these symptoms on raising the blood glucose.

Hypoglycaemia is a disease manifestation and not a diagnosis. There is no completely satisfactory classification of its causes. However, one useful approach is to divide hypoglycaemia into (inappropriate) hyperinsulinaemia, (appropriate) hypoinsulinaemia and reactive hypoglycaemia (Box 12.1).

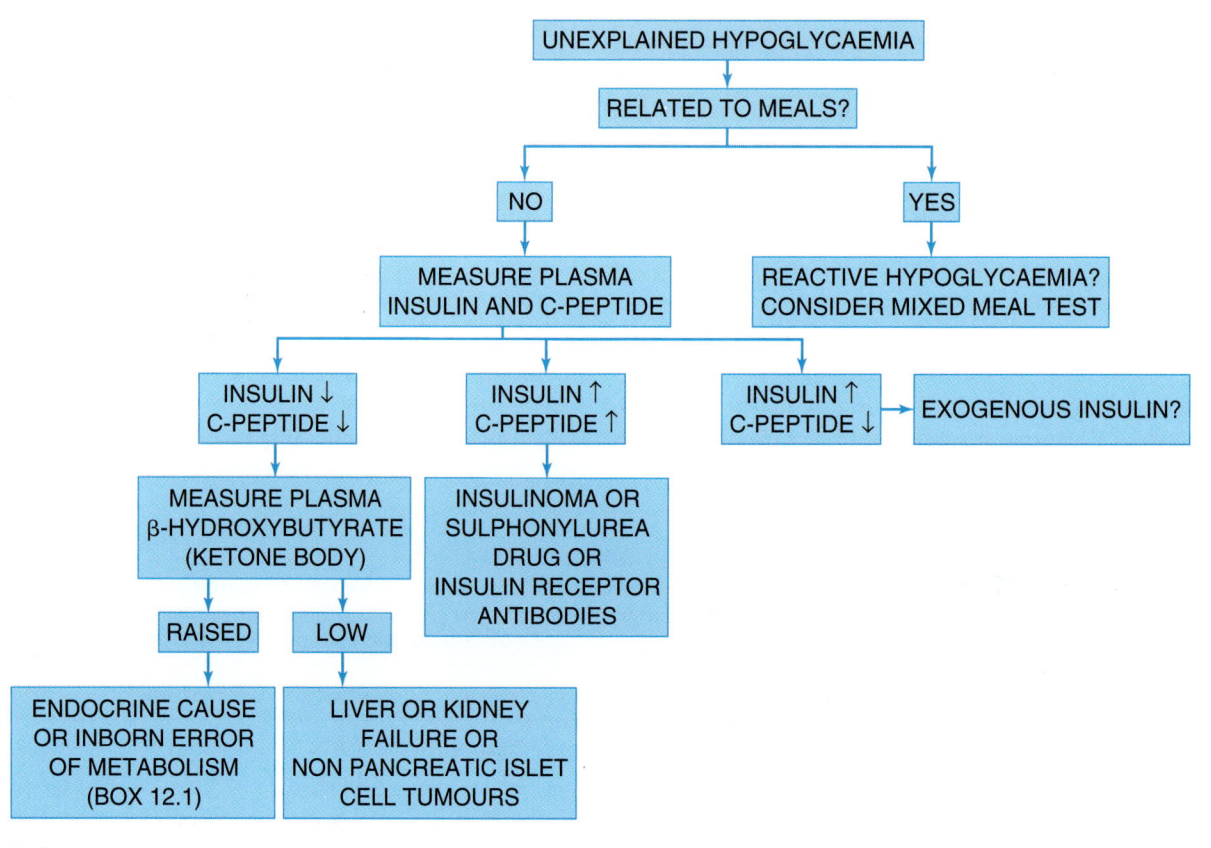

Fig. 12.8 Algorithm for the investigation of hypoglycaemia in adults.

> **Box 12.1 Some causes of hypoglycaemia in adults**
>
> *Hyperinsulinaemia hypoglycaemia*
> **Inappropriately high insulin concentrations due to:**
>   pancreatic tumour – insulinoma
>   hyperplasia of the pancreatic islet cells
>   insulin receptor antibodies
>   autoimmune insulin syndrome
>   exogenous insulin
>   sulphonylureas, meglitinides
>
> *Hypoinsulinaemia hypoglycaemia*
> **Endocrine:**
>   glucocorticoid deficiency/adrenal insufficiency
>   hypothyroidism
>   hypopituitarism
> **Organ failure:**
>   severe liver disease
>   end-stage renal disease
>   severe congestive cardiac failure
>   malaria (particularly if taking quinine)
> **Some non-pancreatic islet cell tumours:**
>   IGF-2-secreting tumours – liver, adrenal, breast
>   mesenchymal, haemangiopericytomas
>   leukaemias, lymphomas, myeloma
>   widespread metastases
>
> *Reactive hypoglycaemia*
> **idiopathic**
> **post-gastric surgery**
> **alcohol induced**

Hypoinsulinaemia hypoglycaemia

Non-pancreatic tumours (non-islet cell tumours)

Although carcinomas (especially of the liver) and sarcomas have been reported to cause hypoglycaemia, this occurs most commonly in association with retroperitoneal tumours of mesenchymal origin, but also with lymphomas, haemangiopericytomas, liver carcinoma and leukaemia. Hypoglycaemia may be the presenting feature. The mechanism is not always clear, but may sometimes be due to the secretion of insulin-like growth factor 2 (IGF-2). The IGF-2 suppresses GH and IGF-1. Tumours secreting IGF-2 are characterized by an increased plasma total IGF-2:IGF-1 ratio and low plasma insulin concentration.

Endocrine causes

Hypoglycaemia may occur in hypothyroidism, pituitary or adrenal insufficiency. However, it is rarely the presenting manifestation of these conditions.

Impaired liver function

The functional reserve of the liver is so great that, despite its central role in the maintenance of plasma glucose concentrations, hypoglycaemia is a rare complication of liver disease. It may complicate very severe hepatitis, hypoxic liver disease associated with congestive cardiac failure or liver necrosis if the whole liver is affected. Plasma IGF-1 concentration may be low.

Renal failure

Renal failure can result in hypoglycaemia as the kidney, like the liver, is a gluconeogenic organ.

Hyperinsulinaemic hypoglycaemia

Insulin or other drugs are probably the commonest causes. It is most important to take a careful drug history. Unless the facts are deliberately concealed by the patient, the offending drug should be easily identifiable. Hypoglycaemia in a diabetic patient may be caused by accidental insulin overdosage, by changing insulin requirements, or by failure to eat after insulin has been given. Self-administration for suicidal purposes or to gain attention is not unknown, and homicidal use is a remote possibility. Sulphonylureas or meglitinides may also induce hypoglycaemia, especially in the elderly.

Hypoglycaemia due to exogenous insulin suppresses insulin and C-peptide secretion. Measurement of plasma C-peptide concentrations may help to differentiate exogenous insulin administration, when C-peptide secretion is inhibited, from endogenous insulin secretion when plasma C-peptide is raised, whether it is from an insulinoma or following pancreatic stimulation by sulphonylurea drugs.

An insulinoma is usually a small, histologically benign primary tumour of the islet cells of the pancreas. It may present at any age. Multiple tumours may occur and may be part of the syndrome of multiple endocrine neoplasia (MEN). As with other functioning endocrine tumours, hormone secretion is inappropriate and usually excessive. C-peptide and proinsulin are released in parallel with insulin, and plasma concentrations are therefore inappropriately high in the presence of hypoglycaemia. Some insulinomas secrete just proinsulin. Attacks of hypoglycaemia occur

> **CASE 4**
>
> A 45-year-old female was being investigated in the endocrine unit because of hypoglycaemic episodes, which manifested as sweating and dizzy attacks and which were relieved by sweet drinks.
>
> Her renal, liver and thyroid functions were all normal. Some of her fasting biochemical results were as follows.
>
> *Plasma*
> Glucose 2.1 mmol/L (5.5–11.1)
> Insulin 168 pmol/L (10–50)
> Insulin C-peptide 998 pmol/L (200–650)
> A urinary sulphonylurea screen was negative.
>
> **DISCUSSION**
> This patient has raised plasma insulin concentrations in the presence of fasting hypoglycaemia. She was subsequently shown to have an insulinoma. Note the raised plasma insulin and C-peptide concentrations in the presence of hypoglycaemia, suggesting the presence of endogenous insulin secretion (exogenous insulin administration would not be expected to be associated with raised C-peptide levels). Her symptoms and their relief by glucose-containing drinks are classical of hypoglycaemic episodes. Insulinomas can be associated with MEN syndrome, which should be excluded.

typically at night and before breakfast, associated with hunger, and may be precipitated by strenuous exercise. Personality or behavioural changes may be the first feature; some patients present initially to psychiatrists.

Insulin antibodies can form in response to exogenous insulin, probably less so for human insulin than for animal types. Sometimes insulin antibodies form despite the patient never having been exposed to exogenous insulin – autoimmune insulin syndrome (AIS). Insulin receptor antibodies may cause hypoglycaemia, although they sometimes lead to insulin resistance and hyperglycaemia.

Reactive (functional) hypoglycaemia

Some people develop symptomatic hypoglycaemia between 2 and 4 hours after a meal or a glucose load. Loss of consciousness is very rare. Similar symptoms may follow a gastrectomy, when rapid passage of glucose into the intestine, and rapid absorption, may stimulate excessive insulin secretion ('late dumping syndrome'). Reactive hypoglycaemia is uncommon and is probably diagnosed too often.

Alcohol-induced hypoglycaemia

Hypoglycaemia may develop between 2 and 10 hours after the ingestion of large amounts of alcohol. It is found most often in malnourished subjects and chronic alcoholics but may occur in young subjects when they first drink alcohol. Hypoglycaemia is probably caused by the suppression of gluconeogenesis during the metabolism of alcohol. Differentiation of hypoglycaemia from alcoholic stupor may be impossible unless the plasma glucose concentration is estimated. It may be necessary to infuse glucose frequently during treatment, until glycogen stores are repleted and plasma glucose concentrations are stable.

See Chapter 26 for a discussion of hypoglycaemia in neonates and children.

Investigation of adult hypoglycaemia

Some of the causes of hypoglycaemia are shown in Box 12.1 and can be divided into hyperinsulinaemic and hypoinsulinaemic groups. The following scheme may be useful in investigating hypoglycaemia. It is important to exclude pseudohypoglycaemia due to in-vitro glucose metabolism, for example an old blood sample or one not collected into fluoride oxalate anticoagulant. Sometimes a cause may be evident from the medical and drug histories and clinical examination.

One of the most important tests in a patient with proven hypoglycaemia is to measure the plasma insulin and C-peptide concentrations when the plasma glucose concentration is low. Plasma for these assays should be separated from cells immediately and the plasma stored at −20 °C until hypoglycaemia has been proven. These tests should differentiate exogenous insulin administration and endogenous insulin production, for example an insulinoma, from other causes of hypoglycaemia.

Raised plasma insulin concentrations and suppressed plasma concentrations of C-peptide suggest exogenous insulin administration (hyperinsulinaemia hypoglycaemia). Conversely, a high plasma insulin and high C-peptide can be seen in sulphonylurea or meglitinide administration, and a urine or plasma drug screen is thus important.

Positive autoantibodies to the insulin receptor or insulin may also evoke hypoglycaemia, such as AIS.

If a sulphonylurea drug screen and an insulin autoantibody screen are negative, raised plasma insulin and C-peptide concentrations are suggestive of an insulinoma.

Some tumours release proinsulin, which can also be assayed. Imaging will also be necessary, such as magnetic resonance imaging or computerized tomography scanning, to localize the tumour and to help exclude MEN syndrome (see Chapter 24).

If both the plasma insulin and C-peptide concentrations are suppressed, the hypoglycaemia (hypoinsulinaemic hypoglycaemia) can then be divided into non-ketotic and ketotic forms. Hypoglycaemia with low plasma ketone concentrations, i.e. β-hydroxybutyrate less than 600 μmol/L, is suggestive of increased insulin or IGF-1 activity such as may occur in non-islet cell tumour hypoglycaemia (NICTH). In NICTH, there is often increased IGF-2 secretion.

Hypoinsulinaemic hypoglycaemia with hypoketonaemia can also be seen in hepatic failure or renal disease. Therefore liver and renal function should be checked. Conversely, hypoinsulinaemia hypoglycaemia with high plasma ketones, i.e. β-hydroxybutyrate more than 600 μmol/L, can be found in hypopituitarism (see Chapter 7) when the plasma GH concentration is usually low. In addition, consider adrenal insufficiency (see Chapter 8) and hypothyroidism (see Chapter 11), in which plasma GH is usually high. High alcohol intake can also present with hypoinsulinaemic hypoglycaemia and raised ketone concentrations.

However, more commonly, the patient has been referred for investigation of previously documented hypoglycaemia or with a history strongly suggestive of hypoglycaemic attacks. If no cause is identified at this point, it may be possible to induce hypoglycaemia by provocation tests, although these are not without the risk of severe hypoglycaemic episodes.

Such tests could be as follows.

- *Overnight fast.* A majority of patients with spontaneous hypoglycaemia manifest one plasma glucose concentration less than 2.5 mmol/L during an overnight (18-hour) fast when assayed on three separate occasions.
- *Exercise test.* Exercise may be used in the induction of insulin-induced hypoglycaemia. Blood is collected at 10-minute intervals during half an hour of intense exercise, for example treadmill, and 30 minutes after stopping. Plasma insulin and C-peptide (and proinsulin, if necessary) are assayed and will be inappropriately high in endogenous hyperinsulinaemia and suppressed appropriately in hypoinsulinaemic hypoglycaemia.
- *Prolonged fast.* The prolonged fast, of up to 48 hours, may be reserved for cases where there is a high index of suspicion of hypoglycaemia that has not been provoked spontaneously or by the above tests. It should be noted that during the prolonged fast the patient must be under close supervision.

Blood should be taken every 6 hours for plasma glucose and insulin estimations and, if symptoms occur, should be assayed for glucose immediately. The test can be stopped if hypoglycaemia is demonstrated. The patient should be fed after the test. If prolonged fasting does not induce hypoglycaemia, endogenous hyperinsulinism is unlikely to be the cause of the symptoms. A few normal individuals may show plasma glucose levels less than 2.5 mmol/L during the test, but they do not exhibit neuroglycopenic symptoms or Whipple's triad.

The insulin provocation test is now rarely used (as it can evoke dangerous hypoglycaemia) when insulin administration fails to suppress plasma insulin and C-peptide in cases of insulinoma.

Reactive hypoglycaemia should not be diagnosed by a prolonged 75 g OGTT, as normal individuals may show false-positive results. However, the mixed meal, based on the sort of foods that evoke the attacks, can be used to investigate postprandial neuroglycopenic symptoms. Capillary blood samples are taken prior to and every half-hour for 6 hours after mixed-meal ingestion. Reactive hypoglycaemia is a possible diagnosis if the patient develops neuroglycopenic symptoms and the capillary plasma glucose concentration is 3.0 mmol/L or less. Note that venous plasma should not be used, as false-positive results may result because postprandial glucose concentrations can be 1–2 mmol/L lower than in capillary blood samples.

Treatment of hypoglycaemia

Milder cases can be managed with oral glucose-containing preparations. Severe hypoglycaemia should be treated by urgent intravenous administration of 10–20 ml of at least 10 per cent (and in adults 20 per cent) glucose solution. Some patients may need to be maintained on a glucose infusion until the cause has been established and treated. Intramuscular glucagon 1 mg can also be used if intravenous access is a problem, but this should not be given in cases of insulinoma.

An insulinoma should be removed surgically. If this is contraindicated for clinical reasons, diazoxide may maintain normoglycaemia.

Laboratory tests

Estimation of plasma or blood glucose

Glucose is measured in the laboratory by specific enzymatic methods. The supply of glucose to cells depends on extracellular (plasma) concentrations. The measurement of plasma glucose concentrations is preferable to that of whole blood. Blood cells, with very low glucose concentrations, 'dilute' glucose, giving results 10–15 per cent lower than in plasma, the actual amount depending on the haematocrit. Capillary blood from a finger prick is used for home glucose monitoring and the results for such samples may fall between those of venous whole blood and venous plasma.

Unless plasma is separated from the blood cells within about an hour of collection, the whole blood sample must be mixed with an inhibitor of glycolysis, such as fluoride. This helps prevent an in-vitro fall in the plasma glucose concentration as glycolysis continues, which may result in pseudohypoglycaemia.

Urinary glucose

Enzyme reagent strips specific for glucose, such as those that use a glucose oxidase method, best detect glycosuria. The directions for use are supplied with the strips. Glycosuria may be due to:

- diabetes mellitus,
- glucose-containing infusion,
- renal glycosuria, which may be inherited as an autosomal dominant trait or in Fanconi's syndrome,
- pregnancy.

False-negative results may occur:

- if the urine contains large amounts of ascorbic acid after the ingestion of therapeutic doses,
- after the injection of tetracyclines, which contain ascorbic acid as a preservative.

False-positive results may occur if the urine container is contaminated with detergent.

Reducing substances in the urine can be detected using copper-containing reagents such as those incorporated in Clinitest tablets. In the neonatal period, the finding of other reducing substances may suggest an inborn error of metabolism, such as galactosaemia (see Chapter 27). It is therefore important to use this test rather than one that is specific for glucose in the screening for such conditions.

Non-glucose reducing substances are identified by chromatography and specific tests. The significance of a Clinitest-positive result varies with the substances, which are as follows.

- *Glucose*.
- *Glucuronates* are relatively common urinary reducing substances. Numerous drugs, such as salicylates and their metabolites, are excreted in the urine after conjugation with glucuronate in the liver.
- *Galactose* is found in the urine in galactosaemia.
- *Fructose* may appear in the urine after very large oral doses of sucrose, or after excessive fruit ingestion, but usually fructosuria is due to one of two rare inborn errors of metabolism, both transmitted as autosomal recessive disorders:
  – essential fructosuria is a harmless condition,
  – hereditary fructose intolerance is characterized by hypoglycaemia that may lead to death in infancy.
- *Lactose*. Lactosuria may occur in:
  – late pregnancy and during lactation,
  – lactase deficiency.
- *Pentoses*. Pentosuria is very rare. It may occur in:
  – alimentary pentosuria, after excessive ingestion of fruits such as cherries and grapes – the pentoses are arabinose and xylose,
  – essential pentosuria, a rare recessive disorder due to a block in glucuronate metabolism characterized by the excretion of xylose – it is harmless.
- *Homogentisic acid* appears in the urine in the rare inborn error alkaptonuria. It is usually recognizable because it forms a blackish precipitate in urine on standing. Urea and creatinine may give weak positive results at high concentrations.

Ketonuria

Most simple urine tests for ketones are more sensitive for detecting acetoacetate than acetone; β-hydroxybutyrate does not always react in these tests. Occasional colour reactions resembling, but not identical to, that of acetoacetate may be given by phthalein compounds when used as a laxative.

Ketostix and Acetest are strips and tablets, respectively, impregnated with ammonium sulphate and sodium nitroprusside.

Remember that raised concentrations of urinary ketones can occur not only in diabetic ketoacidosis but also in alcoholic ketoacidosis or starvation and in some urinary tract infections.

CONCLUSIONS

- Diabetes mellitus is a common medical condition and an understanding of its biochemistry aids its medical management. Type 1 diabetes mellitus is associated with insulin deficiency presenting with weight loss and urinary ketones in young individuals. There is a relationship with autoimmune disease. Treatment is with insulin. Conversely, Type 2 diabetes mellitus is associated with insulin resistance, increased body weight and later age presentation. There may be a strong family history. Treatment involves diet or biguanides or sulphonylureas, although insulin may sometimes be needed.
- Biochemical tests have a major role in the management of diabetes mellitus and in monitoring its complications, such as in the control of blood glucose, HbA_{1c}, plasma lipids and urinary ACR.
- Diabetes mellitus can present with various comas, including hypoglycaemia, diabetic ketoacidosis (type 1), HONK and lactic acidosis.
- Hypoglycaemia can present with neurological impairment and coma. A useful classification is to divide hypoglycaemia into that with high plasma insulin and that with low insulin levels. The causes of hyperinsulinaemia hypoglycaemia include insulinomas and tumours producing insulin-like substances and following insulin administration. The causes of hypoinsulinaemic hypoglycaemia include severe hepatic disease, adrenal insufficiency or pituitary failure.

13 PLASMA LIPIDS AND LIPOPROTEINS

Plasma lipids	198	Disorders of lipid metabolism	206
Fatty acids	199	Investigation of hyperlipidaemias	211
Lipoproteins	200		

Lipids play a critical role in almost all aspects of biological life, they are structural components in cells and are involved in metabolic and hormonal pathways. The importance of having a knowledge of lipid disorders cannot be over-stated, not least because they are common in clinical practice and in some cases associated with atherosclerosis such as coronary heart disease, one of the biggest killers in urbanized societies.

Lipids are defined as organic compounds that are poorly soluble in water but miscible in organic solvents. Lipidology is the study of abnormal lipid metabolism. An understanding of the pathophysiology of plasma lipid metabolism is usefully based on the concept of lipoproteins, the form in which lipids circulate in plasma.

PLASMA LIPIDS

The chemical structures of the four main forms of lipid present in plasma are illustrated in Fig. 13.1.

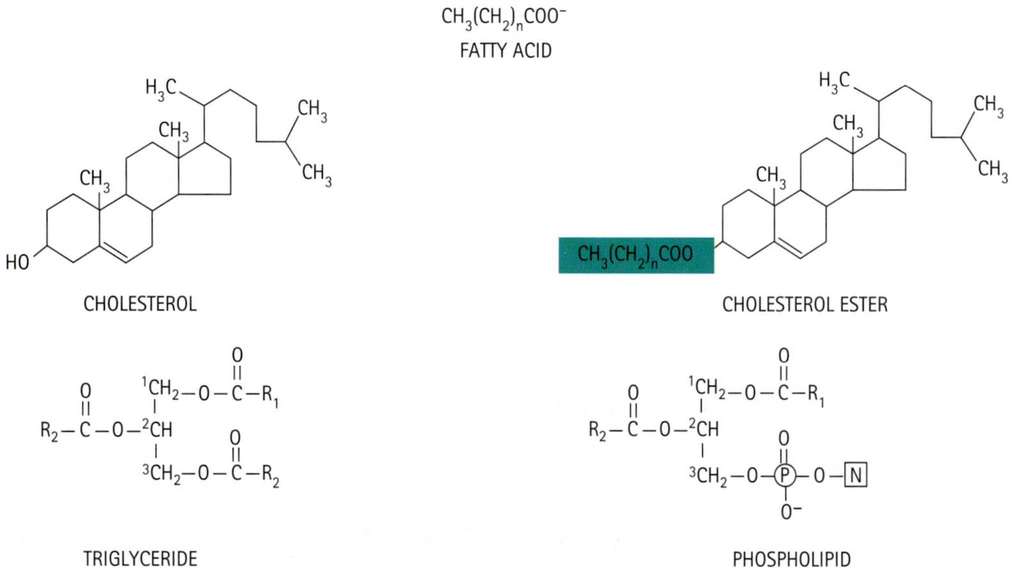

Fig. 13.1 Lipid structures. (P = phosphate; N = nitrogenous base; R = fatty acid.)

FATTY ACIDS

These are straight-chain carbon compounds of varying lengths. They may be saturated, containing no double bonds, mono-unsaturated, with one double bond, or polyunsaturated, with more than one double bond (Table 13.1).

Fatty acids can esterify with glycerol to form triglycerides or be non-esterified or free (NEFA). Plasma NEFAs liberated from adipose tissue by the action of lipase activity are transported to the liver and muscle mainly bound to albumin. The NEFAs provide a significant proportion of the energy requirements of the body. Summary diagrams of fatty acid synthesis and oxidation are shown in Figs 13.2 and 13.3.

A family of nuclear receptors that are activated by fatty acids – called peroxisome proliferator-activated receptors (PPARs) – has been described and implicated in insulin resistance and dyslipidaemia. The PPARs can be subdivided into α-PPARs, which are activated by fibrate drugs, and γ-PPARs, which are activated by thiazolidinedione drugs, for example pioglitazone or rosiglitazone.

Triglycerides are transported from the intestine to various tissues, including the liver and adipose tissue, as lipoproteins. Following hydrolysis, fatty acids are taken up, re-esterified and stored as triglycerides. Plasma triglyceride concentrations rise after a meal, unlike that of plasma cholesterol.

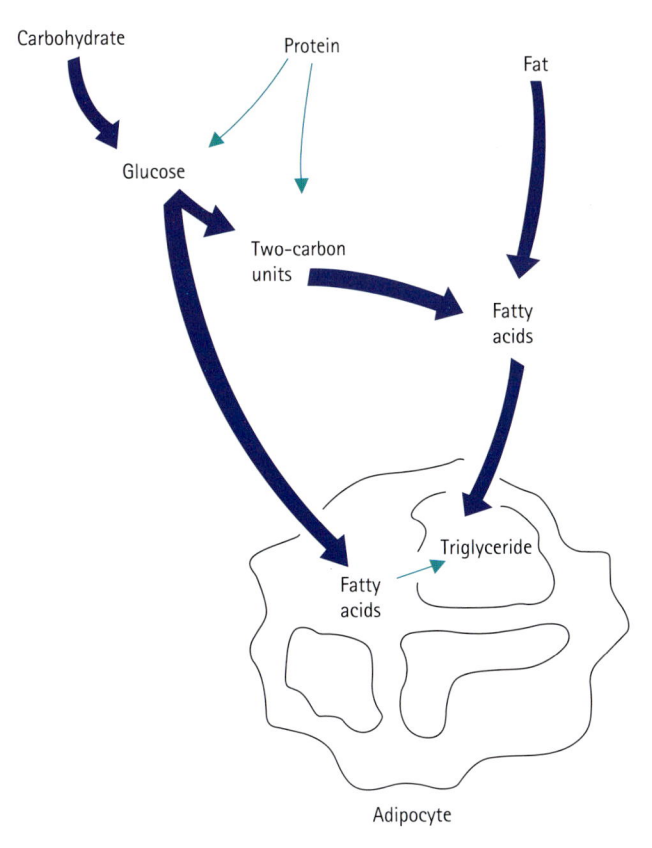

Fig. 13.2 Summary of fatty acid synthesis and adipose tissue substrates. (Reproduced with kind permission from Candlish JK and Crook M, *Notes on Clinical Biochemistry*, Singapore: World Scientific Publishing, 1993.)

Table 13.1 Some of the major fatty acids found in the plasma

Group	Name	Carbon-chain length	Source
Mono-unsaturated	Palmitoleic	C16	Plant oil
	Oleic	C18	Olive oil
Poly-unsaturated	Linoleic	C18	Plant oil
	Linolenic	C18	Plant oil
	Arachidonic	C20	Plant oil
	Eicosapentaenoic	C20	Fish oil
Saturated	Myristic	C14	Coconut oil
	Palmitic	C16	Animal/plant oil
	Stearic	C18	Animal/plant oil

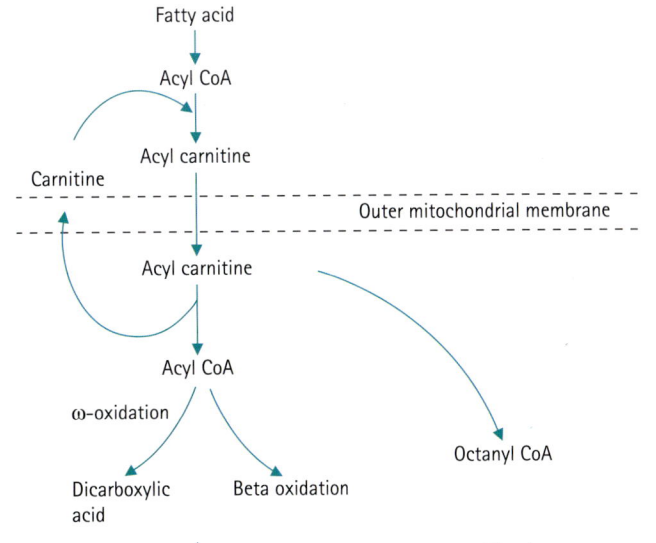

Fig. 13.3 Summary of fatty acid oxidation. (CoA = coenzyme A.) (Reproduced with kind permission from Candlish JK and Crook M, *Notes on Clinical Biochemistry*, Singapore: World Scientific Publishing, 1993.)

Phospholipids are complex lipids, similar in structure to triglycerides but containing phosphate and a nitrogenous base in place of one of the fatty acids. They fulfill an important structural role in cell membranes, and the phosphate group confers solubility on non-polar lipids and cholesterol in lipoproteins.

Cholesterol is a steroid alcohol found exclusively in animals and present in virtually all cells and body fluids. It is a precursor of numerous physiologically important steroids, including bile acids and steroid hormones. A summary of the cholesterol synthetic pathways is shown in Fig. 13.4. The rate-limiting enzyme is 3-hydroxy-3-methylglutaryl coenzyme A reductase (HMG-CoA reductase), which is controlled by negative feedback by the intracellular concentration. About two-thirds of the plasma cholesterol is esterified with fatty acids to form cholesterol esters.

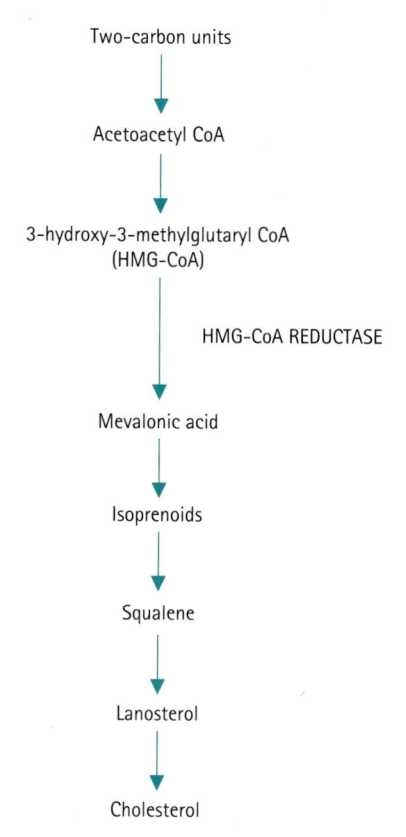

Two-carbon units
↓
Acetoacetyl CoA
↓
3-hydroxy-3-methylglutaryl CoA (HMG-CoA)
↓ HMG-CoA REDUCTASE
Mevalonic acid
↓
Isoprenoids
↓
Squalene
↓
Lanosterol
↓
Cholesterol

Fig. 13.4 Summary of pathways of cholesterol synthesis. (CoA = coenzyme A.) (Reproduced with kind permission from Candlish JK and Crook M, *Notes on Clinical Biochemistry*, Singapore: World Scientific Publishing, 1993.)

LIPOPROTEINS

Because lipids are relatively insoluble in aqueous media, they are transported in body fluids as, often spherical, soluble protein complexes called lipoproteins. Lipids can be derived from food (exogenous) or synthesized in the body (endogenous). The water-soluble (polar) groups of proteins, phospholipids and free cholesterol face outwards and surround an inner insoluble (non-polar) core of triglyceride and cholestrol esters.

Lipoproteins are classified by their buoyant density, which inversely reflects their size. The greater the lipid:protein ratio, the larger their size and the lower the density. Lipoproteins can be classified into five main groups (Table 13.2). The first three are triglyceride rich and, because of their large size, they scatter light, which can give plasma a turbid appearance (lipaemic) if present in high concentrations.

- Chylomicrons are the largest and least dense lipoproteins and transport exogenous lipid from the intestine to all cells.
- Very low-density lipoproteins (VLDLs) transport endogenous lipid from the liver to cells.
- Intermediate-density lipoproteins (IDLs), which are transient and formed during the conversion of VLDL to low-density lipoprotein (LDL), are not normally present in plasma.

Table 13.2 Characteristics of major lipoproteins

Lipoprotein	Source	Composition (% mass)				Apolipoprotein	Electrophoretic mobility
		Pro	Cho	Tg	PL		
Chylomicrons	Gut	1	4	90	5	A, B, C, E	Origin
VLDL	Liver	8	25	55	12	B, C, E	Pre-beta
LDL	VLDL via IDL	20	55	5	20	B	Beta
HDL	Gut/liver	50	20	5	25	A, C, E	Alpha

Pro = protein; Cho = cholesterol; Tg = triglyceride; PL = phospholipid; VLDL = very low-density lipoprotein; LDL = low-density lipoprotein; IDL = intermediate-density lipoprotein; HDL = high-density lipoprotein.

The other two lipoprotein classes contain mainly cholesterol and are smaller in size.

- Low-density lipoproteins are formed from VLDLs and carry cholesterol to cells.
- High-density lipoproteins (HDLs) are the most dense lipoproteins and are involved in the transport of cholesterol from cells back to the liver (reverse cholesterol transport). These lipoproteins can be further divided by density into HDL2 and HDL3.

If a lipaemic plasma sample, for example after a meal, is left overnight at 4 °C, the larger and less dense chylomicrons form a creamy layer on the surface. The smaller and denser VLDL and IDL particles do not rise, and the sample may appear diffusely turbid. The LDL and HDL particles do not contribute to this turbidity because they are small and do not scatter light. Fasting plasma from normal individuals contains only VLDL, LDL and HDL particles.

In some cases of hyperlipidaemia, the lipoprotein patterns have been classified (Fredrickson's classification) according to their electrophoretic mobility. Four principal bands are formed, based on their relative positions, by protein electrophoresis, namely α (HDL), pre-β (VLDL), β (LDL) and chylomicrons (Table 13.3).

Intermediate-density lipoproteins in excess may produce a broad β-band. Some individuals with hyperlipidaemia may show varying electrophoretic patterns at different times.

Ultracentrifugation or electrophoretic techniques are rarely used in routine clinical practice. Instead, the lipoprotein composition of plasma may be inferred from standard clinical laboratory lipid assays. As fasting plasma does not normally contain chylomicrons, the triglyceride content reflects VLDL. Furthermore, generally about 70 per cent of plasma cholesterol is incorporated as LDL and 20 per cent as HDL. The latter particles, because of their high density, can be quantitated by precipitation techniques that can assay their cholesterol content by subtraction.

The Friedewald equation enables plasma LDL cholesterol concentration to be calculated and is often used in clinical laboratories.

$$\text{LDL cholesterol} = \text{total cholesterol} - \text{HDL cholesterol} - \frac{[\text{triglyceride}]}{2.2} \quad (13.1)$$

This equation makes certain assumptions, namely that the patient is fasting and the plasma triglyceride concentration does not exceed 5.0 mmol/L (otherwise chylomicrons make the equation inaccurate).

There has been recent interest in the subdivision of LDL particles into small dense LDL2 and LDL3, which appear to be more atherogenic and more easily oxidized than the larger LDL1 particles. Additionally, another lipoprotein called lipoprotein (a), or Lp(a), has been found. This is similar in lipid composition to LDL but has a higher

Table 13.3 Fredrickson's classification of hyperlipidaemias

Type	Electrophoretic	Increased lipoprotein
I	Increased chylomicrons	Chylomicrons
IIa	Increased β lipoproteins	LDL
IIb	Increased β and pre-β lipoproteins	LDL and VLDL
III	Broad β lipoproteins	IDL
IV	Increased pre-β lipoproteins	VLDL
V	Increased chylomicrons and pre-β lipoproteins	Chylomicrons and VLDL

LDL = low-density lipoprotein; VLDL = very low-density lipoprotein; IDL = intermediate-density lipoprotein.

Table 13.4 The main apolipoproteins and their common functions

Apolipoprotein	Associated lipoprotein	Function
A1	Chylomicrons and HDL	LCAT activator
A2	Chylomicrons and HDL	LCAT activator
B48	Chylomicrons and VLDL	Secretion of chylomicrons/VLDL
B100	IDL, VLDL, LDL	LDL receptor binding
C2	Chylomicrons, HDL, VLDL, IDL	Lipoprotein lipase activator
C3	Chylomicrons, HDL, VLDL, IDL	Lipoprotein lipase inhibitor
E	Chylomicrons, HDL, VLDL, IDL	IDL and remnant particle receptor binding

HDL = high-density lipoprotein; VLDL = very low-density lipoprotein; IDL = intermediate-density lipoprotein; LDL = low-density lipoprotein; LCAT = lecithin-cholesterol acyltransferase.

protein content. One of its proteins, called apolipoprotein (a), shows homology to plasminogen and may disrupt fibrinolysis, thus evoking a thrombotic tendency. The plasma concentration of Lp(a) is normally less than 0.30 g/L and it is thought to be an independent cardiovascular risk factor.

The proteins associated with lipoproteins are called apolipoproteins (apo). ApoA (mainly $apoA_1$ and $apoA_2$) is the major group associated with HDL particles. The apoB series ($apoB_{100}$) is predominantly found with LDL particles and is the ligand for the LDL receptor. Low-density lipoprotein has one molecule of $apoB_{100}$ per particle. Some reports have suggested that the plasma $apoA_1$:apoB ratio may be a useful measure of cardiovascular risk (increased if ratio less than 1) and it is not significantly influenced by the fasting status of the patient. The apoC series is particularly important in triglyceride metabolism and, with the apoE series, freely interchanges between various lipoproteins. Some of the functions of these apolipoproteins are described in Table 13.4.

Lipoprotein metabolism

Exogenous lipid pathways (Fig. 13.5)

Cholesterol and fatty acids released from dietary fats by digestion together with bile are absorbed into intestinal mucosa cells where they are re-esterified to form cholesterol esters and triglycerides. These together with phospholipids and apoA and apoB are then secreted into the lymphatic system as chylomicrons. This secretion is dependent upon $apoB_{48}$. The chylomicrons enter the systemic circulation

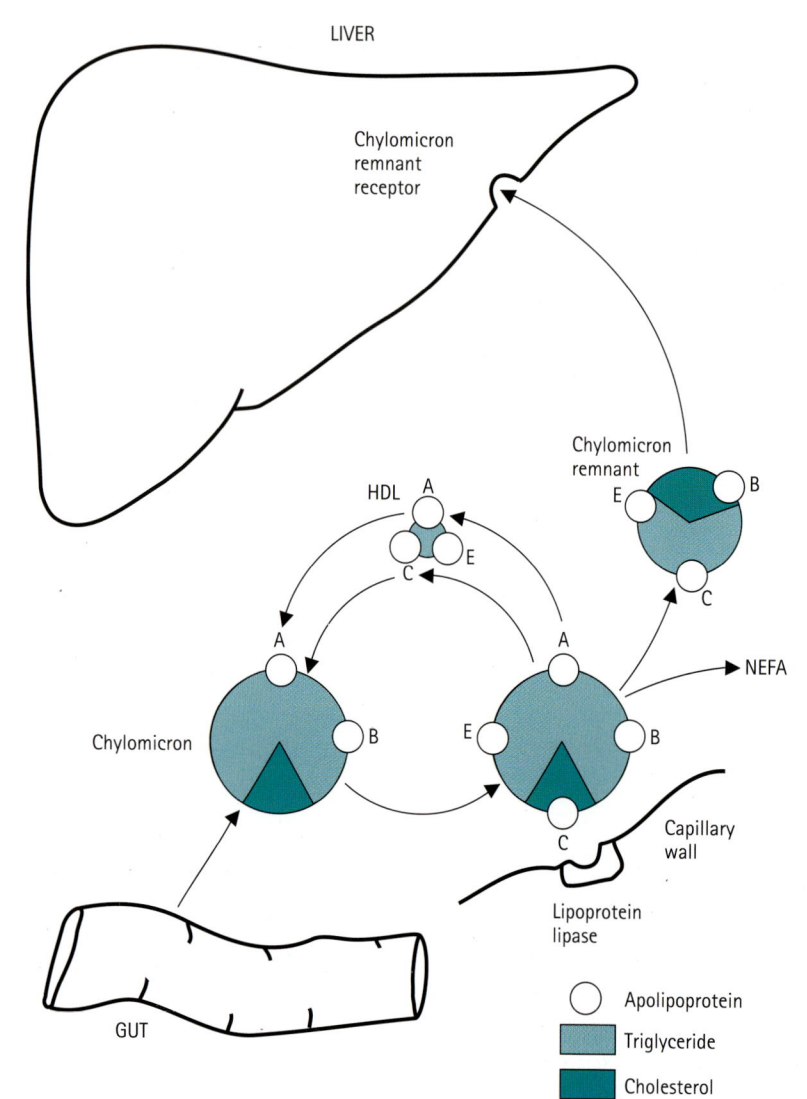

Fig. 13.5 Exogenous lipid pathways. (HDL = high-density lipoprotein; NEFA = non-esterified [free] fatty acid.)

via the thoracic duct. Apolipoprotein C and apoE, both derived from HDL, are added to the chylomicrons in the lymph and plasma.

The enzyme lipoprotein lipase is located on capillary walls and is activated by apoC$_2$ and inhibited by apoC$_3$. It hydrolyses triglyceride to fatty acids and glycerol. The former are taken up by adipose or muscle cells or bound to albumin in the plasma. The glycerol component enters the hepatic glycolytic pathway. During their sojourn within the circulation, the chylomicron particles get smaller and release some apoA and apoC along with phospholipids, which then become incorporated into HDL particles. The chylomicron remnants enriched in apoB and apoE and cholesterol then bind rapidly to hepatic LDL-receptor-related protein, which recognizes the apoE ligand. Within the hepatic cells the cholesterol is utilized and the apolipoproteins catabolized. Thus, ultimately the exogenous pathway delivers triglyceride to adipose tissue and muscle and cholesterol to the liver.

Endogenous lipid pathways (Fig. 13.6)

The liver is the main source of endogenous lipids. Triglycerides are synthesized from fatty acids and glycerol, which may be derived from fat stores or glucose, respectively. Hepatic cholesterol can either be derived from chylomicron remnants via the exogenous pathway or synthesized locally. These lipids are transported from the liver as VLDL.

Very low-density lipoprotein is a large triglyceride-rich particle consisting also of apoB$_{100}$, apoC and apoE. Following hepatic secretion, it incorporates additional apoC from HDL particles within the circulation. Like chylomicrons, VLDL is hydrolysed by lipoprotein lipase in the peripheral tissues, albeit more slowly. The resulting

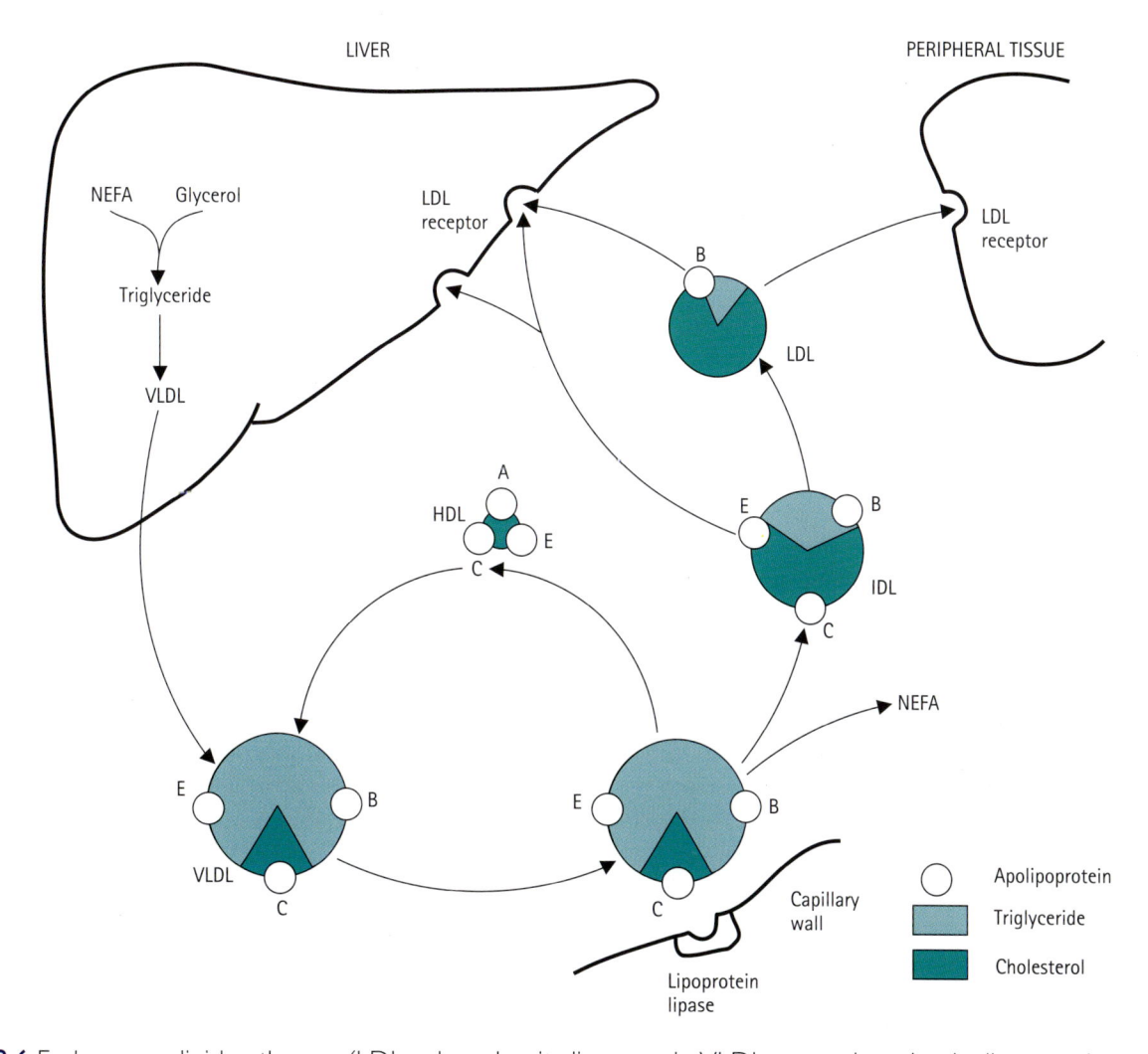

Fig. 13.6 Endogenous lipid pathways. (LDL = low-density lipoprotein; VLDL = very low-density lipoprotein; IDL = intermediate-density lipoprotein; HDL = high-density lipoprotein; NEFA = non-esterified [free] fatty acid.)

VLDL remnant or IDL contains cholesterol and triglyceride as well as apoB and apoE and is rapidly taken up by the liver or converted by the action of hepatic lipase to LDL by losing apoE and triglyceride.

Low-density lipoprotein is a small cholesterol-rich lipoprotein containing only apoB. It represents about 70 per cent of the total plasma cholesterol concentration. It can be taken up by most cells, although mainly the liver by the LDL or B/E receptor which recognizes and binds apoB$_{100}$. Within the cell, the LDL particles are broken down by lysosomes, releasing cholesterol. This cholesterol can be incorporated into cell membranes or in specific tissues such as the adrenal cortex or gonads and utilized in steroid synthesis. Most cells are able to synthesize cholesterol, but to avoid intracellular accumulation, there is a feedback control system reducing the rate of synthesis of the LDL receptors. Although most of the plasma LDL is removed by LDL receptors, if the plasma cholesterol concentration is excessive, LDL particles, by virtue of their small size, can infiltrate tissues by passive diffusion and can even cause damage, as in atheroma formation within arterial walls. An alternative route of removal of LDL is via the reticuloendothelial system, collectively termed the scavenger cell pathway, which only recognizes chemically modified LDL, for example oxidized LDL.

The liver has a central role in cholesterol metabolism:

- it contains most of the LDL receptors,
- it is responsible for most of the endogenous cholesterol synthesis,
- it takes up cholesterol from the diet via lipoproteins,
- it can excrete cholesterol from the body in bile.

Cholesterol is synthesized via a series of enzymatic steps, with HMG-CoA reductase being the rate-limiting enzyme (Fig. 13.4). Suppression of this enzyme may occur if cholesterol synthesis is excessive. Involved in these processes is a family of transcription-regulating proteins called sterol regulatory element binding proteins. Intracellular cholesterol accumulation also reduces the number of hepatic LDL receptors and therefore LDL entry into cells declines and the plasma concentration rises. However, if the dietary intake of cholesterol is excessive, intracellular accumulation can still occur. About 30–60 per cent of the dietary intake of cholesterol (of 1–2 mmol) is absorbed, this amount being increased if the diet is rich in saturated fat. High saturated fat intake can also suppress LDL receptor activity. The richest dietary sources of cholesterol are egg yolks, dairy products and red meat.

Net loss of body cholesterol can occur by bile excretion. Some bile salts are reabsorbed from the intestinal lumen and return to the liver via the enterohepatic circulation. Interruption of this process results in enhanced conversion of cholesterol to bile salts, reduced hepatic cholesterol stores and increased LDL receptors (Fig. 13.7). The rate of LDL receptor synthesis is also increased by thyroxine and oestrogens and decreases with age.

High-density lipoprotein

The transport of cholesterol from non-hepatic cells to the liver involves HDL particles, in a process called reverse cholesterol transport (Fig. 13.8). The HDL is synthesized in both hepatic and intestinal cells and secreted from them as small, nascent HDL particles rich in free cholesterol, phospholipids, apoA and apoE. This cholesterol acquisition is stimulated by adenosine triphosphate-binding cassette protein 1 (ABC1). If the plasma concentration of VLDL or chylomicrons is low, apoC is also carried in HDL, but as the plasma concentrations of these lipoproteins rise, these particles take up apoC from HDL. In addition, HDL can be formed from the surface coat of VLDL and chylomicrons. Various factors control the rate of HDL synthesis, including oestrogens, thus explaining why plasma concentrations are higher in menstruating women compared with menopausal women or men.

The enzyme lecithin-cholesterol acyltransferase (LCAT) is present on HDL and catalyses the esterification of free cholesterol and is activated by apoA$_1$, the predominant apolipoprotein of HDL. Some HDL particles also contain apoA$_2$. Most of this esterified cholesterol is transferred to LDL, VLDL and chylomicron remnants and thus ultimately reaches the liver. Some may be stored within the core of the HDL particle and taken directly to the liver. Cholesterol ester transfer protein (CETP) is involved in these processes.

The HDL particles can be divided into pre-β (or precursor) HDL, HDL2 and HDL3. The HDL2, which is a precursor of smaller HDL3 particles, interconvert as a result of the acquisition of cholesterol by HDL3 through the actions of LCAT and hepatic lipase.

High-density lipoprotein also contains other enzymes, including paroxanase, which may have an antioxidant role. Removal of HDL may occur by endocytosis, although there may be specific receptors such as the murine class B type I scavenger receptor (SR-BI) in liver and steroidogenic tissue, for example adrenals, ovaries and testes. Thus HDL-derived cholesterol can be 'off-loaded' in the liver and secreted in bile or taken up and utilized for steroid synthesis.

In hypertriglyceridaemia there is increased VLDL concentration and, under the action of hepatic lipase, the

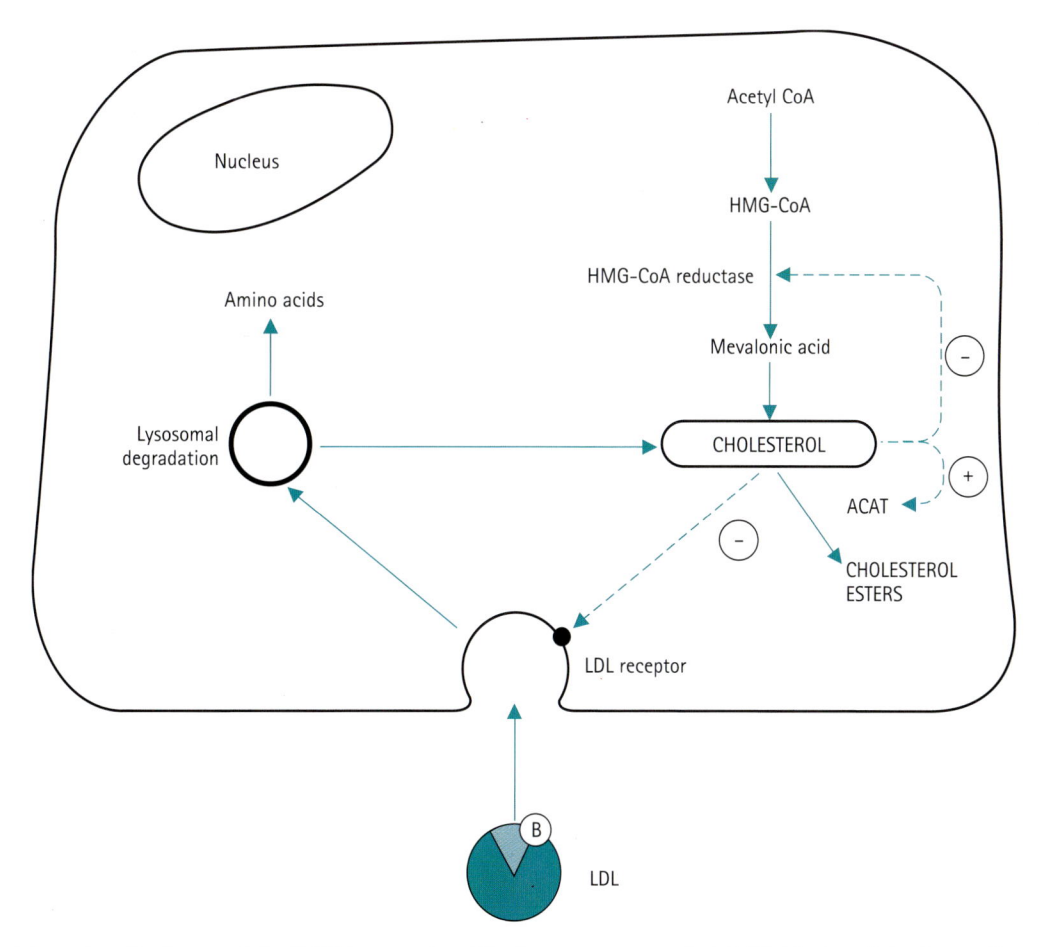

Fig. 13.7 The low-density lipoprotein (LDL) receptor. (CoA = coenzyme A; HMG-CoA = 3-hydroxy-3-methylglutaryl coenzyme A; ACAT = acyl coenzyme A acyl transferase.)

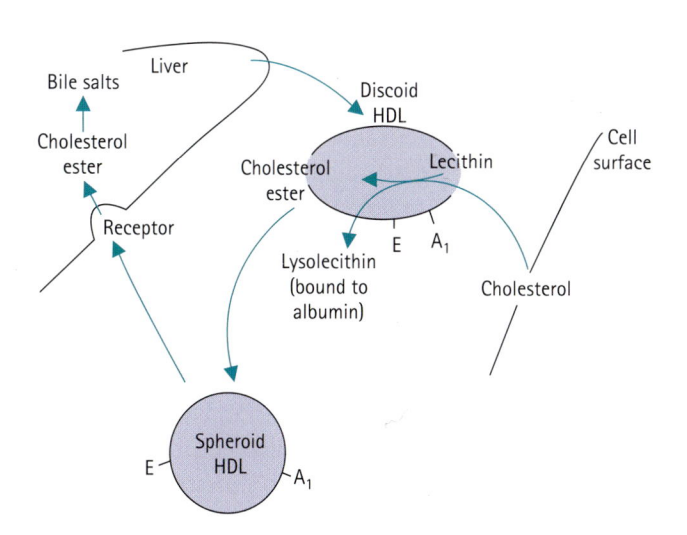

Fig. 13.8 Reverse high-density lipoprotein (HDL) cholesterol transport. (E = apoE; A_1 = apoA_1.) (Reproduced with kind permission from Candlish JK and Crook M, *Notes on Clinical Biochemistry*, Singapore: World Scientific Publishing, 1993.)

HDL becomes overloaded with triglyceride; they reduce in size, losing apoA_1, and the concentration of HDL cholesterol falls. Thus, in hypertriglyceridaemia one often sees an inverse relationship between plasma triglyceride and HDL cholesterol concentrations.

High-density lipoprotein cholesterol is cardioprotective not only because of the reverse cholesterol transport system, which helps to remove cholesterol from the peripheral tissues, but also because of the mechanisms that include increased atherosclerotic plaque stability, protection of LDL from oxidation, and maintaining the integrity of the vascular endothelium.

A plasma HDL cholesterol concentration of less than 1.0 mmol/L confers increased cardiovascular risk and can be raised by various lifestyle changes, such as smoking cessation, regular exercise and weight loss. The fibrate drugs or nicotinic acid are sometimes used if these measures fail (see later). A low HDL cholesterol concentration is associated with diabetes mellitus type 2, obesity and the metabolic syndrome (see Chapter 12). Concentration of plasma non-HDL cholesterol (total cholesterol − HDL cholesterol) may be a better indicator of cardiovascular risk than that of LDL cholesterol.

DISORDERS OF LIPID METABOLISM

The study of hyperlipidaemias has recently gained considerable importance, mainly because of the involvement of lipids in cardiovascular disease. Fredrickson, Levy and Lees first defined the hyperlipidaemias in a classification system based on which plasma lipoprotein concentrations were increased (Table 13.3). Although this so-called Fredrickson's classification helped to put lipidology on the clinical map, it was not a diagnostic classification. It gives little clue as to the aetiology of the disorder; indeed, all of the phenotypes can be either primary or secondary. Furthermore, the Fredrickson type can change as a result of dietary or drug intervention. Nowadays, a more descriptive classification is used for the primary hyperlipidaemias, as follows.

Chylomicron syndrome

This can be due to familial lipoprotein lipase deficiency, an autosomal recessive disorder affecting about 1 in 1 000 000 people. The gene for lipoprotein lipase is found on chromosome 8, and genetic studies have shown insertions or deletions within the gene. Lipoprotein lipase is involved in the exogenous lipoprotein pathway by hydrolysing chylomicrons to form chylomicron remnants, and also in the endogenous pathway by converting VLDL to IDL particles.

Presentation as a child with abdominal pain (often with acute pancreatitis) is typical. There is probably no increased risk of coronary artery disease. Gross elevation of plasma triglycerides due to the accumulation of uncleared chylomicron particles occurs. Lipid stigmata include eruptive xanthomata, hepatosplenomegaly and lipaemia retinalis.

Other variants of the chylomicron syndrome include circulating inhibitors of lipoprotein lipase and deficiency of its physiological activator apoC_2. Apolipoprotein C_2 deficiency is also inherited as an autosomal recessive condition affecting about 1 in 1 000 000 people. The gene for apoC_2 is located on chromosome 19 and mutations resulting in low plasma concentrations have been found.

Treatment of the chylomicron syndrome involves a low-fat diet, aiming for less than 20 g of fat a day if possible, although compliance on such a diet may be difficult. Some clinicians supplement the diet with medium-chain triglycerides and also give 1 per cent of the total calorie intake as linoleic acid.

In cases of apoC_2 deficiency, fresh plasma may temporarily restore plasma apoC_2 levels. To confirm the diagnosis of familial lipoprotein lipase deficiency, plasma lipoprotein lipase can be assayed after the intravenous administration of heparin, which releases the enzyme from endothelial sites. The assay is complicated in that other plasma lipases (hepatic lipase and phospholipase, for example) contribute to the overall plasma lipase activity. Inhibition of lipoprotein lipase can be performed using protamine, high saline concentrations or specific antibodies and its overall activity can be calculated by subtraction.

If apoC_2 deficiency is suspected, the plasma concentrations of this activator can be assayed. Patients may show a type I or V Fredrickson's phenotype. Family members should be investigated.

Familial hypercholesterolaemia

This condition is inherited as an autosomal dominant trait. The inheritance of one mutant gene that encodes for the LDL receptor affects about 1 in every 500 people (more common in Afrikaners and French Canadians), resulting in impaired LDL catabolism and hypercholesterolaemia. At least four types of mutation of the LDL receptor have been described, resulting in reduced synthesis, failure of transport of the synthesized receptor to the Golgi complex within the cell, defective LDL binding or inadequate expression of the LDL receptor at the cell surface.

According to the Simon Broome register, definite familial hypercholesterolaemia is defined as a plasma cholesterol concentration of more than 7.5 mmol/L in an adult (more than 6.7 mmol/L in children under 16 years) or a plasma LDL cholesterol concentration of more than 4.9 mmol/L in an adult *in the presence* of tendon xanthoma. Possible familial hypercholesterolaemia is defined as a plasma cholesterol concentration of more than 7.5 mmol/L in an adult (more than 6.7 mmol/L in children under 16 years) or a plasma LDL cholesterol concentration of more than 4.9 mmol/L in an adult plus a family history of either an elevated plasma cholesterol concentration of more than 7.5 mmol/L in a first-degree or second-degree relative or myocardial infarction below the age of 50 years in a first-degree relative or below the age of 60 years in a second-degree relative.

Typically, patients manifest severe hypercholesterolaemia, with a relatively normal plasma triglyceride

Disorders of lipid metabolism

> ## CASE 1
>
> A 23-year-old female had her plasma lipids checked by her general practitioner because her father had died of a myocardial infarction aged 44 years. Her 24-year-old brother had hyperlipidaemia. Her renal, liver and thyroid function tests were normal, as was her blood glucose.
>
> *Plasma (fasting)*
> Cholesterol 11.4 mmol/L (3.5–5.0)
> Triglyceride 1.1 mmol/L (0.3–1.5)
> HDL cholesterol 1.2 mmol/L (1.0–1.8)
>
> On examination, she had tendon xanthomata on her Achilles tendons and bilateral corneal arci.
>
> ### DISCUSSION
> Note the considerably raised plasma cholesterol concentration. The absence of an obvious secondary hyperlipidaemia in conjunction with the family history of a first-degree relative with premature cardiovascular disease and hyperlipidaemia suggests a genetic hyperlipidaemia. The presence of tendon xanthomata and premature corneal arci supports the diagnosis of familial hypercholesterolaemia. This is an autosomal dominant disorder and a defect of the LDL receptor.

concentration in conjunction with xanthomata, which can affect the back of the hands, elbows, Achilles tendons or the insertion of the patellar tendon into the pretibial tuberosity. Premature cardiovascular disease is often observed, along with corneal arci.

Using the Fredrickson's classification, this condition has also been termed familial type IIa hyperlipoproteinaemia, although some patients may show a type IIb phenotype. Plasma HDL cholesterol concentration can vary in different individuals, although low concentrations may increase the likelihood of cardiovascular disease. It has been shown that in heterozygote familial hypercholesterolaemia there is more likely to be an increased amount of plasma Lp(a) in those subjects with cardiovascular disease.

The diagnosis of familial hypercholesterolaemia is usually obvious from the markedly elevated plasma cholesterol concentration and the presence of tendon xanthomata in the patient or first-degree relation. The diagnosis may not be so clear cut in patients without the lipid stigmata. A functional assay of the LDL receptors has recently been described using cultured lymphocytes, but this has not yet gained wide routine acceptance and DNA analysis is also gaining importance. The response to a lipid-lowering diet is often disappointing and the treatment is usually with the HMG-CoA reductase inhibitors, i.e. the statins.

Homozygous hypercholesterolaemia can be very severe. There is a considerable risk of coronary artery disease, aortic stenosis and early fatal myocardial infarction before the age of 20 years. Florid xanthoma occurs in childhood including tendon, planar and cutaneous types. Atheroma of the aortic root may manifest before puberty, associated with coronary ostial stenosis.

In homozygous familial hypercholesterolaemia, treatment to lower the plasma cholesterol concentration (which can be as high as 20 mmol/L or more) is essential in order to try to reduce the likelihood of sudden death due to coronary artery disease. Plasma exchange, LDL apheresis or heparin extracorporeal LDL precipitation (HELP) can be used in an attempt to remove the plasma LDL particles and thus reduce the plasma cholesterol concentration.

Familial defective apoB$_{3500}$

This condition is due to a mutation in the apoB gene resulting in a substitution of arginine at the 3500 amino acid position for glutamine. Apolipoprotein B is the ligand upon the LDL particle for the LDL receptor. It may be indistinguishable clinically from familial hypercholesterolaemia and is also associated with hypercholesterolaemia and premature coronary artery disease. The treatment is similar to that for heterozygote familial hypercholesterolaemia. The apoB gene is located upon chromosome 2.

Familial combined hyperlipidaemia

In familial combined hyperlipidaemia (FCH), the plasma lipids may not be significantly elevated, plasma cholesterol concentrations often being between 6 mmol/L and 9 mmol/L and plasma triglyceride between 2 mmol/L and 6 mmol/L. The Fredrickson's phenotypes seen in this condition include IIa, IIb and IV. Familial combined hyperlipidaemia may be inherited as an autosomal dominant trait (although others suggest that there may be co-segregation of more than one gene). About 0.5 per cent of the European population is affected, and there is an increased incidence of coronary artery disease in family members. The metabolic defect is unclear, although plasma apoB is often elevated due to increased synthesis; LDL and VLDL apoB concentration is increased. The synthesis of VLDL triglyceride is increased in FCH and there may also be a relationship with insulin resistance.

The diagnosis of FCH is suspected if there is a family history of hyperlipidaemia, particularly if family members show different lipoprotein phenotypes. There is often a family history of cardiovascular disease. However, the diagnosis can be difficult and it sometimes needs to be distinguished from familial hypercholesterolaemia (xanthomata are not usually present in FCH) and familial hypertriglyceridaemia (the IIa and IIb phenotypes are not usually found in familial hypertriglyceridaemia, although they are in FCH). Children with FCH usually show hypertriglyceridaemia and not the type IIa phenotype (unlike the situation found in familial hypercholesterolaemia).

Unlike familial hypertriglyceridaemia, plasma VLDL particles are usually smaller in FCH. Dietary treatment and either the statins or fibrates, as appropriate, are sometimes used.

Familial hypertriglyceridaemia

Familial hypertriglyceridaemia is often observed, with low HDL cholesterol concentration. The condition usually develops after puberty and is rare in childhood. The exact metabolic defect is unclear, although over-production of VLDL or a decrease in VLDL conversion to LDL is likely. The precipitating causes of hypertriglyceridaemia include obesity, high ethanol intake, diabetes mellitus and the use of oestrogens. There may be an increased risk of cardiovascular disease. Acute pancreatitis may also occur, and is more likely when the concentration of plasma triglycerides is more than 10 mmol/L. Some patients show hyperinsulinaemia and insulin resistance. Dietary measures and sometimes lipid-lowering drugs such as the fibrates or omega-3 fatty acids are used to treat the condition.

Type III hyperlipoproteinaemia

This condition is also called familial dysbetalipoproteinaemia or broad β-hyperlipidaemia. The underlying biochemical defect is one of a reduced clearance of chylomicron and VLDL remnants. The name broad β-hyperlipidaemia is sometimes used because of the characteristic plasma lipoprotein electrophoretic pattern that is often observed (the broad β-band that is seen being remnant particles).

An association with type III/broad β-hyperlipidaemia and homozygosity for apoE$_2$ or variants of apoE$_2$ has been described. Apolipoprotein E shows three common alleles, E2, E3 and E4, coded for on chromosome 19, which are important for the binding of remnant particles to the remnant receptor.

The mechanism for the disorder seems to be that apoE$_2$-bearing particles have poor binding to the apoB/E (remnant) receptor and thus are not effectively cleared from the circulation.

It is becoming apparent that it is not just inheriting the apoE$_2$ genotype that is important in developing broad β-hyperlipidaemia. The prevalence of the apoE$_2$/E$_2$ genotype is about 1 in 100 in the general population, yet only about 1 in 5000–10 000 individuals manifest type III

CASE 2

A 43-year-old male attended the vascular surgery outpatients for peripheral vascular disease. He was a non-smoker but had undergone a coronary artery bypass graft the year before. Some of his laboratory results were as follows.

Plasma (fasting)
Cholesterol 8.7 mmol/L (3.5–5.0)
Triglyceride 9.1 mmol/L (0.3–1.5)
HDL cholesterol 0.86 mmol/L (1.0–1.8)
Apolipoprotein E genotype was E$_2$/E$_2$

On examination, he had tuberous xanthomata and palmar striae.

DISCUSSION

The diagnosis was type III hyperlipoproteinaemia (familial dysbetalipoproteinaemia or broad β-hyperlipidaemia). Note the mixed hyperlipidaemia (both cholesterol and triglyceride concentrations raised) in an approximately 1:1 molar ratio and also apoE genotype E$_2$ homozygote (usual is apoE$_3$/E$_3$). The type III hyperlipoproteinaemia is associated with raised concentration of remnant lipoprotein particles, which are particularly atherogenic. Note also the premature peripheral vascular and coronary heart disease.

hyperlipoproteinaemia. A concurrent increase in plasma VLDL concentration also seems necessary for the condition to be expressed, such as might occur in diabetes mellitus, hypothyroidism or obesity. Some patients may show either an autosomal recessive or a dominant mode of inheritance of the condition.

The palmar striae (palmar xanthomata) are considered pathognomonic for the disorder, but tuberoeruptive xanthomata, typically on the elbows and knees, xanthelasma and corneal arcus have also been described in this condition. Peripheral vascular disease is a typical feature of this hyperlipidaemic disorder, as is premature coronary artery disease.

Plasma lipid determination frequently reveals hypercholesterolaemia and hypertriglyceridaemia, often in similar molar proportions with plasma concentrations of around 9–10 mmol/L. Plasma HDL cholesterol concentration is usually low. Plasma LDL concentration may also be low due to the fact that there is reduced conversion from IDL particles, although it may also be normal or elevated.

Plasma lipoprotein electrophoresis can show the classic type III picture with a broad β-band composed of remnant particles, although this is not always present. An association of type III hyperlipoproteinaemia with homozygosity for apoE$_2$ has been described and thus apoE phenotyping or genotyping by a specialized laboratory can be useful, although some patients with broad β-hyperlipidaemia can show other apoE phenotypes or variants.

Another investigation that can be useful in establishing the diagnosis is ultracentrifugation to separate the lipoprotein particles. The cholesterol of the VLDL particles is then quantitated and expressed as a total of the plasma triglyceride concentration. In molar terms, normal individuals show a ratio of less than 0.30, while ratios more than 0.30 are more likely in type III hyperlipoproteinaemia, particularly nearer 0.60.

Treatment consists of dietary measures, correcting the precipitating causes and either the fibrates (first line) or statin drugs.

Polygenic hypercholesterolaemia

This is one of the most common causes of a raised plasma cholesterol concentration. This condition is the result of a complex interaction between multiple environmental and genetic factors. In other words, it is not due to a single gene abnormality and it is likely that it is the result of more than one metabolic defect. There is usually either an increase in LDL production or a decrease in LDL catabolism. The plasma lipid phenotype is usually either IIa or IIb Fredrickson's phenotype. The plasma cholesterol concentration is usually either mildly or moderately elevated. An important negative clinical finding is the absence of tendon xanthomata, the presence of which would tend to rule out the diagnosis. Usually less than 10 per cent of first-degree relations have similar lipid abnormalities, compared with familial hypercholesterolaemia or FCH in which about 50 per cent of first-degree family members are affected. There may also be a family history of premature coronary artery disease. Individuals may have a high intake of dietary fat and be overweight. Treatment involves dietary intervention and sometimes the use of lipid-lowering drugs such as the statins.

Hyperalphalipoproteinaemia

Hyperalphalipoproteinaemia results in elevated plasma HDL cholesterol concentration and can be inherited as an autosomal dominant condition or, in some cases, may show polygenic features. The total plasma cholesterol concentration can be elevated, with normal LDL cholesterol concentration. There is no increased prevalence of cardiovascular disease in this condition; in fact, the contrary probably applies, with some individuals showing longevity. Plasma HDL concentration is thought to be cardioprotective and individuals displaying this should be reassured. Box 13.1 gives the causes of raised plasma HDL cholesterol concentrations.

Secondary hyperlipidaemias

One should not forget that there are many secondary causes of hyperlipidaemia. These may present alone or sometimes concomitantly with a primary hyperlipidaemia. Some of the causes of secondary hyperlipidaemia are listed in Box 13.2. The reader should see the other chapters in this book for details of the relevant diseases.

Box 13.1 Some causes of raised plasma high-density lipoprotein (HDL) cholesterol

Primary
Hyperalphalipoproteinaemia
Cholesterol ester transfer protein deficiency

Secondary
High ethanol intake
Exercise
Certain drugs, e.g. oestrogens, fibrates, nicotinic acid, phenytoin, rifampicin

> **Box 13.2 Some important causes of secondary hyperlipidaemia**
>
> *Predominant hypercholesterolaemia*
> Primary hypothyroidism
> Nephrotic syndrome
> Cholestasis, e.g. primary biliary cirrhosis
> Acute intermittent porphyria
> Anorexia nervosa
> Certain drugs or toxins, e.g. ciclosporin and chlorinated hydrocarbons
>
> *Predominant hypertriglyceridaemia*
> Alcohol excess
> Obesity
> Diabetes mellitus and metabolic syndrome
> Certain drugs, e.g. oestrogens, beta-blockers (without intrinsic sympathomimetic activity), thiazide diuretics, acitretin, protease inhibitors, some neuroleptics and glucocorticoids
> Chronic renal failure
> Some glycogen storage diseases, e.g. von Gierke's type I
> Systemic lupus erythematosus

> **Box 13.3 Causes of low plasma high-density lipoprotein (HDL) cholesterol**
>
> *Primary*
> Familial hypoalphalipoproteinaemia
> ApoA$_1$ abnormalities
> Tangier's disease
> Lecithin-cholesterol acyltransferase deficiency
> Fish-eye disease
>
> *Secondary*
> Tobacco smoking
> Obesity
> Poorly controlled diabetes mellitus
> Insulin resistance
> Chronic renal failure
> Certain drugs, e.g. testosterone, probucol, beta-blockers (without intrinsic sympathomimetic activity), progestogens, anabolic steroids

Other lipid abnormalities

Inherited disorders of low plasma HDL concentration (hypoalphalipoproteinaemia) occur and plasma HDL cholesterol concentration should ideally be more than 1.0 mmol/L. A number of such conditions have been described (such as apoA$_1$ deficiency), many of which are associated with premature cardiovascular disease. In Tangier's disease, individuals have very low levels of HDL, large, yellow tonsils, hepatomegaly and accumulation of cholesterol esters in the reticuloendothelial system. There is a defect in the ABC1 gene involved in HDL transport. The causes of a low plasma HDL cholesterol concentration are shown in Box 13.3.

Defects of apoB metabolism have also been described. In abetalipoproteinaemia or LDL deficiency there is impaired chylomicron and VLDL synthesis. This results in a failure of lipid transport from the liver and intestine. Transport of fat-soluble vitamins is impaired and steatorrhoea, progressive ataxia, retinitis pigmentosa and acanthocytosis (abnormal erythrocyte shape) can result. In hypobetalipoproteinaemia, a less severe syndrome occurs, sometimes due to a truncated form of apoB.

In LCAT deficiency, the accumulation of free unesterified cholesterol in the tissues results in corneal opacities, renal damage, premature atherosclerosis and haemolytic anaemia. The enzyme LCAT catalyses the esterification of free cholesterol. Another condition that is probably due to a defect of LCAT is fish-eye disease, in which there may be low HDL cholesterol concentrations and eye abnormalities.

Lipid-lowering therapy

The help of a dietician is invariably useful in treating dyslipidaemias. Low-saturated fat/reduced cholesterol diets are instigated. Total fat intake should be less than 30 per cent of the total calorie intake, with an increase in mono-unsaturated fat intake up to 20 per cent of total calories. Dietary cholesterol intake should not exceed about 200 mg/day. Five daily portions of fruit and vegetables are advisable. Ideally, patients should aim to achieve their recommended body mass index. Alcohol intake should be less than 14 units/week for females and 21 units/week for males. Increased intake of plant sterols and stanols may lead to competition for cholesterol intestinal absorption, thereby reducing the plasma cholesterol concentration. If diet and lifestyle measures fail, drug therapy may be indicated (Table 13.5).

Bile-salt sequestrants such as colestipol and cholestyramine bind bile salts in the intestinal lumen and thus interrupt their reabsorption and re-utilization. The removal of bile acids stimulates hepatic cholesterol synthesis, which in turn results in an increase in hepatic LDL receptors, resulting in decreased plasma LDL concentration. The side-effects include gastrointestinal symptoms, such as

Table 13.5 Some lipid-lowering drugs and their effects on plasma lipoprotein fractions

Drug	Cho	Tg	HDL	LDL
Statins	↓↓↓	↓	↑	↓↓↓
Fibrates	↓/−	↓↓↓	↑↑	↓/−
Bile-salt-sequestrating agents	↓	↑/−	↑	↓
Ezetimibe	↓↓	↓	↑	↓↓
Nicotinic acid	↓↓	↓↓↓	↑↑↑	↓↓
Omega-3 fats	↓/−	↓↓	↑	↓/−

Cho = cholesterol; Tg = triglyceride; HDL = high-density lipoprotein; LDL = low-density lipoprotein. ↓ = reduced; − = no major change; ↑ = raised.

constipation. To avoid interference with their absorption, these drugs should not be given at the same time as other drugs. They lower plasma cholesterol concentration by about 10–20 per cent; although HDL cholesterol concentration is also modestly raised, triglyceride concentrations can be paradoxically increased. Another agent acting on the gut is ezetimibe, which inhibits intestinal cholesterol uptake specifically.

The rate-limiting enzyme of cholesterol synthesis HMG-CoA reductase is inhibited by HMG-CoA reductase inhibitors, also known as the statins, which can be used to treat hypercholesterolaemia. These agents include lovastatin, simvastatin, pravastatin, atorvastatin, fluvastatin and rosuvastatin. The HDL cholesterol concentration is modestly increased and triglyceride concentration reduced by varying degrees by these agents. The side-effects notably include myalgia, myositis (and rarely rhabdomyolysis) and abnormal liver function.

The fibrate drugs include gemfibrozil, bezafibrate, fenofibrate and ciprofibrate. These drugs have good triglyceride-lowering and HDL-raising abilities, although LDL cholesterol concentration may not be much changed. They are PPARs α-agonists and work on a number of lipid pathways, including increasing lipoprotein lipase activity, reducing apoC_3 and VLDL synthesis and increasing apoA_1 synthesis. The side-effects include myalgia, myositis and gastrointestinal disturbance, and they should not be used in patients with active gallstones or significant renal disease. They can lower plasma alkaline phosphatase concentration, which can be used to monitor drug compliance.

Nicotinic acid and its derivatives have been used to reduce VLDL secretion and LDL concentration and, interestingly, also Lp(a) levels. However, the side-effects include hepatic toxicity, hyperuricaemia, impaired glucose tolerance and flushing.

Omega-3 fatty acids in the form of fish oils or flaxseed oil can lower plasma triglyceride concentrations by reducing VLDL synthesis. They also have an anti-platelet aggregatory action. They can sometimes be used to treat severe hypertriglyceridaemia. However, they show little, if any, LDL-lowering activity. Their side-effects may include gastrointestinal upset or bruising.

Combination drug therapy is sometimes used, for example statin/ezetimibe or statin/nicotinic acid, but is best instigated by an expert with close monitoring, as dangerous side-effects may be increased.

Coronary artery disease and prevention: the importance of lipid lowering

Coronary artery disease remains one of the major causes of morbidity and mortality in the industrial world. Traditionally, however, the major risk factors are hyperlipidaemia, hypertension and smoking, to which can be added diabetes mellitus, a family history of coronary heart disease and obesity.

With primary (the prevention of the occurrence) and secondary (the prevention of further occurrences) coronary heart disease prevention in mind, the usual strategy adopted is to try to reduce the modifiable risk factors. Cardiovascular risk factors tend to cluster together in individuals and interact in such a way that the overall combined effect is greater than the combined risk of individual factors. (See Chapter 22.)

INVESTIGATION OF HYPERLIPIDAEMIAS

Before collecting blood, consider whether the patient is on lipid-lowering therapy, including lipid-containing infusions. Also ensure that the patient fasts overnight for around 12 hours (if safe to do so) and is only allowed water to drink, if required. Although plasma cholesterol concentration is little affected by fasting, triglyceride concentrations rise if not. The patient should be on his or her usual diet for a couple of weeks preceding the test.

Plasma lipids should not be assessed in patients who are acutely ill, for example acute myocardial infarction, as plasma cholesterol concentration may be decreased due to the acute phase response. Wait for about 3 months after the event, although if a sample is taken within 12 hours of an event, a 'true' result may be obtained.

Posture can alter plasma lipid concentrations: in the upright position, plasma cholesterol concentration can be 10 per cent higher than in the recumbent position.

The blood sample should be taken to the laboratory and assayed as soon as possible. The usual fasting lipid profile consists of plasma cholesterol, triglyceride and HDL cholesterol concentrations.

When faced with a hyperlipidaemia, decide whether it is primary or secondary. A family history, clinical features and appropriate blood tests can be useful to help make this decision. Lipid stigmata such as tendon xanthomata or premature corneal arci may point to familial hypercholesterolaemia, and tuberous xanthomata or palmar striae to type III hyperlipoproteinaemia.

Blood glucose concentration is useful to help assess for diabetes mellitus, liver function tests for liver disease such as cholestasis, urinary protein and plasma albumin concentrations for nephrotic syndrome and thyroid function tests for hypothyroidism. It is also important to determine alcohol consumption and medications from the clinical history.

It is generally wise to re-test patients' lipids, a few months apart, as it is recognized that the within-individual variation of lipids can be significant, and reliance cannot be placed on just one set of readings.

It is also useful to assess the patient for other cardiovascular risk factors, including smoking habits, diabetes mellitus, blood pressure, body weight and family history of cardiovascular disease. These should also be managed in their own right. Assessment should also be made of possible atherosclerotic disease, for example does the patient have evidence of coronary, peripheral or carotid artery disease?

If the patient is known to have coronary artery disease, aim for a plasma LDL cholesterol concentration of about 2.0 mmol/L. Statins are first-line drugs for patients with raised LDL cholesterol concentration. Alternatively, there may be a place for a fibrate drug if fasting plasma triglyceride concentrations are raised by more than 5 mmol/L, particularly if there is also a low HDL cholesterol concentration and LDL cholesterol concentration is not much raised. The ideal is to aim for fasting plasma cholesterol concentration of about 4.0 mmol/L, triglyceride concentration less than 1.5 mmol/L and HDL cholesterol concentration more than 1.0 mmol/L.

Severe hypertriglyceridaemia, particularly if the plasma triglyceride concentration is more than 10 mmol/L, is a risk factor for acute pancreatitis. Low-fat diets may help in conjunction with a fibrate (sometimes omega-3 fatty acids are used), aiming ideally for a fasting plasma triglyceride concentration lower than about 1.5 mmol/L.

Remember that severe hypertriglyceridaemia can cause problems with certain assays, for example falsely low plasma amylase concentration or pseudohyponatraemia.

In terms of primary coronary heart disease prevention, the use of a cardiovascular risk factor assessment may be helpful to determine if a lipid-lowering drug is indicated, for example Framingham Study-based calculators.

CASE 3

A 15-year-old female presented to the surgical unit with acute pancreatitis. Some of her laboratory results were as follows.

Plasma (fasting)
Cholesterol 33.4 mmol/L (3.5–5.0)
Triglyceride 69.1 mmol/L (0.3–1.5)
HDL cholesterol 0.9 mmol/L (1.0–1.8)
Amylase <20 U/L (<200)

On examination, she had eruptive xanthomata on her arms and thighs and fundoscopy revealed lipaemia retinalis.

DISCUSSION

This patient has grossly elevated lipid concentrations with severe hypertriglyceridaemia. The blood sample would be lipaemic and some plasma sodium assays may reveal pseudohyponatraemia. She was found to have lipoprotein lipase deficiency when this enzyme was measured before and after heparin administration, which releases the enzyme from capillaries into the circulation. Lipoprotein lipase deficiency can result in the chylomicron syndrome and eruptive xanthomata may be present. Plasma amylase concentration is normally elevated in acute pancreatitis but, due to the gross lipaemia, the assay was unsatisfactory, giving a spuriously low result. The latter is an important practical point and urinary amylase may be preferable or assay of plasma amylase after separation from the lipid fraction under such circumstances.

Close family members should be screened in cases of genetic hyperlipidaemias such as familial hypercholesterolaemia.

Specialist lipid assays may help define the abnormality. The apoE genotype is useful in the diagnosis of type III hyperlipoproteinaemia, as many of these patients are apoE$_2$/E$_2$. Plasma lipoprotein lipase and apoC$_2$ (its activator) assays may be useful in chylomicron syndrome, and LDL receptor DNA studies for familial hypercholesterolaemia. Plasma apoA$_1$ and apoB concentrations and also Lp(a) may help define risk status.

CONCLUSIONS

- Lipids are essential for health, but raised plasma cholesterol and triglyceride concentrations are associated with an increased incidence of cardiovascular disease.
- Conversely, plasma HDL cholesterol is cardioprotective, partly because of its central role in reverse cholesterol transport returning cholesterol from the tissues to the liver.
- There are many cases of secondary hyperlipidaemias, including obesity, alcohol excess, diabetes mellitus, hypothyroidism, chronic renal failure and cholestasis.
- The genetic hyperlipidaemias include familial hypercholesterolaemia, FCH and type III hyperlipoproteinaemia. Familial hypercholesterolaemia results from a defect of the LDL receptor.
- The statins or HMG-CoA reductase inhibitors lower plasma cholesterol concentration and are associated with decreased cardiovascular disease.

14 NUTRITION

Starvation	214	Malnutrition	216
Trauma and sepsis	215	Anorexia nervosa	220
Nutritional assessment	215	Obesity	220

This chapter gives an outline of certain nutritional abnormalities and how they overlap with aspects of chemical pathology. It is not, however, a substitute for a nutrition textbook. The reader may also find Chapters 12 and 13 (on carbohydrate and lipid disorders, respectively), Chapter 15 (on vitamin/trace elements) and Chapter 16 (on gastrointestinal function) relevant. Nutrition is an important topic, as about 1 billion of the world's population are overweight yet, ironically, at the same time approximately 1 billion are malnourished or starving.

Adequate nutrition is essential for a variety of reasons, including optimal cardiovascular function, muscle strength, respiratory ventilation, protection from infection, wound healing and psychological well-being.

The principles of carbohydrate and lipid metabolism and gastrointestinal digestion and absorption all have important implications in the management of nutrition, and of intravenous (parenteral) nutrition in particular. These principles, including those of fluid and electrolyte homeostasis, must be fully understood in order to manage patients receiving parenteral nutrition.

Daily energy loss as heat is about 120 kJ (30 kcal) per kilogram of body weight in a normal adult. In addition there is a daily protein turnover of about 3 g/kg body weight (about 0.5 g of nitrogen), of which about 0.15 g of nitrogen/kg body weight is excreted (1 g of nitrogen is derived from about 6.25 g of protein). These losses are usually balanced by dietary intake of equivalent amounts of energy, as carbohydrate, fat and protein. Glucose provides 4 kcal/g, and fat 9 kcal/g.

Excess energy is stored as glycogen and triglyceride. If expenditure exceeds intake, these energy stores are drawn upon. In a well-nourished adult, enough energy is stored as hepatic glycogen to last at least a day, and therefore postoperative patients without complications do not need intravenous feeding. Once this store has been depleted, energy is derived from triglyceride, and later from body tissue components such as the proteins of cells, including those of muscle. This may cause severe ketosis from the metabolism of fats and ketogenic amino acids and increase nitrogen turnover and loss. The daily energy and nitrogen requirements are not constant, as we will now see.

STARVATION

During starvation the body tries to maintain blood glucose levels in the acute phase and in the longer term to preserve body protein mass.

Hepatic glycogen stores are largely consumed within 24 hours. The obligatory glucose requirements of the brain, erythrocytes and other organs are met by gluconeogenesis. During the first week or so of acute starvation, up to 150 g of protein is utilized to achieve this. Insulin levels decrease, resulting in amino acid (mainly alanine) release from protein, glycogen conversion to glucose, and adipocyte fatty acid release for energy needs. Plasma insulin concentration is reduced, but concentrations of glucagon, glucocorticoids, catecholamines and growth hormone are raised. Thus, blood glucose concentrations are generally maintained despite starvation.

In later starvation, ketone bodies replace glucose as the predominant brain fuel (ketoadaptive phase) and a metabolic acidosis may result. The ketone bodies also inhibit muscle protein degradation and the flow of alanine into the circulation. There is thus a decrease in urinary nitrogen excretion, a decline in hepatic gluconeogenesis and increased brain oxidation of ketone bodies whilst plasma amino acid concentrations decrease. Plasma insulin is reduced, as are glucagon, glucocorticoids, catecholamines and growth hormone.

Starvation results in initial rapid weight loss, due mostly to protein breakdown and diuresis. The latter is partly due to increased renal tubule urea load and results in renal loss of calcium, phosphate and potassium. Continuing starvation results in a slower decline in body weight, as after the gluconeogenic phase, fat is catabolized. This is associated with water conservation about 3–5 days later. The basal metabolic rate (BMR) decreases and the kidney becomes the most important gluconeogenic organ, using glutamine to synthesize glucose.

Feeding converts the situation to an anabolic state. The level of ketone bodies falls, along with a decline in urinary nitrogen. Thus positive nitrogen balance can be achieved with fat gain.

TRAUMA AND SEPSIS

In the face of trauma, including burns, the body strives for wound healing and the evoked response is directly related to the severity of the injury. Two phases have been described.

- *Early ebb* or *shock phase*. Here, in an attempt to survive, there is a decrease in body energy expenditure to conserve resources. Plasma insulin concentration is reduced but concentrations of glucagon, glucocorticoids, catecholamines and growth hormone are raised. There is reduced oxygen consumption and decreased glucose oxidation.
- *Later flow* or *hypermetabolic phase*. Should blood volume be restored and circulation satisfactory, then the flow phase may take place. Concentrations of hormones, such as glucagon, glucocorticoids, catecholamines and growth hormone, increase, as may that of insulin. Consequently, gluconeogenesis (which may lead to hyperglycaemia) occurs and also proteolysis. Urinary nitrogen loss can range from more than 25 g/day in severe burns to 10 g/day in the case of an uncomplicated surgical procedure. Accelerated muscle proteolysis results in a loss of lean body mass. Furthermore, there is increased fat catabolism, and lipolysis provides the predominant non-protein source of energy in traumatized patients.

Resting energy expenditure increases after trauma or sepsis, by 20 per cent in long bone fracture to 100 per cent in severe burns and trauma. Most adults require 1750–2500 kcal/day. Indeed, even in malnourished patients, more than 2500 kcal/day is rarely needed, as their BMR is lower. Only in severely traumatized patients such as those with major burns is 3000 kcal/day necessary. Most patients need 11–16 g nitrogen/day; rarely is 20 g nitrogen/day needed (protein requirement = 6.25 × nitrogen requirement.)

NUTRITIONAL ASSESSMENT

In many cases, patient weight is suitable to assess nutritional status, with a loss of 10 per cent or more being suggestive of possible malnutrition. However, this can be inaccurate if there are significant changes in body water and does not provide adequate information about body fat or protein stores.

A good dietary history is essential for helping to assess nutritional status. Ask about food intake, including type of food and frequency.

Examination of the patient is also essential, including weight and height. Body mass index (BMI) is a useful indicator of nutrition, with the main exceptions being patients with oedema or dehydration.

Other tests include the following.

- *Fat assessment*. Measurement of triceps skin-fold thickness using suitable calipers may be useful but is dependent on operator technique, the presence of oedema and skin pliability.
- *Skeletal muscle protein*.
  - Arm muscle circumference (AMC) can be calculated from the mid-arm circumference and triceps skin-fold thickness by the following equation:

  $$\text{AMC (cm)} = \text{mid-arm circumference (cm)} - (0.314 \times \text{skin-fold thickness}) \text{ (mm)} \quad (14.1)$$

  Operator technique may result in inaccuracies in mid-arm circumference measurement.
  - Hand-grip strength gives indirect evidence of body protein status by looking at muscle strength.
- *Biochemical tests*.
  - Measurement of circulating visceral proteins has been used to assess the impairment of hepatic protein production indirectly. Various plasma proteins have been used.
    Albumin: this protein has a plasma half-life of about 20 days but is a poor index of nutritional status as it is influenced by degree of hydration,

loss from the body, for example gastrointestinal or renal, hepatic well-being and intravascular/extravascular movement (see Chapter 19).

Transferrin: this has a shorter half-life, of about 9 days, and may be a better guide to nutritional status, although it is dependent upon iron status. Other plasma proteins or peptides that have been studied as potential markers of nutritional status include retinol-binding protein, IGF-1 and fibronectin.

- Poor nutrition may cause impaired immunological function with decreased lymphocyte count and abnormalities of delayed hypersensitivity.
- Urinary creatinine-to-height ratio: lean body mass is associated with urinary creatinine excretion, but this test has the problem of requiring accurate urine collection.
- 24-hour urinary urea excretion (mmol/L) $\times$ 0.034 approximates to urinary nitrogen excretion. This can be used as a guide to nitrogen and thus protein requirements.
- Complex laboratory tests are available, such as the assessment of total body fat by impedance measurement, or total body nitrogen to assess protein status. However, these are usually only used in research settings and not in routine clinical practice.
- Laboratory tests may also show fatty acid deficiencies (see Chapter 13) and/or vitamin and trace element abnormalities (see Chapter 15).

Prognostic nutritional index

The prognostic nutritional index (PNI) has been devised as a marker of nutritional status and incorporates a number of the components discussed above including plasma albumin and transferrin concentration, skin fold thickness and lymphocyte function.

Subjective global assessment

This looks at a number of subjective weightings on key variables, including weight loss, gastrointestinal disorders, functional capacity and physical signs of deficiency. Weighting A is well nourished, B moderately nourished and C poorly nourished.

MALNUTRITION

This starts with reduced intake or nutrient loss. Eventually the stores of nutrients are depleted, which leads to biochemical and metabolic consequences and eventually clinical symptoms and signs.

Kwashiorkor occurs in individuals with visceral protein loss associated with impaired immunological function, although other nutritional components are satisfactory. Visceral proteins are decreased, but body weight, mid-arm circumference and triceps skin-fold thickness are relatively normal. Conversely, marasmus is generalized malnutrition with reduction in weight, mid-arm circumference and skin-fold thickness, although visceral proteins are relatively normal.

Do not forget that patients can be malnourished on the hospital ward, particularly the elderly and those who are severely ill, post-surgical or in intensive care.

Nutritional support or artificial nutrition

Nutritional support can take many forms. For example, in coeliac disease (Chapter 16), a gluten-free diet is important, and for lactose intolerance, specific dietary restriction of lactose is required.

Normally, however, whole nutritional support should be considered:

- when the patient has lost 10 per cent or more of body weight and continues to lose weight because of inadequate intake,
- if the disease process is thought likely to result in impaired nutritional intake for 10 days or more.

Malnutrition is associated with increased mortality and morbidity and prolonged hospital stay and should be remedied promptly. It may be possible to encourage eating and, if necessary, enhance it by supplements. However, sometimes patients are not able to eat, and artificial nutrition becomes necessary. The average daily adult requirements are shown in Table 14.1.

Approximations based on the Harris–Benedict equation give an estimate of the total energy requirements. The daily BMR in kilocalories is:

- for *males*,

$$(66.5 + 13.8W + 5.0H - 6.8A) \times \text{activity factor} \times \text{injury factor} \quad (14.2)$$

- for *females*,

$$(655.1 + 9.6W + 1.9H - 4.7A) \times \text{activity factor} \times \text{injury factor} \quad (14.3)$$

where W = weight (kg), H = height (cm) and A = age (years). The activity factor, for example when confined to

Table 14.1 Average daily adult nutritional requirements[a]

Water	30–35 mL
Energy	20–35 cal
Protein	0.8–1.5 g
Carbohydrate	2–5 g
Fat	1–3 g
Sodium	1–2 mmol
Potassium	1–2 mmol
Calcium	0.1–0.3 mmol
Phosphate	0.2–0.4 mmol
Magnesium	0.1–0.3 mmol
Vitamins plus trace elements	

[a]All units are expressed as per kilogram of body weight. It is important to note that these values are extremely variable depending upon individual circumstances.

bed = 1.2. The injury factor after a minor operation = 1.4 and with major sepsis = 1.6.

If the patient cannot take food orally, there are two main alternatives depending on the presenting indications: enteral or parenteral nutrition.

Enteral nutrition

If the gastrointestinal tract is functioning, enteral feeding is usually indicated. This is the most effective and natural route, and is preferable because it is more physiological and has fewer complications. The indications for enteral nutrition may include:

- dysphagia,
- coma or delirious state,
- postoperative,
- persistent anorexia.

There are various enteral routes available:

- nasogastric,
- nasoduodenal,
- nasojejunal.

The complications of enteral nutrition include tube complications, poor gut absorption and biochemical disturbances (these may be similar to those seen in parenteral nutrition – see below). More specific complications of enteral nutrition include aspiration pneumonia and diarrhoea.

Parenteral nutrition

If possible, all patients should be fed orally or enterally, both of which are simpler than parenteral feeding and generally cause fewer complications. The basic rule is that if the gut works, use it. However, if oral or enteral feeding is contraindicated, for example when there is intestinal obstruction or fistula, short bowel syndrome, ileus or persistent vomiting, parenteral feeding may be indicated.

Parenteral nutrition can be given through a peripheral vein or through a central venous catheter into a large vessel. The amount of energy that can be given into a peripheral vein is limited because glucose and amino acid solutions are hyperosmolar and cause irritation to small vessel walls, sometimes causing thrombophlebitis. Thus peripheral parenteral feed osmolarity should usually be less than about 600 mmol/kg. Hyperosmolar solutions infused through a central venous catheter minimize the risk of thrombophlebitis, which is more likely via a peripheral line.

The choice depends partly on the length of time for which parenteral feeding is required, as the peripheral route is only used for short periods, usually of 1–2 weeks. Some experts use a glyceryl trinitrate patch at the site of insertion of peripheral catheters to facilitate insertion and reduce thrombophlebitis. The insertion of central venous catheters requires expertise to ensure correct positioning of the catheter, and strict attention must be paid to aseptic technique to reduce the risk of line infection.

The regimen depends on the clinical condition of the patient and the volume that can safely be infused.

Energy source

The energy source can be either glucose-containing or fat-containing fluids, although usually a combination of the two is given. At least 50 per cent of the energy requirements should be provided as glucose/lipid. Giving energy as glucose and fat minimizes the use of amino acids for gluconeogenesis and reduces urinary nitrogen loss.

Glucose. Severe illness may cause insulin resistance, and the administration of large amounts of glucose may be inadvisable unless exogenous insulin is given. Glucose infusion should not be stopped suddenly; insulin must be stopped first or hypoglycaemia may occur. Glucose should preferably be infused throughout the 24 hours.

Fat. The fat particles are similar to chylomicrons. Provided that some carbohydrate is given at a constant rate, there is no risk of significant ketoacidosis. A grossly lipaemic plasma may interfere with some laboratory analyses, particularly that of plasma sodium. If lipaemia persists, it indicates that the rate of administration is faster than the rate at which the fat can be metabolized, and the infusion should be slowed. Rarely, fat overload can occur. The administration of fat protects against essential fatty acid deficiency.

Nitrogen supplementation

Nitrogen supplements containing amino acids are needed to replace the daily nitrogen loss and to promote tissue healing. The assessment of nitrogen requirements may be difficult. A normal adult patient needs about 9 g of nitrogen/day, but this increases as the catabolic rate increases, for example up to 20 g of nitrogen/day in stress and infection. During the catabolic phase, the body cannot use administered nitrogen efficiently, and much of it is excreted in the urine as urea or free amino acids. About 840 kJ (200 kcal) of energy per gram of nitrogen are needed by a normal adult to synthesize protein from amino acids. This proportion decreases slightly as the catabolic rate and nitrogen requirements increase. Protein intake should be about 10–15 per cent of total calorie requirement.

The essential amino acids are arginine, histidine, isoleucine, leucine, threonine, lysine, methionine, phenylalanine, tryptophan and valine. These should constitute about 25 per cent of the total amino acids. The essential amino acids tend to have more complex structures such as aromatic rings or long side-chains; they can be synthesized by bacteria and plants, but not by humans. Arginine and histidine may become essential only under certain circumstances. The following is a useful mnemonic to remember these essential amino acids: **a**ny **h**elp **i**n **l**earning **t**hese **li**ttle **m**olecules **p**roves **t**ruly **v**aluable.

Glutamine, although not an essential amino acid, is an important energy source for the cells of the immune system and gut. There are data indicating that the addition of glutamine to parenteral feeds may benefit certain patients, such as those on intensive care.

If glomerular function is normal, estimation of the 24-hour urinary nitrogen output can be used as a rough guide to replacement. However, once tissue repair predominates, the use of amino acid increases (anabolic phase) and urinary nitrogen loss may fall suddenly; this indicates an increased, not a decreased, need for nitrogen. Conversely, during the catabolic phase, increasing nitrogen intake may result in an increased urinary loss because it cannot be used.

Vitamin, mineral and trace element supplementation

This must be given during long-term parenteral feeding, in addition to meeting the nitrogen and energy requirements. Urinary trace metal loss is high during the catabolic phase, but falls as anabolism becomes predominant. If parenteral feeding has been very prolonged, deficiencies may become apparent and weight gain may be impaired if supplements are not given.

Daily parenteral nutrition solutions are sometimes prepared in 3 L bags that contain the appropriate daily energy, glucose, lipid, nitrogen, vitamin and trace element requirements in addition to electrolytes, calcium, phosphate and magnesium. Intravenous feeding should not be stopped suddenly; the patient should gradually be weaned on to oral or enteral feeding.

Monitoring of parenteral feeding

Some clinical and metabolic complications associated with long-term parenteral feeding are shown in Box 14.1. One of the most important complications is infection of the central line and careful nursing attention is therefore essential. It is also important to review the patient's fluid balance. The biochemical investigations that may be used to prevent the onset of these complications are discussed below.

Initially, measurement of the daily plasma sodium, potassium, bicarbonate and urea/creatinine concentrations helps in the assessment of water and electrolyte needs and renal function. Plasma glucose concentrations must be monitored carefully, as patients may develop stress-related glucose intolerance with hyperglycaemia, consequent cell

---

Box 14.1 Some clinical and metabolic complications of long-term parenteral nutrition

Complications of central line, e.g.:
   malposition
   infection
   thrombosis
   air embolus
Hyperglycaemia/hypoglycaemia
Acid–base disturbances
Electrolyte disorders
Fluid overload
Hypophosphataemia
Metabolic bone disease
Liver disease
Biliary sludging
Essential vitamin and mineral deficiencies
Aluminium and manganese toxicity
Misinterpretation of laboratory results associated
   with lipid infusion
Gut atrophy
Essential fatty acid deficiency
Fat overload syndrome

dehydration and polyuria or rebound hypoglycaemia if glucose infusion is stopped suddenly.

Plasma albumin, protein, calcium, phosphate and magnesium concentrations should be measured to detect possible metabolic complications. The full blood count, including haemoglobin, white cells and platelets, as well as clotting, should also be monitored.

A cholestatic type of liver disorder associated with biliary sludging may develop in some patients receiving intravenous nutrition; thus liver function tests also need to be monitored. The plasma alkaline phosphatase activity increases, with a later rise in plasma transaminase activities. Unless significant symptoms occur, such as severe jaundice, this is not necessarily an indication to stop parenteral feeding because liver dysfunction usually resolves when the parenteral feeding is stopped.

Plasma concentrations of trace elements, in particular zinc, selenium, manganese and copper, should be measured initially every 2 weeks, as well as ferritin, vitamin B_{12} and folate. Some patients may not clear the fat in the parenteral feed and this can be assessed by measuring the plasma triglyceride concentration.

Estimation of 24-hour urinary nitrogen output may help to assess nitrogen use and the amount that should be replaced. If urea excretion increases quantitatively when nitrogen intake is increased, this indicates that the nitrogen cannot be used, and thus should *not* be increased. If nitrogen loss falls while supplements are being given, this indicates that anabolism is increasing, and supplements *should be* increased until urinary excretion increases. Once the patient has been established on long-term feeding, the frequency of monitoring can be reduced.

Re-feeding syndrome

This potentially lethal condition can be defined as severe electrolyte and fluid shifts associated with metabolic abnormalities in malnourished patients undergoing re-feeding, whether this is oral, enteral or parenteral.

It can be associated with significant morbidity and mortality. Clinical features include fluid balance abnormalities, abnormal glucose metabolism, hypophosphataemia (see Chapter 6), hypomagnesaemia and hypokalaemia. In addition, thiamine deficiency can occur. The conditions associated with the re-feeding syndrome are shown in Box 14.2.

Prior to re-feeding, electrolyte disorders should be corrected and the circulatory volume carefully restored. In practice, this may delay the administration of nutrition but it can usually be accomplished within the first 12–24 hours.

Vitamin and trace element deficiencies should also be corrected and, specifically, thiamine should be given before re-feeding is instigated. Further thiamine may be

> **Box 14.2 Factors that increase the risk of the re-feeding syndrome**
>
> Kwashiorkor or marasmus
> Anorexia nervosa
> Chronic malnutrition, e.g. associated with carcinoma or old age
> Chronic alcoholism
> Prolonged fasting
> Cancer treatment
> Surgery

CASE 1

A 64-year-old male with an inoperable oesophageal carcinoma had been unable to eat solid foods for about 2 months. A day after he had been commenced on total parenteral nutrition, the following blood results were obtained.

Plasma
Sodium 136 mmol/L (135–145)
Potassium 2.7 mmol/L (3.5–5.0)
Urea 2.7 mmol/L (2.5–7.0)
Creatinine 70 μmol/L (70–110)
Corrected calcium 2.23 mmol/L (2.15–2.55)
Phosphate 0.21 mmol/L (0.80–1.35)
Magnesium 0.32 mmol/L (0.70–1.0)

DISCUSSION

The patient has biochemical features of the re-feeding syndrome, with hypokalaemia, hypophosphataemia and hypomagnesaemia. Considerable care is needed when feeding patients after prolonged absence of food to avoid these dangerous biochemical features. Other complications may include thiamine deficiency and fluid balance disturbance.

necessary until the patient is stabilized. Some preparations containing thiamine have been associated with anaphylaxis and therefore facilities for treating this should be readily at hand.

The calorie repletion should be slow, at approximately 20 kcal/kg per day or on average 1000 kcal/day initially. However, this may not meet the patient's fluid, sodium, potassium or vitamin requirements unless these are specifically addressed. The usual protein requirement is about 1.2–1.5 g/kg per day, or about 0.17 g nitrogen/kg per day. Gradual introduction of calories, particularly over the first week of re-feeding, may be prudent until the patient is metabolically stable.

ANOREXIA NERVOSA

In this condition, which is more common in females, there are psychological problems with body self-image and self-inflicted starvation. In some respects this condition can resemble hypopituitarism with amenorrhoea resulting from decreased luteinizing hormone and follicle-stimulating hormone release. However, instead of the loss of axillary and pubic hair, as in hypopituitarism, there is additional lanugo hair. There may be severe weight loss and elevated growth hormone and cortisol concentrations. Severe hypokalaemia, hypomagnesaemia and hypophosphataemia are also seen, particularly if the re-feeding syndrome ensues. Strangely, hypercholesterolaemia may also occur.

OBESITY

It may seem strange to talk about obesity in the same chapter as malnutrition and starvation. However, about 20 per cent of the European population is obese, with higher prevalence figures in other populations such as African Americans and Pacific Islanders.

An estimated 230 million Europeans try a diet. The average person gains about 800 g during their lifetime, which could be prevented by cutting their dietary intake by about 100 calories/day, for example one or two average-sized biscuits.

Although these definitions rely on BMI, an alternative approach is to measure the waist circumference, with 88 cm for females and 102 cm for males being indicative of central obesity (Table 14.2).

The reason for this epidemic of obesity is partly the decrease in physical activity seen in sedentary societies combined with the increased intake of calorie-dense food such as saturated fat. However, there may also be underlying genetic or molecular mechanisms, which are reviewed briefly here.

Table 14.2 Classification of body mass index (BMI)

BMI (kg/m^2)	WHO classification	Common description
<18.5	Underweight	Thin
18.5–24.9	Normal	Normal
25.0–29.9	Grade 1	Overweight
30.0–39.9	Grade 2	Obese
>40.0	Grade 3	Morbid obesity

WHO = World Health Organization.

Leptin, a 16-kDa protein that is expressed in adipocytes, is an afferent signal that relays the magnitude of the fat stores to the central nervous system, primarily the hypothalamus, and plasma levels correlate with the adipose tissue mass. In the *ob/ob* mouse, there is defective leptin production associated with obesity and insulin resistance. Leptin administration causes weight loss in *ob/ob* mice partly by reducing food intake. In times of starvation, leptin levels decline. Adiponectin is another adipose-released hormone that is thought to sensitize tissues to insulin.

Neuropeptide Y is a potent stimulator of food intake the production of which is inhibited by leptin. Pro-opiomelanocortin is also involved in obesity and is cleaved to form adrenocorticotrophin and α-melanocyte-stimulating hormone (MSH) (see Chapter 7). The latter acts on the melanocorticortin-4 receptor (MC4-R) in the hypothalamus, which in turn increases energy expenditure and reduces food intake. Agouti protein, which is also expressed in hair follicles, antagonizes the actions of MSH by blocking MC4-R. Obese humans paradoxically have high levels of leptin, presumably because of tissue resistance to it. A minority of cases of obesity may be due to mutations in leptin receptors. Also involved in obesity is the β-3-adrenoreceptor, which mediates adipose metabolism by the sympathetic nervous system.

Obesity is associated with numerous medical problems, including type 2 diabetes mellitus, hyperlipidaemia, hypertension, coronary artery disease and stroke. There are various treatment strategies for obesity. Remember that energy balance and weight gain are extremely tightly regulated and it only needs an excess of 100 kcal/day, such as a chocolate biscuit, to result in a 4 kg gain in a year.

Increased physical activity and reduced calorie intake, sometimes combined with psychotherapy or behavioural

> **CASE 2**
>
> A 49-year-old male presented to his general practitioner wanting to lose weight. His blood pressure was raised, at 168/98 mmHg, and his BMI was 40.4 kg/m². His fasting blood glucose was 6.0 mmol/L and plasma lipids showed cholesterol 6.3 mmol/L, triglyceride 4.8 mmol/L and high-density lipoprotein (HDL) cholesterol 0.67 mmol/L.
>
> The GP requested an oral glucose tolerance test (OGTT), which had the following results.
>
> Time 'zero' before the OGTT: fasting venous plasma glucose 5.9 mmol/L.
>
> Two hours after oral 75 g anhydrous glucose load: plasma glucose 9.4 mmol/L.
>
> **DISCUSSION**
>
> This patient shows grade 3 obesity, which is associated with hypertension, mixed hyperlipidaemia and impaired glucose tolerance. This is an increasing problem, particularly in industrialized societies.

therapy, are the cornerstone of treatment, although many people fail to act on the advice given. Some new drug therapies are available, but these should not be viewed as a universal panacea for obesity as there are no short-cut easy answers and they may have side-effects. One such drug is orlistat, a pancreatic lipase inhibitor that causes reduced small intestine fat absorption. Another is sibutramine, which inhibits the reuptake of noradrenaline (norepinephrine) and 5-hydroxytryptamine, resulting in a reduction in appetite. Other therapeutic possibilities are neuropeptide Y antagonists, leptin analogues and β-3-adrenoreceptor agonists. Surgical options such as gastric banding have also been used for some resistant cases.

> **CONCLUSIONS**
>
> - Daily energy loss as heat is about 120 kJ (30 kcal) per kilogram of body weight in a normal adult. In addition, there is a daily protein turnover of about 3 g/kg body weight (about 0.5 g of nitrogen), of which about 0.15 g of nitrogen/kg body weight is excreted (1 g of nitrogen is derived from about 6.25 g of protein). These losses are usually balanced by dietary intake of equivalent amounts of energy, as carbohydrate, fat and protein. Glucose provides 4 kcal/g; fat provides 9 kcal/g.
> - During starvation, the body tries to maintain blood glucose levels in the acute phase and in the longer term to preserve body protein mass.
> - Kwashiorkor occurs in individuals with visceral protein loss associated with impaired immunological function, although other nutritional components are satisfactory. Visceral proteins are decreased, but body weight, mid-arm circumference and triceps skin-fold thickness are relatively normal. Conversely, marasmus is generalized malnutrition with reduction in weight, mid-arm circumference and skin-fold thickness, although relatively normal visceral proteins.
> - Enteral or parenteral feeding may be necessary for patients needing nutritional support.
> - Although about 1 billion of the world's population are malnourished, approximately 1 billion are overweight. Obesity is increasing, particularly in Western urbanized societies.

15 VITAMINS, TRACE ELEMENTS AND METALS

Vitamin deficiencies	222	Trace metals	230
Vitamin excess	222	Metal poisoning	232
Classification of vitamins	222		

This chapter looks at vitamins and trace elements, and might usefully be read in conjunction with Chapter 14 ('Nutrition'). It also discusses certain metals that are important in disease states.

At one time, vitamins were thought to be amines and hence the term 'vitamines' was coined for substances that are essential for life but needed in only minute amounts. Vitamins are now known to be organic compounds, not necessarily amines, which are essential for normal growth and development. They must be included in the diet because the body either cannot synthesize them at all or cannot do so in amounts sufficient for its needs.

Trace elements are inorganic compounds that, like vitamins, are essential for health and needed only in small amounts, known as the reference nutrient intake. A normal mixed diet should provide adequate amounts of vitamins and trace elements and thus supplementation is not usually necessary.

Testing for vitamin and trace element deficiency should be carried out as soon as the diagnosis is suspected; the results of laboratory tests usually revert rapidly to normal once the patient has resumed eating a normal diet, for example after admission to hospital, and it may then be impossible to confirm the original diagnosis. Where the diagnosis is difficult, a trial of the micronutrient may be the most reliable and simplest method of assessment.

VITAMIN DEFICIENCIES

These may have the following causes.

- *Inadequate intake*. Deficiencies are rarely seen in affluent populations except in:
  - individuals with an inadequate dietary intake or unusual diet,
  - chronic alcoholism,
  - patients with anorexia nervosa,
  - patients on parenteral or enteral nutrition.
- *Inadequate absorption*, for example malabsorption states.
- *Excess loss*, for example via gastrointestinal or renal tract.
- *Enhanced utilization*, for example sepsis or trauma.

VITAMIN EXCESS

Some vitamins (notably A and D) are toxic if taken in excess, and over-dosage has recently become more common, possibly because of the increased availability of these compounds in over-the-counter preparations.

CLASSIFICATION OF VITAMINS

Vitamins are classified into two groups on the basis of their solubilities: fat soluble and water soluble. The distinction is of clinical importance because steatorrhoea may be associated with a deficiency of fat-soluble vitamins, with relatively little clinical evidence of lack of most of the water-soluble vitamins except B_{12} and folate.

Fat-soluble vitamins

The principal fat-soluble vitamins are:

- A (retinol),
- D (calciferol),
- E (alpha-tocopherol),
- K (2-methyl-1,4-naphthoquinone).

Each of these has more than one active chemical form, but variations in structure are minimal and in this chapter each vitamin is considered as a single substance.

Vitamin A (retinol)

Sources

Precursors of vitamin A (the carotenes) are found in the yellow and green parts of plants and are especially abundant in carrots. The active vitamin is formed by the hydrolysis of beta-carotene in the intestinal mucosa; each molecule can produce two molecules of vitamin A, which are absorbed as retinol esters and stored in the liver. Retinol is transported to tissues bound to the α-globulin retinol-binding protein (RBP).

Vitamin A is stored in animal tissues, particularly the liver, and is also present in milk products and eggs.

Functions

Rhodopsin (visual purple), the retinal pigment that is necessary for vision in poor light (scotopic vision), consists of a protein (opsin) combined with vitamin A. Rhodopsin decomposes in bright light. It is partly regenerated in the dark, but, because this is not quantitatively complete, vitamin A is needed to maintain retinol levels. Vitamin A is also essential for normal mucopolysaccharide synthesis and mucus secretion.

Clinical effects of vitamin A deficiency

The clinical effects of vitamin A deficiency include the following.

- *Due to rhodopsin deficiency.*
  - 'Night blindness' (nyctalopia): deficiency is associated with poor vision in dim light, especially when the eyes have recently been exposed to bright light.
- *Due to deficient mucus secretion* leading to drying and squamous metaplasia of ectodermal tissue.
  - Skin secretion is diminished and there may be hyperkeratosis of hair follicles. Dry, horny papules (follicular hyperkeratosis) are found mainly on the extensor surfaces of the thighs and forearms. Squamous metaplasia of the bronchial epithelium has also been reported and may be associated with a tendency to develop chest infections.
  - The conjunctiva and cornea become dry and wrinkled, with squamous metaplasia of the epithelium and keratinization of the tissue (xerosis conjunctivae and xerophthalmia). Bitot's spots are elevated white patches, composed of keratin debris, found in the conjunctivae. Prolonged deficiency leads to keratomalacia, with ulceration and infection and consequent scarring of the cornea, causing blindness.
  - Poor bone growth in the skull, leading to cranial nerve compression.
  - Anaemia, which responds to vitamin A but not to iron therapy.

Causes of vitamin A deficiency

Hepatic stores of vitamin A are large and therefore clinical signs only develop after many months, or even years, of dietary deficiency. Such prolonged deficiency is very rare in affluent communities. In steatorrhoea, clinical evidence of vitamin A is rare, although plasma concentrations may be low. Deficiency is relatively common in poor countries, especially in children, and can cause blindness.

Diagnosis and treatment of vitamin A deficiency

The diagnosis is usually made on the basis of clinical criteria; very low plasma vitamin A concentrations usually confirm deficiency. In conditions such as non-cirrhotic liver disease, in which plasma concentrations of RBP are low, concentrations of vitamin A may be decreased despite normal liver stores. In cirrhosis of the liver, the stores may be very low.

Laboratory tests for the diagnosis of vitamin A deficiency consist of testing for plasma retinol concentration. Retinol-binding protein is also low in vitamin A deficiency, but this may also occur in protein deficiency and the acute phase response.

Vitamin A deficiency can be treated with retinyl palmitate. High doses of vitamin A should be given to treat xerophthalmia and advanced skin lesions. 'Night blindness' and early retinal and corneal changes often respond rapidly to treatment, although corneal scarring may be irreversible.

Hypervitaminosis A

Vitamin A in large doses is toxic. Acute intoxication has been reported in Arctic regions as a result of eating polar bear liver, which has very high vitamin A content. More commonly, over-dosage is due to the excessive use of vitamin preparations.

In acute poisoning, symptoms include nausea and vomiting, abdominal pain, drowsiness and headache. Pregnant women are usually advised not to eat liver, which is a storage organ for many vitamins, to avoid the risk of fetal damage.

Chronic hypervitaminosis A is associated with fatigue, insomnia, bone pain, loss of hair, desquamation and discoloration of the skin, hepatomegaly, headaches, abdominal pain, bone and joint pain, benign intracranial hypertension, osteoporosis and weakness.

Additionally, a very high intake of carrots or orange juice can lead to carotenaemia, which can mimic jaundice except that plasma bilirubin is normal.

Vitamin D (calciferol)

The metabolism and functions of vitamin D, the effects and treatment of its deficiency and hypocalcaemia are discussed in Chapter 6, as are disorders of bone, including rickets and osteomalacia.

Over-dosage may cause hypercalcaemia. In chronic over-dosage, stores of cholecalciferol are large and therefore hypercalcaemia may persist, or even progress, for several weeks after ingestion of the vitamin is stopped.

Vitamin E (alpha-tocopherol)

Vitamin E acts as an anti-oxidant, and deficiency can have many clinical sequelae.

Vitamin E deficiency

The common causes of vitamin E deficiency are poor intake and fat malabsorption, for example cystic fibrosis. Low plasma concentrations may also be seen in the rare hypobetalipoproteinaemia or abetalipoproteinaemia, in which there are low concentrations of the lipoproteins that are involved in carrying some of the fat-soluble vitamins (see lipid metabolism, Chapter 13).

The clinical features of vitamin E deficiency include increased haemolysis, a possibly increased risk of atherosclerosis and, in low-birth-weight babies, retrolental fibroplasias and intraventricular haemorrhages.

Laboratory tests for deficiency consist of measurement of plasma vitamin E levels (alpha-tocopherol is the most active form). Sometimes increased erythrocyte haemolysis can be measured in the laboratory as an index of vitamin E deficiency.

It has been proposed that supplementation of dietary anti-oxidants such as vitamins A, C and E may protect against atherosclerosis by reducing low-density lipoprotein (LDL) oxidation. However, the results of some intervention trials have been disappointing, having failed to show any significant reduction in cardiovascular events for those on anti-oxidant supplementation.

Vitamin E excess is rare.

Vitamin K

Vitamin K is needed for the synthesis of prothrombin and coagulation factors VII, IX and X in the liver, and deficiency is accompanied by a bleeding tendency with a prolonged prothrombin time. Clinically, vitamin K is sometimes given to reverse the actions of the anticoagulant warfarin in patients in whom it is causing bleeding problems, as evidenced by a prolonged prothrombin time or International Normalized Ratio. Vitamin K is also involved in bone mineralization.

Vitamin K can be synthesized by bacteria in the ileum, from where it can be absorbed; thus dietary deficiency is unlikely. However, deficiency may occur:

- in patients with steatorrhoea: the vitamin, whether taken in the diet or produced by intestinal bacteria, cannot be absorbed normally;
- after the administration of some broad-spectrum antibiotics, which may alter the intestinal bacterial flora and so reduce the synthesis of vitamin K, especially in children.

If vitamin K deficiency occurs, it can be corrected by parenteral administration.

In the newborn, plasma vitamin K concentrations are lower than in adults because very little can be transported across the placenta, the neonatal gut is only gradually colonized by bacteria capable of synthesizing vitamin K and protein synthesis has not yet reached full adult capacity, particularly in premature infants.

Deficiency may be severe enough to cause haemorrhagic disease of the newborn, a condition that may present within 2–3 days of birth.

Laboratory tests for vitamin K deficiency are usually indirect, involving measurement of the prothrombin time. Although one can measure blood vitamin K or its metabolites in specialized laboratories, this is rarely indicated.

Excess vitamin K is rare and may sometimes cause haemolytic anaemia.

Water-soluble vitamins

The water-soluble vitamins are:

- the B complex:
  - thiamine (B_1)
  - riboflavine (B_2)
  - nicotinamide (niacin)
  - pyridoxine (B_6)
  - folate (pteroylglutamate)
  - the vitamin B_{12} complex (cobalamins)
  - biotin and pantothenate (probably of no clinical significance in humans),
- ascorbate (vitamin C).

Thiamine, folate, vitamin B_{12} and ascorbate are actively absorbed from the intestinal tract and the rest diffuse passively through the intestinal mucosal wall.

The vitamin B complex

Most of these vitamins act as enzyme cofactors and many are synthesized by colonic bacteria. As the absorption of water-soluble vitamins from the large intestine is poor, probably most of those synthesized within the colon are unavailable to the body.

Clinical deficiency is rare in affluent communities. When deficiency does occur, it is usually multiple, involving most of the B group, and is associated with protein malnutrition; for this reason it may be difficult to decide which signs and symptoms are specific for an individual vitamin and which are part of a general malnutrition syndrome (Fig. 15.1).

Thiamine (B_1)

Sources and causes of deficiency
Humans cannot synthesize thiamine. It is found in many dietary components; wheat germ, oatmeal and yeast are particularly rich sources. Adequate amounts are present in a normal diet and deficiency is most common in alcoholics and in patients with anorexia nervosa.

Functions
Thiamine is a component of thiamine pyrophosphate, which is an essential cofactor for decarboxylation of 2-oxoacids; one such reaction is the conversion of pyruvate to acetyl Coenzyme A (see Chapter 12). In thiamine deficiency, pyruvate cannot be metabolized and accumulates in the blood. Thiamine pyrophosphate is also an essential cofactor for transketolase in the pentose-phosphate pathway.

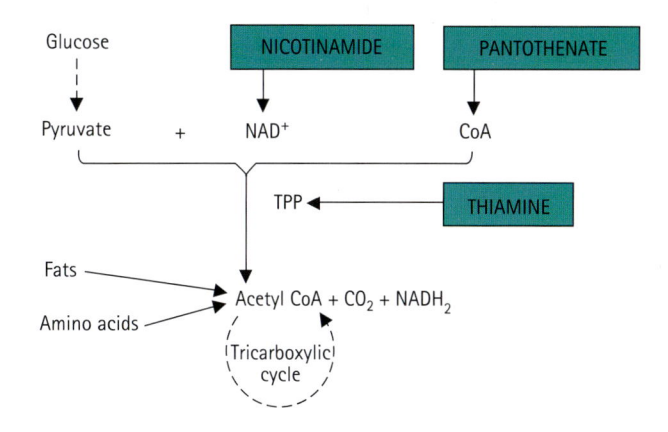

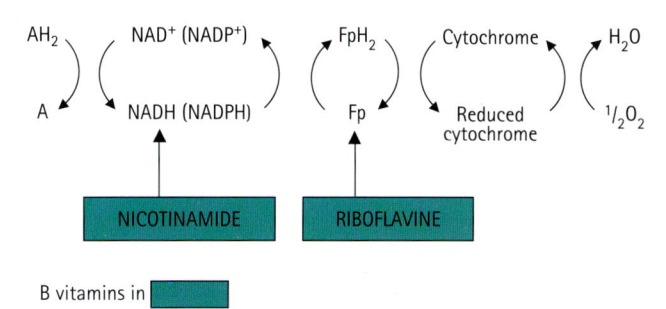

Fig. 15.1 Some biochemical interrelations of the B vitamins. (NAD = nicotinamide adenine dinucleotide; CoA = coenzyme A; TPP = thiamine pyrophosphate; A = substrate [e.g. pyruvate]; AH_2 = reduced substrate [e.g. lactate]; Fp = flavoprotein.)

Clinical effects of thiamine deficiency
Deficiency is usually due to excess ethanol intake with high carbohydrate but poor vitamin intake, although it can also be seen in intensive care patients with high carbohydrate intake. One of the commonest causes worldwide is a diet high in un-enriched white flour or rice. The level of thiaminase, which breaks down thiamine, is high in raw fish.

Deficiency of thiamine causes beriberi, in which anorexia, emaciation, neurological lesions (motor and sensory polyneuropathy, amnesia, encephalopathy called Wernicke–Korsakoff syndrome) and cardiac arrhythmias may occur. This form is called 'dry' beriberi (shoshin) and is associated with low cardiac output. In 'wet' beriberi there is peripheral oedema, sometimes associated with cardiac failure.

Beriberi may be aggravated by a high-carbohydrate diet, possibly because this leads to an increased rate of glycolysis and therefore of pyruvate production.

Laboratory diagnosis of thiamine deficiency

Probably the most reliable test for thiamine deficiency is the estimation of erythrocyte transketolase activity, with and without added thiamine pyrophosphate. Reduced activity, if due to thiamine deficiency, becomes normal after the addition of the cofactor. This test is rarely indicated and of little use once a normal diet, or vitamin supplementation, has been started because plasma concentrations are rapidly corrected. Other tests may be useful, including the measurement of both blood and urinary thiamine concentrations, and a raised blood pyruvate concentration is indicative.

Riboflavine (B$_2$)

Sources

Riboflavine is found in large amounts in yeasts and germinating plants such as peas and beans, and in smaller amounts in fish, poultry and meat, especially offal.

Functions

Riboflavine is present in many naturally occurring flavoproteins, in most of which it is incorporated in the form of flavine mononucleotide (FMN) and flavine adenine dinucleotide (FAD). Both FMN and FAD are reversible electron carriers in biological oxidation systems, which are, in turn, oxidized by cytochromes.

Clinical effects of riboflavine deficiency

The causes of riboflavine deficiency include poor intake, malabsorption, alcoholism and increased metabolic rate in severe illness. Riboflavine deficiency (ariboflavinosis) causes a rough, scaly skin, especially on the face, cheilosis (red, swollen, cracked lips), angular stomatitis and similar lesions at the mucocutaneous junctions of the anus and vagina (oro-genital syndrome), and a swollen, tender, red tongue that is described as magenta coloured. Congestion of conjunctival blood vessels may be visible if the eye is examined with a slit lamp.

Laboratory diagnosis of riboflavine deficiency

Riboflavine acts as a cofactor for glutathione reductase. The finding of a low erythrocyte activity of this enzyme, which increases by about 30 per cent after the addition of FAD, suggests riboflavine deficiency. A low urinary riboflavine concentration may also be a useful marker of deficiency. The treatment for deficiency is to give riboflavine. Riboflavine excess is very rare.

Nicotinamide (niacin)

Sources

Nicotinamide can be formed in the body from nicotinic acid. Both substances are plentiful in animal and plant foods although much of that in plants is bound in an unabsorbable form. Some nicotinic acid can also be synthesized in humans from tryptophan. Probably both dietary and endogenous sources are necessary to provide enough nicotinamide for normal metabolism.

Functions

Nicotinamide is the active constituent of nicotinamide adenine dinucleotide (NAD$^+$) and its phosphate (NADP$^+$), which are important cofactors in oxidation–reduction reactions. Reduced NAD$^+$ and NADP$^+$ are, in turn, re-oxidized by flavoproteins, and the functions of riboflavine and nicotinamide are closely linked. The NAD$^+$ and NADP$^+$ and their reduced forms are essential for glycolysis and oxidative phosphorylation, and for many synthetic processes.

Clinical effects of nicotinamide deficiency

It may be difficult to distinguish between the clinical features due to coexistent deficiencies, such as of pyridoxine, and those specifically due to nicotinamide. However, nicotinamide deficiency is probably the most important factor precipitating the clinical syndrome of pellagra. The mnemonic 'three Ds' – dementia, dermatitis, diarrhoea – may help in remembering the symptoms.

- Dementia, with delusions, may be preceded by irritability and depression.
- Dermatitis is a sunburn-like erythema, especially severe in areas exposed to the sun, which may progress to pigmentation and thickening of the skin; 'pellagra' literally means 'rough skin'.
- Diarrhoea is due to widespread inflammation of the mucosal membranes of the gastrointestinal tract; anorexia may aggravate weight loss.

Other features include achlorhydria, stomatitis and vaginitis.

Causes of nicotinamide deficiency

Dietary deficiency of nicotinamide, like that of the other B vitamins, is rare in affluent communities.

Hartnup disease is due to a rare inborn error of metabolism involving the renal, intestinal and other cellular transport mechanisms for the monoamino-monocarboxylic amino acids, including tryptophan. Subjects with the disorder may present with a pellagra-like rash that can be cured by giving nicotinamide daily. If the endogenous supply of tryptophan is reduced, dietary nicotinic acid is probably insufficient to supply the body's needs over long periods of time; under these circumstances, only a slight reduction of intake may precipitate pellagra. A similar clinical picture has been reported as a rare complication of the carcinoid syndrome, when tryptophan is diverted to the synthesis of large amounts of 5-hydroxytryptamine.

Nicotinic acid (but not nicotinamide) may reduce the hepatic secretion of very low-density lipoprotein (VLDL) and therefore plasma concentrations of VLDL and LDL (see Chapter 13).

Laboratory diagnosis of nicotinamide deficiency
If a normal diet has not been started, the diagnosis can sometimes be made by measuring urinary n-methyl-nicotinamide concentration, which is low in deficiency. Treatment is usually with nicotinamide.

Pyridoxine (B_6)

Functions
Pyridoxal phosphate, formed in the liver from pyridoxine, pyridoxal and pyridoxamine, is a cofactor mainly for the transaminases, and for decarboxylation of amino acids.

Sources of pyridoxine and causes of deficiency
Pyridoxine (pyridoxol), its aldehyde (pyridoxal) and amine (pyridoxamine) are widely distributed in food; dietary deficiency is very rare. The antituberculous drug isoniazid (isonicotinic hydrazide) and possibly also L-dopa have been reported to produce the picture of pyridoxine deficiency, probably by competing with it in metabolic pathways. Other causes of deficiency include alcoholism, malabsorption and inborn errors.

Clinical effects
Deficiency may cause roughening of the skin, peripheral neuropathy and a sore tongue. A rare hypochromic microcytic anaemia, with increased iron stores (sideroblastic anaemia), responds to large doses of pyridoxine even when there is no evidence of vitamin deficiency ('pyridoxine-responsive' anaemia).

Laboratory diagnosis of pyridoxine deficiency
Pyridoxal phosphate is needed for the conversion of tryptophan to nicotinic acid, and this pathway is impaired in pyridoxine deficiency. Xanthurenic acid is the excretion product of 3-hydroxykynurenic acid, the metabolite before the 'block'; in pyridoxine deficiency, it is found in abnormally high amounts in the urine after an oral tryptophan load. The urinary metabolite of pyridoxal phosphate, 4-pyridoxic acid, may also be measured.

Increase in the activity of erythrocyte aspartate transaminase after the addition of pyridoxal phosphate may be measured. The more severe the pyridoxine deficiency, the greater the increase in enzyme activity after addition of the vitamin.

Excess pyridoxine can occur with over-dose regularly greater than 10 mg/day and may lead to a peripheral neuropathy.

Biotin and pantothenate

It is not clear whether lack of these two vitamins produces a clinical deficiency syndrome.

Biotin is produced by intestinal bacteria. It is also present in eggs, but large amounts of raw egg white in experimental diets have caused loss of hair and dermatitis that are thought to be due to biotin deficiency. Probably the protein avidin, present in egg white, combines with biotin and prevents its absorption. Biotin is a cofactor in carboxylation reactions.

Pantothenate is a component of coenzyme A, which is essential for fat and carbohydrate metabolism. The vitamin is widely distributed in foodstuffs.

Folate and vitamin B_{12}

Both folate and vitamin B_{12} are essential for the normal maturation of erythrocytes; deficiency of either causes macrocytosis or megaloblastic anaemia. Their effects are so closely interrelated that they are usually considered together. A fuller discussion of the haematological diagnosis and treatment of megaloblastic anaemia will be found in haematology textbooks.

Folate is present in green vegetables and some meats. It is easily destroyed during cooking, and dietary deficiency may occasionally occur. Folate is absorbed throughout the small intestine and, in contrast to most of the other B vitamins (except B_{12}), clinical deficiency is relatively common in intestinal malabsorption syndromes, especially in the 'contaminated bowel' syndrome. In these conditions, and during pregnancy and lactation, low red-cell folate concentrations may be associated with megaloblastic anaemia or macrocytosis. Low maternal folate intake is also associated with neural tube defects in the fetus.

The active form of the vitamin is tetrahydrofolate, which is essential for the transfer of one-carbon units; it is particularly important in purine and pyrimidine, and therefore DNA and RNA, synthesis. Methotrexate, a cytotoxic analogue of folate, competes with it for metabolism and therefore inhibits DNA synthesis.

The vitamin B_{12} group includes several cobalamins, found in animal products but not in green vegetables. Dietary deficiency is rare. The cobalamins are transported

CASE 1

A 67-year-old female saw her general practitioner because of tiredness and paraesthesiae in her feet as well as anaemia. On examination, there was evidence of a sensory peripheral neuropathy. A number of blood tests were requested, and the abnormal results are shown below.

Plasma
Vitamin B_{12} 90 ng/L (150–600)
Folate 2.8 µg/L (2.0–3.8)
Strongly positive parietal cell antibodies.

A full blood count showed mean cell volume (MCV) of 102 fL (82–98); concentrations of haemoglobin, white cells and platelets were all low (pancytopenia).

DISCUSSION
The diagnosis is vitamin B_{12} deficiency resulting in pernicious anaemia. Note the raised MCV, as macrocytosis is a feature of vitamin B_{12} deficiency, as is a pancytopenia. Symptoms suggestive of a neuropathy may occur. There is an abnormality of vitamin B_{12} intestinal absorption and positive parietal cell antibodies.

in plasma by a specific carrier protein, transcobalamin II. Deoxyadenosyl-cobalamin and methylcobalamin have, like folate, coenzyme activity in nucleic acid synthesis.

Hydroxycobalamin is the form most commonly used in treatment, and both it and cyanocobalamin are converted to cofactor forms in the body. All forms are absorbed mainly in the terminal ileum, combined with intrinsic factor derived from the gastric parietal cells. In pernicious anaemia, antibodies to gastric parietal cells or to intrinsic factor cause malabsorption of vitamin B_{12}. The Schilling test has been used to diagnose pernicious anaemia.

Schilling test procedure
A small dose of radiolabelled vitamin B_{12} is given orally and its excretion is measured in the urine. A flushing dose of non-radiolabelled vitamin is given parenterally at the same time as, or just after, the labelled dose to ensure quantitative urinary excretion. Haematological tests, such as the examination of blood and bone marrow films, should have been completed before the vitamin B_{12} is given.

Interpretation. If malabsorption of the vitamin is due to pernicious anaemia, administration of the labelled vitamin with intrinsic factor restores normal absorption; if it is due to intestinal disease, for example ileal resection or bacterial overgrowth, malabsorption persists. Intrinsic factor and parietal antibodies should be tested, as these may be positive in pernicious anaemia (see Chapter 16).

Deficiency of vitamin B_{12}, like that of folate, causes megaloblastic anaemia. However, unlike that of folate, it can cause subacute combined degeneration of the spinal cord. Although the megaloblastic anaemia of vitamin B_{12} deficiency can be reversed by folate, this treatment should never be given in pernicious anaemia because it does not improve, and may even aggravate, the neurological lesions.

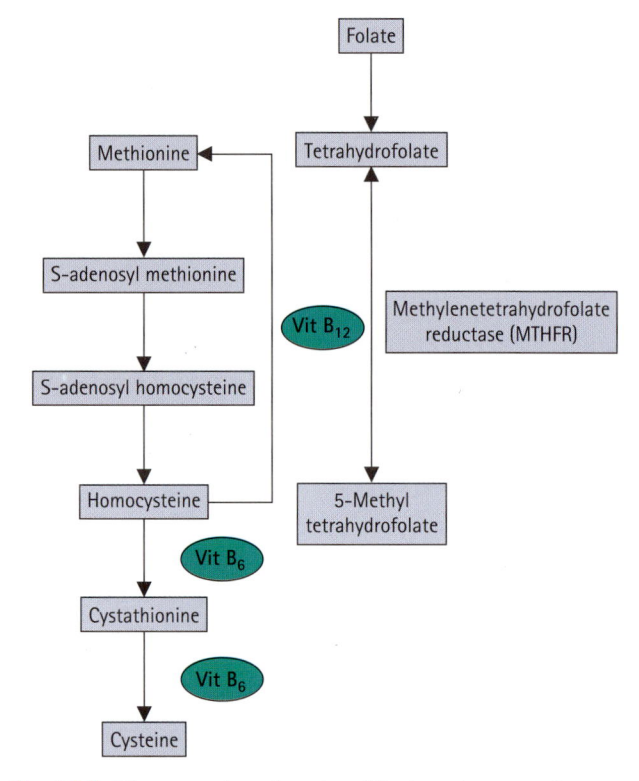

Fig. 15.2 Diagram showing simplified pathways of homocysteine metabolism.

It has recently become established that homocysteine, a sulphur-containing amino acid, is an independent cardiovascular risk factor. Both folate and vitamin B_{12} regulate the enzyme methylenetetrahydrofolate reductase and methionine synthase, respectively, whilst vitamin B_6 is a cofactor of the enzyme cystathionine synthase (Fig. 15.2). Supplementation with folate and/or vitamin B_{12} may lower homocysteine plasma levels (see also Chapter 22).

Table 15.1 The biochemical functions and clinical deficiency syndromes associated with the B vitamins

Name	Synonym	Biochemical function	Clinical deficiency syndrome
Thiamine	Vitamin B_1	Cocarboxylase (as thiamine pyrophosphate)	Beriberi (neuropathy) Wernicke–Korsakoff syndrome
Riboflavine	Vitamin B_2	In flavoproteins (electron carriers as FAD and FMN)	Ariboflavinosis (affecting skin and eyes)
Nicotinamide	Niacin	In NAD^+ and $NADP^+$ (electron carriers)	Pellagra (dermatitis, diarrhoea dementia)
Pyridoxine	Vitamin B_6	Cofactor in decarboxylation and deamination (as phosphate)	Pyridoxine responsive anaemia Dermatitis
Biotin		Carboxylation cofactor	Failure to thrive in infants
Pantothenate		In Coenzyme A	Failure to thrive in infants
Folate	Pteroyl glutamate	Metabolism of purines and pyrimidines	Megaloblastic anaemia Raised homocysteine Neural tube defects in fetus
Cobalamins	Vitamin B_{12} group	Cofactor in synthesis of nucleic acid	Megaloblastic anaemia Subacute combined degeneration of the spinal cord Raised homocysteine

The known biological functions and the clinical syndromes associated with deficiencies of the B vitamins are summarized in Table 15.1. Generally, deficiencies of this group cause lesions of skin, mucous membranes and the nervous system.

Ascorbate (vitamin C)

Sources

Ascorbate is found in fruit, particularly citrus fruits, and vegetables. It is added to other foods as a preservative. It cannot by synthesized by humans.

Functions

Ascorbate can be reversibly oxidized in biological systems to dehydroascorbate and, although its functions in humans are not clear, it probably acts as a hydrogen carrier and antioxidant as well as being involved in collagen synthesis.

Causes of ascorbate deficiency

Deficiency of ascorbate causes scurvy, which was common on long sea voyages before the eighteenth century when fresh fruit and vege-tables were unavailable.

Dehydroascorbate is easily and irreversibly oxidized and loses its biological activity in the presence of oxygen; this reaction is catalysed by heat.

Deficiency occurs most commonly in the elderly, especially those who do not eat fresh fruit and vegetables. It can also occur in iron overload.

Clinical effects of ascorbate deficiency

Many of the signs and symptoms of scurvy are related to deficient collagen formation and include the following.

- Fragility of vascular walls causing a bleeding tendency, often with a positive Hess test, petechiae and ecchymoses, swollen, tender, spongy, bleeding gums and, sometimes, haematuria, epistaxis and retinal haemorrhages. In infants, subperiosteal bleeding and haemarthroses are extremely painful and may lead to permanent joint deformities.
- Poor wound healing.
- Deficiency of bone matrix causing osteoporosis and poor healing of fractures. In children, bone formation is impaired at the epidiaphysial junctions, which look 'frayed' radiologically and can mimic non-accidental injury. The enzyme procollagen hydroxylase is mediated by vitamin C and is important for the intracellular matrix. In children thereare tender limbs due to poor osteoid, costochondral bleeding (scorbutic rosary) and ground-glass bone X-ray appearance.

- Anaemia, possibly due to impaired erythropoiesis and poor iron absorption. The anaemia is aggravated by bleeding.

These signs and symptoms are often cured by the administration of ascorbate.

Diagnosis of ascorbate deficiency

Laboratory confirmation of the clinical diagnosis of ascorbate deficiency can only be made *before* therapy has started. Once ascorbate has been given, it is difficult to prove that deficiency was previously present. Although the assay of leucocyte ascorbate was thought to be more reliable in confirming the diagnosis than that of plasma, levels probably alter in parallel; plasma assay is technically more satisfactory, but chemical estimations are rarely indicated. There is also an oral vitamin C loading test that may show a low urinary excretion of vitamin C in deficiency states. Treatment of deficiency is with vitamin C.

Ascorbate excess

Excess vitamin C is rare, but may increase oxalate levels and the likelihood of renal oxalate calculi.

TRACE METALS

Inorganic micronutrients, or trace metals, are essential for normal health and, by definition, make up less than 0.01 per cent of the body's dry weight.

Zinc

Zinc is a cofactor for certain enzymes, for example polymerases, carbonic dehydratase and alkaline phosphatase. Zinc deficiency may result in a number of clinical states, including growth retardation, alopecia, dermatitis, diarrhoea, poor wound healing, infertility and increased risk of infections.

The causes of zinc deficiency are acrodermatitis enteropathica, poor intake, for example parenteral nutriton, increased utilization and high levels of dietary phytates. Useful laboratory tests for deficiency include the measurement of plasma or urinary zinc levels. The plasma zinc-carrying protein metallothionine may also prove useful. Note that plasma zinc levels may be low during an acute-phase response, as the zinc is also partly bound to albumin, which is a negative acute-phase reactant.

Zinc toxicity is rare, usually occurring after inappropriate administration, and may result in pulmonary oedema, jaundice and oliguria.

Copper

Copper functions as an enzyme co-factor, for example cytochromes. Copper deficiency may cause cardiac arrhythmias, neutropenia, hypochromic anaemia and, in children, bony problems such as subperiosteal haematomas.

The causes of deficiency include poor intake, for example long-term parenteral nutrition. Menke's disease is an inborn error of copper transport resulting in low plasma copper concentrations and abnormal hair that has a characteristic 'kink' appearance.

Laboratory tests for deficiency include the measurement of plasma copper. Copper is carried on the protein caeruloplasmin, the level of which may be increased due to an acute-phase response, oestrogens or pregnancy. Copper deficiency can be treated with certain copper salts, but care is needed in case there is an effect on zinc and iron absorption.

Copper excess can lead to toxicity, causing renal problems, fits, haemolysis and hypotension. Wilson's disease, in which copper excess and decreased caeruloplasmin occur, is an inborn error of metabolism.

Wilson's disease

Some plasma copper is loosely bound to albumin, but most is incorporated in the protein caeruloplasmin. Copper is mainly excreted in bile. There are two defects of copper metabolism in Wilson's disease:

- impaired biliary excretion leads to deposition in the liver,
- deficiency of caeruloplasmin results in low plasma copper concentrations. Most is in a loosely bound form and is therefore deposited in tissues; more than normal is filtered at the glomeruli and urinary copper excretion is increased.

Excessive deposition of copper in the eyes, basal ganglia of the brain, liver and renal tubules produces:

- Kayser–Fleischer rings at the edges of the cornea due to deposition of copper in Desçemet's membranes,
- neurological symptoms due to degeneration of the basal ganglia,
- liver damage leading to cirrhosis,
- renal tubular damage with any or all of the associated biochemical features, including aminoaciduria (Fanconi syndrome).

Diagnosis

Most patients have low plasma caeruloplasmin (less than 0.2 g/L) and copper concentrations (less than

> **CASE 2**
>
> A 21-year-old male was referred to the neurology out-patients' department because of dysarthria and leg weakness. A number of investigations were organized and some of the pertinent results are as follows.
>
> Urine analysis showed amino-aciduria.
>
> *Plasma*
> Alanine transaminase 98 U/L (<42)
> Bilirubin 12 µmol/L (<20)
> Alkaline phosphatase 367 U/L (<250)
> Albumin 44 g/L (35–45)
> Gamma-glutamyl transferase 234 U/L (<55)
> Caeruloplasmin 0.08 g/L (0.2–0.6)
> Copper 10 µmol/L (11–20)
>
> **DISCUSSION**
> The patient was found to have Wilson's disease presenting with neurological sequelae, abnormal liver function tests and renal tubular damage leading to amino-aciduria. The concentration of copper-binding protein caeruloplasmin is low. Urinary free copper concentration would be expected to be high.

12 µmol/L) and high urinary copper excretion (more than 1.2 µmol/ day).

The penicillamine test is sometimes used in the diagnosis of Wilson's disease and is based on the principle that penicillamine solubilizes copper and enhances copper urinary excretion. Post-oral penicillamine dose urinary copper excretion is more than 25 µmol/day and indicative of Wilson's disease.

Low plasma caeruloplasmin concentrations may also occur during the first few months of life due to malnutrition, and in the nephrotic syndrome due to urinary loss. Raised plasma caeruloplasmin concentrations are found in active liver disease, in women taking oral contraceptives, during the last trimester of pregnancy and non-specifically when there is tissue damage due, for example, to inflammation or neoplasia. These may account for the rare finding of 'normal' plasma caeruloplasmin concentrations in patients with Wilson's disease.

Histological examination, with the demonstration of an increased copper content, of a liver biopsy specimen is often necessary to confirm the diagnosis.

Wilson's disease has a recessive mode of inheritance, but reduced plasma caeruloplasmin concentrations may be demonstrable in heterozygotes. The distinction between presymptomatic homozygotes and heterozygotes is important because the former can be treated.

Treatment with copper-chelating agents such as D-penicillamine may reduce tissue copper concentrations.

Selenium

The main function of selenium is to mediate the activity of the enzyme glutathione peroxidase, which acts as an anti-oxidant.

Deficiency can be caused by poor intake and is most commonly seen in certain areas of China. Patients on artificial nutrition, for example parenteral support, are also more susceptible. Selenium deficiency may also cause cardiomyopathy (Keshan disease), osteoarthropathy (Kaschin–Beck disease), myopathy, macrocytosis and anaemia.

Diagnostic laboratory tests for selenium deficiency include the measurement of urinary or blood selenium or finding decreased erythrocyte glutathione peroxidase activity.

Manganese

This is an enzyme cofactor, for example of superoxide dismutase. Deficiency is associated with vitamin K deficiency and may be seen in patients who are being fed artificially.

Manganese excess can occur, for example in miners of manganese ores, and can result in Parkinson-like disease and defects of the basal ganglia. Sometimes parenteral nutrition regimens may cause raised plasma manganese concentration. Manganese is mainly biliary excreted and therefore toxicity may occur with hepatic dysfunction or cholestasis.

Chromium

Chromium is an insulin cofactor. Chromium deficiency can occur on long-term parenteral nutrition, leading to glucose intolerance and neuropathy.

Toxicity is associated with gastrointestinal problems, lung cancer and hepatitis.

Molybdenum

Molybdenum is a cofactor of xanthine oxidase and other enzymes.

Deficiency can occur on long-term parenteral nutrition and may lead to tachycardia, central scotomas, 'night blindness' and coma.

Cobalt

This is important for vitamin B_{12} metabolism. Toxicity is rare and has been described in dialysis patients and heavy drinkers of beer that is contaminated with cobalt, leading to cardiomyopathy.

METAL POISONING

It would be highly unusual to have a deficiency of the following metals, although, for completeness, metal poisoning is included in this chapter.

Mercury

Mercury poisoning can occur from organic or inorganic salts or elemental mercury vapour. Acute toxicity may result in a metallic taste and respiratory distress, nausea and vomiting. More chronic features include neuropathy and renal dysfunction.

Acute toxicity can be treated with dimercaprol-chelating agents, which increase excretion via urine and bile. In chronic exposure, N-acetyl penicillamine has been used to chelate mercury.

The diagnosis of mercury poisoning can be established from urinary or blood mercury levels. Sometimes hair mercury levels can be used to monitor long-term exposure.

Aluminium

Aluminium toxicity, although rare, is well described in patients with renal impairment. Contamination of the water used in dialysis fluid has been implicated in renal osteodystrophy and dialysis dementia. Dialysis water is now usually treated to decontaminate aluminium. Toxicity has also been seen in individuals with excess oral intake, such as of aluminium-containing antacids for dyspepsia. Aluminium exposure is diagnosed by plasma aluminium measurements.

Desferrioxamine has been used to chelate aluminium in toxicity.

Cadmium

Cadmium toxicity can occur in industrial workers exposed to cadmium fumes. Clinical features include nephrotoxicity, hepatotoxicity and bone disease. Cadmium exposure can be assessed from the levels in blood and urine. Renal tubular damage can be monitored by raised urinary β_2-microglobulin concentration.

Lead

For a discussion of lead poisoning, see Chapter 21.

CONCLUSIONS

- Vitamins are essential for biochemical processes and can be divided into those that are fat soluble and water soluble. The former include vitamin A, D, E and K; the latter are vitamins B and C.
- Vitamin A and E deficiencies are more common in developing countries. Vitamin D deficiency can result in rickets or osteomalacia (discussed in Chapter 6). Vitamin K deficiency can cause bleeding problems with prolonged prothrombin time.
- Vitamin B_1 (thiamine) deficiency is associated with beriberi and Wernicke–Korsakoff's syndrome.
- Vitamin B_{12} deficiency can be seen in pernicious anaemia.
- Vitamin C deficiency causes scurvy.
- Trace elements are also essential, such as zinc, copper, manganese and selenium. Deficiencies can occur, usually if the patient has poor dietary intake.
- Trace element excess can occur, for example in Wilson's disease, in which plasma caeruloplasmin concentration is low, resulting in excess unbound copper.

16 THE GASTROINTESTINAL TRACT

Physiology and biochemistry of normal digestion	233	Pancreatic disorders	239
Gastric function	234	Malabsorption syndromes	239
Normal intestinal absorption	234	Laboratory investigation of abdominal pain	248
Normal pancreatic function	238		

Gastrointestinal disorders present relatively commonly to doctors, and biochemical laboratory tests have important roles in their investigation. This chapter looks at gastrointestinal pathophysiology and how chemical pathology tests may be useful in diagnosis and treatment.

PHYSIOLOGY AND BIOCHEMISTRY OF NORMAL DIGESTION

The major functions of the gastrointestinal tract are the digestion and absorption of nutrients. Additionally, it synthesizes certain hormones along its length that act locally (paracrine hormones), so controlling gut motility and the release of digestive enzymes and secretions. The gastrointestinal tract handles about 8–9 L of fluid per day, with the majority of this derived from endogenous secretions. Fluid reabsorption by the gastrointestinal tract (mainly the small intestine) is highly efficient (98 per cent), with only 100–200 mL lost daily in the stools.

Digestion and absorption depend on food and the products of its digestion being diluted with a large volume of fluid, mostly an ultrafiltrate of extracellular fluid filtered through the 'tight junctions' between epithelial cells, mainly in the duodenum. Some is reabsorbed in the proximal jejunum, along the osmotic gradient created by reabsorption of the products of digestion; a large amount remains in the lumen to be reclaimed more distally.

A small amount of the nutrients from desquamated intestinal cells also enters the lumen; most is reabsorbed. Almost all the fat in normal faeces is of endogenous origin, which is relevant when interpreting the results of a faecal fat estimation. A much smaller volume of fluid enters the lumen by active secretion. As a result, the pH and the electrolyte and enzyme concentrations change during the passage of fluid through the tract in such a way that the conditions for enzyme activity are near optimal for digestion. Adjustment of pH and electrolyte concentrations occurs in the distal ileum and colon; sodium reabsorption (and therefore water reabsorption) is enhanced by aldosterone in the colon. The colon can metabolize undigested carbohydrates into short-chain fatty acids such as butyrate, propionate and acetate. These are an important energy source for the colon.

Disturbances of water, electrolyte and hydrogen ion homeostasis may occur in small intestinal or colonic disease. If there is loss of fluid and electrolytes from the upper intestinal tract because of vomiting or because the function of intestinal cells is so perturbed that the amount of fluid and electrolytes entering the distal parts exceeds the reabsorptive capacity, similar changes may occur (see also Chapter 2).

Digestive enzymes usually act on complex molecules such as protein, polysaccharides and fat. This process starts in the mouth, where food is broken down by mastication and is mixed with saliva containing α-amylase. In the stomach, acid fluid is added and the low pH initiates protein digestion by pepsin. The stomach also secretes intrinsic factor, essential for vitamin B_{12} absorption from the terminal ileum. However, most digestion takes place in the duodenum and upper jejunum, where alkaline fluid is added to the now liquid intestinal contents. Pancreatic enzymes digest proteins to small peptides and amino acids, polysaccharides to monosaccharides, disaccharides and oligosaccharides, and fat to monoglycerides and fatty acids.

GASTRIC FUNCTION

The main components of gastric secretion are hydrochloric acid, pepsin and intrinsic factor, all of which are important for normal digestion and absorption. Loss of hydrochloric acid by vomiting, as in pyloric stenosis, may cause a metabolic alkalosis (Chapter 4). Gastric secretion may be stimulated by the following.

- The *vagus nerve*, which in turn responds to stimuli from the cerebral cortex, normally resulting from the sight, smell and taste of food. Hypoglycaemia can stimulate gastric secretion and so can be used to assess the completeness of a vagotomy.
- *Gastrin*, which is carried by the bloodstream to the parietal cells of the stomach; its action is mediated by histamine. Gastrin secretion is inhibited (by negative feedback) by acid in the pylorus. Calcium also stimulates gastrin secretion and this may explain the relatively high incidence of peptic ulceration in patients with chronic hypercalcaemia.

Histamine stimulates gastric secretion after binding to specific cell-surface receptors, of which there are at least two types:

- those for which antihistamines compete with histamine (H1 receptors): these are found on smooth muscle cells;
- those on which antihistamines have no effect: these H2 receptors are found on gastric parietal cells.

Hypersecretion of gastric juice may cause duodenal ulceration. However, there is overlap between the amount of acid secreted in normal subjects and in those with duodenal ulceration. The estimation of gastric acidity is of very limited diagnostic value. In the very rare Zollinger–Ellison syndrome, acid secretion is very high due to excessive gastrin produced by a gastrinoma – a tumour more usually involving the pancreas or duodenum (see later).

Drugs such as ranitidine and cimetidine compete with histamine for the H2 receptors, so directly reducing acid secretion. Proton pump inhibitors such as omeprazole and lansoprazole have to some degree surpassed these agents.

Hyposecretion of gastric juice occurs most commonly in association with pernicious anaemia, due to the formation of antibodies to the parietal cells of the gastric mucosa.

Extensive carcinoma of the stomach and chronic gastritis may also cause gastric hyposecretion. Plasma gastrin concentrations are raised, because reduced acid secretion causes the loss of negative feedback inhibition.

Tests of gastric function involving the measurement of acid secretion have largely been superseded by endoscopic examination of the stomach and duodenum and by histological examination of the biopsy material obtained.

Post-gastrectomy syndromes

There may be some degree of malabsorption after gastrectomy. Rapid passage of the contents of the small gastric remnant into the duodenum may be associated with the following.

The *early dumping syndrome*. Soon after a meal, the patient may experience abdominal discomfort and feel faint and nauseated. These symptoms may be caused by the rapid passage of hypertonic fluid into the duodenum. Before this abnormally large load can be absorbed, water passes along the osmotic gradient from the extracellular space into the lumen. The reduced plasma volume causes faintness and the large volume of fluid causes abdominal discomfort.

The *late dumping syndrome* (or post-gastrectomy hypoglycaemia). If a meal containing a high glucose concentration passes quickly into the duodenum, glucose absorption is very rapid, stimulating a surge in insulin secretion. The resultant 'overswing' of plasma glucose concentration may cause hypoglycaemic symptoms, typically occurring about 2 hours after a meal. This is a form of reactive hypoglycaemia (see Chapter 12).

Both these dumping syndromes can be minimized if frequent, small, low-carbohydrate meals are taken.

NORMAL INTESTINAL ABSORPTION

There are three phases of digestion and absorption: the luminal phase, mucosal phase and post-absorptive phase.

Absorption depends on:

- the presence of nutrient in an absorbable form (and therefore on normal digestion),
- the integrity and large surface area of absorptive cells,
- a normal ratio of the rate of absorption to the rate of passage of contents through the intestinal tract.

The absorptive area of the small intestine is very large. The mucosa forms macroscopically visible folds, increasing the area considerably. Microscopically, these folds are covered with villi lined with absorptive cells (enterocytes), which increase the area about eight-fold. A large number of minute projections (microvilli) cover the surface of each enterocyte, separated by microvillous spaces. These increase the absorptive area about a further twenty-fold. The absorptive area is significantly reduced if the villi are flattened, as they are, for example, in gluten-sensitive enteropathy.

Absorption also depends on whether a molecule is:

- *water soluble*, so that it can be absorbed either by active transport against a physicochemical gradient or by passive diffusion along gradients,
- *lipid soluble*, enabling it to diffuse across the lipid membranes of the enterocytes.

The release of intestinal secretions and the control of gut motility are, in part, controlled by a series of peptide hormones produced in the mucosa of the gastrointestinal tract. Like other hormones, their release is under feedback control by either the product or the physiological response of the target tissue.

Cells that synthesize gut peptides are scattered throughout the length of the gastrointestinal tract, although the secretory cells are often concentrated in one segment of the tract. Many of these peptides are present in other organs, particularly the brain, where they probably act as neurotransmitters.

- *Gastrin* is released from the gastrin-secreting G-cells in the gastric antrum in response to distension and to protein. It stimulates the contraction of the stomach muscles and the secretion of gastric acid. Acid inhibits gastrin release by negative feedback.
- *Cholecystokinin* stimulates contraction of the gall bladder and the release of pancreatic digestive enzymes.
- *Secretin* stimulates the release of pancreatic fluid rich in bicarbonate.
- *Pancreatic* polypeptide inhibits pancreatic secretion,
- *Vasoactive* intestinal polypeptide (VIP) and motilin regulate gut motility.

Carbohydrate absorption

Polysaccharides, such as starch, consist either of straight chains of glucose molecules joined by 1:4 linkages, called amylose, or of branch chains, in which the branches are joined by 1:6 linkages, called amylopectin. Salivary and pancreatic α-amylases hydrolyse starch to 1:4 disaccharides such as maltose (glucose + glucose). Pancreatic amylase is quantitatively the more important. A few larger branch-chain saccharides (limit dextrans) remain undigested.

Disaccharides (maltose, sucrose [glucose + fructose] and lactose [glucose + galactose]) are hydrolysed to their constituent monosaccharides by the appropriate disaccharidases, β-galactosidases (lactase) and α-glucosidases (maltase, sucrase), located on the surface of enterocytes ('brush border'), especially in the proximal jejunum. Sucrase also hydrolyses the 1:4, and isomaltase the 1:6, linkages of limit dextrans.

Monosaccharides are actively absorbed in the duodenum and proximal jejunum. Unlike for fructose, a common active process absorbs glucose and galactose. Carbohydrate absorption depends on:

- the presence of *amylase*, and therefore on normal pancreatic function (polysaccharides only),
- the presence of *disaccharidases* on the luminal membrane of intestinal cells (disaccharides),
- *normal intestinal mucosal cells* with normal active transport mechanisms (monosaccharides).

Polysaccharides can be absorbed only if all three mechanisms are functioning.

Xylose absorption test

This can be used to test the integrity of the intestinal mucosa. Xylose is a pentose that, like glucose, can be absorbed without digestion (by facilitated diffusion), but the metabolism of which is not hormone controlled; therefore, unlike glucose, it is not affected by insulin secretion.

An oral dose of xylose is absorbed by normally functioning upper small intestinal cells. Metabolism of the absorbed pentose is very slow and, because it is freely filtered by the glomeruli, most of it appears in the urine. In the xylose absorption test, either the amount excreted in the urine during a fixed period or, in children, the plasma concentration at a defined time after the dose is measured.

Intestinal disease (for example blind loops) or impaired mucosal surface area (as in coeliac disease) may impair xylose absorption and therefore reduces excretion. Pancreatic disease does not affect either process. Therefore this test can distinguish between pancreatic insufficiency and conditions affecting the intestinal mucosa.

Unfortunately, there are several sources of error in the xylose test.

- Xylose is absorbed mostly from the upper small intestine and absorption may therefore be normal despite significant ileal dysfunction, for example in Crohn's disease.

- The urine test depends on accurate collections over a short time interval and therefore even more significant errors may occur than in 24-hour collections.
- Mildly impaired renal function decreases glomerular filtration of xylose and may give falsely low results in the urine tests, or a falsely high plasma concentration. This is a common cause of misleading results in the elderly. The xylose absorption test should not be performed if glomerular function is even only marginally impaired.
- Both plasma concentrations and urine excretion depend partly on the volume of distribution of the absorbed xylose. In oedematous or very obese patients, results may be falsely low.

A possible scheme for carrying out the xylose test is now discussed.

Procedure

A dose of 5 g of xylose is preferable to one of 25 g because a high xylose concentration within the intestinal lumen may, like a large dose of glucose, have an osmotic effect that causes symptoms and affects the results.

- The patient fasts overnight.
- *08.00 hours.* The bladder is emptied and the specimen discarded. Then 5 g of xylose dissolved in 200 mL of water is given orally. All specimens passed between 08.00 hours and 10.00 hours are put into a bottle labelled Number 1.
- *10.00 hours.* The bladder is emptied and the specimen is put into Bottle 1, which is now complete. All specimens passed between 10.00 hours and 13.00 hours are put into a bottle labelled Number 2.
- *13.00 hours.* The bladder is emptied and the specimen is put into Bottle 2, which is now complete. Both bottles are sent to the laboratory for analysis.

Interpretation

In the normal subject, more than 1.5 g xylose should be excreted during the 5 hours. About 50 per cent or more of the total excretion should occur during the first 2 hours. In mild intestinal malabsorption, the total 5-hour excretion may be normal, but delayed absorption is reflected in a 2:5-hour ratio of less than 40 per cent. In pancreatic malabsorption, the result should be normal.

Protein absorption

Protein in the intestinal lumen is derived from the diet, intestinal secretions and desquamated mucosal cells. Dietary protein is broken down by gastric pepsin and in the duodenum by trypsin and other proteolytic enzymes secreted in pancreatic juice; pancreatic trypsinogen is converted to active trypsin by enterokinase located on the brush border. The products of digestion are small peptides and amino acids. Many peptides are further hydrolysed by peptidases on the brush border.

Amino acids are actively absorbed in the small intestine. Small peptides are absorbed by an active transport mechanism, independently of amino acids and, with a few exceptions, are hydrolysed intracellularly. Protein absorption depends on the presence of pancreatic proteolytic enzymes (and therefore on normal pancreatic function) and an intestinal mucosa with normal active transport mechanisms.

Lipid absorption

Digestion of fats

Triglycerides are the main form of dietary fat and are esters of glycerol with three, usually different, fatty acids. They are insoluble in water. Cholesterol, in the intestinal lumen, is derived from bile salts and from the diet; only about 30 per cent of the dietary cholesterol is absorbed (see Chapter 13).

Primary bile acids are synthesized in the liver from cholesterol, conjugated with the amino acid glycine or taurine in the liver, and then enter the intestinal lumen in the bile. In the alkaline duodenal fluid their sodium salts act as detergents, emulsifying and so facilitating the digestion and absorption of fats. Most of the bile salts are actively reabsorbed in the distal ileum, although some enter the colon where they are converted by bacteria to secondary bile salts, some of which are absorbed. The absorbed bile salts are recirculated to the liver and resecreted into the bile (the enterohepatic circulation).

Some bacteria within the gut lumen contain enzymes that catalyse the deconjugation of bile salts; unconjugated bile salts emulsify fat less effectively than conjugated ones and this may contribute to fat malabsorption. Triglycerides are emulsified by bile salts within the duodenum. They are hydrolysed by pancreatic lipase at the glycerol/fatty acid bond, primarily in positions 1 and 3. The end products are mainly 2-monoglycerides, some diglycerides and free fatty acids. Colipase, a peptide coenzyme secreted by the pancreas, is essential for lipase activity. It anchors lipase at the fat/water interface, prevents the inhibition of the enzyme by bile salts and reduces its pH optimum from about 8.5 to about 6.5; the latter is the pH in the upper intestinal lumen.

Micelle formation

Monoglycerides and free fatty acids aggregate with bile salts to form water-miscible micelles. The micelles also contain free cholesterol liberated by the hydrolysis of cholesterol esters in the lumen and phospholipids, as well as fat-soluble vitamins (A, D, E and K). The diameter of the negatively charged micelles is between 100 and 1000 times smaller than that of the emulsion particles. Both their small size and their charge allow them to pass through the narrow microvillous spaces.

Within enterocytes, triglycerides are resynthesized from monoglycerides and fatty acids, and cholesterol is re-esterified. Triglycerides, cholesterol esters and phospholipids, together with fat-soluble vitamins, combine with apolipoproteins manufactured in enterocytes to form chylomicrons. These are suspended in water and pass into the lymphatic circulation.

Some short-chain and medium-chain free fatty acids pass directly through the intestinal cells into the portal bloodstream.

The absorption of lipids and fat-soluble vitamins depends on:

- an adequate absorptive area of the intestinal mucosa for chylomicron formation,
- the presence of bile salts,
- the digestion of triglycerides by lipase and therefore on normal pancreatic function.

Faecal fat estimation test

Faecal fat excretion should represent the difference between the fat absorbed and that entering the gastrointestinal tract from the diet and from the body. The absorption of fat and, more importantly, the addition of fat to the intestinal contents occur throughout the small intestine. A single 24-hour collection of faeces gives very inaccurate results for two reasons: the transit time from the duodenum to the rectum is variable and rectal emptying is variable and may not be complete.

Consecutive 24-hour collections give faecal fat results that may vary by several hundred per cent. The longer the period of collection, the more accurate the calculated daily mean result; ideally, stools should be collected for a minimum of 3 days. Collecting between 'markers' (usually dyes or radio-opaque pellets taken orally) may increase the test's precision. The dye can be visually detected and the pellets can be detected by radiological visualization of the stools. Neither a barium enema nor a barium meal should be performed for a few days before or during the collection because barium interferes with the estimation.

Interpretation

A mean daily fat excretion of more than 18 mmol (5 g) indicates steatorrhoea. The result is not affected by diet within very wide limits, because in the normal subject almost all the fat is of endogenous origin. However, if the patient is on a very low-fat diet, mild steatorrhoea may be undetected.

It has been suggested by some experts that the faecal fat test is too inaccurate for clinical use and should be abandoned.

The triolein breath test

The triolein breath test has also been used to assess fat absorption. Absorbed fat is ultimately metabolized to CO_2 and water. If ^{14}C-labelled triglyceride (triolein) is given by mouth, the ratio of $^{14}CO_2$ to unlabelled CO_2 can be measured in expired air. A low ratio usually indicates impaired fat absorption. The assay uses expensive isotopes and requires special expertise. Although the results correlate with faecal fat measurements, these limitations have prevented its widespread adoption.

Vitamin B_{12} absorption

Vitamin B_{12} can be absorbed only when it has formed a complex with intrinsic factor, a glycoprotein secreted by the parietal cells of the stomach (see Chapter 15). This complex is resistant to proteolytic digestion and binds to specific cell receptors in the distal ileum, from where it is absorbed. Some intestinal bacteria need vitamin B_{12} for growth and may prevent its absorption by competing for it with intestinal cells. Intestinal bacterial overgrowth is associated with intestinal strictures, diverticula and 'blind loops'. Vitamin B_{12} absorption therefore depends on normal gastric secretion of intrinsic factor, intestinal mucosa in the distal ileum and intestinal bacterial flora.

Absorption of other water-soluble vitamins

Most of the other water-soluble vitamins (C and the B group except B_{12}) are absorbed in the upper small intestine, probably by specific transport mechanisms. Clinical deficiencies of all but folate are relatively uncommon in the malabsorption syndromes, probably because their absorption does not depend on that of fat. Folate deficiency may be caused by intestinal malabsorption, inadequate intake or increased use by intestinal bacteria (see Chapter 15).

Calcium and magnesium absorption

Calcium is absorbed mainly from the duodenum and upper jejunum in the free ionized form; this is enhanced by the vitamin D metabolite 1,25-dihydroxycholecalciferol, which influences both active transport and passive diffusion. Calcium absorption is impaired by the formation of insoluble salts with free fatty acids and with phosphate. Much of the faecal calcium is endogenous in origin, being derived from intestinal secretions (see Chapter 6).

An active process that may be shared with calcium also absorbs magnesium. Calcium and magnesium absorption depends on:

- a low concentration of fatty acids and phosphate in the intestinal lumen,
- the absorption and metabolism of vitamin D, and therefore on normal fat absorption,
- normal intestinal mucosal cells.

Iron absorption

Iron is absorbed in the duodenum and upper jejunum in the ferrous form (Fe^{2+}). Absorption is increased by anaemia of any kind and probably also by vitamin C. Some of the iron absorbed into intestinal cells enters the plasma, but some is lost into the lumen with desquamated cells (see Chapter 21).

NORMAL PANCREATIC FUNCTION

Pancreatic secretions can be divided into endocrine and exocrine components. The endocrine function and insulin and glucagon that control the plasma glucose concentration are discussed in Chapter 12. The exocrine secretions are made up of two components, the alkaline pancreatic fluid and the digestive enzymes. The alkaline fluid is primarily responsible for neutralizing gastric acid secretions, thus providing an optimal environment for duodenal digestive enzyme activity. These enzymes include the proteases trypsin, elastase and chymotrypsin, and amylase and lipase. Some of the proteases are secreted as precursors and are converted to the active form within the intestinal lumen.

Gut peptides control pancreatic secretion and are released from the duodenum in response to a rise in the hydrogen ion concentration or to the presence of food. They include secretin (which stimulates the release of a high volume of alkaline fluid) and cholecystokinin (which stimulates the release of a fluid rich in enzymes).

Tests of exocrine pancreatic function

Plasma enzymes

Plasma enzyme measurements are of limited value in assessing exocrine function. They include the following.

Amylase

This enzyme consists of two forms, of salivary gland and pancreatic origin, respectively. In acute pancreatitis, total plasma amylase activity is usually significantly increased due to release from damaged cells.

Plasma amylase is discussed more fully in Chapter 18 in the context of enzymology. Typically, plasma amylase activity increases about five-fold in acute pancreatitis, but plasma enzyme activities of up to, and even above, this value may be reached in a number of other disorders, in particular after gastric perforation.

Occasionally, the plasma enzyme activity in acute pancreatitis may not be very high and usually falls rapidly as the enzyme is excreted in the urine. Consequently, a high plasma amylase activity is only a rough guide to the presence of acute pancreatitis, and normal or only slightly raised values do not exclude the diagnosis. Plasma amylase concentrations can be spuriously low or normal in acute pancreatitis evoked by severe hypertriglyceridaemia. In such circumstances a raised urinary amylase concentration may facilitate diagnosis or clearing the plasma lipaemia by centrifugation prior to assay. Haemorrhagic pancreatitis or chronic pancreatitis can also show a normal plasma amylase concentration.

Lipase

This enzyme is more specific for the pancreas and can be useful to measure if the source of a raised plasma amylase concentration is not obvious. Lipase has a longer half-life than amylase and thus may be useful in the late diagnosis of acute pancreatitis, when amylase activity can fall within the reference range.

Trypsin

This may be used to screen for cystic fibrosis (see later and Chapter 27) during the first 6 weeks of life. Blockage of pancreatic ductules by sticky mucous secretion causes high plasma trypsin concentrations. After about 6 weeks, plasma concentrations may fall as pancreatic insufficiency develops; normal levels do not exclude the diagnosis.

Duodenal enzymes

Measurement of pancreatic enzymes and the bicarbonate concentration in duodenal aspirates before and after stimulation with cholecystokinin and secretin is not very suitable for routine use because of the difficulty in positioning the duodenal tube and in quantitative sampling of the secretions.

'Tubeless tests' have been developed that avoid the need for intubation and that overcome the difficulties of invasive sample collection.

The PABA test

A synthetic peptide, labelled with p-aminobenzoic acid (PABA), is taken orally. After PABA has been split from the peptide by chymotrypsin, it is absorbed and excreted in the urine. Urinary excretion of PABA is significantly reduced in chronic pancreatitis. Abnormal results may occur if there is renal glomerular dysfunction, liver disease or malabsorption, even in the presence of normal pancreatic function. The effect of these conditions is assessed by repeating the test with unconjugated PABA, which eliminates the need for digestion before absorption.

The pancreolauryl test

A similar, but technically simpler, test uses oral fluorescein dilaurate. Fluorescein is released and absorbed and the amount excreted in a timed urine sample is measured as an indirect measure of pancreatic function.

Faecal enzymes

A low faecal elastase determination is a useful screening test for pancreatic malabsorption. This can be assayed in a small 'pea'-sized faecal sample. Similarly, faecal chymotrypsin can also be measured.

PANCREATIC DISORDERS

The absence of pancreatic secretions may, by impairing digestion, cause malabsorption. However, there are two pancreatic diseases that are only rarely associated with malabsorption.

Acute pancreatitis

Acute pancreatitis due to the necrosis of pancreatic cells is associated with the release of enzymes into the retroperitoneal space and bloodstream. The presence of pancreatic juice in the peritoneal cavity causes severe abdominal pain and shock. A vicious circle is set up as the released enzymes digest more pancreatic cells. Acute pancreatitis may be idiopathic, but may follow gallstones, obstruction of the pancreatic duct or regurgitation of bile along this duct. Other predisposing factors include excess alcohol ingestion and trauma to the pancreas. Hypercalcaemia and hypertriglyceridaemia may also evoke acute pancreatitis, as can certain drugs such as opiates.

The severity of an acute attack of pancreatitis can be assessed by the Ranson or Glasgow criteria (Table 16.1).

Table 16.1 The Ranson/Glasgow criteria for assessing the severity of an acute attack of pancreatitis

At presentation	During first 48 hours
Age >55 years	Plasma urea rise >10 mmol/L
White blood count >16 × 10^9/L	Plasma calcium <2.0 mmol/L
Plasma glucose (in non-diabetic) >10 mmol/L	PaO_2 < 8 kPa
	Plasma albumin <32 g/L
	Haematocrit fall >10%
Plasma aspartate transaminase >250 U/L	Fluid sequestration >6 L
Plasma lactate dehydrogenase >350 U/L	

The mortality rate amongst patients with more than seven of these criteria is near 100%.

Carcinoma of the pancreas

This tends to present late. Lesions at the head of the organ may cause obstructive jaundice; extensive gland destruction may cause late-onset diabetes mellitus. The concentration of the tumour marker CA19-9 may be raised in pancreatic carcinoma (see Chapter 24).

MALABSORPTION SYNDROMES

Generalized malabsorption may result from either intestinal or pancreatic disease.

- In intestinal malabsorption, fat digestion is usually normal, but absorption of the products of digestion is impaired.
- In pancreatic malabsorption, the absorptive capacity is normal, but fat cannot be digested because there is deficiency of digestive enzymes.

> ## CASE 1
>
> A 57-year-old male presented to the surgeons in the casualty department with an acute abdomen, severe epigastric pain and nausea. On examination, he was found to be hypotensive and showing abdominal guarding. Some of his laboratory test results are as follows.
>
> *Plasma*
> Sodium 135 mmol/L (135–145)
> Potassium 5.0 mmol/L (3.5–5.0)
> Bicarbonate 25 mmol/L (24–32)
> Urea 10.5 mmol/L (2.5–7.0)
> Creatinine 140 µmol/L (70–110)
> Glucose 17.5 mmol/L (3.5–5.5)
> 'Corrected' calcium 1.89 mmol/L (2.15–2.55)
> Triglyceride 1.3 mmol/L (<2.3)
> Amylase 2567 U/L (<200)
>
> ### DISCUSSION
> The very high plasma amylase concentration supports the diagnosis of acute pancreatitis, which was confirmed by computerized tomography (CT) imaging. The scan also showed the presence gallstones, which were thought to be the cause of the acute pancreatitis. Note the hypocalcaemia, impaired renal function and hyperglycaemia, which can be associated with this condition. High alcohol intake is another cause of acute pancreatitis, as can be hypercalcaemia, hypertriglyceridaemia, trauma and certain drugs.

Steatorrhoea

Malabsorption is usually, but not always, associated with impaired fat absorption (steatorrhoea). No biochemical test is sensitive enough for the early detection, or precise enough for the differential diagnosis, of steatorrhoea; endoscopy and ultrasound have reduced the need for laboratory tests. However, biochemical tests are important in detecting and monitoring the treatment of the metabolic effects of prolonged and severe malabsorption.

Steatorrhoea has been discussed above and can be defined as a daily faecal fat excretion consistently more than 18 mmol (5 g) of fat, measured as fatty acids. This is usually associated with a faecal stool weight greater than 60 g. Unequivocal steatorrhoea can only be demonstrated when the disease is extensive and has usually already been elucidated by radiological or histopathological means. Gross steatorrhoea causes foul-smelling, bulky, pale, greasy stools, which are difficult to flush away in the toilet.

Mechanisms of malabsorption

Reduction of absorptive areas or generalized impairment of transport mechanisms

Villous atrophy
Malabsorption may be caused by a reduction of the absorptive area because of flattened intestinal villi, demonstrated by microscopic examination of a mucosal biopsy specimen, and by the following.

- Coeliac disease (gluten-sensitive enteropathy) is caused by sensitivity to the protein α-gliadin, present in gluten in wheat and rye. The condition is characterized by villous atrophy, mainly in the proximal small intestine, which is usually reversible following gluten withdrawal from the diet. Clinical symptoms usually become evident at about 1 year of age with failure to thrive and diarrhoea, but may present at any age. Antibodies to α-gliadin or endomysium (the latter probably reflects tissue transglutaminase) may be detected in plasma and their measurement can be used in diagnosis and to monitor compliance with a gluten-free diet. The long-term prognosis is good, although patients have an increased susceptibility to developing lymphomas and hyposplenism. Exclude immunoglobulin A (IgA) deficiency, as some assays for coeliac screening look at IgA antibodies, which may be falsely negative in IgA deficiency (see Chapter 19).
- Tropical sprue, in which villous atrophy does not respond to a gluten-free diet. There may be a bacterial cause because the condition sometimes responds to broad-spectrum antibiotics and folate supplements.
- Extensive surgical resection or fistulae of the small intestine may so reduce the absorptive area as to cause malabsorption. Normally the small bowel spans from 260 to 800 cm. Any disease, trauma, radiation or vascular event that leaves less than 200 cm of viable small bowel remaining puts the patient at risk of developing short-gut syndrome. The short-gut syndrome can present with malabsorption, diarrhoea and malnutrition. Electrolyte disturbances may include severe hypokalaemia and hypomagnesaemia as well as fluid depletion. Intestinal failure can be defined as a

> **CASE 2**
>
> A 31-year-old hairdresser presented to the gastroenterologists with weight loss of about 15 kg in 1 year, frequent diarrhoea and abdominal distension. There was a family history of coeliac disease.
>
> On examination, she was found to have abdominal tenderness and looked pale. Her blood count showed a haemoglobin level of 8.9 g/dL and she had a low plasma folate concentration. Her anti-gliadin and anti-endomysial antibodies were strongly positive. A jejunal biopsy was reported as near-total villous atrophy.
>
> **DISCUSSION**
>
> The clinical history and clinical features are typical of coeliac disease. Note also the folate deficiency. Her symptoms improved on a gluten-free diet, with gain in weight and normalization of her haemoglobin.

condition in which there is inability of the intestine to absorb nutrients and water sufficiently.
- Infiltration or inflammation of the small intestinal wall, for example caused by Crohn's or Whipple's disease or small intestinal lymphoma, may impair absorption. Malabsorption may be aggravated by alteration of the bacterial flora due to reduced intestinal motility.

Increased rate of transit through the small intestine

Food passes through the intestine more rapidly than usual in the following circumstances.

- After gastrectomy, when normal mixing of food with fluid, acid and pepsin does not occur in the stomach, resulting in impaired enzyme activity within the small intestine. An increased rate of transit through the duodenum may contribute to the malabsorption. However, post-gastrectomy malabsorption is rarely severe, although iron deficiency is a relatively common complication.
- In carcinoid syndrome, which is a rare condition associated with excessive production of 5-hydroxytryptamine (serotonin) by tumours of argentaffin cells usually arising in the small intestine, or by their metastases, for example in the liver. It may occasionally present with malabsorption, which is probably the result of increased intestinal motility due to the concomitant release of the gut peptide substance P (see Chapter 24).

Impaired digestive enzyme activity

Failure of digestive enzyme secretion

Pancreatic dysfunction may cause malabsorption by reducing the secretion of digestive enzymes. The following are some important examples.

- Chronic pancreatitis. Commonly due to alcohol excess, this is not always associated with steatorrhoea or malabsorption. It rarely follows a severe attack of acute pancreatitis, but is more likely after repeated acute or subacute attacks. Diabetes mellitus requiring insulin may occur due to islet cell damage. There may be steatorrhoea due to the impairment of lipase activity because of bile salt deficiency. Pancreatic lipase activity can be reduced by up to 75 per cent before chemical steatorrhoea occurs.

  Low plasma trypsin levels are relatively specific for chronic pancreatitis, but malabsorption does not tend to occur until more than 90 per cent of the pancreas has been destroyed. Similarly, there may also be low faecal elastase or chymotrypsin concentrations. Direct pancreatic enzyme tests are sometimes needed to detect the disease in its early stages.

  Direct invasive tests require specialist expertise and involve collecting duodenal aspirates by a tube in a cannulated pancreatic duct, sometimes in conjunction with endoscopic retrograde cholangiopancreatography (ERCP) after stimulation by exogenous secretin or cholecystokinin. Other tests may be used to diagnose chronic pancreatitis, including abdominal X-ray (calcification of pancreas is a useful sign), computerized axial tomography (CAT) or magnetic resonance imaging (MRI) scanning, endoscopic ultrasonography (EUS) or magnetic resonance cholangiopancreatography (MRCP).
- Cystic fibrosis. This is an autosomal, recessively inherited disorder of chloride transport affecting exocrine glandular secretions. It may present in the newborn with intestinal symptoms, such as meconium ileus (failure to pass the first faeces containing bile, intestinal debris and mucus), or in early childhood with recurrent respiratory infections; however, it may not be diagnosed until the patient is an adult. Thick, viscous

> **CASE 3**
>
> A 32-year-old female with known cystic fibrosis presented to the general physicians with copious pale, floating and offensive-smelling stools and diabetes mellitus. The results of some of her laboratory tests are as follows.
>
> *Plasma*
> Sodium 135 mmol/L (135–145)
> Potassium 2.8 mmol/L (3.5–5.0)
> Urea 2.7 mmol/L (2.5–7.0)
> Creatinine 80 μmol/L (70–110)
> Glucose 13.9 mmol/L (3.5–5.5)
>
> A stool sample revealed very low elastase activity with a faecal fat content of 65 mmol/day (less than 18).
>
> **DISCUSSION**
> The diagnosis was considered to be steatorrhoea secondary to cystic fibrosis because of pancreatic insufficiency. Note the hypokalaemia (due to prolonged diarrhoea) and hyperglycaemia (secondary to pancreatic endocrine malfunction).

pancreatic and bronchial secretions may cause malabsorption and chronic lung disease, respectively. Cirrhosis of the liver and sterility may develop. The diagnosis is made clinically and by measuring the sweat electrolyte concentrations; the chloride and sodium concentrations are usually more than 60 mmol/L. The detection of albumin in meconium or a raised plasma trypsin concentration during the first 6 weeks of life may be used to screen for the disorder.

More than 200 different mutations have been identified; the commonest, which has a prevalence of about 70 per cent, shows a 3 base pair (bp) deletion in codon 508 of the cystic fibrosis chloride channel gene. Prenatal diagnosis is available in some countries using chorionic villus sampling at 8–10 weeks, but is usually only offered if the gene defect has already been established within the family following the identification of an affected child (see Chapter 30).

Inactivation of pancreatic enzymes by acid
The increased intestinal hydrogen ion activity in the Zollinger–Ellison syndrome may inactivate pancreatic lipase and cause precipitation of bile salts within the gut lumen, so resulting in malabsorption (see later and also Chapter 24).

Differential diagnosis of generalized intestinal and pancreatic malabsorption
(Table 16.2)

The diagnosis of malabsorption is usually made by clinical, haematological, histological and radiological means, and supplemented by biochemical tests. Malabsorption of fat occurs both in generalized intestinal and in pancreatic disease.

Anaemia is rarer in pancreatic than in intestinal malabsorption because iron, vitamin B_{12} and folate do not depend

Table 16.2 Differential diagnosis and investigation of causes of steatorrhoea

	Upper small intestinal disease	Pancreatic disease	Contaminated bowel syndrome
Anaemia	Dimorphic picture (mixed megaloblastic and iron deficiency common)	Rare	Megaloblastic common
Plasma glucose	Low/normal	May be raised[a]	Normal
Intestinal biopsy or other cause	Flattened villi	Normal	Normal
Xylose absorption	Reduced	Normal	Usually normal
Pancreolauryl test or PABA test	Normal	Abnormal	Normal
Faecal elastase	Normal	Reduced	Normal

[a] If endocrine function of pancreas abnormal. PABA = p-aminobenzoic acid.

on pancreatic enzymes for absorption. The blood and bone marrow films typically show a mixed iron deficiency and megaloblastic picture.

Polysaccharide absorption is impaired in both conditions but hypoglycaemia is rare. In pancreatic malabsorption, in which neither disaccharidase activity nor active monosaccharide absorption is affected, both monosaccharides and disaccharides can be absorbed. Hyperglycaemia suggests that pancreatic disease is the cause of malabsorption.

Failure of absorption of specific substances (non-generalized malabsorption)

Altered intestinal bacterial flora may cause malabsorption of vitamin B_{12} and fat. This can occur in the following conditions.

- Contaminated bowel ('blind loop') syndrome, which is caused by bacterial proliferation due to impaired intestinal motility and stagnation of intestinal contents. It occurs when the 'blind loops' are the result of surgery or in the presence of small intestinal diverticula. Some bacteria may cause malabsorption by catalysing the deconjugation of bile salts. Since more vitamin B_{12} and folate may be used by the bacteria, megaloblastic anaemia is common. A metabolic acidosis, D-lactic acidosis, may also occur. Treatment with broad-spectrum antibiotics may, by altering the small intestinal bacterial flora, cause a similar syndrome.

    Abnormal bacterial growth may sometimes be diagnosed by the following.
    - Culture of organisms from a specimen collected into a special anaerobic microbiological medium after intubation of the upper small intestine. However, the test is invasive and cultures may be falsely negative.
    - The xylose breath test, in which $^{13}C/^{14}C$-labelled xylose is given orally. In the intestine, xylose is bacterially degraded and the released labelled CO_2 can be measured in the breath. This test may be more sensitive than the ^{14}C-glycocholate breath test, in which ^{14}C-glycocholate is taken orally. The intestinal bacteria split the cholate from the labelled glycine, which is absorbed and metabolized; $^{14}CO_2$ is measured in the expired air. False-positive results may occur in patients with disorders of the terminal ileum.
    - Increased urinary indican concentration, which entails the assay of bacterial-derived metabolites (usually of tryptophan) in the urine but may not be specific and is now rarely measured.

- Biliary obstruction causes malabsorption of fat and of fat-soluble substances by preventing the secretion of bile salts into the intestinal lumen; steatorrhoea results. The diagnosis is usually clinically obvious due to the presence of jaundice. Retention of bile salts, such as may occur in primary biliary cirrhosis, may cause pruritus.

- Local diseases or surgery of the small intestine may cause selective malabsorption of substances absorbed predominantly at those sites. Diseases involving the terminal ileum, such as Crohn's disease or tuberculosis, may impair the absorption of bile salts and vitamin B_{12}. Vitamin B_{12} absorption may also be impaired because of intrinsic factor deficiency caused either by damage to gastric parietal cells in pernicious anaemia or by total gastrectomy or extensive malignant infiltration of the stomach. Malabsorption of vitamin B_{12} may be demonstrated using the Schilling test (see Chapter 15).

- Disaccharidase deficiency may occur in generalized disorders of the intestinal wall because the enzymes are localized on the brush border of the enterocyte. This deficiency is relatively unimportant compared with that due to general malabsorption. Tests for these syndromes are therefore useful only in the absence of steatorrhoea, when selective rather than generalized malabsorption of carbohydrate may be present.

    The symptoms of disaccharidase deficiency are due to the effects of unabsorbed, osmotically active sugars in the intestinal lumen. They include faintness, abdominal discomfort and severe diarrhoea after ingestion of the offending disaccharide (compare with the 'dumping syndrome'). Diarrhoea may be severe enough to cause volume depletion in infants. Stools are typically acid because bacteria metabolize sugars to acids. Unabsorbed sugars may be detectable in the faeces, and some disaccharides, which may be absorbed intact, may be detectable in the urine.

    Lactase deficiency may be caused by several disorders.
    - Acquired lactase deficiency or lactose intolerance is commoner than the congenital form and is probably the commonest type of disaccharidase deficiency. It may not present until childhood, or even adult life, possibly in genetically predisposed individuals. It may also present secondary to other intestinal disorders, such as coeliac disease and inflammatory bowel disease.
    - Lactase deficiency associated with prematurity may resemble the congenital form. However, the

sensitivity to breast milk usually disappears when lactase is synthesized within a few days of birth.
- Congenital lactase deficiency (autosomal recessive) is very rare. Infants present with severe diarrhoea or colicky abdominal pain soon after the introduction of milk feeds. The syndrome is treated by removing milk and milk products from the diet.

Sucrase and isomaltase deficiency usually coexist. Congenital sucrase–isomaltase deficiency is more common than congenital lactase deficiency. Acquired sucrase–isomaltase deficiency and maltase deficiency of any kind is very rare.

The diagnosis of disaccharidase deficiency may be confirmed by:
- estimating the relevant enzymes in intestinal biopsy tissue: this is the most reliable test and no others may be needed, although it is invasive;
- measuring the plasma glucose concentration, as in the glucose tolerance test, after giving an oral load of the particular disaccharide. If the disaccharide cannot be hydrolysed, the constituent monosaccharides cannot be absorbed and the concentrations of plasma glucose rise very little. The result should be compared with that of a glucose tolerance test. If this is also flat, the abnormal response to disaccharides is not diagnostic. If the patient experiences typical symptoms, or if disaccharides are excreted in the urine when the offending sugar is given, the comparison need not be made.

A relatively simple and sensitive test for carbohydrate malabsorption is the hydrogen breath test. Patients are given an oral solution of lactose. In lactase deficiency, unabsorbed lactose is digested by colonic flora, which results in an elevated breath hydrogen content in expired air. Bacterial bowel overgrowth can do the same, but the two conditions can be distinguished by using oral glucose instead of lactose.

Protein-losing enteropathy

In many cases of malabsorption, protein is lost through the gut due to failure to digest and absorb that entering it in intestinal secretions and by cell desquamation. Isolated protein-losing enteropathy is a very rare syndrome in which absorption is normal but the intestinal wall is abnormally permeable to large molecules, a condition similar to that of the glomeruli in the nephrotic syndrome. It occurs in a variety of conditions in which there is ulceration of the bowel or abnormal lymphatic drainage. The clinical picture is largely due to hypoalbuminaemia.

If there is no evidence of generalized malabsorption and the disorder is suspected, the diagnosis can be made after the intravenous administration of a radiolabelled protein such as albumin or transferrin by measuring its recovery in a timed stool collection. Alternatively, the concentration of α_1-antitrypsin, a protein resistant to proteolytic degradation, can be measured in a known weight of faeces; gastrointestinal bleeding may cause false-positive results. Typically, the serum protein electrophoretic pattern is similar to that found in the nephrotic syndrome; the relatively high molecular weight components of the α_2-fraction are retained and all other fractions are reduced (see Chapter 19).

Metabolic consequences of malabsorption

The following findings may occur after very prolonged disease but are not necessary for the diagnosis of malabsorption. This section is best read in conjunction with Chapter 14 (nutrition) and Chapter 15 (vitamins).

Fat-soluble vitamin deficiency may be a consequence of impaired fat absorption due to steatorrhoea.

- Vitamin A deficiency can sometimes be demonstrated.
- Vitamin D deficiency causes impaired calcium absorption and sometimes leads to rickets or osteomalacia.
- Vitamin E deficiency may lead to neurological symptoms.
- Vitamin K deficiency may cause bleeding problems.

Amino acid and peptide malabsorption occurs in intestinal disease, due to impaired intestinal transport mechanisms; in pancreatic disease, the digestion of protein is severely impaired. In either case, prolonged disease may cause generalized muscle and tissue wasting and osteoporosis and reduced concentration of all plasma proteins: the low plasma albumin concentration may cause oedema, and reduced antibody formation (immunoglobulins) may predispose to infection.

Anaemia is less likely in pancreatic than in intestinal malabsorption; iron, vitamin B_{12} and folate do not depend on pancreatic enzymes for absorption. The blood and bone marrow films typically show a mixed iron deficiency and megaloblastic picture. Anaemia may be aggravated by protein deficiency.

The presenting clinical features in severe and long-standing generalized malabsorption, whether intestinal or pancreatic, may include:

- bulky, fatty stools, with or without diarrhoea,
- generalized wasting and malnutrition (protein deficiency),

> **CASE 4**
>
> A 60-year-old female with a medical history of numerous attacks of acute pancreatitis secondary to high alcohol intake noticed that her stools had turned paler, associated with abdominal discomfort and weakness. In addition she experienced paraesthesiae of her hands and polydipsia.
>
> Abdominal examination confirmed the abdominal discomfort and a plain abdominal X-ray showed pancreatic calcification. Some of her laboratory tests were as follows.
>
> *Plasma*
> 'Corrected' calcium 1.80 mmol/L (2.15–2.55)
> Phosphate 0.56 mmol/L (0.70–1.0)
> Alkaline phosphatase 544 U/L (<250)
> Albumin 28 g/L (35–45)
> Glucose (fasting) 17 mmol/L (3.5–5.5)
>
> **DISCUSSION**
> The patient has obvious features of malabsorption with hypocalcaemia due to vitamin D deficiency. The latter is a fat-soluble vitamin, and hypocalcaemia can evoke neurological symptoms. She also has hypoalbuminaemia and diabetes mellitus secondary to pancreatic insufficiency. Multiple attacks of acute pancreatitis can lead to chronic pancreatitis. She required insulin for her diabetes mellitus, calcium and vitamin D supplementation for her hypocalcaemia, and oral pancreatic extract (Creon) to replace her pancreatic enzymes.

- oedema (hypoalbuminaemia due to protein deficiency),
- osteoporosis and osteomalacia (protein and calcium deficiency),
- tetany (hypocalcaemia due to vitamin D and calcium deficiency),
- recurrent infections (immunoglobulin deficiency).

Investigation strategy for suspected malabsorption

This proposed scheme is for the investigation of suspected malabsorption.

- Malabsorption may be suspected if the patient presents with:
  - a history of chronic diarrhoea of unknown origin,
  - a history of weight loss,
  - clinical, radiological, haematological and/or biochemical findings suggestive of malnutrition with no obvious cause.
- Has the patient a history that may suggest alteration in the intestinal bacterial flora?
  - Have they been on long-term broad-spectrum antibiotics and what other relevant medications are they taking?
  - Has there been gastrointestinal surgery that may have resulted in 'blind loops'?
  - Ask about foreign travel or possibly contaminated drinking water. If so, consider the possibility of tropical sprue or other infective origin.
- What is the appearance of the stool?
  - Bulky, pale, greasy stools suggest steatorrhoea.
  - Constipation with hard, dry stools makes the diagnosis of malabsorption less likely.
  - Watery stools, especially if bloodstained, suggest colonic disease such as ulcerative colitis.
    The possibility of purgative or laxative abuse must always be considered in this context: consider measuring the stool osmality gap to see if the diarrhoea is secretory or osmotic.
    Is there a relationship to the type of food eaten, for example gluten-containing products? Check coeliac screen antibodies.
- Are there plasma electrolyte abnormalities, especially hypokalaemia and hypomagnesaemia? Signs of extracellular volume depletion without obvious evidence of malnutrition favour colonic disease as a cause of diarrhoea rather than a small intestinal malabsorption syndrome. Check also for an acid–base disturbance as well as hypoalbuminaemia, hypoproteinaemia or hypogammaglobulinaemia.
- Anaemia is more likely to be due to intestinal than to pancreatic disease.
  - A hypochromic, microcytic picture may be the result of blood loss at any level of the gastrointestinal tract.
  - A normochromic, normocytic picture is a non-specific finding in any chronic disease.
  - A dimorphic (mixed iron deficiency and macrocytic) picture is very suggestive of intestinal malabsorption.

- Low red cell folate and/or plasma vitamin B_{12} concentrations suggest intestinal malabsorption.
- If doubt remains, faecal fat estimation may help. However, because of the difficulty of obtaining an accurately timed faecal collection, only very high results are of unequivocal significance; in such cases steatorrhoea will probably be obvious visually. For this reason many hospital laboratories no longer perform this test. In any case, normal faecal fat does not exclude malabsorption, as carbohydrate absorption may be impaired.
- A new test that is looking promising is the stool elastase assay, which measures elastase activity in a small piece of stool. Low stool elastase levels are indicative of malabsorption of pancreatic origin.
- The xylose absorption test is sometimes helpful in distinguishing pancreatic malabsorption from intestinal problems. If it is unequivocally normal, an upper intestinal lesion is unlikely. Such a result does not, however, exclude ileal or pancreatic disease, contaminated bowel syndrome, or even some cases of coeliac disease.
- A pancreolauryl test or PABA test if available may also help confirm the presence of pancreatic insufficiency. Some authorities suggest the gold standard test for assessing pancreatic function is the secretin–pancreozymin test, but this is invasive and requires specialist skill.
- If any or all of the above investigations suggest steatorrhoea, a cause should be sought. The following are the most definitive tests.
    - Endoscopy, with histological examination of an intestinal biopsy specimen. Flattened villi suggest: coeliac disease, tropical sprue.
    - *Giardia lamblia* may be detected microscopically and stool culture is useful in case of other organisms.
    - Radiological examination may detect abnormal intestinal mucosa.
- The diagnosis of chronic pancreatitis and of causes of pancreatic malabsorption may also need imaging techniques such as ERCP or MRCP. Tests such as abdominal ultrasound or CT scanning may help, especially if pancreatic carcinoma is suspected. Plain abdominal X-ray may show pancreatic calcification.
- If steatorrhoea is obvious on clinical grounds and after visual inspection of the stool, and if the intestinal histological picture is normal, the most likely possibilities are:
    - localized intestinal disease, such as Crohn's disease,
    - contaminated small bowel ('blind loop') syndrome,
    - pancreatic disease such as chronic pancreatitis.

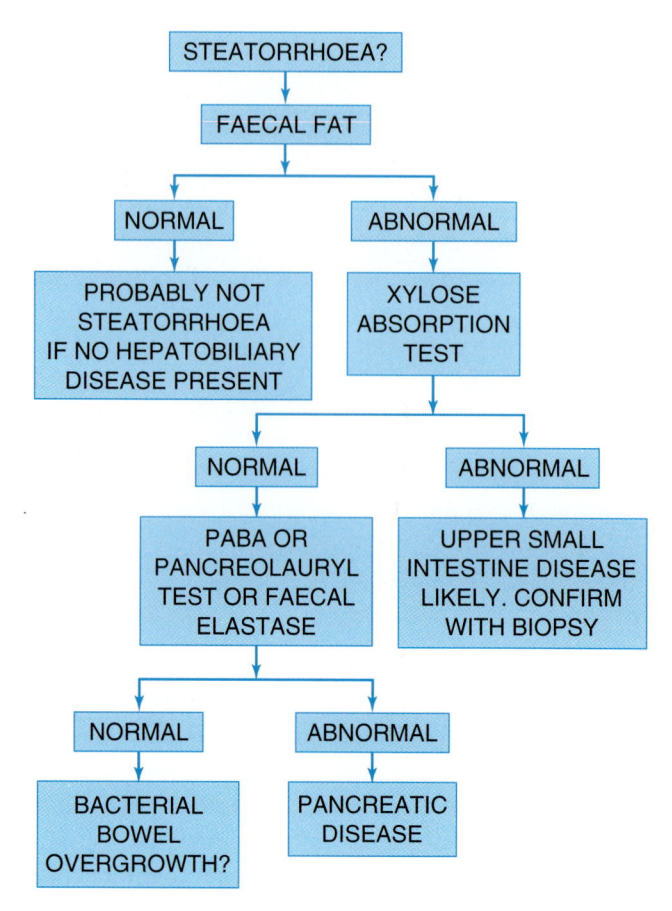

Fig. 16.1 Algorithm for the biochemical investigation of Steatorrhoea (imaging and endoscopy investigations may also be required). (PABA = p-amino benzoic acid.)

- Intestinal malabsorption may need further anatomical delineation. Ileal disease may require a Schilling test or ^{14}C-radiolabelled glycocholic acid test. Bacterial intestinal overgrowth may require one of the breath tests.

Figure 16.1 gives a summary algorithm for the investigation of steatorrhoea (see also Box 16.1).

Laboratory tests to identify some metabolic complications of malabsorption

Laboratory investigations of plasma can be carried out to identify some of the complications of generalized malabsorption:

- plasma electrolytes may show hypernatraemia and impaired renal function if there is significant water loss,
- plasma potassium and magnesium may reveal the presence of hypokalaemia and hypomagnesaemia,

> **Box 16.1 Some causes of malabsorption**
>
> *Luminal phase abnormalities*
> Abnormal hydrolysis of nutrients:
>   pancreatic insufficiency
>   rapid gut transit
>   enzyme inactivation by gastric hypersecretion
>   enzyme deficiencies, e.g. enterokinase or trypsin
>   decreased bile acid secretion, e.g. hepatic disease, biliary obstruction
>   intestinal stasis, e.g. scleroderma, obstruction, blind loops
> Abnormal luminal processing:
>   bacterial overgrowth
>   lack of intrinsic factor, e.g. vitamin B_{12} deficiency
>
> *Mucosal phase abnormalities*
> Brush-border abnormality, e.g. lactase or sucrase-isomaltase deficiency
> Glucose–galactose malabsorption, Hartnup disease
> Acquired defects:
>   gut resection
>   poor absorbing surface, e.g. coeliac disease, sprue, radiation damage, gut infiltrations such as lymphoma
>   infection such as acquired immunodeficiency syndrome, giardiasis, Whipple's disease
>
> *Post-absorptive phase abnormalities*
> Lymphatic obstruction, e.g. intestinal lymphangiectasia
> Lymphoma
> Protein-losing enteropathy

Other gastrointestinal conditions in which biochemical tests may be useful

Purgative or laxative abuse

Some individuals abuse purgatives and laxatives, and may have psychiatric problems, including Munchausen syndrome. Stool samples can be screened for purgatives such as senna or phenolphthalein by thin layer chromatography. Also look out for associated hypokalaemia due to gastrointestinal potassium loss resulting from this (see Chapter 5).

Diarrhoea fluid can be classified into two types: osmotic and secretory. The former could be due to lactose intolerance, or osmotic laxatives containing magnesium or lactulose. The latter could be the result of infections, inflammatory bowel disease, carcinoid syndrome or VIPoma, to name but a few. The osmolality of faecal water can be calculated from:

$$2\ [\text{sodium} + \text{potassium}] \qquad (16.1)$$

If the measured osmolality is greater than the calculated osmolality, an osmotically active constituent is likely to be present, suggestive of osmotic diarrhoea (see Chapter 2).

Helicobacter pylori infection

Helicobacter pylori is found in up to 50 per cent of European adults. It has gained importance recently as it is associated with peptic ulcer, gastric adenocarcinoma and non-Hodgkin's lymphoma of the stomach. There are many laboratory tests for this organism, including microscopy, bacterial culture and the direct urease test using gastric mucosa biopsies. Non-invasive tests include blood, stool or saliva IgG antibody studies to detect *Helicobacter pylori* infection, or breath tests that look at labelled carbon, which is released by this urea-splitting organism. The latter test is useful in determining whether the organism has been eradicated.

Inflammatory bowel disease

In inflammatory bowel disease such as Crohn's disease elevated faecal calprotectin may occur. Calprotectin is a calcium-binding protein secreted by neutrophils.

Colorectal carcinoma

Colorectal carcinoma is one of the most prevalent cancers. Screening has been shown to reduce mortality, but direct visualization by colonoscopy is invasive, costly and requires skilled personnel.

At present, faecal occult blood tests are being used for screening purposes, as the tumour often releases blood

- there may sometimes be a metabolic acidosis, which may be due to D-lactic acidosis (if bacterial overgrowth), or a hyperchloraemic acidosis (see Chapter 4).

Investigations may also reveal the following.

- Anaemia: haematological investigations such as ferritin, folate and vitamin B_{12}.
- Rickets/osteomalacia: plasma calcium with albumin, phosphate and alkaline phosphatase activity.
- Abnormal bleeding (vitamin K deficiency): clotting studies such as prolonged prothrombin time.
- Low plasma immunoglobulin (hypogammaglobulinaemia) or low plasma cholesterol (hypocholesterolaemia) concentrations.

into the gastrointestinal tract. This can be observed by point of care testing or laboratory tests that analyse the blood in small faecal samples. However, false positives can occur in people with a high meat intake.

Future screening tests may look at altered faecal DNA derived from the tumour. Plasma carcinoembryonic antigen can be used to monitor the treatment of colorectal carcinoma. (See Chapter 24 for tumour markers.)

Tumours of the enteropancreatic system secreting gut hormones

(It is suggested that this section is read in conjunction with Chapter 24.) These tumours are very rare. They are usually found in the pancreatic islets and cause well-recognized clinical and pathological syndromes.

Gastrinomas

Gastrinomas, usually in the pancreatic islets, secrete large quantities of gastrin despite high gastric hydrogen ion levels, and may cause the Zollinger–Ellison syndrome. About 60 per cent of gastrinomas are malignant. Of the remaining 40 per cent, only about a third (13 per cent of the total) are single, resectable adenomas, the rest being multiple. The very high rate of gastric acid secretion causes ulceration in the stomach and proximal small intestine with severe diarrhoea; inhibition of pancreatic lipase activity by the low pH may cause steatorrhoea. This syndrome may be associated with benign, and usually non-functioning, adenomas elsewhere, for example in the anterior pituitary, parathyroid and thyroid glands and in the adrenal cortex (multiple endocrine neoplasia [MEN1] syndrome). The diagnosis depends on the following.

- Fasting plasma gastrin concentrations are up to 30 times the upper reference limit in Zollinger–Ellison syndrome. Plasma concentrations more than 1000 µg/L with acid hypersecretion strongly support this diagnosis.
  However, high plasma gastrin concentrations may also be caused by hypochlorhydria, for example atrophic gastritis, pernicious anaemia or post-vagotomy. H2 blockers and proton pump inhibitors are usually stopped prior to sampling.
- The Zollinger–Ellison syndrome basal gastric acid output may be more than 15 mmol/hour, with large gastric secretory volumes and gastric pH of less than 2.0.
- In cases in which basal plasma gastrin concentrations are equivocal, the secretin test may be useful. Intravenous secretin (2 units/kg body weight) raises plasma gastrin concentration to more than 200 µg/L within 10 minutes if a gastrinoma is present.

- Imaging techniques such as CT, MRI and endoscopic ultrasound may be useful, and also somatostatin receptor scintigraphy to localize tumours and metastases.

Glucagonomas

Glucagonomas usually arise from the α-cells of the pancreatic islets. The presenting clinical feature is a bullous rash, known as necrolytic migratory erythema, often accompanied by psychiatric disturbances, thromboembolism, glossitis, weight loss, impaired glucose tolerance, anaemia and a raised erythrocyte sedimentation rate. Diagnosis may be confirmed by finding a very high plasma glucagon concentration.

VIPomas

VIPomas are extremely rare tumours, usually of the pancreatic islet cells, that secrete VIP, a hormone that increases intestinal motility. They cause a syndrome in which there is very profuse, watery diarrhoea – the Verner–Morrison or watery diarrhoea, hypokalaemia and achlorhydria syndrome. Plasma concentrations of VIP are high.

LABORATORY INVESTIGATION OF ABDOMINAL PAIN

In some cases, a clinical history and examination with imaging techniques such as abdominal X-ray, ultrasound, CT or even laparotomy may reveal a diagnosis. However, sometimes biochemical tests may help, particularly in the following situations.

- Plasma amylase or lipase concentration may be raised in acute pancreatitis (see Chapter 18).
- Gallstones may present with abnormal liver function tests, in particular plasma bilirubin and alkaline phosphatase. They may sometimes be associated with jaundice (see Chapter 17).
- Diabetes ketoacidosis can present with an acute abdomen and therefore hyperglycaemia and urinary ketones are present (see Chapter 12).
- Hypercalcaemia is another cause of abdominal pain (see Chapter 6).
- Severe hypokalaemia can evoke a paralytic ileus and intestinal obstruction (see Chapter 5).
- Sickle-cell disease or crisis can be investigated by haemoglobin studies for HbS.

- Acute porphyria can present as an acute abdomen (see Chapter 21).
- Addison's disease can present as an adrenal crisis (see Chapter 8).
- Heavy metal poisoning, for example lead, can cause abdominal pain (see Chapter 21).
- Ectopic pregnancy can be detected by a raised concentration of plasma β-human chorionic gonadotrophin (see Chapter 10).
- Raised plasma C-reactive protein concentration may indicate sepsis, but may also occur in inflammatory bowel disease such as Crohn's disease (see Chapter 19).

Clinical biochemistry laboratory tests can also be used in the management of abdominal pain, for example postoperatively. Plasma urea and electrolytes and creatinine as well as chloride and bicarbonate concentrations are useful, particularly if intravenous fluids are given or an acid–base disturbance is suspected.

CONCLUSIONS

- The routine hospital chemical pathology laboratory has a role in the investigation of gastrointestinal disorders but the tests carried out in the laboratory do not replace more specialized invasive tests such as endoscopy or radiology.
- Normal intestinal, hepatic and pancreatic function is essential for digestion and absorption.
- The gut is not merely an absorbing surface, but also secretes hormones and is controlled by both humoral and neural pathways.
- Malabsorption can be due to various pathologies, which should be sought and which can present as abdominal discomfort, weight loss and steatorrhoea. Vitamin deficiencies may result, as can hypoalbuminaemia and hypogammaglobulinaemia.
- Acute pancreatitis is a potentially lethal condition; its diagnosis is supported by the presence of elevated plasma amylase or lipase.
- Intestinal failure, for example gastrointestinal fistula or short gut, can result in severe fluid loss and electrolyte disturbance.
- Abdominal pain is common and some of its causes are biochemical.
- The gastrointestinal tract is the source of various tumours, the diagnosis and treatment of which can be assisted by biochemical tests.

17 LIVER DISORDERS AND GALLSTONES

Functions of the liver	250	Bile and gallstones	263
Biochemical tests for liver disease	253	Investigation of suspected liver disease	264
Diseases of the liver	255		

This chapter looks at the chemical pathology of liver and gall bladder disorders. These are common in clinical practice, and liver function tests constitute one of the most frequently requested clinical biochemistry laboratory profiles.

FUNCTIONS OF THE LIVER

The liver has essential synthetic and excretory functions and can be thought of as a large 'metabolic factory'. It also detoxifies and, like the kidneys, excretes the end products of metabolism. The main blood supply to the liver is via the portal vein. The liver is made up of hexagonal lobules of cells (Fig. 17.1). Rows of hepatocytes radiate from the central hepatic vein and are separated by sinusoidal spaces, along the walls of which are interspersed hepatic macrophages, the Kupffer cells. These phagocytic cells are part of the reticuloendothelial system and have an important detoxifying function. At the corners of each lobule are the portal tracts that contain branches of the hepatic artery, the portal vein and bile ducts. Blood flows from the portal tracts towards the central hepatic vein. Therefore:

- hypoxia and toxins that are metabolized in the liver cause damage to the centrilobular area first;
- toxins that do not depend on hepatic metabolism primarily affect the periphery of the lobule.

Almost all nutrients from the gastrointestinal tract pass through the sinusoidal spaces prior to entering the systemic circulation. The hepatic architecture may be disturbed in cirrhosis (fibrosis).

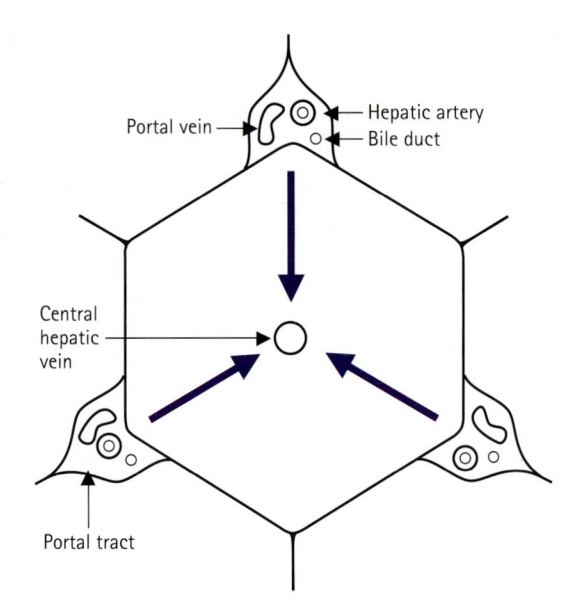

Fig. 17.1 Diagrammatic representation of a cross-section of a hepatic lobule showing the relation between the central hepatic vein and the portal tracts. Blood flows towards the central vein, as indicated by the arrows.

General metabolic functions

When the glucose concentration is high in the portal vein, it is converted to glycogen and the carbon skeletons of fatty acids, which are transported to adipose tissue as very low-density lipoprotein (VLDL). During fasting, the systemic plasma glucose concentration is maintained by the breakdown of glycogen (glycogenolysis) or by the synthesis of glucose from substrates such as glycerol, lactate and amino acids (gluconeogenesis). Fatty acids reaching the liver from fat stores may be metabolized in the tricarboxylic acid cycle, converted to ketones or incorporated into triglycerides (see Chapter 13).

Synthetic functions

Hepatocytes synthesize:

- *plasma proteins*, excluding immunoglobulins and complement,
- most *coagulation factors*, including fibrinogen and factors II (prothrombin), V, VII, IX, X, XI, XII and XIII. Of these, prothrombin (II) and factors VII, IX and X cannot be synthesized without vitamin K,
- *primary bile acids*,
- the *lipoproteins*, such as VLDL and high-density lipoprotein (HDL) (see Chapter 13).

The liver has a very large functional reserve. Deficiencies in synthetic function can only be detected if liver disease is extensive. Before a fall in plasma albumin concentration is attributed to advanced liver disease, extrahepatic causes must be excluded, such as the loss of protein through the kidney, gut or skin, or across capillary membranes into the interstitial space, as in even mild inflammation or infection (see Chapter 19).

Prothrombin levels, assessed by measuring the prothrombin time, may be reduced because of impaired hepatic synthesis, whether due to failure to absorb vitamin K or to hepatocellular damage. If hepatocellular function is adequate, parenteral administration of vitamin K may reverse the abnormality.

Excretion and detoxification

The excretion of bilirubin is considered in more detail below. Other substances that are inactivated and excreted by the liver include the following.

- *Cholesterol*, which is excreted in the bile either unchanged or after conversion to bile acids.
- *Amino acids*, which are deaminated in the liver. Amino groups, and the ammonia produced by intestinal bacterial action and absorbed into the portal vein, are converted to urea.
- *Steroid hormones*, which are metabolized and inactivated by conjugation with glucuronate and sulphate and excreted in the urine in these water-soluble forms.
- Many *drugs*, which are metabolized and inactivated by enzymes of the endoplasmic reticulum system; some are excreted in the bile.
- *Toxins*, the reticuloendothelial Kupffer cells in the hepatic sinusoids are well placed to extract toxic substances that have been absorbed from the gastro-intestinal tract.

Efficient excretion of the end products of metabolism and of bilirubin depends on:

- normally functioning liver cells,
- normal blood flow through the liver,
- patent biliary ducts.

Formation and excretion of bilirubin
(Fig. 17.2)

At the end of their lifespan, red blood cells are broken down by the reticuloendothelial system, mainly in the spleen. The released haemoglobin is split into globin, which enters the general protein pool, and haem, which is converted to bilirubin after the removal of iron, which is re-used (see Chapter 21).

About 80 per cent of bilirubin is derived from haem within the reticuloendothelial system. Other sources include the breakdown of immature red cells in the bone marrow and of compounds chemically related to haemoglobin, such as myoglobin and the cytochromes. Less than 300 µmol of bilirubin is produced daily from the breakdown of erythrocytes, whilst the normal liver is able to conjugate up to about 1 mmol/day, and therefore hyperbilirubinaemia is an insensitive index of parenchymal hepatic disease.

Bilirubin is normally transported to the liver bound to albumin. In this form it is called unconjugated bilirubin, which is lipid soluble and therefore, if not protein bound, can cross cell membranes, including those forming the blood–brain barrier. In this form it is potentially toxic; however, at physiological concentrations it is all protein bound.

In the adult, about 300 µmol per day of bilirubin reaches the liver, where it is transferred from plasma albumin, through the permeable vascular sinusoidal membrane. The hepatocytes can process a much greater load than this. Bilirubin is bound to ligandin (Y protein). From there it is actively transported to the smooth endoplasmic reticulum, where it is conjugated with glucuronate by a process catalysed by uridine diphosphate glucuronyl transferase.

Bilirubin monoglucuronide passes to the canalicular surfaces of the hepatocytes, where, after the addition of a second glucuronate molecule, it is secreted by active processes into the bile canaliculi. This process is largely dependent on the active secretion of bile acids from

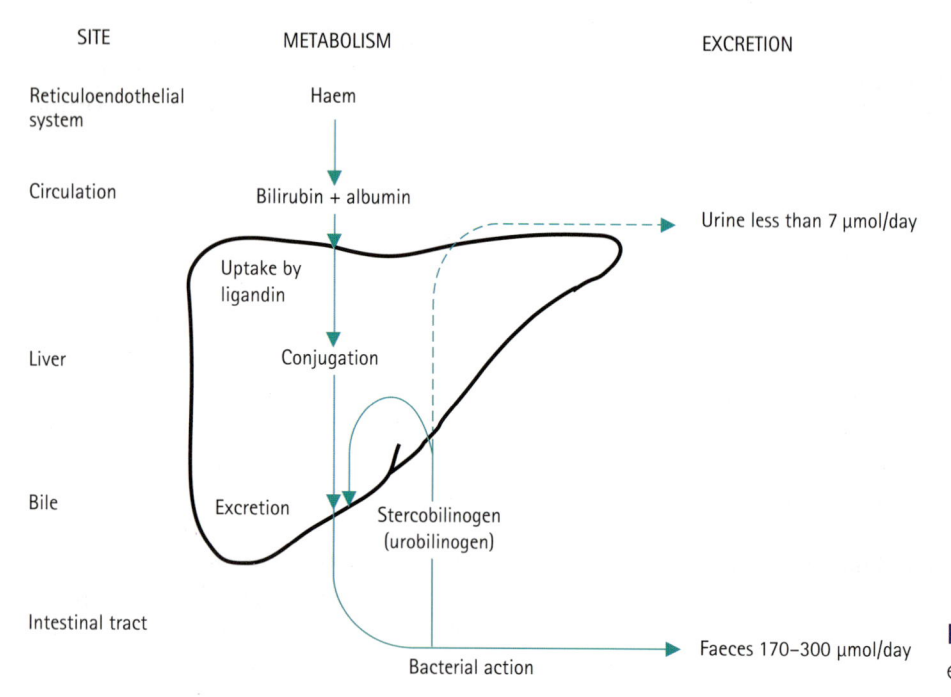

Fig. 17.2 Metabolism and excretion of bilirubin.

hepatocytes. These energy-dependent steps are the ones most likely to be impaired by liver damage (hypoxia and septicaemia) and by increased pressure in the biliary tract. Other anions, including drugs, may compete for binding to ligandin, thus impairing bilirubin conjugation and excretion. Novobiocin inhibits glucuronyl transferase, thus exacerbating unconjugated hyperbilirubinaemia.

Bilirubin is often assayed by the Van den Bergh reaction, which allows conjugated (direct-reacting) and unconjugated (indirect-reacting) bilirubin to be distinguished.

Bilirubin metabolism and jaundice

Jaundice usually becomes clinically apparent when the plasma bilirubin concentration reaches about 50 μmol/L (hyperbilirubinaemia), about twice the upper reference limit. It occurs when bilirubin production exceeds the hepatic capacity to excrete it. This may be because:

- an increased rate of bilirubin production exceeds normal excretory capacity of the liver (prehepatic jaundice);
- the normal load of bilirubin cannot be conjugated and/or excreted by damaged liver cells (hepatic jaundice);
- the biliary flow is obstructed, so that conjugated bilirubin cannot be excreted into the intestine and is regurgitated into the systemic circulation (posthepatic jaundice).

Retention of bilirubin in plasma: jaundice

Unconjugated hyperbilirubinaemia occurs if there is:

- a marked increase in the bilirubin load as a result of haemolysis, or of the breakdown of large amounts of blood after haemorrhage into the gastrointestinal tract or, for example, under the skin due to extensive bruising; in cases of haemolysis, plasma bilirubin rarely exceeds 75 μmol/L;
- impaired binding of bilirubin to ligandin or impaired conjugation with glucuronate in the liver.

In some pathological conditions, plasma unconjugated bilirubin levels may increase so much that they exceed the protein-binding capacity. The lipid-soluble, unbound bilirubin damages brain cells (kernicterus). This is most likely to occur in newborn, particularly premature, infants in whom the hepatic conjugating mechanisms are immature. In addition, the proportion of unbound, unconjugated bilirubin, and therefore the risk of cerebral damage, increases if:

- plasma albumin concentration is low,
- unconjugated bilirubin is displaced from binding sites, for example by high levels of free fatty acids or drugs such as salicylates or sulphonamides.

Unconjugated bilirubin is normally all protein bound, is not water soluble and therefore cannot be excreted in the urine. Patients with unconjugated hyperbilirubinaemia do not have bilirubinuria ('acholuric jaundice').

Conjugated bilirubinaemia is one of the earliest signs of impaired hepatic excretion. In most cases of jaundice in adults, both conjugated and unconjugated fractions of bilirubin are increased in plasma but conjugated bilirubin predominates. Conjugated bilirubin is water soluble, is less strongly protein bound than the unconjugated form, and therefore can be excreted in the urine. Bilirubinuria is always pathological. Dark urine may be an early sign of some forms of hepatobiliary disease.

Conjugated bilirubin enters the gut lumen in bile; it is broken down by bacteria in the distal ileum and the colon into a group of products known as stercobilinogen (faecal urobilinogen). Some is absorbed into the portal circulation, most of which is re-excreted in bile (enterohepatic circulation). A small amount enters the systemic circulation and is excreted in the urine as urobilinogen, which can be oxidized to a coloured pigment, urobilin.

Urobilinogen

Urobilinogen, unlike bilirubin, is often detectable in the urine of normal people by testing with commercial strip tests, particularly if the urine, and therefore the urobilinogen, is concentrated. Urinary urobilinogen concentration is increased in the following situations.

- When haemolysis is very severe: large amounts of bilirubin enter the intestinal lumen and are converted to stercobilinogen. An increased amount of urobilinogen is formed and absorbed. If the hepatic capacity to re-secrete it is exceeded, it is passed in the urine.
- When liver damage impairs re-excretion of normal amounts of urobilinogen into the bile.

The colourless, unabsorbed stercobilinogen is oxidized to stercobilin, a pigment that contributes to the brown colour of faeces. Pale stools may, therefore, suggest biliary obstruction associated with an absence of urinary urobilinogen.

BIOCHEMICAL TESTS FOR LIVER DISEASE

Several biochemical tests comprise what are called the liver function tests. Different tests can give different information about hepatic dysfunction.

Hepatocyte damage

Strictly speaking, changes in plasma enzyme activity generally indicate liver cell membrane damage rather than hepatic function capacity. Because these enzymes are also present in other tissues, changes in plasma activities may reflect damage to those tissues rather than to the liver (see Chapter 18).

Aminotransferases (alanine and aspartate)

A rise in plasma aminotransferase activities is a sensitive indicator of damage to cytoplasmic and/or mitochondrial membranes. Plasma enzyme activities rise when the membranes of only very few cells are damaged. Liver cells contain more aspartate aminotransferase (AST) than alanine aminotransferase (ALT), but ALT is confined to the cytoplasm, in which its concentration is higher than that of AST.

In inflammatory or infective conditions, such as viral hepatitis, the cytoplasmic membrane sustains the main damage; leakage of cytoplasmic contents causes a relatively greater increase in plasma ALT than AST activities.

In infiltrative disorders in which there is damage to both mitochondrial and cytoplasmic membranes, there is a proportionally greater increase in plasma AST than ALT activity.

The relative plasma activities of ALT and AST may help to indicate the type of cell damage. The former is more specific for hepatic disease; AST may be present in skeletal muscle and is more sensitive than ALT.

Raised plasma transaminase concentrations are indicative of hepatocyte damage, but do not necessarily reveal its mechanism. However, aminotransferase levels greater than this suggest primary hepatocyte damage such as drug/toxin-induced or viral hepatitis.

Hepatic synthetic function

The measurement of plasma albumin and prothrombin time may be used to assess function. The hepatic synthetic and secretory capacities are large; only severe and usually prolonged liver disease, for example cirrhosis, demonstrably impairs albumin and prothrombin synthesis.

Albumin

Hypoalbuminaemia is such a common finding in many severe illnesses that it is a less specific indicator of impaired synthetic capacity than a prolonged prothrombin time. A plasma albumin concentration below the lower reference limit may imply hepatic disease chronicity. However, there are many other causes of a low plasma albumin concentration not due to hepatic disease (see Chapter 19).

Table 17.1 Typical biochemical features of certain hepatic disorders

	Plasma albumin	Bilirubin	ALT	ALP	GGT
Acute alcoholic hepatitis	–	↑	↑	↑	↑↑
Acute viral hepatitis	–	↑↑	↑↑	↑	↑↑
Chronic viral hepatitis	– or ↓	↑ or –	↑	↑ or –	↑
Cirrhosis	↓	↑ or –	↑	↑	↑
Gilbert's syndrome	–	↑	–	–	–
Primary biliary cirrhosis	– or ↓	↑↑	↑	↑↑	↑↑
Tumour secondaries	–	↑ or –	↑	↑↑	↑↑

↑ = raised; – = normal; ↓ = reduced.
ALT = alanine aminotransferase; ALP = alkaline phosphatase; GGT = gamma-glutamyltransferase.

Prothrombin time

The prothrombin time may be prolonged due to cholestasis; fat-soluble vitamin K cannot be absorbed normally if fat absorption is impaired due to intestinal bile salt deficiency. The abnormality is then corrected by parenteral administration of the vitamin. A prolonged prothrombin time may also result from severe impairment of synthetic ability if the liver cell mass is greatly reduced; in such cases it is *not* corrected by parenteral administration of vitamin K.

Hepatic excretory function

A high plasma conjugated bilirubin concentration indicates impaired hepatic excretory function; this may be accompanied by a high plasma alkaline phosphatase (ALP) activity, as we will now see. Jaundice has been described above.

Other tests for liver disease

Alkaline phosphatase

Alkaline phosphatase is derived from a number of different tissues, including the liver, the osteoblasts in bone and the placenta. Plasma activities rise in cholestatic liver disease because ALP synthesis is increased and the enzyme within the biliary tract is regurgitated into plasma. A raised ALP concentration in the presence of a raised γ-glutamyltransferase (GGT) concentration implies that the ALP is of hepatic origin.

Gamma-glutamyltransferase

Gamma-glutamyltransferase is an enzyme derived from the endoplasmic reticulum of the cells of the hepatobiliary tract. As this reticulum proliferates, for example in response to the prolonged intake of alcohol and of drugs such as phenobarbitone and phenytoin, synthesis of the enzyme is induced and plasma GGT activity increases. Therefore, raised plasma activities do not necessarily indicate hepatocellular damage, but may reflect enzyme induction.

Biochemical tests can be used to investigate hepatic disorders, the mechanisms underlying which can be divided into three main groups; these often coexist, but one usually predominates in any particular condition (Table 17.1).

- Liver-cell damage is characterized by the release of enzymes (AST and ALT) from damaged hepatocytes. Plasma ALT and AST activities are increased.
- Cholestasis is characterized by retention of conjugated bilirubin and of ALP, and by increased ALP synthesis at the sinusoidal surface. Plasma conjugated bilirubin levels and ALP activities are increased.
- Reduced mass of hepatocytes, if considerable, is characterized by a reduction in albumin and prothrombin synthesis. The plasma albumin concentration is reduced and the prothrombin time is prolonged.

Urine tests useful in suspected hepatic disease

Fresh urine analysis may confirm the presence of bilirubin (conjugated hyperbilirubinaemia) and urobilinogen.

Ictostix includes stabilized, diazotized 2,4-dichloraniline, which reacts with bilirubin to form azobilirubin. These reagents are incorporated in multiple test sticks. The test will detect about 3 μmol/L of *bilirubin*. Drugs, such as large doses of chlorpromazine, may give false-positive results.

Urobilistix includes paradimethylaminobenzaldehyde, also incorporated in multiple test sticks, which reacts with *urobilinogen*. Urobilistix does not react with porphobilinogen. This test will detect urobilinogen in urine from some normal subjects. False-positive results may occur after taking drugs such as *p*-aminosalicylic acid and some sulphonamides.

Bile acid measurement in obstetric cholestasis

Raised total plasma bile acid concentrations in the third trimester of pregnancy associated with pruritus are suggestive of obstetric cholestasis, which can lead to both maternal and fetal morbidity and mortality. Elevation of plasma ALT concentration may follow the increase in the concentration of plasma bile salts (see Chapter 10).

New hepatic function tests

Due to the very large hepatic reserve, tests for impairment of metabolic (including synthetic and secretory) function are relatively insensitive indicators of liver disease.

There are a number of new tests that are being devised to improve the accuracy of the diagnosis of hepatic disorders. Tests of hepatocellular activity have been proposed, such as galactose elimination capacity, the aminopyrine breath test, indocyanine green clearance, and monoethylglycinexylidide production. All these tests are indirect measures of hepatic activity that rely on measuring compounds or their metabolites after they have been acted on by the liver. As yet, they do not have a place in routine clinical diagnosis.

DISEASES OF THE LIVER

Cholestasis

Cholestasis may be either:

- *intrahepatic*, in which bile secretion from the hepatocytes into the canaliculi is impaired, due to:
  - viral hepatitis,
  - drugs such as chlorpromazine or toxins such as alcohol,
  - inflammation of the biliary tract (cholangitis),
  - autoimmune disease (primary biliary cirrhosis),
  - cystic fibrosis,
- *extrahepatic*, due to obstruction to the flow of bile through the biliary tract by:
  - biliary stones,
  - inflammation of the biliary tract,
  - pressure on the tract from outside by malignant tissue, usually of the head of the pancreas,
  - biliary atresia (rare).

It is essential to distinguish between intrahepatic and extrahepatic causes of cholestasis, as surgery may be indicated for the latter but is usually contraindicated for intrahepatic lesions. The biochemical findings may be similar.

- Bilirubin concentrations in plasma may be normal if only part of the biliary system is involved by intrahepatic lesions such as cholangitis, early primary biliary cirrhosis or primary or secondary tumours. The unaffected areas can secrete bilirubin.
- Alkaline phosphatase activity is a sensitive test for cholestasis. Increased synthesis of ALP in the affected ducts increases the activity of this enzyme in plasma. If this is the only abnormal finding, it must be shown to be of hepatic origin before it is assumed to indicate liver disease.

Patients with prolonged and more widespread cholestasis may present with severe jaundice and pruritus due to the deposition of retained bile salts in the skin; the plasma bilirubin concentration may be more than 800 μmol/L. More rarely, there is bleeding due to malabsorption of vitamin K, with consequent prothrombin deficiency. Cholesterol retention may cause hypercholesterolaemia. Dark urine and pale stools suggest biliary retention of conjugated bilirubin.

The jaundice caused by extrahepatic obstruction due to malignant tissue is typically painless and progressive, but there may be a history of vague persistent back pain and weight loss. By contrast, intraluminal obstruction by a gallstone may cause severe pain, which, like the jaundice, is often intermittent. Gallstones may not always cause such symptoms. If a large stone lodges in the lower end of the common bile duct, the picture may be indistinguishable from that of malignant obstruction.

Although most of the findings are directly attributable to cholestasis, biliary back-pressure may damage hepatocytes, and plasma aminotransferase activities may increase. Unless the cause is clinically obvious, evidence of dilated ducts due to extrahepatic obstruction should be sought using tests such ultrasound, computerized tomography (CT) scanning or cholangiography.

Primary biliary cirrhosis

This is a rare autoimmune disorder that occurs most commonly in middle-aged women. Destruction and proliferation of the bile ducts produce a predominantly cholestatic picture, with pruritus and a plasma ALP activity that may be very high. Jaundice develops late in most patients. Mitochondrial antibodies are detectable in the plasma of more than 90 per cent of cases; the plasma IgM concentration is usually raised. Patients may also manifest

> ### CASE 1
>
> A 52-year-old female was referred to the hepatology clinic because of jaundice, pruritus, hepatomegaly, xanthelasma and the following abnormal liver test results.
>
> *Plasma*
> Bilirubin 93 µmol/L (<20)
> Alanine aminotransferase 111 U/L (<42)
> Alkaline phosphatase 826 U/L (<250)
> Albumin 34 g/L (35–45)
> Gamma-glutamyltransferase 764 U/L (<55)
> She had a positive test result for anti-mitochondrial antibodies.
>
> **DISCUSSION**
> Subsequent studies, including liver biopsy, showed the patient to have primary biliary cirrhosis. Note the predominant cholestatic biochemical picture with raised plasma ALP and GGT concentrations. This condition is associated with hyperlipidaemia, hence the xanthelasma, and is more common in middle-aged females with other autoimmune disorders. There may also be raised plasma IgM concentration and osteoporosis and osteomalacia.

hypercholesterolaemia, xanthelasma (see Chapter 13), other autoimmune disorders and osteoporosis.

Parenteral nutrition

Prolonged parenteral nutrition may be associated with a progressive increase in plasma ALP activity and a subsequent rise in the plasma aminotransferase concentrations. The cause is not known, although biliary sludging may occur and the biochemical changes may return to normal when the parenteral feeding is discontinued. Cyclical parenteral nutrition may help the situation when patients are fed intermittently (see Chapter 14).

Acute hepatitis

The biochemical findings in acute hepatitis are predominantly those of cell membrane damage with an increase in plasma ALT activity greater than that of AST. There may be a superimposed cholestatic picture and, in very severe cases, impaired prothrombin synthesis.

Viral hepatitis

Viral hepatitis may be associated with many viral infections, such as infectious mononucleosis (Epstein–Barr virus), rubella and cytomegalovirus. However, the term is most commonly used to describe three principal types of viral infection in which the clinical features of the acute illness are very similar, although with a different incubation period.

Hepatitis A ('infectious hepatitis'), transmitted by the faecal–oral route as a food-borne infection, is relatively common in schools and other institutions and has an incubation period of between 15 and 45 days. Relapses may occur, but it rarely progresses to chronic hepatitis.

Hepatitis B ('serum hepatitis') is transmitted by blood products and other body fluids; it occurs more sporadically than hepatitis A. It has a longer incubation period, of between 40 and 180 days. Some patients may be anicteric; some may develop fulminant hepatitis or chronic active hepatitis and later cirrhosis and hepatocarcinoma. They may become asymptomatic carriers of the disease.

Hepatitis C (non-A, non-B hepatitis), which may be the result of sexual transmission or the transfusion of blood products, has an incubation period of between 15 and 50 days. It may progress to cirrhosis.

In all types there may be a 3–4-day history of anorexia, nausea and tenderness or discomfort over the liver before the onset of jaundice. Some patients remain anicteric. Plasma aminotransferase activities are very high from the onset of symptoms; they peak about 4 days later, when jaundice becomes detectable, but may remain elevated for several months. Once jaundice appears, some of the initial symptoms improve.

In the early stages there is often a cholestatic element, with pale stools due to reduced intestinal bilirubin, and dark urine due to a rise in plasma conjugated bilirubin concentration; unconjugated bilirubin concentrations also increase due to impaired hepatocellular conjugation.

Plasma bilirubin concentrations rarely exceed 350 µmol/L and the plasma ALP activity is only moderately raised, or even normal. If hepatocellular damage is severe and extensive, the prothrombin time may be increased and, in cases with cholestasis, malabsorption of vitamin K may be a contributory factor.

Serological findings

Testing for viral antigens, or for antibodies synthesized in response to the virus, can be used to diagnose viral hepatitis.

CASE 2

A 22-year-old female intravenous drug addict was referred to the hepatology clinic because of the following abnormal liver test results.

Plasma
Bilirubin 93 μmol/L (<20)
Alanine aminotransferase 761 U/L (<42)
Alkaline phosphatase 306 U/L (<250)
Albumin 44 g/L (35–45)
Gamma-glutamyltransferase 324 U/L (<55)

Urinary bilirubin positive.

Further investigations, including hepatitis screen, showed her to be hepatitis B positive.

DISCUSSION

Note the grossly elevated plasma aminotransferase concentrations, indicative of extensive hepatocyte damage.

Intravenous drug addicts are at increased risk of hepatitis B infection. The urinary bilirubin is positive, as the hyperbilirubinaemia is predominantly conjugated, i.e. water soluble.

Hepatitis A viral (HAV) antibodies of the IgG class are detectable in the plasma of patients at the onset of symptoms. The presence of an IgM anti-HAV antibody is suggestive of previous infection. Most cases of hepatitis A recover completely.

Hepatitis B viral (HBV) infection, during the prodromal illness, can be diagnosed by the presence in the plasma of a viral surface antigen (HB_sAg) and a core antigen (Hb_e), an internal component of the virus. These antigens are short lived. During the next few weeks, an antibody response occurs, with the appearance of plasma antibodies to the viral core (anti-HB_c), to HB_e and finally to the surface antibody (anti-HB_s), which may be used to document previous infection (Fig. 17.3).

The presence of the HB_e antigen correlates with infectivity, and its disappearance is a good prognostic sign; HB_sAg may persist, especially in patients with an impaired immune response, and indicates chronicity associated with raised plasma aminotransferase activities.

Hepatitis C viral (HCV; non-A, non-B hepatitis) infection is often diagnosed by exclusion. Anti-HCV antibodies may be detected in plasma about 12 weeks after exposure to the virus in about 50 per cent of patients.

Alcoholic hepatitis

Alcoholic hepatitis occurs in heavy drinkers, often after a period of increased alcohol intake. Although the clinical features may mimic acute viral hepatitis, the plasma aminotransferase activities and bilirubin concentration are not usually as markedly elevated, although GGT may be.

There is no perfect laboratory marker of alcohol abuse. A raised mean corpuscular red cell volume (MCV), hypertriglyceridaemia, hyperuricaemia and GGT are clues, but are not specific. Increased plasma desialylated or

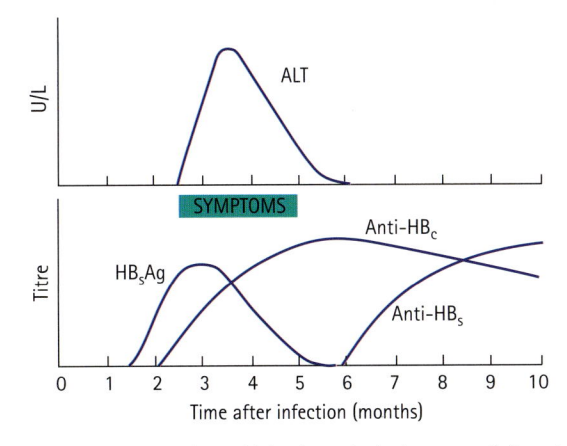

Fig. 17.3 Serological and biochemical changes following infection with hepatitis B virus. (ALT = alanine aminotransferase; HB_sAg = viral surface antigen; Anti HB_c = antibody to the viral core; Anti HB_s = antibody to viral surface.)

carbohydrate-deficient transferrin or raised plasma sialic acid levels have been proposed as markers of alcohol abuse, as sialic acid metabolism may be perturbed in the presence of high concentrations of alcohol. Note that the consumption of more than 80 g a day of alcohol may raise GGT concentration, not necessarily by hepatic damage, but by enzyme induction.

Drugs and other toxins

Various drugs and other toxins are hepatotoxic, sometimes directly and sometimes due to a hypersensitivity reaction; in the latter case, the damage is not dose related. The clinical picture may resemble that of acute viral hepatitis. *A drug history is an essential part of the assessment of a patient presenting with liver disease.* Table 17.2 lists some of these agents.

Table 17.2 Some drug effects on the liver

	Hepatic necrosis	Acute hepatitis-like reaction	Chronic hepatitis	Cholestasis
Carbamazepine				+
Chlorambucil		+		+
Chlorpromazine				+
Cytotoxic drugs	+a			
Erythromycin				+
Ferrous sulphate	+a			
Halothane	+	+		+
Indometacin				+
Isoniazid		+	+	
Methotrexate			+	
Methyldopa	+	+	+	+
Nitrofurantoin		+	+	+
Paracetamol	+a		+	
Phenothiazines				+
Phenylbutazone		+		+
Phenytoin		+		
Salicylate (aspirin)	+a			
17-Alpha-alkylated steroids (oral contraceptives)				+
Statins, e.g. simvastatin		+		
Valproate	+			+

a Indicates that the damage is dose dependent and predictable.

Chronic hepatitis

The finding of persistent, (usually only slightly) raised plasma aminotransferase activities, sometimes with chronic or recurrent symptoms suggesting liver disease, may be due to several disorders. It may be the only abnormal biochemical finding.

Chronic persistent hepatitis

This is a term used to describe the finding of raised plasma aminotransferase activities without clinical signs or symptoms and without a significant change in activity over many years. The activities rarely exceed three times the upper reference limits. Jaundice is unusual.

Chronic active hepatitis

This is caused by active hepatocellular destruction with episodes of relapses and remissions. It may progress to cirrhosis. It occurs at any age, but is most common in women.

It may:

- be associated with, or a consequence of, viral infections such as HBV or HCV or may be drug induced,
- be part of an autoimmune process that sometimes involves more than one organ,
- have no obvious cause.

The earliest findings that differentiate it from chronic persistent hepatitis are an increasing plasma IgG concentration, perhaps detected by a rising plasma γ-globulin concentration, and the presence of smooth muscle and antinuclear antibodies. As the disease progresses, more cells are destroyed and the plasma AST activity may rise to or exceed that of ALT; slight jaundice may develop. If there is significant hepatocellular destruction, the plasma albumin concentration falls.

Cirrhosis

Cirrhosis is the end-result of many inflammatory and metabolic diseases involving the liver, including prolonged

> **CASE 3**
>
> A 50-year-old known alcoholic male attended the general medical clinic because of ascites and the following abnormal liver test results.
>
> *Plasma*
> Bilirubin 52 μmol/L (<20)
> Alanine aminotransferase 76 U/L (<42)
> Alkaline phosphatase 271 U/L (<250)
> Albumin 18 g/L (35–45)
> Gamma-glutamyltransferase 324 U/L (<55)
>
> Urinary bilirubin and protein normal.
>
> **DISCUSSION**
> The abnormal liver test results and hypoalbuminaemia together with ascites supported the diagnosis of cirrhosis, secondary to his alcohol problem. Hypoalbuminaemia may be due to many disorders, such as gross proteinuria, but in the presence of hepatic disease suggests a reduction in hepatic synthetic capacity typical of cirrhosis.

toxic damage usually due to alcohol. In 'cryptogenic cirrhosis', the cause is unknown. The fibrous scar tissue distorts the hepatic architecture, and regenerating nodules of hepatocytes disrupt the blood supply, sometimes increasing the pressure in the portal vein, causing portal hypertension. Blood may be shunted from the portal into the hepatic vein, bypassing the liver.

In the early stages there may be no abnormal biochemical findings. During phases of active cellular destruction, the plasma AST, and sometimes ALT, activities rise. In advanced cases, the biochemical findings are mostly associated with a reduced functioning cell mass. The vascular shunting allows antigenic substances, which have been absorbed from the intestine, to bypass the normal hepatic sinusoidal filtering process, and to stimulate increased synthesis of IgG and IgA, producing the typical serum protein electrophoretic pattern of β-γ fusion (see Chapter 19).

Portal hypertension and impaired lymphatic drainage lead to the accumulation of fluid in the peritoneal cavity (ascites). This may be aggravated by hypoalbuminaemia, which may also cause peripheral oedema. In advanced cirrhosis, the findings of hepatocellular failure develop.

There are a number of causes of ascites including cirrhosis, malignancy or infection, nephrotic syndrome, hypothyroidism, pancreatitis and cardiac failure. Primary hepatocellular carcinoma may develop in a cirrhotic liver.

The Child–Pugh classification system is a way of grading the severity of cirrhosis in the face of portal hypertension (Table 17.3). Survival for grade C is less than one year.

Hepatocellular failure and hepatic encephalopathy

Liver damage severe enough to cause obvious clinical signs of impaired hepatocellular function may be caused by severe hepatitis or advanced cirrhosis, or follow an overdose of a liver toxin such as paracetamol (acetaminophen). The biochemical findings may include any or all of those of acute hepatitis. Jaundice is progressive. In the final stage, the number of hepatocytes, and so the *total* amount of aminotransferases released, may be so reduced that plasma activities fall despite continuing damage to the remaining cells. This finding should not be interpreted as a sign of recovery. Other features may include the following.

Table 17.3 Severity of hepatic failure

Grade	Plasma bilirubin (μmol/L)	Plasma albumin (g/L)	Ascites/ encephalopathy	INR
A	Normal	>35	None	<1.7
B	34–50	28–35	Mild	1.7–2.3
C	>50	<28	Severe	>2.3

- Hypovolaemia and hypotension, which are due to loss of circulating fluid in ascites and in the oedema fluid formed because of hypoalbuminaemia, and which may be aggravated by vomiting. The resultant low renal blood flow may have two consequences:
  - secondary hyperaldosteronism, causing electrolyte disturbances, especially hypokalaemia, and sometimes dilutional hyponatraemia;
  - renal circulatory insufficiency, causing oliguria, a high plasma creatinine concentration and uraemia despite reduced urea synthesis.
- Impaired hepatic deamination of amino acids, causing accumulation of amino acids in plasma with overflow amino-aciduria and sometimes hyperammonaemia. If the reduced formation of urea from amino acids is not balanced by renal retention due to

the decrease in glomerular filtration rate (GFR), the plasma urea concentration may be low.
- Impairment of hepatic gluconeogenesis may cause hypoglycaemia.

Treatment of end-stage liver disease

Liver transplantation may be the only possible treatment for end-stage liver disease. Complications include graft failure, hepatic artery thrombosis, infection and acute and chronic rejection. Both acute rejection (which occurs in up to 80 per cent of recipients) and chronic rejection (occurring in about 10 per cent of cases) are associated with a rise in plasma bilirubin concentration and ALP activity; chronic rejection may be irreversible. The indications for hepatic transplantation may include prolonged prothrombin time and plasma bilirubin more than 300 μmol/L.

Hepatic infiltration and malignant disease

Invasion of the liver by secondary carcinoma, or infiltration by lymphoma or granulomas such as sarcoidosis, may be associated with abnormal biochemical tests. Sometimes the only abnormal finding is raised plasma AST activity; the ALT concentration may also be raised to a lesser extent or there may be GGT concentration elevation. The picture may reflect cholestasis, with or without jaundice.

Metabolic function is rarely demonstrably impaired. If a primary hepatocellular carcinoma develops, either in a cirrhotic liver or de novo, the plasma aminotransferase and ALP activities usually rise rapidly, and plasma α-fetoprotein concentrations are often very high; this latter finding is *not* diagnostic of primary hepatic malignancy (see Chapter 24).

Metabolic liver disease

A group of rare metabolic disorders, most of which are inherited, is associated with liver disease, especially cirrhosis.

Haemochromatosis

Idiopathic haemochromatosis is a genetically determined disorder in which slightly increased intestinal absorption of iron over many years produces large iron deposits of parenchymal distribution, including the liver (see Chapter 21).

Alpha$_1$-antitrypsin deficiency

Alpha$_1$-antitrypsin deficiency (see Chapter 19) is associated with neonatal hepatitis that progresses to cirrhosis in childhood. Often there is basal emphysema.

Galactosaemia

This autosomal recessive disorder, due most commonly to a deficiency of galactose-1-phosphate uridyltransferase, may cause cirrhosis of the liver if untreated. Liver transplantation may be indicated if hepatocellular carcinoma, a complication of cirrhosis, develops (see Chapter 27).

Wilson's disease

This is a rare, recessively inherited disorder caused by reduced biliary excretion of copper and by impaired hepatic incorporation of copper into caeruloplasmin. The symptoms are due to the excessive accumulation of copper in the liver, brain and kidneys and present with evidence of acute liver failure, chronic hepatitis or cirrhosis in children or in young adults (see also Chapter 14).

CASE 4

A 70-year-old male with known colonic carcinoma, operated on 2 years previously, was found by his general practitioner to have the following liver test results.

Plasma
Bilirubin 33 μmol/L (<20)
Alanine aminotransferase 62 U/L (<42)
Alkaline phosphatase 408 U/L (<250)
Albumin 35 g/L (35–45)
Gamma-glutamyltransferase 527 U/L (<55)

Urinary bilirubin negative.

An abdominal ultrasound scan showed multiple space-occupying lesions within the liver.

DISCUSSION

The patient was eventually found to have widespread hepatic secondaries from his colonic tumour and died a few months later. The combination of raised plasma ALP and GGT concentrations is suggestive of hepatic space-occupying lesions, particularly in the absence of major cholestasis.

Reye's syndrome

This rare disorder presents as acute hepatitis, associated with marked encephalopathy, severe metabolic acidosis and hypoglycaemia in children typically between the ages of 3 and about 12 years. There is acute fatty infiltration of the liver. The plasma aminotransferase activities are high, but plasma bilirubin levels are only slightly raised.

The aetiology is uncertain, but the condition may be precipitated by viral infections, such as influenza A or B, drugs such as salicylates and sodium valproate, and certain toxins; it has been recommended that children should not be given aspirin. One possible mechanism is that there is uncoupling of mitochondrial oxidative phosphorylation. A number of inherited metabolic disorders, particularly those involving fatty acid oxidation, may present with a Reye-like syndrome in children under the age of about 3 years.

Non-alcoholic steatotic hepatitis or fatty liver

Non-alcoholic steatotic hepatitis (NASH) is associated with insulin resistance (see Chapter 12). The concentration of plasma aminotransferases is usually raised and may relate to body mass index. In some cases, NASH may lead to fibrosis and cirrhosis. It is important to exclude other liver disorders, and hepatic ultrasound may show increased echogenicity. The biochemical features of NASH may improve with dietary measures and treatment of hyperlipidaemia (see Chapter 13).

Hepatorenal syndrome

This syndrome occurs when cirrhosis presents in conjunction with renal dysfunction. It is thought to be due to impaired renal perfusion due to vasoconstriction of renal arteries. Usually the creatinine clearance is less than 40 mL/min, plasma creatinine is greater than about 150 μmol/L, with a urine volume of less than 500 mL/day and urinary sodium less than 10 mmol/L.

Haemolytic jaundice

There are many causes of haemolysis, including sickle-cell anaemia, thalassaemia and spherocytosis, and it can also be drug or autoimmune induced. In adults, unconjugated hyperbilirubinaemia is usually mild because of the large reserve of hepatic secretory capacity. The plasma bilirubin concentration is usually less than 70 μmol/L. Erythrocytes contain a high concentration of AST and lactate dehydrogenase (LD1 and LD2) (see Chapter 18). Blood reticulocytes may be raised, with abnormal blood film and low plasma haptoglobin concentration. A haemolytic component may be seen in alcoholic hepatitis known as Zieve's syndrome. Urinary bilirubin concentration is usually not raised in haemolysis (acholuric jaundice).

Jaundice in the newborn

Red-cell destruction, together with immature hepatic processing of bilirubin, may cause a high plasma level of unconjugated bilirubin in the newborn; so-called physiological jaundice is common. Normal full-term babies may show jaundice between days 2 and 8 of life.

Physiological jaundice rarely exceeds 100 μmol/L. Jaundice on the first day of life is invariably pathological, as are levels of bilirubin exceeding the aforementioned limits or if the hyperbilirubinaemia is conjugated. As a result of haemolytic disease, the plasma concentration of unconjugated bilirubin may be as high as 500 μmol/L and may exceed the plasma protein-binding capacity; free unconjugated bilirubin may be deposited in the brain, causing kernicterus. Neonatal jaundice and its treatment are discussed more fully in Chapter 26.

The inherited hyperbilirubinaemias

There is a group of inherited disorders in which either unconjugated or conjugated hyperbilirubinaemia is the only detectable abnormality.

Unconjugated hyperbilirubinaemia

Gilbert's syndrome

This is a relatively common (3–7 per cent of the population) familial condition, which may be present at any age but usually develops after the second decade. Plasma unconjugated bilirubin concentrations are usually between 20 μmol/L and 40 μmol/L and rarely exceed 80 μmol/L. They fluctuate, and may rise during intercurrent illness, dehydration, menstruation and fasting. The condition is probably harmless but must be differentiated from haemolysis and liver disease. It often becomes evident when plasma bilirubin concentrations fail to return to normal after an attack of hepatitis, or during any mild illness, which, because of the jaundice, may be misdiagnosed as hepatitis.

Mutations in the hepatic uridine diphosphate glucoronyl transferase (UGT) gene have been observed. Hepatic UGT activity is decreased to approximately 30 per cent of normal in individuals with Gilbert's syndrome. Decreased activity

> **CASE 5**
>
> A healthy 43-year-old male, on no medication, had the following results of tests performed during a private healthcare screening programme.
>
> *Plasma*
> Bilirubin 43 μmol/L (<20)
> Unconjugated bilirubin 36 μmol/L (<5)
> Alanine aminotransferase 21 U/L (<42)
> Alkaline phosphatase 126 U/L (<250)
> Albumin 40 g/L (35–45)
> Gamma-glutamyltransferase 24 U/L (<55)
>
> Urinary bilirubin negative.
> Normal full blood count, reticulocytes and blood film.
>
> **DISCUSSION**
> The raised concentration of plasma bilirubin is predominantly unconjugated. There is no evidence of haemolysis and the other liver function tests are normal. A likely diagnosis is of Gilbert's syndrome. This is a common condition and its diagnosis is based on the exclusion of liver disease and haemolysis in the presence of a modest concentration of unconjugated hyperbilirubinaemia.

has been attributed to an expansion of thymine–adenine (TA) repeats in the promoter region of the *UGT-1A1* gene, the principal gene encoding this enzyme.

Diagnosis of Gilbert's syndrome is by exclusion of haemolysis and other hepatic disorders. Prolonged fasting (48 hours with calories restricted to 300 kcal/day) may result in an increase of plasma bilirubin concentration by 90 per cent, with unconjugated bilirubin concentration increasing by about 110 per cent if Gilbert's syndrome is present. Increases are also seen after the administration of 50 mg intravenous nicotinic acid. However, these dynamic tests are not without side-effects and are rarely used.

Crigler–Najjar syndrome

This is due to a rare deficiency of hepatic UGT, and is a more serious condition. It usually presents at birth. The plasma unconjugated bilirubin may increase to concentrations that exceed the binding capacity of albumin and so cause kernicterus. The defect may be *complete* (Type I) and inherited as an autosomal recessive condition or, *partial* (Type II) and inherited as an autosomal dominant condition.

In Type II drugs that induce enzyme synthesis, such as phenobarbitone, may reduce plasma bilirubin concentration.

Conjugated hyperbilirubinaemia

Dubin–Johnson syndrome

This is probably harmless and is due to defective excretion of conjugated bilirubin, but not of bile acids. It is characterized by slightly raised plasma conjugated bilirubin levels that tend to fluctuate. Because the bilirubin is conjugated, it may be detectable in the urine. Plasma

> **Box 17.1 Some of the causes of jaundice**
>
> *Conjugated hyperbilirubinaemia*
> Drugs, e.g. see Table 17.2
> Infections, e.g. hepatitis, cytomegalovirus, Epstein–Barr virus, sepsis
> Damage to bile ducts, e.g. primary biliary cirrhosis, sclerosing cholangitis
> Alcohol, haemochromatosis, Wilson's disease
> Gallstones, cholangiocarcinoma, bile duct strictures, pancreas tumours
> Metabolic disorders, e.g. α_1-antitrypsin, Reye's syndrome, fatty liver, pregnancy liver
> Diffusion infiltration, e.g. sarcoid, lymphoma, amyloid
> Inborn errors, e.g. Dubin–Johnson syndrome, Rotor syndrome
>
> *Unconjugated hyperbilirubinaemia*
> Physiological jaundice of the newborn
> Gilbert's syndrome
> Crigler–Najjar syndrome
> Haemolysis

ALP activities are normal. There may be hepatomegaly and the liver is dark brown in appearance due to the presence of a pigment with the staining properties of lipofuscin. The diagnosis may be confirmed by the characteristic staining of a specimen obtained by liver biopsy.

Rotor syndrome

Rotor syndrome is similar in most respects to the Dubin–Johnson syndrome, but the liver cells are not pigmented (Box 17.1).

BILE AND GALLSTONES

Bile acids and bile salts

Four bile acids are produced in humans. Two of these, cholic acid and chenodeoxycholic acid, are synthesized in the liver from cholesterol and are called primary bile acids. They are secreted in bile as sodium salts, conjugated with the amino acid glycine or taurine (primary bile salts). These are converted by bacteria within the intestinal lumen to the secondary bile salts, deoxycholate and lithocholate, respectively (Fig. 17.4).

Secondary bile salts are partly absorbed from the terminal ileum and colon and are re-excreted by the liver (enterohepatic circulation of bile salts). Therefore bile contains a mixture of primary and secondary bile salts.

Deficiency of bile salts in the intestinal lumen leads to impaired micelle formation and malabsorption of fat (see Chapter 13). Such deficiency may be caused by cholestatic liver disease (failure of bile salts to reach the intestinal lumen) or by ileal resection or disease (failure of reabsorption causing a reduced bile-salt pool).

Formation of bile

Between 1 L and 2 L of bile are produced daily by the liver. This hepatic bile contains bilirubin, bile salts, phospholipids and cholesterol, as well as electrolytes in concentrations similar to those in plasma. Small amounts of protein are also present.

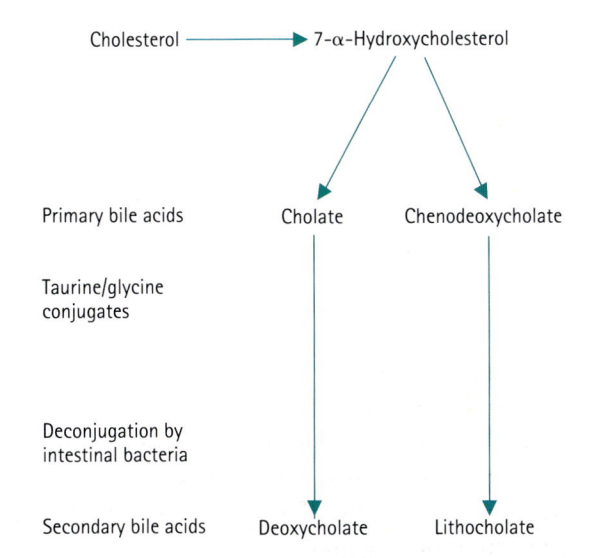

Fig. 17.4 Synthesis of bile acids in the liver and their conversion to secondary bile salts in the intestine.

In the gall bladder there is active reabsorption of sodium, chloride and bicarbonate, together with an isosmotic amount of water. Consequently, gall bladder bile is ten times more concentrated than hepatic bile; sodium is the major cation and bile salts the major anions. The concentrations of other non-absorbable molecules, such as conjugated bilirubin, cholesterol and phospholipids, also increase.

Gallstones

Although most gallstones contain all biliary constituents they consist predominantly of one. Only about 10 per cent contain enough calcium to be radio-opaque and in this way differ from renal calculi.

Pigment stones

Pigment stones are found in such chronic haemolytic states as hereditary spherocytosis. Increased breakdown of haemoglobin increases bilirubin formation and therefore biliary secretion. The stones consist mostly of bile pigments, with variable amounts of calcium. They are small, hard and dark green or black, and are usually multiple. Rarely, they contain enough calcium to be radio-opaque.

Cholesterol stones

Cholesterol is most likely to precipitate if bile is supersaturated with it; further precipitation on a nucleus of crystals causes progressive enlargement. Not all patients with a high biliary cholesterol concentration suffer from bile stones. Changes in the relative concentrations of different bile salts may favour precipitation. The stones may be single or multiple. They are described as mulberry-like and are either white or yellowish; the cut surface appears crystalline.

There is no clear association between hypercholesterolaemia and the formation of cholesterol gallstones, although both may be more common in obese individuals. However, there may be an increased incidence in patients taking some lipid-lowering drugs, such as the fibric acid derivatives.

Mixed stones

Most gallstones contain a mixture of bile constituents, usually with a cholesterol nucleus as a starting point. They are multiple, faceted, dark-brown stones with a hard shell and a softer centre and may contain enough calcium to be radio-opaque.

Consequences of gallstones

Gallstones may remain silent for an indefinite length of time and be discovered only at laparotomy for an unrelated condition. They may, however, lead to various clinical consequences.

- *Biliary colic.*
- *Acute cholecystitis*: obstruction of the cystic duct by a gallstone causes chemical irritation of the gall bladder mucosa by trapped bile and secondary bacterial infection.
- *Chronic cholecystitis* may also be associated with gallstones.
- *Obstruction of the common bile duct* occurs if a stone lodges in it. The patient may present with biliary colic, obstructive jaundice (Table 17.4), which is usually intermittent, or acute pancreatitis if the pancreatic duct is also occluded.
- Rarely, gallstones may be associated with *gallstone ileus* or *carcinoma of the gall bladder*.

Treatment of gallstones

The commonest treatment for symptomatic gallstones is cholecystectomy, either open or laparoscopic. The following are some alternative approaches.

- *Dissolving the gallstone*: the bile acid ursodeoxycholic acid reduces the relative saturation of bile with cholesterol and so facilitates dissolving cholesterol stones, particularly small, uncalcified ones.
- *Shock-wave lithotripsy*: the stone is shattered into tiny fragments and can then pass through the cystic duct.

Table 17.4 Some causes of obstructive jaundice or cholestasis

Dilated ducts/ mechanical obstruction (extrahepatic)	Undilated ducts/non-mechanical obstruction (intrahepatic)
Gallstones	Primary biliary cirrhosis
Pancreatic carcinoma	Primary sclerosing cholangitis
Pancreatic duct stricture	Cholestatic drug reaction
Cholangiocarcinoma	
Parasite infections	

INVESTIGATION OF SUSPECTED LIVER DISEASE

The commonly available biochemical laboratory tests for the diagnosis of liver disease involve the measurement of plasma levels of:

- bilirubin – excretory function,
- aminotransferases (ALT and/or AST) – hepatocellular damage,
- alkaline phosphatase – cholestasis,
- albumin and/or prothrombin time – synthetic function,
- gamma-glutamyltransferase – enzyme induction or hepatocellular damage.

The initial selection of investigations depends on the age of the patient, the history and clinical features.

Jaundice as a presenting feature
(Fig. 17.5)

Whereas a patient with chronic liver disease may present with jaundice, the differential diagnosis of jaundice with bilirubinuria (due to conjugated bilirubin) in a previously well patient is usually between acute hepatocellular damage and cholestasis. A suggested scheme is as follows. (For neonatal jaundice, see Chapter 26.)

- When taking the history pay special attention to:
  - recent exposure to hepatitis or infectious mononucleosis; including a sexual and occupational history,
  - recent administration of blood or blood products,
  - medication and alcohol intake (see Table 17.2),
  - intravenous drug abuse or tattoos,
  - associated symptoms such as abdominal pain, pruritus, weight loss or anorexia and nausea,
  - recent changes in the colour of the urine or stools,
  - recent foreign travel.
- On clinical examination, look for:
  - severity of jaundice,
  - hepatomegaly and splenomegaly,
  - signs of liver decompensation such as liver flap, 'liver palms', spider naevi, ascites etc.
- Measure plasma bilirubin and unconjugated/conjugated bilirubin fractions.
  Predominantly unconjugated hyperbilirubinaemia with plasma conjugated bilirubin levels less than

Investigation of suspected liver disease

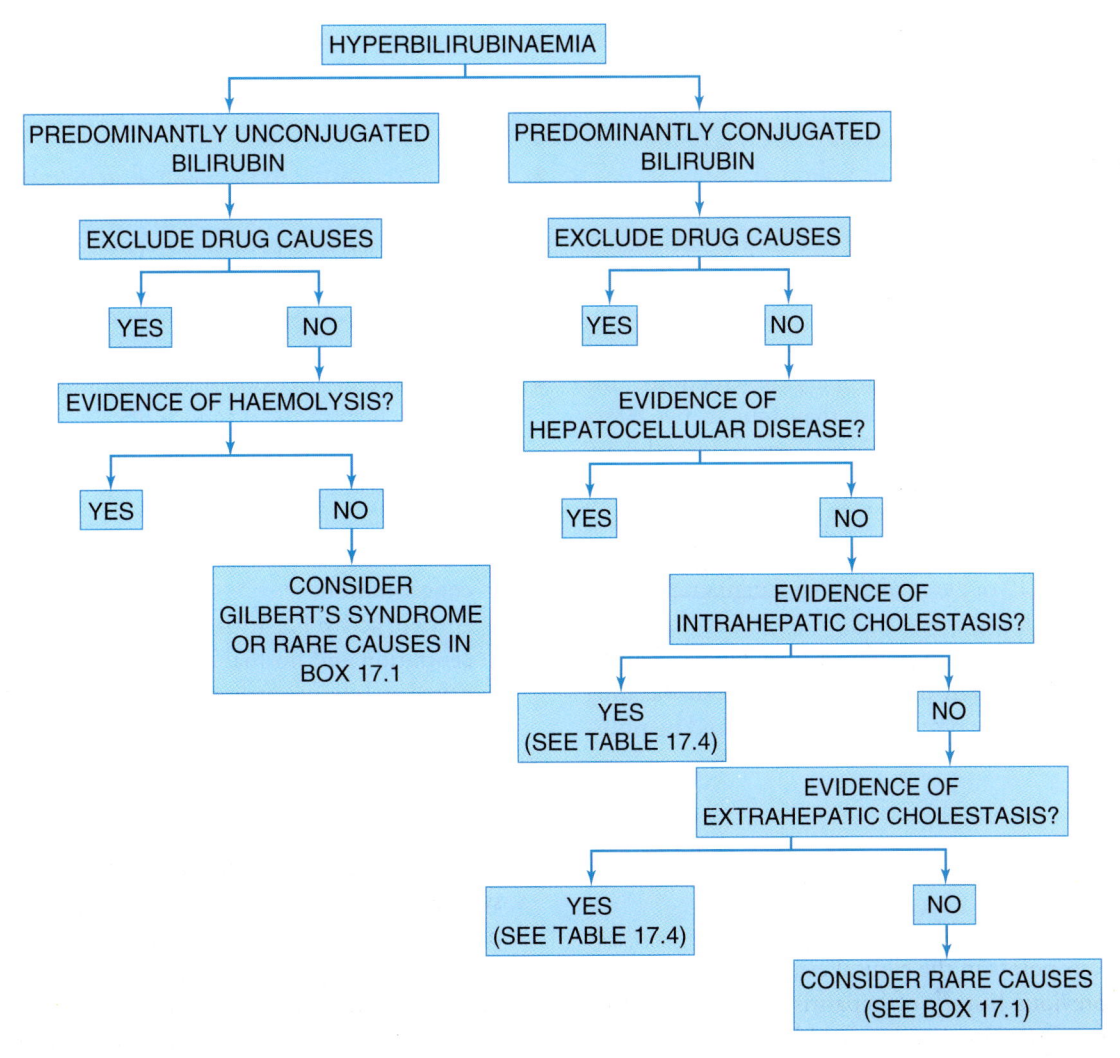

Fig. 17.5 Algorithm for the investigation of jaundice in an adult.

about 10 per cent of the total, and with little or no bilirubinuria, may suggest haemolysis as a cause. Haemolysis is supported by a raised reticulocyte count, reduced plasma haptoglobin and raised plasma lactate dehydrogenase concentrations.

If haemolysis is excluded, consider Gilbert's syndrome provided other liver tests are normal and other hepatic disorders have been excluded.

- A *fresh* urine sample should be examined. This test may show the presence of bilirubin if conjugated hyperbilirubinaemia is present. Dark-yellow or brown urine suggests biliary obstruction. An absence of urinary urobilinogen is seen in biliary obstruction. Reagent strips are available for testing for bilirubin and urobilinogen in urine.
- Pale stools suggest biliary obstruction as a cause of jaundice.
- Whatever the results of the urine and stool inspection and testing, request plasma aminotransferase, ALP and GGT assays.
  - In hepatitis, there is a predominant increase in the concentrations of plasma aminotransferases; usually the plasma ALT activity is higher than the AST activity. If hepatitis or infectious mononucleosis is suggested by the history, request serological tests.
  - In cholestasis, there is predominant elevation of the plasma ALP and GGT activities. Bile duct dilatation should be sought using ultrasound or other radiological tests:
    if the bile ducts are dilated, there is obstruction that may require surgery;
    if the plasma ALP activity is high but dilated ducts are not demonstrated, there is probably intrahepatic cholestasis.

- Other tests, such as ferritin and iron saturation (?haemochromatosis), and autoantibody (such as smooth muscle, p-anti-neutrophil cytoplasmic antigen, mitochondrial, nuclear antibodies) and immunoglobulin levels, may also be indicated.
- If acute alcoholic hepatitis is suspected, contributory evidence may be the finding of a disproportionately high plasma GGT activity compared with those of the aminotransferases. There may also be macrocytosis, hypertriglyceridaemia and hyperuricaemia.
- In obstructive jaundice (biliary obstruction), the plasma ALP is usually more than four to five times and GGT more than ten times normal. Liver/biliary ultrasound is useful to distinguish between obstructive jaundice with dilated biliary ducts or undilated ducts. Endoscopic retrograde cholangiopancreatography (ERCP) or percutaneous cholangiography may be indicated.
- If the diagnosis is in doubt, a liver biopsy may be indicated, although there may be a risk of bleeding and therefore the prothrombin time should be measured beforehand.

Suspected liver disease showing abnormal plasma hepatic enzymes

- Relevant points in the clinical evaluation are:
  - a previous history of hepatitis, intravenous drug use, occupational and sexual history,
  - alcohol intake and medication history, for example paracetamol,
  - the presence, or history, of other autoimmune disorders,
  - jaundice, pruritus or features of malabsorption,
  - family history of liver disease.
- Request tests for plasma bilirubin, aminotransferases (ALT and AST), albumin, GGT and ALP.
  - A raised plasma ALT activity higher than that of the AST may be due to reversible alcoholic hepatitis, to chronic persistent hepatitis, or to early chronic active hepatitis.
  - A raised plasma AST activity higher than that of ALT may be due to cirrhosis or severe chronic active hepatitis.
  - A high plasma ALP activity with raised GGT concentration suggests cholestasis.
  - Aminotransferase levels of more than ten times normal suggest primary hepatocyte damage, as in viral hepatitis or caused by drugs/toxins.
- An alcohol-related aetiology is supported by a macrocytosis and plasma GGT concentration, but neither test is fully diagnostic. See above.
- Check hepatitis serology, for example A, B and C.
- Detectable plasma mitochondrial or smooth-muscle antibodies are suggestive of primary biliary cirrhosis or chronic active hepatitis, respectively.
- A raised plasma ferritin concentration with high iron saturation (see Chapter 21) may reveal haemochromatosis.
- Plasma protein electrophoresis and immunoglobulin assay may help in the diagnosis of:
  - cirrhosis – high plasma IgG and IgA concentrations causing β-γ fusion on the electrophoretic strip,
  - alcoholic cirrhosis – may present with raised IgA concentration,
  - chronic active hepatitis – a high plasma IgG concentration and normal IgA,
  - primary biliary cirrhosis – a high plasma IgM concentration.

  A low plasma albumin concentration (hypoalbuminaemia) in the face of abnormal liver function tests can be seen in cirrhosis implying chronicity.
- A prolonged prothrombin time implies poor hepatic synthetic capacity, for example clotting factors, and is prognostic in paracetamol overdose. It is also important if a liver biopsy is considered.
- Significant infiltration of the liver by tumour cells, or by granulomas such as sarcoidosis (possibly with raised plasma angiotensin-converting enzyme concentration), may occur. In this situation raised plasma AST activity may be the most sensitive test, despite a normal plasma ALT activity. Hepatic space-occupying lesions may additionally present with raised GGT and ALP concentrations, and a liver ultrasound is useful to detect these.
- Fatty livers may be revealed by liver ultrasound with increased echogenicity. This may be associated with hypertriglyceridaemia, obesity and type 2 diabetes mellitus or impaired glucose regulation.
- If primary hepatocellular carcinoma is suspected, the plasma α-fetoprotein level may also be high.
- Low plasma copper and caeruloplasmin concentrations may suggest Wilson's disease (see Chapter 15), and plasma α_1-antitrypsin deficiency can result in cirrhosis (see Chapter 19).
- Radionuclide scans or other imaging procedures (CT or MRI) may be useful. A liver biopsy may be indicated to clarify a histological diagnosis.

CONCLUSIONS

- The liver has an enormous synthetic capacity and is involved in numerous metabolic pathways, including vitamin storage, amino acid deamination, bile salt and cholesterol synthesis, and the production of various proteins such as clotting factors and hormones.
- Compounds 'released' from the liver into the plasma can be used as markers of liver damage, including bilirubin, ALT, AST, GGT and ALP.
- Hyperbilirubinaemia can be due to raised unconjugated or conjugated bilirubin concentration. The former may be due to haemolysis and the latter to hepatic or extrahepatic causes.
- Raised plasma aminotransferase concentrations suggest hepatocyte damage and raised hepatic ALP concentration is associated with cholestasis.
- Plasma GGT is a sensitive marker of hepatic damage but its concentration can also be raised as a result of enzyme induction, hypertriglyceridaemia and increased alcohol intake.
- A prolonged prothrombin time and low plasma albumin concentration may both reflect reduced hepatic synthetic capacity.

18 PLASMA ENZYMES IN DIAGNOSIS (CLINICAL ENZYMOLOGY)

Assessment of cell damage and proliferation	268	Normal plasma enzyme activities	270
Factors affecting results of plasma enzyme assays	269	Plasma enzyme patterns in disease	278

This chapter discusses the principles of clinical enzymology, which have already been encountered in some of the preceding chapters. Enzymology can be defined as the assay of an enzyme(s) in body fluids, usually blood, that can be used diagnostically or to monitor a clinical condition.

An enzyme is a protein that catalyses one or more specific biochemical reactions. It is usually easier to measure enzyme *activity* in body fluids, by monitoring changes in either substrate or product concentrations, than to measure enzyme protein concentration directly, although this is sometimes done. However, measurement of the enzyme protein concentration is more specific and less prone to analytical variation.

Generally, enzymes are present in cells at much higher concentrations than in plasma. Some occur predominantly in cells of certain tissues, where they may be located in different cellular compartments such as the cytoplasm or the mitochondria. 'Normal' plasma enzyme concentrations reflect the balance between the rate of synthesis and release into plasma during cell turnover, and the rate of clearance from the circulation.

The enzyme activity in plasma may be:

- *higher than normal*, due to the proliferation of cells, an increase in the rate of cell turnover or damage or in enzyme synthesis (induction), or to reduced clearance from plasma;
- *lower than normal*, due to reduced synthesis, congenital deficiency or the presence of inherited variants of relatively low biological activity – examples of the latter are the cholinesterase variants.

Sometimes macroenzymes are found, that is to say, a high-molecular-weight form of a native enzyme. Often these are enzymes complexed with immunoglobulins and are more common in individuals with autoimmune disease. It is important to recognize macroenzymes as they can sometimes cause diagnostic confusion.

As we will now see, changes in plasma enzyme activities may be useful to detect and localize tissue cell damage or proliferation, or to monitor the treatment and progress of disease.

ASSESSMENT OF CELL DAMAGE AND PROLIFERATION

Plasma enzyme levels depend on the extent of cell damage and the rate of release from damaged cells, which, in turn, depends on the rate at which damage is occurring.

In the absence of cell damage, the rate of release depends on the degree of induction of enzyme synthesis and the rate of cell proliferation.

These factors are balanced by the rate of enzyme clearance from the circulation.

Acute cell damage, for example in viral hepatitis, may cause very high plasma aminotransferase activities that reduce as the condition resolves. By contrast, the liver may be much more extensively involved in advanced cirrhosis but the *rate* of cell damage is often low, and consequently plasma enzyme activities may be only slightly raised or within the reference range. In very severe liver disease, plasma enzyme activities may even fall terminally when the number of hepatocytes is grossly reduced (see Chapter 17).

Relatively small enzymes, such as amylase, can be cleared by the kidneys. Thus, plasma amylase activity may be high as a result of renal glomerular impairment rather than pancreatic damage. However, most enzymes are large proteins and may be catabolized by plasma proteases before being taken up by the reticuloendothelial system.

In health, each enzyme has a fairly constant and characteristic biological half-life, a fact that may be used to assess the time since the onset of an acute illness. After a myocardial infarction, for example, plasma levels of creatine kinase (CK) and aspartate aminotransferase (AST) fall to normal before those of lactate dehydrogenase (LDH), which has a longer half-life (see Chapter 22).

Localization of damage

Most of the enzymes commonly measured to assess tissue damage are present in nearly all body cells, although their relative concentrations in certain tissues may differ. Measurement of the plasma activity of an enzyme known to be in high concentration within cells of a particular tissue may indicate an abnormality of those cells, but the results will rarely enable a specific diagnosis to be made. For example, if there is circulatory failure after a cardiac arrest, very high plasma concentrations of enzymes originating from many tissues may occur because of hypoxic damage to cells and reduced rates of clearance.

The distribution of enzymes within cells may differ. Alanine aminotransferase (ALT) and LDH are predominantly located in cytoplasm, and glutamate dehydrogenase in mitochondria, whereas AST occurs in both these cellular compartments. Different disease processes in the same tissue may affect the cell in different ways, causing alteration in the relative plasma enzyme activities.

The diagnostic precision of plasma enzyme analysis may be improved by the following.

Serial enzyme estimations. The rate of change of plasma enzyme activity is related to a balance between the rate of entry and the rate of removal from the circulation. A persistently raised plasma enzyme activity is suggestive of a chronic disorder or, occasionally, impaired clearance.

Isoenzyme determination. Some enzymes exist in more than one form; these isoenzymes may be separated by their different physical or chemical properties. If they originate in different tissues, such identification will give more information than the measurement of plasma total enzyme activity; for example, CK may be derived from skeletal or cardiac muscle, but one of its isoenzymes is found predominantly in the myocardium.

Estimation of more than one enzyme. Many enzymes are widely distributed, but their relative concentrations may vary in different tissues. For example, although both ALT and AST are abundant in the liver, the concentration of AST is much greater than that of ALT in heart muscle.

Non-specific causes of raised plasma enzyme activities

Before attributing a change in plasma enzyme activity to a specific disease process, it is important to exclude the presence of factitious or non-specific causes.

Slight rises in plasma AST activities are common, non-specific findings in many illnesses. Moderate exercise, or a large intramuscular injection, may lead to a rise in plasma CK activity; isoenzyme determination may identify skeletal muscle as the tissue of origin.

Some drugs, such as the anticonvulsants phenytoin and phenobarbitone, may induce the synthesis of the microsomal enzyme γ-glutamyltransferase (GGT), and so increase its plasma activity in the absence of disease.

Plasma enzyme activities may be raised if the rate of clearance from the circulation is reduced. In the absence of hepatic or renal disease, this may occur if, for example, the plasma enzyme forms:

- macromolecules (aggregates), such as in macroamylasaemia,
- complexes with immunoglobulins, as occasionally occur with LDH, alkaline phosphatase (ALP) or CK.

FACTORS AFFECTING RESULTS OF PLASMA ENZYME ASSAYS

Analytical factors

The total concentration of all plasma enzyme proteins is less than 1 g/L. The results of enzyme assays are not usually expressed as concentrations, but as activities. Changes in concentration may give rise to proportional changes in catalytic activity, but the results of such measurements depend on many analytical factors, including:

- substrate concentration,
- product concentration,

- enzyme concentration,
- reaction temperature,
- reaction pH,
- presence of activators or inhibitors.

The definition of 'international units' does not take these factors into account, and the results from different laboratories, which are apparently expressed in the same units, may not be directly comparable. Therefore, plasma enzyme activities must be interpreted in relation to the reference ranges from the issuing laboratory.

Non-disease factors

Examples of non-disease factors affecting enzyme activities include the following.

Age

Plasma AST activity is moderately higher during the neonatal period than in adults. Plasma ALP activity of bony origin is higher in children than in adults and peaks during the pubertal bone growth spurt before falling to adult levels. A second peak occurs in the elderly.

Sex

Plasma GGT activity is higher in men than in women. Plasma CK activity is also higher in males.

Race/ethnicity

Plasma CK activity is higher in Africans and Afro-Caribbeans than in Caucasians.

Physiological conditions

Plasma ALP activity rises during the last trimester of pregnancy because of the presence of the placental isoenzyme. Several enzymes, such as AST and CK, rise moderately in plasma during and immediately after labour or strenous exercise.

Plasma enzyme activities should therefore be interpreted in relation to the sex, race/ethnicity and age-matched reference ranges of the issuing laboratory.

NORMAL PLASMA ENZYME ACTIVITIES

Individual enzymes of clinical importance are considered in the following section. Applications of their assays in defined clinical situations are discussed later in the chapter and in other chapters in this book.

Aminotransferases

The aminotransferases (ALT and AST) are enzymes involved in the transfer of an amino group from a 2-amino acid to a 2-oxoacid; they need the cofactor pyridoxal phosphate for optimal activity. They are widely distributed in the body. (See Chapter 17, which deals with hepatic disease, for further details.) The aminotransferases are used as part of the biochemical liver profile.

Aspartate aminotransferase

Aspartate aminotransferase (glutamate oxaloacetate aminotransferase, GOT) is present in high concentrations in cells of cardiac and skeletal muscle, liver, kidney and erythrocytes. Damage to any of these tissues may increase plasma AST levels.

Causes of raised plasma AST activities

- *Artefactual*: due to in-vitro release from erythrocytes if there is haemolysis or if separation of plasma from cells is delayed.
- *Physiological*: during the neonatal period (about 1.5 times the upper adult reference limit).
- *Marked increase* (may be greater than five to ten times the upper reference limit, URL):
  - circulatory failure with 'shock' and hypoxia,
  - myocardial infarction,
  - acute viral or toxic hepatitis.
- *Moderate to slight increase* (usually less than five times URL):
  - cirrhosis (may be normal sometimes),
  - infectious mononucleosis (due to liver involvement),
  - cholestatic jaundice,
  - malignant infiltration of the liver (may be normal),
  - skeletal muscle disease,
  - after trauma or surgery (especially after cardiac surgery),
  - severe haemolytic episodes (of erythrocyte origin),
  - various drugs.

Note that AST is not specific for hepatic disease.

Alanine aminotransferase

Alanine aminotransferase (glutamate pyruvate aminotransferase, GPT) is present in high concentrations in liver and, to a lesser extent, in skeletal muscle, kidney and heart.

Causes of raised plasma ALT activities

- *Marked increase* (may be greater than five to ten times URL):
  - circulatory failure with 'shock' and hypoxia,
  - acute viral or toxic hepatitis.
- *Moderate to slight increase* (usually less than five times URL):
  - cirrhosis (may be normal sometimes),
  - infectious mononucleosis (due to liver involvement),
  - liver congestion secondary to congestive cardiac failure,
  - cholestatic jaundice,
  - surgery or extensive trauma and skeletal muscle disease (much less affected than AST),
  - certain drugs.

Note that ALT is more specific for hepatic disease than AST.

Lactate dehydrogenase

Lactate dehydrogenase catalyses the reversible interconversion of lactate and pyruvate. The enzyme is widely distributed in the body, with high concentrations in cells of cardiac and skeletal muscle, liver, kidney, brain and erythrocytes; measurement of plasma total LDH activity is therefore a non-specific marker of cell damage.

Causes of raised plasma total LDH activity

- *Artefactual*: due to in-vitro haemolysis or delayed separation of plasma from whole blood.
- *Marked increase* (may be greater than five to ten times URL):
  - circulatory failure with 'shock' and hypoxia,
  - myocardial infarction (see Chapter 22),
  - some haematological disorders: in blood diseases such as megaloblastic anaemia, acute leukaemias and lymphomas, very high levels (up to 20 times the URL in adults) may be found. Smaller increases occur in other disorders of erythropoiesis, such as thalassaemia, myelofibrosis and haemolytic anaemias, renal infarction or, occasionally, during rejection of a renal transplant.
- *Moderate to slight increase* (usually less than five times URL):
  - viral hepatitis,
  - malignancy of any tissue,
  - skeletal muscle disease,
  - pulmonary embolism,
  - infectious mononucleosis,
  - certain drugs.

Isoenzymes of LDH

Five main isoenzymes can be detected by electrophoresis and are referred to as LDH_1 to LDH_5. LDH_1, the fraction that migrates fastest towards the anode, predominates in cells of cardiac muscle, erythrocytes and kidney. The slowest moving isoenzyme, LDH_5, is the most abundant form in the liver and in skeletal muscle.

Whereas in many conditions there is an increase in all fractions, the finding of certain patterns is of diagnostic value.

- Predominant elevation of LDH_1 and LDH_2 (LDH_1 more than LDH_2) occurs after myocardial infarction, in megaloblastic anaemia and after renal infarction.
- Predominant elevation of LDH_2 and LDH_3 occurs in acute leukaemia; LDH_3 is the main isoenzyme elevated as a result of malignancy of many tissues.
- Elevation of LDH_5 occurs after damage to the liver or skeletal muscle.

It is rarely necessary to quantify LDH isoenzyme activity. A rise in LDH_1 is most significant in the diagnosis of myocardial infarction. However, as LDH_1 and, to a lesser extent LDH_2 and LDH_3, can use 2-hydroxybutyrate as well as lactate as substrate, some laboratories assay hydroxybutyrate dehydrogenase (HBD) as an index of LDH_1 activity. Lactate dehydrogenase is sometimes used in the delayed diagnosis of a myocardial infarct (troponin has largely taken over this role from LDH) and also as a marker for certain tumours, for example lymphomas, and to help determine haemolysis (see Chapters 17 and 22).

Creatine kinase

Creatine kinase is most abundant in cells of cardiac and skeletal muscle and in brain, but also occurs in other tissues such as smooth muscle.

Isoenzymes of CK

Creatine kinase consists of two protein subunits, M and B, which combine to form three isoenzymes, BB (CK-1), MB (CK-2) and MM (CK-3).

- *CK-MM* is the predominant isoenzyme in skeletal and cardiac muscle and is detectable in the plasma of normal subjects.
- *CK-MB* accounts for about 35 per cent of the total CK activity in cardiac muscle and less than 5 per cent

in skeletal muscle; its plasma activity is always high after myocardial infarction. The use and limitations of CK–MB estimation are considered in Chapter 22. It may be detectable in the plasma of patients with a variety of other disorders in whom the total CK activity is raised, but this accounts for less than 6 per cent of the total CK activity.

- *CK-BB* is present in high concentrations in the brain and in the smooth muscle of the gastrointestinal and genital tracts. Increased plasma activities may occur during parturition. Although they have also been reported after brain damage, for example trauma or cerebrovascular accident, and in association with malignant tumours of the bronchus, prostate and breast, measurement is not of proven value for diagnosing these conditions. In malignant disease, plasma total CK activity is usually normal.

There are also other forms of CK. One is a mitochondrial form seen in hepatic disease, certain tumours and critically ill patients. There are also type 1 and type 2 macroenzyme forms of CK. Type 1 macroenzyme is associated with autoimmune disease such as rheumatoid arthritis and is thought to be CK complexed with IgG; type 2 macroenzyme is an oligomer of mitochondrial CK.

Causes of raised plasma CK activities

- *Artefactual*: due to in-vitro haemolysis, using most methods.
- *Physiological*:
  - neonatal period (slightly raised above the adult URL),
  - during and for a few days after parturition,
  - plasma CK is generally higher in Africans compared with Caucasians.
- *Marked increase* (may be greater than five to ten times URL):
  - dermatomyositis and polymyositis,
  - 'shock' and circulatory failure,
  - myocardial infarction,
  - muscular dystrophies,
  - rhabdomyolysis (the breakdown of skeletal muscle),
  - necrotizing fasciitis.
- *Moderate to slight increase* (usually less than five times URL):
  - muscle injury,
  - infections, for example viral,
  - after surgery (for about a week),
  - physical exertion – there may be a significant rise in plasma activity after only moderate exercise, muscle cramp or following an epileptic fit,
  - after an intramuscular injection,
  - hypothyroidism (thyroxine may influence the catabolism of the enzyme),
  - alcoholism (possibly partly due to alcoholic myositis),
  - some cases of cerebrovascular accident and head injury,
  - malignant hyperpyrexia,
  - certain drugs, for example statins, ciclosporin, cocaine,
  - glycogen storage diseases,
  - carnitine palmityl transferase deficiency.

CASE 1

A 45-year-old male was prescribed a 3-hydroxyl-3-methylglutaryl coenzyme A reductase inhibitor (statin) by his general practitioner because of hypercholesterolaemia. A week after commencement on the drug, he complained of severe muscle aches. The following are the results of the tests requested by his general practitioner.

Plasma
Creatine kinase 14200 U/L (<250)
Bilirubin 12 μmol/L (<20)
Alanine aminotransferase 22 U/L (<42)
Asparate aminotransferase 98 U/L (<45)
Alkaline phosphatase 113 U/L (<250)
Albumin 40 g/L (35–45)

Urine was positive for myoglobin.

DISCUSSION
The grossly elevated CK activity supports the diagnosis of rhabdomyolysis. This is a rare complication of statin drug usage. It is important also to monitor renal function, as the myoglobin released from muscle is nephrotoxic. Intracellular ions such as potassium are also released from the muscle into the circulation, resulting in hyperkalaemia. Note that the plasma AST concentration is raised, as this can be found in muscle as well as liver tissue.

Plasma CK activity is raised in all types of muscular dystrophy, but not usually in neurogenic muscle diseases such as poliomyelitis, myasthenia gravis, multiple sclerosis or Parkinson's disease.

Rhabdomyolysis can be defined as an acute increase in plasma CK concentration greater than ten times the upper limit of normal with a normal CK-MB fraction. Severe muscle breakdown results in grossly elevated plasma CK concentrations, sometimes up to 100 000 U/L. This can be due to trauma, severe exertion, alcohol, heat, electrolyte disturbances and drugs such as statins.

Plasma myoglobin (another muscle protein) is elevated and, being of low molecular weight, is filtered through the renal glomeruli and can precipitate out in the renal tubules, resulting in acute renal failure.

Urinary myoglobin can be inferred by the red-brown colour and positive urine dipstick test for haem in the absence of erythrocytes as judged by microscopy. Intravascular volume expansion with saline and sometimes mannitol-alkaline diuresis my help reduce the risk of this. Rhabdomyolysis is associated with hyperkalaemia and hyperphosphataemia due to the release of intracellular ions from myocytes, and calcium can be sequestered, resulting in hypocalcaemia.

Aldolase

This glycolytic enzyme has been measured in plasma as a marker of muscle disease. However, generally it offers no major advantage over CK and is now rarely used.

Amylase

Amylase (molecular weight 45 kDa) breaks down starch and glycogen to maltose. It is present at a high concentration in pancreatic juice and in saliva and may be extracted from other tissues, such as the gonads, Fallopian tubes, skeletal muscle and adipose tissue. Being of relatively low molecular weight, it is excreted in the urine.

Estimation of plasma amylase activity is mainly requested to help in the diagnosis of acute pancreatitis, in which the plasma activity may be very high. However, it may also be raised in association with other intra-abdominal and extra-abdominal conditions that cause similar acute abdominal pain; thus a high result is not a specific diagnostic marker for acute pancreatitis (Fig. 18.1; see also Chapter 16). If the plasma amylase activity fails to fall after an attack of acute pancreatitis, there may be leakage of pancreatic fluid into the lesser sac (a pancreatic pseudocyst). Plasma levels may be near normal in chronic or haemorrhagic pancreatitis.

Causes of raised plasma amylase activity

- *Marked increase* (may be greater than five to ten times URL):
  - acute pancreatitis,
  - severe glomerular impairment,
  - diabetic ketoacidosis,
  - perforated peptic ulcer, especially if there is perforation into the lesser sac.
- *Moderate to slight increase* (usually less than five times URL).
  - Other acute abdominal disorders: perforated peptic ulcer,

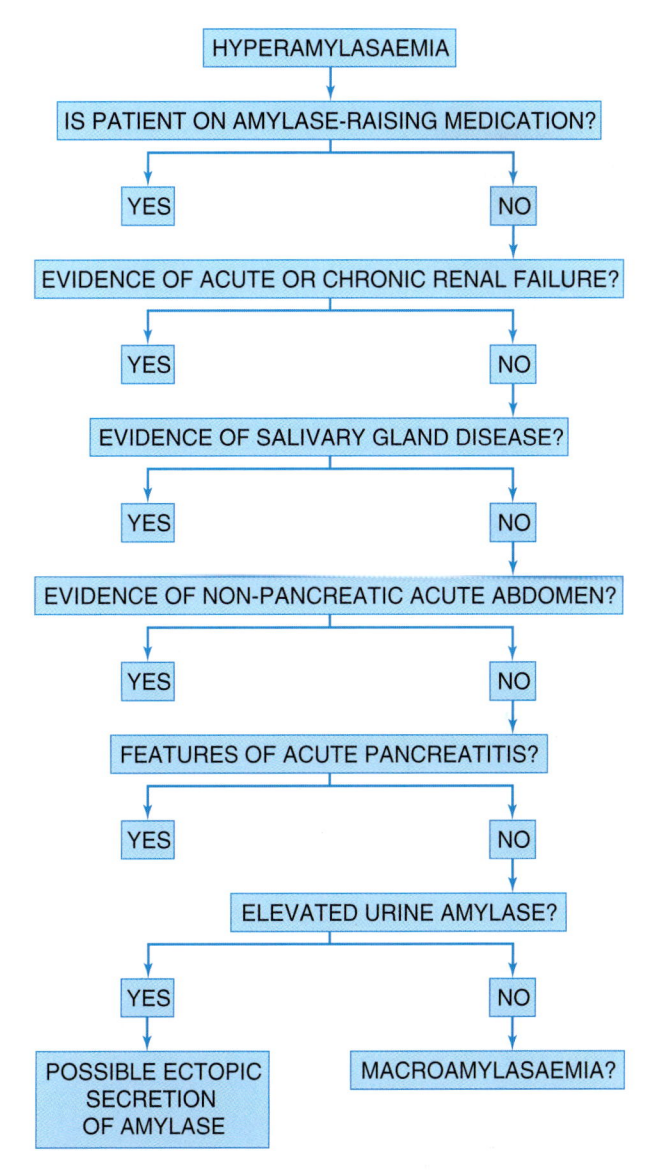

Fig. 18.1 Algorithm for the investigation of a raised plasma amylase.

acute cholecystitis,
intestinal obstruction,
abdominal trauma,
ruptured ectopic pregnancy,
- Salivary gland disorders:
mumps,
salivary calculi,
Sjögren's syndrome,
after injection of contrast medium into salivary ducts for sialography.
- Miscellaneous causes:
morphine administration (spasm of the sphincter of Oddi),
myocardial infarction (occasionally),
acute alcoholic intoxication,
macroamylasaemia,
ectopic production from tumour.

Macroamylasaemia

In some patients, high plasma amylase activity is due to low renal excretion of a macroenzyme form, despite normal glomerular function. The condition is symptomless and it is thought that the enzyme is bound to IgA, giving a complex of molecular weight about 270 kDa. This harmless condition may be confused with other causes of hyperamylasaemia. If amylase and creatinine are assayed in simultaneous plasma and urine samples, an amylase clearance to creatinine clearance ratio can be calculated. If the result is multiplied by 100, a ratio of less than 0.02 is suggestive of macroamylasaemia.

Isoenzymes of amylase

Plasma amylase is derived from the pancreas and salivary glands. It is rarely necessary to identify the isoenzyme components in plasma, but they can be distinguished by electrophoretic techniques, or by using an inhibitor derived from wheat germ. Possible indications for isoenzyme determination include:

- the coexistence of mumps or renal failure, which complicate the interpretation of high activities due to acute pancreatitis;
- the possibility of chronic pancreatic disease, in which low activities may be found.

Some laboratories now measure plasma-specific 'pancreatic' amylase activity.

Lipase

Sometimes, when it is difficult to interpret plasma amylase results, it may be useful to measure plasma lipase instead. This enzyme is also derived from the pancreas but is more specific for pancreatic pathology. In addition, lipase has a longer half-life than amylase and therefore may be more useful in the diagnosis of late-presenting acute pancreatitis.

Alkaline phosphatase

The ALPs are a group of enzymes that hydrolyse organic phosphates at high pH. They are present in most tissues but are in particularly high concentration in the osteoblasts

---

CASE 2

A 23-year-old male was investigated in the gastroenterology clinic because his plasma amylase was 445 U/L (less than 200) and some of his blood results were as follows.

Plasma
Sodium 139 mmol/L (135–145)
Potassium 4.0 mmol/L (3.5–5.0)
Bicarbonate 26 mmol/L (24–32)
Urea 4.5 mmol/L (2.5–7.0)
Creatinine 100 μmol/L (70–110)
Glucose 4.5 mmol/L (3.5–5.5)
'Corrected' calcium 2.39 mmol/L (2.15–2.55)

No other investigations revealed any abnormality, including upper gastrointestinal endoscopy and abdominal ultrasound. A urine determination did not find any measurable amylase.

DISCUSSION
The question here is what is the explanation for the raised plasma amylase concentration? Amylase is normally present in the urine because of its relatively small molecular size. Its absence in urine and serum amylase electrophoretic studies confirmed macroamylasaemia. This is a large form of amylase, usually IgA bound, that is not renally cleared.

of bone and the cells of the hepatobiliary tract, intestinal wall, renal tubules and placenta.

In adults, plasma ALP is derived mainly from bone and liver in approximately equal proportions; the proportion due to the bone fraction is increased when there is increased osteoblastic activity that may be physiological (Fig. 18.2).

Causes of raised plasma ALP activity

- *Physiological*.
  - During the last trimester of pregnancy, the plasma total ALP activity rises due to the contribution of the placental isoenzyme. Plasma ALP concentration may increase by up to five times and usually returns to normal levels by 1 month post-partum.
  - In preterm infants, plasma total ALP activity is up to five times the URL in adults, and consists predominantly of the bone isoenzyme.
  - In children, the total activity is about 2.5 times (and increases to up to five times) this upper limit during the pubertal bone growth spurt. There is a gradual increase in the proportion of liver ALP with age.
  - In the elderly, the plasma bone isoenzyme activity may increase slightly.
- *Bone disease*:
  - rickets and osteomalacia (see Chapter 6),
  - Paget's disease of bone (may be very high),
  - secondary malignant deposits in bone,
  - osteogenic sarcoma (only if very extensive),
  - primary hyperparathyroidism with extensive bone disease (usually normal but may be slightly elevated),
  - secondary hyperparathyroidism.
- *Liver disease*:
  - intrahepatic or extrahepatic cholestasis (see Chapter 17),
  - space-occupying lesions, tumours, granulomas and other causes of hepatic infiltration.
- Inflammatory bowel disease or intestinal obstruction: the gut ALP isoenzyme can be increased.
- *Malignancy:* bone or liver involvement or direct tumour production.

A placental-like, so-called 'Regan' isoenzyme may occasionally be identified in plasma in patients with malignant

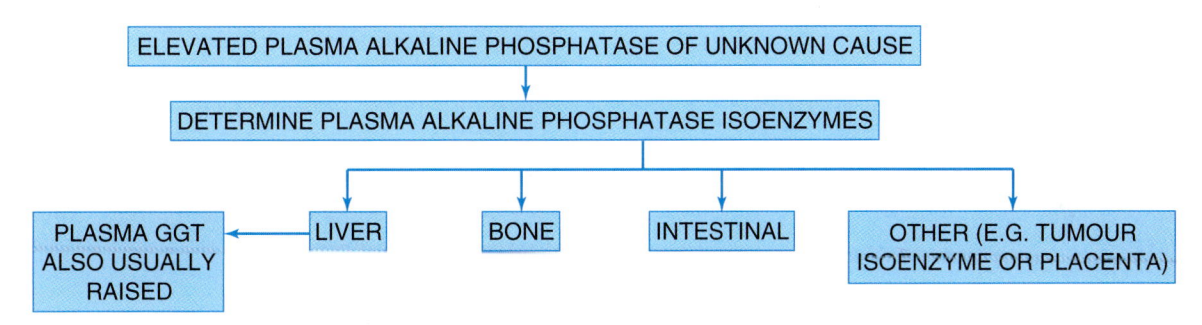

Fig. 18.2 Algorithm for the investigation of a raised plasma alkaline phosphatase.

CASE 3

A 64-year-old male with lung carcinoma attended the oncology clinic. Some of his blood results were as follows.

Plasma
Bilirubin 10 μmol/L (<20)
Alanine aminotransferase 23 U/L (<42)
Alkaline phosphatase 426 U/L (<250)
Gamma-glutamyltransferase 50 U/L (<55)
Albumin 36 g/L (35–45)
'Corrected' calcium 2.22 mmol/L (2.15–2.55)

Phosphate 1.11 mmol/L (0.80–1.35)
A liver ultrasound and bone scan were normal.

DISCUSSION
The question here is what is the source of the raised ALP concentration? The normal GGT concentration makes a hepatic source unlikely. Similarly, the normal plasma calcium concentration and bone scan do not make a bone source likely either. However, ALP isoenzymes showed the presence of a Regan isoenzyme, thought to be ectopically released from his lung carcinoma.

disease, especially carcinoma of the bronchus. There is also a Nago isoenzyme released by certain tumours.

Transient very high levels of ALP (up to 30 times URL) have been recorded in children, but the clinical significance of this finding is unknown. This has been called transient hyperphosphatasaemia and may be either the bone or the liver isoenzyme. It may be associated with abdominal symptoms and usually resolves within a few months.

Plasma total ALP activity is not usually increased in myelomatosis, despite the X-ray appearance of multiple 'punched-out' osteolytic lesions. The lesions are in the marrow cavity, not the bone substance, and osteoblastic activity is not stimulated. However, ALP activity may be raised if there is liver involvement or, more rarely, if there is healing of very extensive pathological fractures.

Possible causes of low plasma ALP activity

A low plasma ALP concentration is less usual, but may be caused by the following.

- *Arrested bone growth*:
  - achondroplasia,
  - hypothyroidism,
  - severe vitamin C deficiency.
- *Hypophosphatasia*, an autosomal recessive disorder, associated with rickets or osteomalacia.
- *Treatment of hyperlipidaemia with a fibrate drug*, for example bezafibrate. This observation can be useful to determine drug compliance of fibrates.

Isoenzymes of ALP

Bone disease with increased osteoblastic activity and liver disease with involvement of the biliary tracts are the commonest causes of an increased total ALP activity.

Rarely, the cause is not apparent and further tests may be helpful. The isoenzymes originating from the cells of bone, liver, intestine and placenta may be separated by electrophoresis, but interpretation may be difficult if the total activity is only marginally raised. The placental and 'Regan' isoenzymes are more stable at 65 °C than the bone, liver and intestinal isoenzymes, and heat inactivation may help to differentiate the heat-stable from the heat-labile fraction.

The placental isoenzyme does not cross the placenta and is therefore not detectable in the plasma of the newborn.

Acid phosphatase

Acid phosphatase (ACP) is found in cells of the prostate, liver, erythrocytes, platelets and bone. The main indications for estimation are to help diagnose prostatic carcinoma and to monitor its treatment. Estimation has been largely replaced by the measurement of plasma prostate-specific antigen (PSA), a protein derived from the prostate (see Chapter 24). This test is more specific and sensitive for diagnosis and monitoring treatment and has essentially rendered the plasma ACP assay obsolete in the diagnosis and management of prostatic carcinoma.

Haemolysed blood samples should also be avoided, as ACP is found in erythrocytes. Normally, ACP drains from the prostate, through the prostatic ducts and into the urethra, and very little can be detected in plasma. In extensive prostatic carcinoma, particularly if it has spread extensively or has metastasized, plasma ACP activity rises, probably because of the increased number of prostatic ACP-containing cells. Another problem with plasma ACP is that its concentration can increase after rectal examination.

Isoenzymes of ACP

The release of ACP from blood cells in vitro may occur even in unhaemolysed samples and many methods have been devised in an attempt to measure only the prostatic fraction, without complete success. One method makes use of the fact that L-tartrate inhibits prostatic ACP; the assay is performed with and without the addition of L-tartrate; the difference in activity between the results (the tartrate-labile fraction) is mainly prostatic ACP. Other methods measure the prostatic enzyme protein concentration directly by immunoassay.

Causes of raised plasma ACP activity

- *Tartrate labile*:
  - artefactually following rectal examination, acute retention of urine or passage of a catheter, due to pressure on prostatic cells,
  - disseminated carcinoma of the prostate.
- *Total*:
  - artefactually in a haemolysed specimen, or following rectal examination, acute retention of urine or passage of a catheter,
  - disseminated carcinoma of the prostate,
  - Paget's disease of bone,
  - some cases of metastatic bone disease, especially with osteosclerotic lesions,
  - Gaucher's disease (probably from Gaucher cells),
  - occasionally in thrombocythaemia or polycythaemia.

The assay is not of major diagnostic value in these conditions, although there is current research looking at the potential use of bone-derived ACP as a marker of osteoclastic activity in osteoporosis.

Gamma-glutamyltransferase

Gamma-glutamyltransferase occurs mainly in the cells of liver, kidneys, pancreas and prostate. Plasma GGT activity is usually higher in males than in females.

Causes of raised plasma GGT activity

- Induction of enzyme synthesis, without cell damage, by drugs or alcohol. Many drugs (most commonly the anticonvulsants, phenobarbitone and phenytoin) and alcohol induce proliferation of the endoplasmic reticulum.
- Cholestatic liver disease, when changes in GGT activity usually parallel those of ALP. In the cholestatic jaundice of pregnancy, plasma GGT activities may not increase.
- Hepatocellular damage, such as that due to infectious hepatitis; measurement of plasma aminotransferase activities is a more sensitive indicator of such conditions.

Slightly raised activities (up to about two to three times URL) are particularly difficult to interpret. Very high plasma GGT activities, out of proportion to those of the aminotransferases, may be due to:

- alcoholic hepatitis,
- induction by anticonvulsant drugs or by alcohol intake,
- cholestatic liver disease,
- hypertriglyceridaemia,
- fatty liver.

A patient should never be labelled an alcoholic because of a high plasma GGT activity alone. (For a fuller description of liver disease see Chapter 17.)

Plasma cholinesterase and suxamethonium sensitivity

There are normally two isoenzymes of cholinesterase:

- cholinesterase ('pseudocholinesterase'), found in plasma and synthesized mainly in the liver;
- acetylcholinesterase, found predominantly in erythrocytes and nervous tissue.

Causes of decreased plasma cholinesterase activity

- Hepatic parenchymal disease (reduced synthesis).
- Ingestion, or absorption through the skin, of such anticholinesterases as organophosphates.
- Inherited abnormal cholinesterase variants, with low biological activity.
- Pregnancy.

Causes of increased plasma cholinesterase activity

- Recovery from liver damage (actively growing hepatocytes).
- Nephrotic syndrome.

Suxamethonium sensitivity

The muscle relaxants suxamethonium (succinyl choline; 'scoline') and mivacurium are usually broken down by plasma cholinesterase, and this limits the duration of their action. Giving these agents to patients with a low

---

CASE 4

A 23-year-old female had her wisdom teeth removed under general anaesthesia, with suxamethonium as an inducing agent. Postoperatively she required prolonged mechanical ventilation for 4 hours. Some of her laboratory test results were as follows.

Plasma
Cholinesterase 782 U/L (600–1400)
Dibucaine number 63 (76–83)
Fluoride number 51 (56–66)

DISCUSSION

The patient has had an anaesthetic reaction. Although the plasma cholinesterase activity is within the reference range, further cholinesterase studies showed low dibucaine and fluoride numbers. The data are suggestive of a variant cholinesterase (UA). This metabolizes suxamethonium more slowly than the 'normal' cholinesterase enzyme, resulting in prolonged post-operative apnoea.

cholinesterase activity (usually due to an enzyme variant) may result in a prolonged period of apnoea ('scoline apnoea'); such patients may need prolonged ventilatory support after an operation.

The abnormal cholinesterase variants may be classified by measuring the percentage inhibition of the enzyme activity by dibucaine (dibucaine number) or by fluoride (fluoride number). A low dibucaine number and/or fluoride number with or without low plasma activity is suggestive of a cholinesterase variant, for example A, K, J or silent gene types.

The identification of patients susceptible to suxamethonium, and of their affected relatives, is important. Close blood relatives should be traced and investigated to identify their genotype, and so to predict the chance of future anaesthetic risk. All affected individuals should carry a warning card or a 'Medic Alert' bracelet and should notify the anaesthetist if they require an anaesthetic.

Reduced red cell acetylcholinesterase activity can be useful as a measure of exposure to organophosphates, for example certain pesticides, and this activity can be used to monitor people at risk of organophosphate exposure.

Angiotensin-converting enzyme

Angiotensin-converting enzyme (ACE) is a dipeptidyl carboxypeptidase and cleaves dipeptides from the free carboxy end of various polypeptides, including angiotensin I and bradykinin. One of its actions is releasing angiotensin II by cleaving the dipeptide histidyl-leucine from angiotensin I. The major site of ACE production is the pulmonary endothelium.

This enzyme can be measured in plasma as a marker of disease activity in sarcoidosis. It can be elevated in other lung conditions and therefore is not specific for sarcoidosis. High plasma ACE levels may decline on treatment with steroids.

Tryptase

Classic allergy such as bronchospasm and urticaria generally produces allergen-specific IgE to certain agents, with IgE-producing mast-cell degranulation.

Tryptase is a serine protease found in mast cells. In cases of mast cell degranulation, as occurs in systemic anaphylaxis, tryptase levels rise within 1 hour and remain elevated for 4–6 hours. In patients with life-threatening systemic reactions to diverse allergens (such as venoms, latex and drugs), the finding of elevated plasma tryptase levels (more than 1 μg/L) between 1 and 6 hours after the event is highly sensitive and specific for confirming mast-cell degranulation as the cause of the event.

PLASMA ENZYME PATTERNS IN DISEASE

Myocardial infarction

The diagnosis of a myocardial infarction is usually made on the clinical presentation and electrocardiographic findings and confirmed by the characteristic changes in plasma enzyme activities or troponins. The latter now appear to have superseded enzyme analysis in this context (see Chapter 22).

Liver disease

Plasma enzyme changes in liver disease are discussed in Chapter 17 and are important in the diagnosis of various liver disorders.

Muscle disease

In the muscular dystrophies, for example Duchenne's, plasma levels of the muscle enzyme CK (isoenzyme CK-MM) and also of LDH and the aminotransferases (mainly AST) are increased as a result of leakage from the diseased cells. Results of plasma CK estimation are more specific than LDH and AST for muscle disease.

Points to consider in the interpretation of CK levels in Duchenne's muscular dystrophy are:

- activities are highest (may be greater than five to ten times the URL) in the early stages of the disease; later, when much of the muscle has wasted, they are lower and may even be normal;
- activities are higher following muscular activity immediately after rest (because of the release of CK built up in muscle during rest) than after prolonged activity.

The clinical diagnosis of the Duchenne type of muscular dystrophy can be confirmed by measuring the plasma CK activity, examining a muscle biopsy specimen and by DNA analysis in the majority of cases (see Chapter 30).

Carriers of the disorder can often be detected by DNA analysis of the dystrophin gene and by finding raised plasma CK activities. The rise is only moderate, and non-specific causes of raised enzyme activities must be excluded.

Less marked changes in plasma CK, LDH and AST are found in some patients with the other muscle disorders described above.

Enzymes in malignancy

Plasma total enzyme activities may be raised, or an abnormal isoenzyme detected, in several neoplastic disorders.

- Plasma prostatic (tartrate-labile) ACP activity rises in some cases of malignancy of the prostate gland, but plasma PSA determination has now essentially replaced its clinical use.
- Malignancies may be associated with a non-specific increase in plasma LDH and, occasionally, aminotransferase activity.
- Plasma aminotransferase and ALP estimations may be of value to monitor the treatment of malignant disease. Raised ALP levels may indicate secondary deposits in liver or in bone. Liver deposits may also cause an increase in plasma LDH or GGT concentration.
- Tumours occasionally produce a number of enzymes, such as the 'Regan' ALP or Nago isoenzyme, LDH_1 (HBD) or CK-BB, assays of which may be used as an aid to diagnosis or for monitoring treatment.

Haematological disorders

Very high activities of LDH may be found in megaloblastic anaemias and leukaemias and in other conditions in which bone marrow activity is abnormal. Typically there is much less change in the plasma AST than in the LDH activities. Severe in-vivo haemolysis produces changes in both AST and LDH activities, which mimic those of myocardial infarction.

It should be evident that enzymology is important in diagnostic processes. (The reader is also referred to Chapter 16 on gastrointestinal disorders, Chapter 17 concerning liver function tests, Chapter 22 on cardiovascular chemical pathology and Chapter 24 on tumour markers.) Enzymes can also be measured in other body fluids, such as faeces, i.e. elastase (see Chapter 16), and pleural fluid, for example adenosine deaminase (see Chapter 23).

CONCLUSIONS

- Enzymes can be measured in body fluids, mainly plasma, to aid the clinical diagnosis and management of certain conditions. This is called clinical enzymology.
- Enzymes may exist as isoenzymes (molecular variants of enzymes), which may be present in different tissues. Examples are ALP (hepatic, bone, intestinal and placental isoenzymes) and CK (striated muscle, MM; brain, BB; and cardiac muscle, MB).
- Certain aminotransferases (AST and ALT) and also GGT can be used in the investigation of hepatic disease.
- Clinical enzymology has limitations, as generally plasma enzyme activity lacks specificity. Isoenzyme determination or measuring a number of enzymes may increase diagnostic accuracy.
- Some enzymes may complex with larger molecules, such as immunoglobulins, forming macroenzymes.

19 PROTEINS IN PLASMA AND URINE

| Plasma proteins 280 | Blood sampling for protein estimations 299 |
| Proteins in urine 295 | |

PLASMA PROTEINS

Plasma albumin and total protein are often included as part of a biochemistry department's assay profile, and other more specialized plasma proteins such as C-reactive protein (CRP) may also be measured in certain circumstances. There are also a number of clinical conditions that involve abnormalities of plasma and urinary proteins, some of which are discussed in this chapter.

Metabolism of proteins

The amount of protein in the vascular compartment depends on the balance between the rate of synthesis and catabolism or loss. However, also important is the relative distribution between the intravascular and extravascular compartments, as the concentration depends on the relative amounts of protein and water in the vascular compartment. Therefore, abnormal concentrations do not necessarily reflect defects in protein metabolism.

Protein synthesis

Hepatocytes synthesize many plasma proteins; those of the complement system are also made by macrophages. Immunoglobulins are mainly derived from the B lymphocytes of the immune system.

Protein catabolism and loss

Most plasma proteins are taken up by pinocytosis into capillary endothelial cells or mononuclear phagocytes, where they are catabolized. Small-molecular-weight proteins are lost passively through the renal glomeruli and intestinal wall. Some are reabsorbed, either directly by renal tubular cells or after digestion in the intestinal lumen; others are catabolized by renal tubular cells.

Functions of plasma proteins

Peptide hormones and blood clotting factors contribute quantitatively relatively small, but physiologically important, amounts of plasma protein. Some plasma proteins originate from cell breakdown.

Control of extracellular fluid distribution

The distribution of water between the intravascular and extravascular compartments is influenced by the colloid osmotic effect of plasma proteins, predominantly albumin (see Chapter 2).

Transport

Albumin and specific binding proteins transport hormones, vitamins, lipids, bilirubin, calcium, trace metals and drugs. Combination with protein allows poorly water-soluble substances to be transported in plasma. The protein-bound fraction of many of these substances is physiologically inactive, unlike the unbound fraction.

Inflammatory response and control of infection

The immunoglobulins and the complement proteins form part of the immune system and the latter, together with a group of proteins known as acute-phase reactants, for example CRP, are involved in the inflammatory response.

Methods of assessing plasma proteins

Plasma proteins may be expressed either as concentrations (for example g/L) or as activities of those proteins that have defined functions, such as clotting times for prothrombin or enzyme activity (see Chapter 18). The distinction is important when abnormal forms of protein are present at normal concentration but with impaired function, such as C1 inhibitor (see p. 286).

Total plasma proteins

Acute changes in proteins are more likely to be due to loss from, or gain by, the vascular compartment of protein-free fluid than of protein. Only marked changes of major constituents, such as albumin and immunoglobulins, are likely to alter total protein concentrations significantly.

Plasma total protein concentrations may be misleading for other reasons. They may be normal in the presence of quite marked changes in the constituent proteins. For example a fall in plasma albumin concentration may be approximately balanced by a rise in immunoglobulin concentrations. Also, most individual proteins apart from albumin contribute little to the total protein concentration; therefore, quite a large percentage change in the concentration of one may not cause a detectable change in the total protein concentration.

Raised plasma total protein concentrations may be due to loss of protein-free fluid, or excessive stasis during venepuncture, or a major increase in the concentration of one or more of the immunoglobulins, including paraproteins.

Low plasma total protein concentrations may be due to dilution, for example if blood is taken near the site of an intravenous saline infusion, hypoalbuminaemia or severe immunoglobulin deficiency.

Qualitative methods for studying plasma and urinary proteins

Electrophoresis

Electrophoresis is a technique that separates compounds such as proteins according to their different electrical charges. It is usually performed by applying a small amount of serum to a strip of cellulose acetate or agarose and passing a current across it for a standard time. In this way, five main groups of proteins – namely albumin and the α_1, α_2, β and γ globulins – may be distinguished after protein staining and may be visually compared with those in a normal control serum. Each of the globulin fractions contains several proteins (Fig. 19.1).

Changes in electrophoretic patterns are most obvious when the concentrations of protein such as albumin that are usually high are abnormal, there are parallel changes in several proteins in the same fraction or a band not present in normal serum is visible.

The following description applies to the normal appearance, in adults, of the principal bands seen after electrophoresis on cellulose acetate.

- *Albumin*, usually a single protein, makes up the most obvious band.
- *Alpha$_1$-globulins* consist almost entirely of α_1-antitrypsin and α_1-antichymotrypsin.
- *Alpha$_2$-globulins* consist mainly of α_2-macroglobulin and haptoglobin.
- *Beta-globulins* often separate into two; β_1 consists mainly of transferrin with a contribution from low-density lipoprotein (LDL), and β_2 consists of the C3 component of complement.
- *Gamma-globulins* are immunoglobulins; some immunoglobulins are also found in the α_2 and β regions.

If plasma rather than serum is used, fibrinogen appears as a distinct band in the β–γ region. This may make interpretation difficult. Blood should be allowed to clot and serum used, rather than plasma, if electrophoresis is to be performed.

Electrophoretic patterns in disease (Fig. 19.2)

Some abnormal electrophoretic patterns are characteristic of a particular disorder or group of related disorders, while others indicate non-specific pathological processes. For example, the α_2 band, which contains haptoglobin, may be reduced if there is in-vivo haemolysis and may split into two if in-vitro haemolysis has occurred.

Parallel changes in all protein fractions

Reduction may occur in severe malnutrition, sometimes due to malabsorption, unless accompanied by infection and haemodilution. An increase may occur in haemoconcentration.

The acute-phase pattern

Tissue damage of any kind triggers the sequence of biochemical and cellular events associated with inflammation. The biochemical changes include the stimulation of synthesis of the so-called acute-phase proteins, with a rise in the

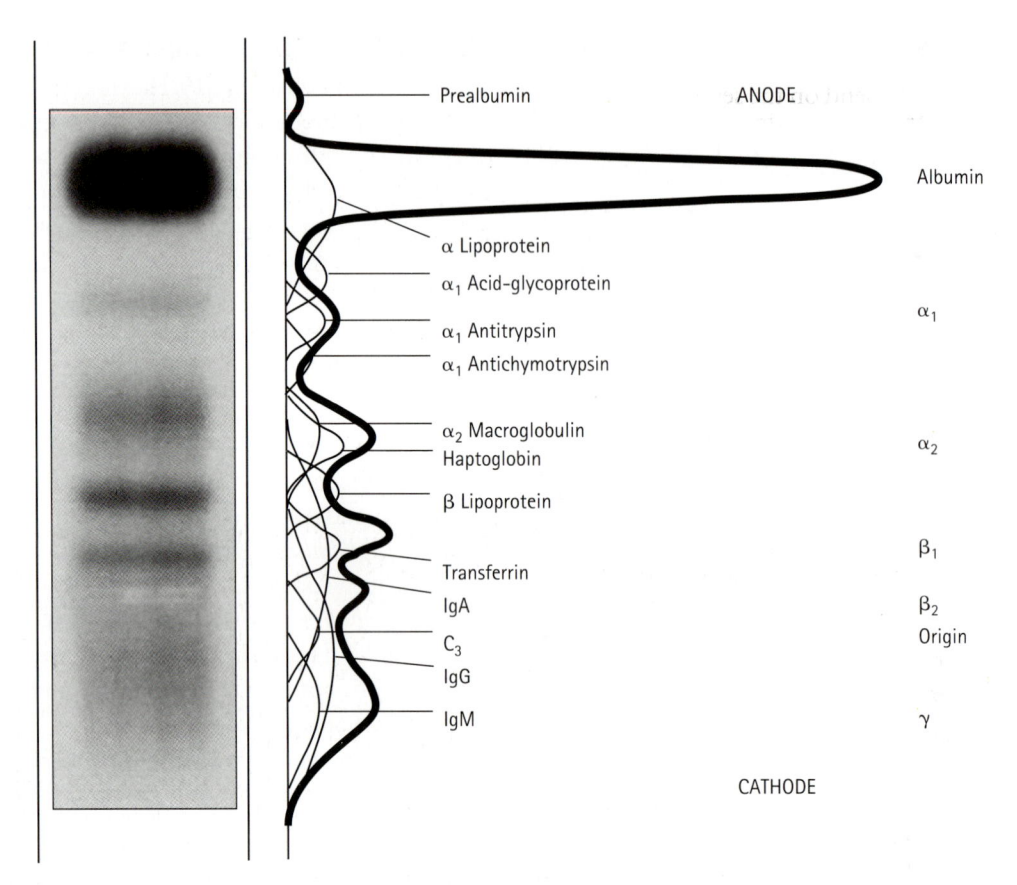

Fig. 19.1 The normal serum electrophoretic pattern. In this example the globulin has separated into β_1 and β_2 fractions. This finding is not uncommon, especially in stored specimens.

α_1-globulin and α_2-globulin fractions. The plasma concentrations of these proteins reflect the activity of the inflammatory response, and their presence is responsible for the rise in the erythrocyte sedimentation rate (ESR) and increased plasma viscosity characteristic of such a response.

Chronic inflammatory states

In chronic inflammation, the usual increase in immunoglobulin synthesis may be visible as a diffuse rise in γ-globulin. If there is an active inflammatory reaction, the increased density in the γ-globulin region is associated with an increase in the α_1 and α_2 fractions of the acute-phase response.

Cirrhosis of the liver

The changes in the concentrations of plasma proteins in liver disease are discussed in Chapter 17. They are usually 'non-specific', but in cirrhosis a characteristic pattern is sometimes seen. Albumin and often α_1-globulin concentrations are reduced and the γ-globulin concentration is markedly raised, with apparent fusion of the β and γ bands because of an increase in plasma IgA concentrations.

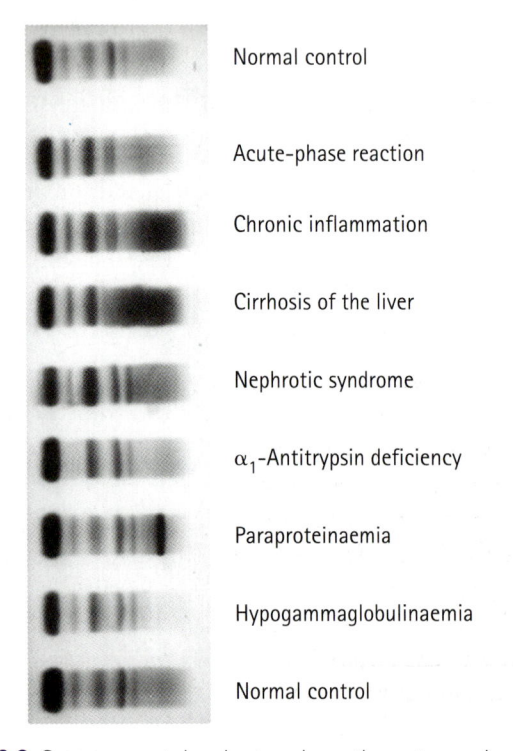

Fig. 19.2 Serum protein electrophoretic patterns in disease.

Nephrotic syndrome

Plasma protein changes depend on the severity of the renal lesion. In early cases, a low plasma albumin concentration may be the only abnormality, but the typical pattern in established cases is reduced albumin, α_1-globulin and sometimes γ-globulin bands and an increase in α_2-globulin concentration due to a relative or absolute increase in the high-molecular-weight α_2-macroglobulin. If the syndrome is due to conditions such as systemic lupus erythematosus (SLE), the γ-globulin concentration may be normal or raised.

Alpha$_1$-antitrypsin deficiency

The α_1 band consists almost entirely of α_1-antitrypsin and its absence or an obvious reduction in its density suggests α_1-antitrypsin deficiency. Occasionally, α_1-antitrypsin variants may present with a split α_1 band.

Other protein abnormalities

Hypogammaglobulinaemia shows reduced plasma γ-globulins and is discussed in the sections on immunoglobulins.

Multiple myeloma and paraproteinaemia may show a band(s) on the electrophoretic strip and are also discussed later.

Albumin

Albumin, with a molecular weight of about 65 kDa, is synthesized by the liver. It has a normal plasma biological half-life of about 20 days. About 60 per cent in the extracellular fluid is in the interstitial compartment. However, the concentration of albumin in the smaller intravascular compartment is much higher because of the relative impermeability of the blood vessel wall. This concentration gradient across the capillary membrane is important in maintaining plasma volume (see Chapter 2).

There are several inherited abnormalities of albumin synthesis:

- the *bisalbuminaemias*, in which two forms of albumin are present; there are usually no clinical consequences;
- *analbuminaemia*, in which there is deficient synthesis of the protein; clinical consequences are slight, and oedema, although present, is surprisingly mild.

An abnormally high plasma albumin concentration is found only artefactually in a sample taken with prolonged venous stasis or after loss of protein-free fluid.

Causes of hypoalbuminaemia

A low plasma albumin concentration may be due to dilution or to redistribution. True albumin deficiency may be caused by a decreased rate of synthesis, or by an increased rate of catabolism or loss from the body.

Dilutional hypoalbuminaemia

Dilutional hypoalbuminaemia may, as in the case of total protein, result from artefactual changes due to taking blood from the arm into which an infusion is flowing, administration of an excess of protein-free fluid or fluid retention, usually in oedematous states or during late pregnancy.

Redistribution of albumin

Redistribution of albumin from plasma into the interstitial fluid space results from:

- *recumbency*: plasma albumin concentrations may be 5–10 g/L lower in the recumbent than in the upright position because of the redistribution of fluid;
- *increased capillary membrane permeability*: this is the usual cause of the rapid fall in plasma concentration found in many circumstances, for example postoperatively and in most illnesses.

The slight fall in plasma albumin concentration found in mild illness may be due to a combination of the above two factors.

Decreased synthesis of albumin

Normally, about 4 per cent of the body albumin is replaced each day. Hepatic impairment, such as cirrhosis, causes hypoalbuminaemia if the rate of synthesis of new amino acids is inadequate to replace those deaminated during metabolism; most of the amino nitrogen is then lost as urinary urea. Hypoalbuminaemia may therefore be due to:

- *malnutrition*, resulting in an inadequate supply of dietary nitrogen;
- *malabsorption*, resulting in impaired absorption of dietary peptides and amino acids;
- *impairment of synthesis*, due to chronic liver dysfunction, for example cirrhosis.

Increased loss of albumin from the body

Due to its relatively low molecular weight, significant amounts of albumin and other low-molecular-weight proteins are lost in conditions associated with increased membrane permeability. The plasma concentration of albumin is higher than that of the other proteins and its loss is therefore more obvious. Albumin loss may occur through:

- the *skin*, because of extensive burns or skin diseases such as psoriasis; a large part of the interstitial fluid is subcutaneous;
- the *intestinal wall*, in protein-losing enteropathy;
- the *glomeruli*, in the nephrotic syndrome.

Increased catabolism of albumin

Catabolism (and therefore nitrogen loss) is increased in many illnesses, including sepsis and hyperthyroidism. This may worsen the hypoalbuminaemia due to other causes.

Consequences of hypoalbuminaemia

The following may occur.

- *Fluid distribution*: albumin is quantitatively the most important protein contributing to the plasma colloid osmotic pressure. Oedema may occur in severe hypoalbuminaemia (see Chapter 2).
- *Binding functions*: albumin binds calcium, bilirubin and free fatty acids. (See Chapter 6 for a discussion of albumin-corrected calcium.)

A number of drugs, such as salicylates, penicillin and sulphonamides, may become albumin bound. The albumin-bound fractions are physiologically and pharmacologically inactive. A marked reduction in plasma albumin, by reducing the binding capacity, may increase the plasma free concentration of those substances leading to toxic effects.

Albumin-bound drugs may, if administered together, compete for binding sites, thus increasing free concentrations; an example of this is the simultaneous administration of salicylates and the anticoagulant warfarin, potentiating the effect of the latter (see Chapter 25).

The acute phase response

The body responds to tissue damage and to the presence of infecting organisms or other foreign substances by a complex, inter-related series of cellular and humoral responses. These act together to initiate and control the inflammatory reaction and so to remove damaged tissues and foreign substances. Defence mechanisms can be separated into two main groups.

- The *inflammatory response*: this is non-specific, requires changes in the permeability of membranes and depends on humoral factors such as acute-phase reactants, complement or cytokines released in response to inflammation and on a phagocytic cellular response dependent on the function of polymorphonuclear leucocytes and monocytes.
- The *immune response*: in this type of response, cellular or humoral factors act on specific foreign organisms. It depends on the function of lymphocytes, which can be differentiated into:
  - *B-lymphocytes*, activated by antigens and by lymphokines, which develop into plasma cells in the bone marrow and synthesize and secrete immunoglobulins;
  - *T-lymphocytes*, which, in the thymus, acquire a range of surface antigens that play a vital role in T-cell function after migration to other lymphoid tissue. These include cytotoxicity and delayed hypersensitivity. They also have a regulatory function as either helper or suppressor cells. Each group can be further subdivided using antibodies against the cell surface markers; this is known as cluster differentiation (CD) (Fig. 19.3).

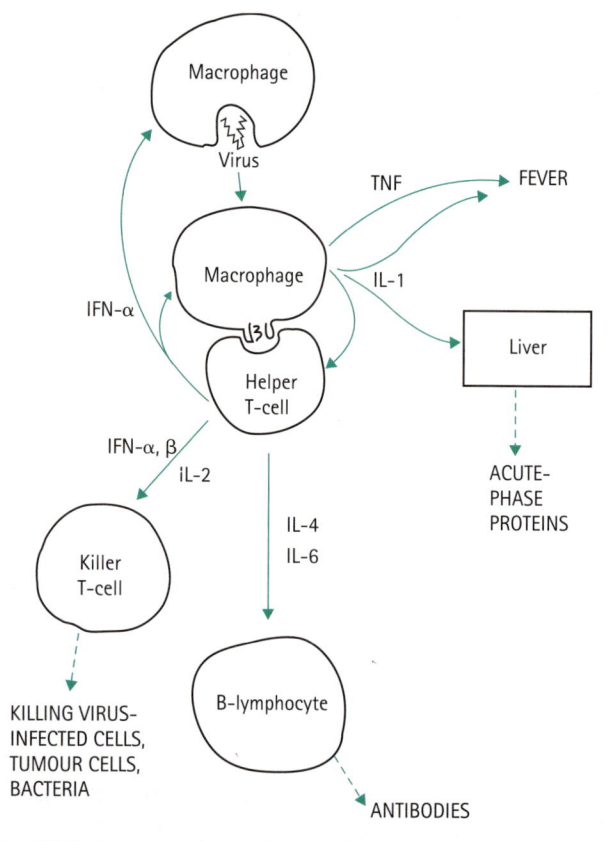

Fig. 19.3 Some of the actions of the cytokines. (TNF = tumour necrosis factor; IFN = interferon; IL = interleukin.) (Reproduced with kind permission from Candlish JK and Crook M, *Notes on Clinical Biochemistry*, Singapore: World Scientific Publishing, 1993.)

The inflammatory response and the ability to kill foreign organisms may be impaired if there is deficiency of either cellular or humoral components.

Acute-phase proteins

The innate or natural immune system, which is phylogenetically older than so-called acquired or adaptive immunity, is a rapid first-line defence mechanism based on non-lymphoid tissue components. The acute-phase response is part of this system and results in pronounced changes in the concentration of plasma proteins in response to a variety of stresses, including infection, tissue injury and inflammation. The concentration of some of these proteins increases (positive acute-phase proteins), such as CRP, fibrinogen and plasma amyloid A, whereas that of others decreases (negative acute-phase proteins), such as albumin and transferrin. (See Fig. 19.4.)

The non-specific changes in plasma protein concentrations occurring in response to acute or chronic tissue damage are caused by increased protein synthesis in the liver in response to peptide mediators or cytokines.

Cytokines regulate the immune and inflammatory responses. They are classified, depending on their principal biological functions, into groups such as interleukins (IL), interferons (IFN) and tumour necrosis factors (TNF).

They activate receptors on adjacent cells (paracrine) or on the same cell (autocrine), but those involved in the inflammatory response, such as IL-1, IL-6 and TNF-α, affect distant (endocrine) organs.

The acute-phase reactants include the following.

- *Activators* of other inflammatory pathways such as CRP, so called because it reacts with the C-polysaccharide of pneumococci. This protein combines with bacterial polysaccharides or phospholipids released from damaged tissue to become an activator of the complement pathway. Plasma concentrations of CRP rise rapidly in response to acute inflammation and its assay is particularly useful in the early detection of acute infection.
- *Inhibitors*, such as α_1-antitrypsin, which control the inflammatory response and so minimize damage to host tissue.
- *Scavengers*, such as haptoglobin, which binds haemoglobin released by local in-vivo haemolysis during the inflammatory response.

The concentrations of plasma fibrinogen and of several complement components also increase. An acute-phase response increases blood viscosity and therefore the ESR. The plasma albumin concentration falls and secondary decreases of complement and haptoglobin occur if they are used up excessively. Haptoglobin may be undetectable if much haemoglobin is released from red cells due to intravascular haemolysis or haemorrhage into tissues.

The non-specific nature of the response means that the measurement of individual acute-phase proteins is rarely helpful as an aid to diagnosis. The demonstration of a rise in plasma CRP concentration is more sensitive and specific than measurement of the ESR and is most often raised in bacterial infections and in other acute inflammatory conditions (Fig. 19.4).

Clinically, plasma CRP is used in the following circumstances.

- *To detect an infection*: plasma CRP concentrations are not usually increased in viral infections, but the highest levels are seen in bacterial infections. It has a particular place in diagnosing neonatal infections. In immunosuppressed patients, the usual systemic response to infection such as neutrophil leucocytosis and fever may not be present, and therefore a raised plasma CRP concentration of greater than 10 mg/L suggests infection.
- *As a guide to the severity of connective tissue disease activity*: such conditions include rheumatoid arthritis, juvenile chronic polyarthritis (Still's disease) and polymyalgia rheumatica. Systemic lupus erythematosus

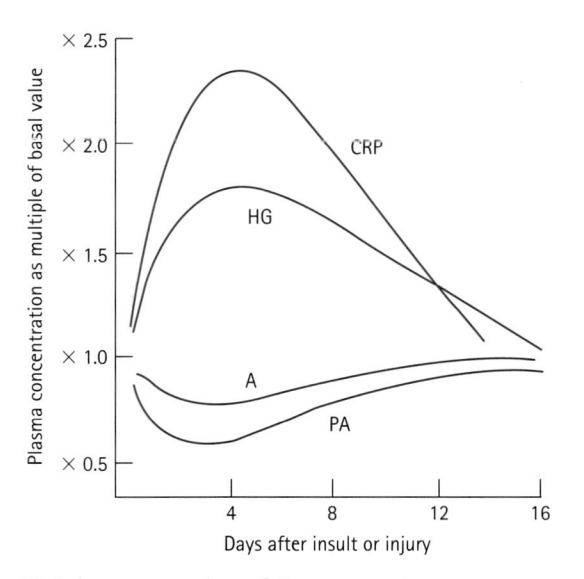

Fig. 19.4 Some proteins of the acute-phase response. (CRP = C-reactive protein; HG = haptoglobulin; A = albumin; PA = prealbumin. The latter pair can be termed negative acute-phase proteins.) (Reproduced with kind permission from Candlish JK and Crook M, *Notes on Clinical Biochemistry*, Singapore: World Scientific Publishing, 1993.)

shows less of a CRP rise, but this may be useful to distinguish infection in SLE from an acute disease flare-up (plasma concentrations more than 60 mg/L indicate the former).
- *In the diagnosis of inflammatory bowel disease*: plasma CRP levels more than 50 mg/L are more indicative of Crohn's disease than ulcerative colitis.
- *As an indicator of cardiovascular risk*: raised plasma CRP concentrations using a high-sensitivity assay are a strong cardiovascular risk factor (see Chapter 22), as subclinical inflammatory processes have been implicated in atherosclerosis. Plasma levels less than 1 mg/L constitute low cardiovascular risk; patients with levels more than 3 mg/L are at high risk of cardiovascular disease.

Procalcitonin is a 14-kDa protein encoded by the *Calc-1* gene. Blood levels of procalcitonin are increased in systemic inflammation and procalcitonin has been proposed as a possibly better marker of bacterial sepsis than CRP.

Complement

Macrophages and hepatocytes synthesize a group of proteins called the complement system, which is part of the innate immune system. Sequential activation reduces complement plasma concentrations, but in many instances this is compensated for by increased synthesis of acute-phase reactants. The products of activation attract phagocytes to the area of inflammation (chemotaxis), which, by increasing the permeability of the capillary wall to both cellular and chemical components, allows them to reach affected cells. Activation of the complete complement pathway on foreign cell surfaces results in their lysis and, together with immunoglobulins, some of the complement components act as opsonins, which enhance phagocytosis. Due to inhibitors, complement usually circulates in an inactive form.

Clinically, the most important of the complement proteins is C3. Two main pathways are concerned with its activation (Fig. 19.5). Activation of either results in low plasma C3 concentrations.

Classical pathway

In the classical pathway, C3 is activated by the products of a pathway initiated by the activation of C1, usually by antigen-bound IgG or IgM (immune complexes), by protein within the cell walls of many strains of *Staphylococcus aureus*, or by CRP. C4 (and C2) are used during the resultant sequence of events, which also activates the alternative pathway via C3; plasma C3 and C4 concentrations fall. Once the formation of immune complexes stops, plasma C3 and C4 concentrations are restored. The enzyme C1q esterase inhibits the serine protease C1 (which is composed of C1q, C1r and C1s).

Alternative pathway

In the alternative pathway, which is the more important of the two, C3 is activated by IgA immune complexes, and substances such as lipopolysaccharides and peptidoglycans in the walls of certain bacteria and viruses, factor B and properdin are involved. C3b is formed, which in turn activates more C3. Other products of C3b cause vasodilatation and cell lysis. The cyclical process is self-perpetuating and plasma C3 concentrations fall. If the initial stimulus is removed, inhibitors such as those formed in the acute-phase reaction control the reaction and C3 concentrations return to normal; factors H and I inhibit the enzyme C3 convertase. The alternative pathway is most important in the absence of preformed antibodies.

Recently, a third pathway of C3 activation has been described involving mannose-binding lectin, one of the colectin proteins. After C3 activation, the terminal complement system consists of other activated proteins such as C5–9, collectively known as the membrane attack complex. This is involved in puncturing cell membranes.

In immune-complex disease, such as SLE, circulating immune complexes persist. The products of C3, released by continued activation of the classical pathway, may damage blood vessels, joints and the kidneys. Plasma concentrations of both C3 and C4 are low. Persistently low plasma C3 concentrations may help to distinguish chronic mesangiocapillary glomerulonephritis, with a poor prognosis, from the less serious and self-limiting acute post-streptococcal glomerulonephritis, in which plasma C3 concentrations return to normal within a few months.

Normal cellular response to infection

Two types of phagocytic cells help to combat infection. *Polymorphonuclear neutrophil leucocytes* migrate into sites of acute inflammation and represent a non-specific first line of defence against pyogenic bacteria. *Mononuclear phagocytes* circulate in blood as monocytes. They migrate to sites of chronic inflammation, where they develop into macrophages. Under T-cell control, macrophages are activated and develop a greatly enhanced ability to phagocytose and digest pathogenic organisms.

The most important functions of T-cells in the inflammatory response are the initiation and maintenance of chronic cellular inflammatory responses to invading organisms and the control of immune inflammation by providing helper and suppressor influences on other cells. B-cells need the co-operation of T-cells (helper cells) to make antibodies to complex antigens.

T-cell modulation of inflammatory and immune responses is mediated by chemical messengers called lymphokines. T-cells also have a cytotoxic function directed towards destroying the body's own cells infected by intracellular pathogens such as viruses.

Immune response

Immunoglobulins

Immunoglobulins, synthesized by B lymphocytes, are incorporated into cell membranes, where they act as antigen receptors. On exposure to a specific antigen in the presence of T-helper cells, these B lymphocytes proliferate and differentiate into plasma cells synthesizing and secreting immunoglobulins.

Structure

The basic immunoglobulin is a Y-shaped molecule (depicted schematically in Fig. 19.6).

Usually four polypeptide chains are linked by disulphide bonds. There are two heavy (H) and two light (L) chains in each unit. The H chains in a single unit are identical and determine the immunoglobulin class of the protein. Heavy chains γ, α, μ, δ and ϵ occur in IgG, IgA, IgM, IgD and IgE respectively. The L chains are of two types, κ and λ. In a single molecule, the L chains are of the same type, although the immunoglobulin class as a whole contains both types.

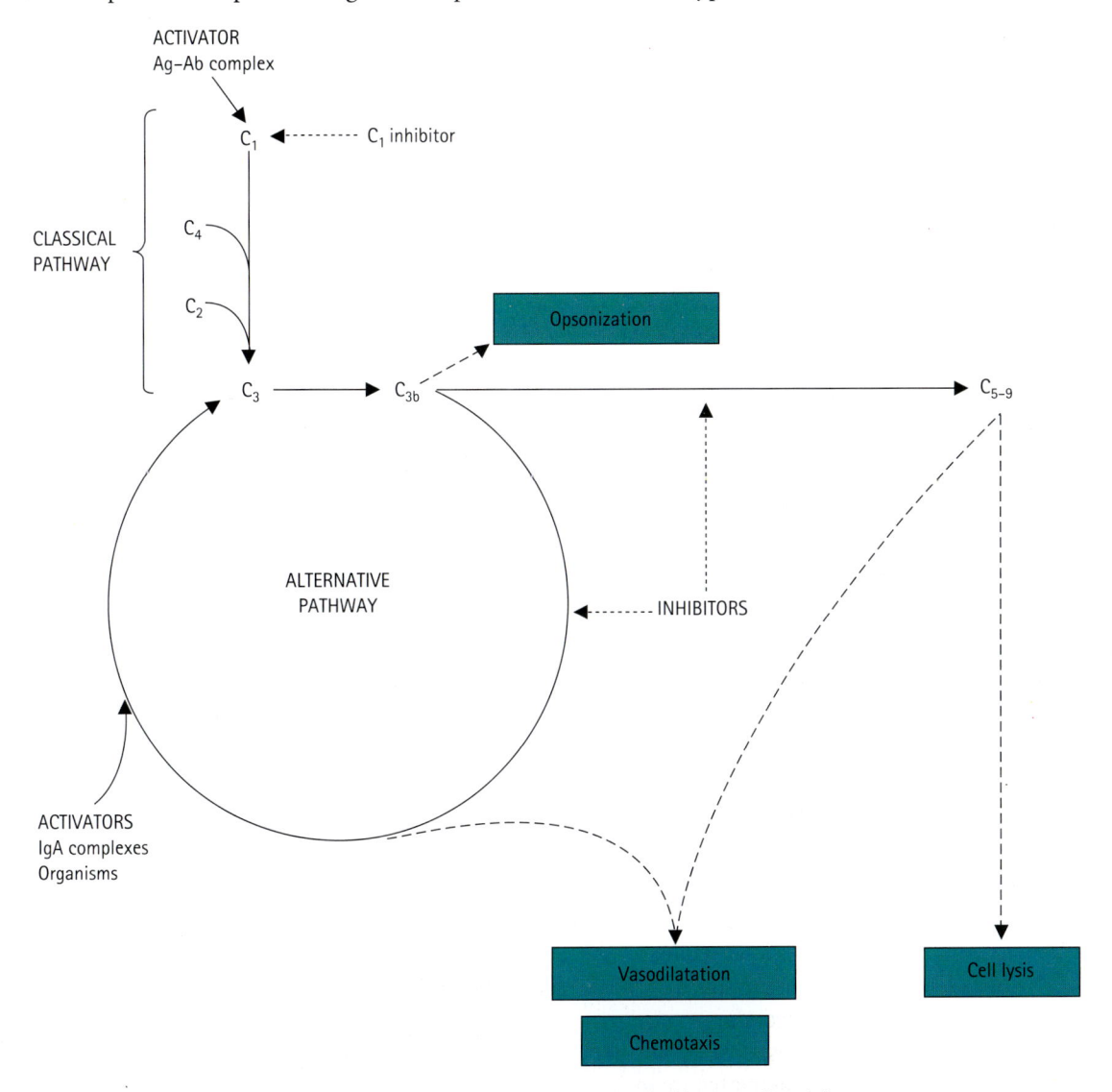

Fig. 19.5 The complement pathway, much simplified. (Ag = antigen; Ab = antibody.)

There are two antigen-combining sites per monomer, together known as the F(ab)₂ piece. These lie at the ends of the arms of the Y; both H and L chains are necessary for full antibody activity. The amino acid composition of this part of the chain varies in different units (variable region). When the F(ab)₂ site combines with antigen, conformational changes are transmitted through the hinge region of the heavy chain and the Fc segment of the molecule becomes activated and reacts with Fc receptors on a number of immune cell types resulting in immune activation.

The rest of the H and L chains is less variable (constant region, which includes the Fc segment). The activated Fc segments of the H chains are responsible for such properties as the ability to bind complement or actively to cross the placental membrane. The H chains are associated with a variable amount of carbohydrate; IgM has the highest content.

Some immunoglobulin molecules contain more than one basic unit bound together by 'J' chains; for example, the IgM molecule consists of five units. Because of the variation in size and therefore in density, the classes can be separated by ultracentrifugation. They are classified by their Sedimentation coefficient (Svedberg units/S), the S value of a protein increasing with increasing size. The S values of immunoglobulins, together with their most important functions and properties, are shown in Table 19.1.

Normal immunoglobulin response to infection

In response to infection, each plasma cell produces an immunoglobulin of a single class.

IgG

Immunoglobulin G concentrations rise slightly later in response to soluble antigens such as bacterial toxins. Due to their relatively low molecular weight, they can diffuse into the interstitial fluid to fight against tissue infection. Within a few weeks of the initial infection, raised plasma concentrations of all immunoglobulins may be demonstrated and may be detectable as a diffusely increased γ zone on the electrophoretic strip. There are four subclasses (IgG 1–4) in humans.

IgM

Immunoglobulin M is synthesized first in response to particulate antigens such as blood-borne organisms. Due to the relatively large size of IgM, it mostly remains in the

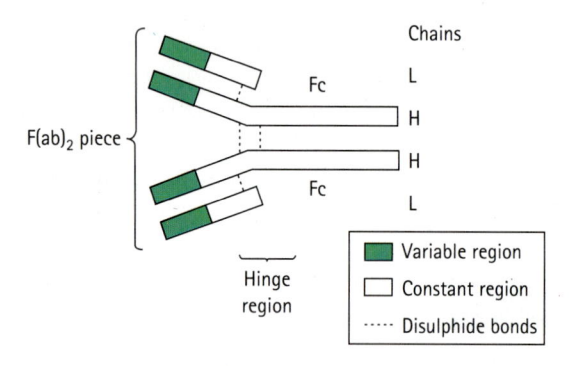

Fig. 19.6 Diagram of an immunoglobulin monomer. (L = light; H = heavy.)

Table 19.1 The properties and functions of the plasma immunoglobulins

	IgG	IgA	IgM	IgE	IgD
Molecular weight (kDa)	160	160	1000	200	190
Sedimentation coefficient (Svedberg units)	7S	7S	19S	8S	7S
% total plasma Ig	73	19	7	0.001	1
Complement activation	Yes	Yes	Yes	No	No
Placental transfer	Yes	No	No	No	No
Mean adult concentration (g/L)	10	2	1	0.0003	0.03
Adult levels reached	3–5 years	15 years	9 months	15 years	15 years
Major function	Protects extravascular tissue space Secondary response to antigen Inactivates toxin	Protects body surfaces as secretory IgA (11S)	Protects blood stream Primary response to antigen Bacterial lysis	Mast cell activation	?

vascular compartment. This, together with the speed of synthetic response, makes it the first line of defence amongst immunoglobulins against invading organisms. The fetus can synthesize IgM, and high plasma concentrations at birth usually indicate that there has been an intrauterine infection.

IgA

Immunoglobulin A is synthesized predominantly submucosally and is present in intestinal and respiratory secretions, sweat, tears and colostrum. It is affected more than other immunoglobulins in diseases of the gastrointestinal and respiratory tracts. Secretory IgA is a dimer, in which two subunits are joined by a peptide 'J' chain, and has a 'secretory piece' synthesized by epithelial cells.

Infections, particularly if chronic, activate B lymphocytes and cause a polyclonal immunoglobulin response. However, immunoglobulin estimation adds little to the observation of increased γ-globulin visible in the serum electrophoretic pattern.

In certain conditions (some of which are listed in Table 19.2), one or more immunoglobulin class predominates.

Although there is considerable overlap, individual immunoglobulin estimation may occasionally help in the diagnosis of some of these conditions.

Immunoglobulin response to allergy

IgE

Immunoglobulin E is synthesized by plasma cells beneath the mucosae of the gastrointestinal and respiratory tracts and in the lymphoid tissue of the nasopharynx. Circulating IgE is rapidly bound to cell surfaces, particularly those of mast cells and basophils; plasma concentrations are therefore very low.

The combination of antigen with this cell-bound antibody stimulates cells to release biologically active mediators and accounts for such immediate hypersensitivity reactions as occur in hay fever, the severest form of hypersensitivity being anaphylactic shock.

Raised plasma IgE concentrations are found in several diseases with an allergic (atopic) component, such as some cases of eczema, asthma due to allergens ('extrinsic') and parasitic infestation (Table 19.3).

The diagnosis of an allergic disorder is usually made from the history, but skin testing and the measurement of plasma IgE concentrations may be needed. In skin testing, a small drop of dilute allergen is injected subcutaneously; a positive 'wheal and flare' develops within a few minutes (immediate hypersensitivity). *This test is contraindicated in patients with a history of eczema or anaphylaxis*, and plasma IgE may be assessed to detect specific allergens.

Table 19.2 Some abnormalities of plasma immunoglobulins in disease

Predominant class of immunoglobulin (Ig) increased	Examples of clinical conditions
IgG	Autoimmune diseases, e.g. systemic lupus erythematosus and chronic active hepatitis
IgA	Diseases of the intestinal tract, e.g. Crohn's disease Diseases of the respiratory tract, e.g. tuberculosis, bronchiectasis
IgM	Primary biliary cirrhosis Haemoprotozoan infections, e.g. malaria At birth, indicating intrauterine infections Viral hepatitis and some acute viral infections
IgG, IgA, IgM	Chronic bacterial infections, sarcoidosis, acquired immunodeficiency syndrome

Table 19.3 Diseases associated with increased serum IgE

Allergic disease (type 1 hypersensitivity)	'Extrinsic' asthma Hay fever Atopic eczema Urticaria-angioedema Anaphylaxis
Allergic disease arising secondary to immunodeficiency or immunosuppression	Some genetic defects Other primary T-cell deficiencies and acquired immunodeficiency syndrome
Direct response to infections	Mainly parasitic helminths (e.g. echinococcosis, ascariasis and toxocariasis)

Deficiencies of components of the inflammatory response and of proteins of the immune system

Deficiencies of the inflammatory or immune response of the host defence system may result in an increased risk of infection and lack of immune regulation. Plasma immunoglobulins reflect only the humoral phase of the immune system; their measurement does not assess cellular immunity. *Normal plasma immunoglobulin concentrations do not exclude an immune deficiency state*; they may, in fact, be raised, as in the acquired immunodeficiency syndrome (AIDS). The human immunodeficiency virus binds to CD4 cells and becomes internalized.

As a general rule, any patient with a severe, protracted, unusual or recurrent infection should be investigated for an underlying deficiency in 'defence' mechanisms.

B cell and immunoglobulin deficiency

Dysgammaglobulinaemia

Dysgammaglobulinaemia is defined as an abnormality in the structure or distribution in the class(es) of immunoglobulins.

The plasma globulin concentration may be reduced or normal.

Immunoglobulin G subclass deficiency may be associated with certain recurrent respiratory tract infections.

Hypogammaglobulinaemia

Hypogammaglobulinaemia can be defined as a decrease in plasma immunoglobulins. Total plasma protein concentration is usually low.

A marked reduction in plasma immunoglobulin concentrations may be detectable as obvious hypogammaglobulinaemia in the serum electrophoretic pattern, but usually measurement of individual proteins is needed to make a diagnosis. The effects of deficiencies of individual immunoglobulins are related to their functions and distribution.

- *IgA deficiency* may be symptomless, or may be associated with recurrent, mild respiratory tract infections or intestinal diseases.
- *IgG deficiency* may result in recurrent pyogenic infections of tissue spaces, especially in the lungs and skin, by toxin-producing organisms such as staphylococci and streptococci.
- *IgM deficiency* frequently predisposes to septicaemia.

Primary immunoglobulin deficiency is less common than that which is secondary to other disorders.

Various classifications have been proposed for these deficiencies, some of which are discussed below.

Transient immunoglobulin deficiency

In the newborn infant, circulating IgG is derived from the mother by active placental transfer. Plasma concentrations decrease over the first 3–6 months of life and then gradually rise as endogenous IgG synthesis increases. In some infants, onset of synthesis is delayed and 'physiological hypogammaglobulinaemia' may persist for several months.

During pregnancy, most of the IgG transfer across the placenta takes place in the last 3 months. Severe deficiency may therefore develop in very premature babies because the concentration of IgG derived from the mother falls before the endogenous concentration rises.

Primary immunoglobulin deficiency

Primary IgA deficiency in plasma, saliva and other secretions is relatively common, with an incidence of about 1 in 500 of the population. Most cases are symptom free.

Several rare syndromes, usually familial, have been described. In infantile sex-linked agammaglobulinaemia (Bruton's disease), which occurs only in males, there is almost complete absence of B-cells and circulating immunoglobulins, while cellular (T-cell) immunity is normal. Other syndromes have varying degrees of immunoglobulin deficiency and impaired cellular immunity and can occur in either sex.

Secondary immunoglobulin deficiency

Low plasma immunoglobulin concentrations are most common in patients with malignant disease, particularly of the haemopoietic and immune systems, and often precipitated by chemotherapy or radiotherapy; they are an almost invariable finding in patients with myelomatosis (immune paresis). In severe protein-losing states, such as the nephrotic syndrome or protein-losing enteropathy, low plasma immunoglobulin concentrations (especially of IgG) are due partly to the loss of relatively low-molecular-weight immunoglobulins and partly to increased catabolism. Other causes are shown in Box 19.1.

T-cell deficiency

Patients with T-cell deficiency present with severe, protracted infections caused by viruses, fungi or rarely detected

> **Box 19.1 Some causes of hypogammaglobulinaemia**
>
> *Primary*
> Bruton's or Swiss-type agammaglobulinaemia
>
> *Secondary*
> Protein-losing states, e.g. nephrotic syndrome, major burns and protein-losing enteropathy
> Malnutrition
> Diabetes mellitus
> Cushing's syndrome
> Malignancy, including chronic lymphocytic leukaemia, lymphomas, paraproteinaemia
> Chronic renal failure
> Chronic infections
> Drugs such as steroids, azathioprine, cyclophosphamide
> Irradiation

organisms such as *Pneumocystis carinii* and *Cryptococcus*. It is important to identify T-cell deficiencies, because the administration of live vaccines and blood products is then contraindicated. T-cell deficiency may be classified as:

- *primary* (congenital) deficiencies, which are rare, often severe and usually present soon after birth; they range from total or partial T-cell depletion to loss of function;
- *secondary* (acquired) deficiencies, associated with metabolic disorders such as diabetes mellitus, malnutrition, drug abuse, auto-immunity, malignancy and immunosuppressive treatment or radiation; secondary T-cell deficiency is relatively common, often mild and presents at any age.

In severe combined immunodeficiency (SCID) syndrome, T-cell function is affected, often also with B-cell abnormalities. This syndrome can be caused by a number of genetic conditions that interfere with lymphocyte development and function, including SCID-X1, a defect of the γ-chain of interleukin receptors, and adenosine deaminase deficiency, which allows a lymphocyte toxic build-up of adenosine diphosphate, guanosine triphosphate and deoxyadenosine triphosphate.

T-cells may be decreased in number or may function abnormally. The total lymphocyte count may be normal despite severe T-lymphocytopenia, such as occurs in acquired deficiencies, or malignancy, as in chronic lymphocytic leukaemia. T-cell function may be assessed by determining cell-surface markers and therefore changes in the different T-cell subsets. Changes in the ratio of helper to suppressor cells occur in many conditions, but are profound in AIDS, in which the virus specifically affects the CD4 cell population and numbers can go below 200 cells/mm^3.

Deficiencies of other proteins of the inflammatory response

Other proteins involved in complement activation or as acute-phase reactants may be deficient in addition to immunoglobulins. The most clinically significant are discussed below.

Complement deficiency

Complement deficiencies, for example of C5–9, are very rare, although they may predispose individuals to infections, for example meningococcal. C1, C2 and C4 deficiency are associated with SLE. Mannose-binding lectin deficiency increases the risk of *Neisseria meningitidis* and *Streptococcus pneumoniae* infection. C5 deficiency may lead to Leiner's disease, associated with diarrhoea, seborrhoeic dermatitis and wasting.

In hereditary angioneurotic oedema, C1 esterase inhibitor is deficient or of low activity. The condition is characterized by episodes of increased capillary permeability and consequent oedema of the subcutaneous tissues and mucous membranes of the upper respiratory or gastrointestinal tract. Laryngeal oedema may be fatal. Plasma C1 esterase inhibitor concentration or activity can be measured.

Complement deficiences can be assessed by measuring individual complement components and also CH50 (a measure of the complement activity).

Alpha$_1$-antitrypsin deficiency

Alpha$_1$-antitrypsin normally controls the proteolytic action of lysosomal enzymes from phagocytes (protease inhibitors, PI), and is an acute-phase reactant. Plasma concentrations rise 2–3 days after trauma or acute infection.

There are more than 50 genetic variants of α$_1$-antitrypsin, inherited as autosomal co-dominant alleles. The most common allele is *PIM* with a genotype *MM*. At least seven of the phenotypes are associated with low functional plasma α$_1$-antitrypsin concentrations, the most important of which is *PI* null, are associated with complete deficiency of the protein. Others include *PIS* and *PIZ*, in which protein accumulates in the liver because it cannot be secreted after synthesis, and *PIM Duarte*, in which plasma concentrations of the protein may be normal but there is deficient functional activity.

Alpha$_1$-antitrypsin deficiency may be suspected after serum electrophoresis if the α_1 band is much reduced, absent or split; the condition may present clinically with the following.

- *Hepatic cirrhosis*, occurring in 10–20 per cent of subjects, such as *PIZ* homozygotes, in whom the protein cannot be secreted by hepatocytes. The condition may present as hepatitis in the neonatal period or as cirrhosis in children or young adults (see Chapter 17).
- *Pulmonary disease*: the unopposed action of proteases from phagocytes in the lung may, by destroying elastic tissue, cause basal panlobular emphysema in adults, aged between 30 and 40 years, who are homozygous for the abnormal alleles. The condition may be exacerbated by cigarette smoking, air pollution or infection.

The diagnosis of α_1-antitrypsin deficiency can usually be confirmed by demonstrating that the plasma α_1-antitrypsin concentration is low; the phenotype or genotype should then be identified. Blood relations should be investigated and all those with abnormal plasma concentrations should receive genetic counselling and be advised not to smoke.

B-cell disorders

Each B-cell clone is highly specialized and synthesizes a single class and type of immunoglobulin. The normal B-cell response to an antigenic stimulus, such as infection, is synthesis of a range of different immunoglobulins by groups (clones) of cells. This is known as a *polyclonal* response and causes a diffuse hypergammaglobulinaemia in the electrophoretic pattern. If one of these cells proliferates to form a clone of like cells, a single protein will be produced in excess. The *monoclonal* proliferation of B-cells is often, but not always, malignant.

Paraproteinaemia

The term paraprotein refers to the appearance of an abnormal, narrow dense band on the electrophoretic strip. It is found most commonly in the γ region, but may be anywhere from the α_2 to the γ region. Paraproteins can often be shown to be monoclonal.

Causes of paraproteinaemia

Although the presence of a paraprotein is strongly suggestive of a malignant process, it is not diagnostic. Paraproteins may be found in the following malignant conditions:

- *myelomatosis*, which accounts for most of the cases of malignant paraproteinaemia,
- *macroglobulinaemia* (Waldenström's macroglobulinaemia),
- *B-cell lymphomas*, including chronic lymphatic leukaemia,
- sometimes in *SLE, chronic inflammation* or *infection*,
- *cryoglobulinaemia*.

The consequences of malignant B-cell proliferation

Some of the clinical and laboratory findings are similar in all malignant B-cell tumours. Whether they occur depends on the concentration of paraprotein, the presence or absence of immune paresis and the presence of Bence-Jones protein (BJP). However, malignant tumours of B-cells can exist without all or, rarely, any of these findings.

Consequences of paraproteins

Unless the concentration of paraprotein is very high, these findings may not be present. Very high plasma concentrations, which are suggestive of malignancy, may be associated with a very elevated ESR or CRP and also with the following.

- In-vivo effects of increased plasma viscosity with sluggish blood flow in small vessels. This may result in retinal-vein thrombosis with impairment of vision, cerebral thrombosis, or even peripheral gangrene (hyperviscosity syndrome).
- An increased blood viscosity that may be noticeable during venepuncture; it may also be difficult to prepare blood films. Hyperviscosity is most common in macroglobulinaemia but may occur in myelomatosis.
- A high plasma total protein concentration despite a normal or low plasma albumin concentration; the difference between the total plasma protein concentration and albumin concentration is termed the globulin concentration.
- Spurious hyponatraemia (pseudohyponatraemia) may occur due to the space-occupying effect of the protein and the effect on indirect ion electrodes (see Chapter 2).
- Bence-Jones protein is usually, but not invariably, found in the urine of patients with malignancy of B-cells (Fig. 19.7); it can also be found in the absence

paraprotein, is reduced or absent and concentrations of the other immunoglobulins are low (Fig. 19.7).

Other findings in patients with malignant B-cell tumours are:

- *normochromic normocytic anaemia*, a common presenting feature of any malignant disease;
- *haemorrhages*, perhaps due to complexing of coagulation factors by the paraprotein;
- *Raynaud's phenomenon*, which may occur if the paraprotein is a cryoglobulin;
- *hypercalcaemia* may also be present.

Beta$_2$-microglobulin is a low-molecular-weight protein (11.8 kDa) that forms part of the human lymphocyte antigen on the surface of all nucleated cells. The protein is readily filtered by glomeruli, and plasma concentrations are normally low. In myelomatosis the plasma β_2-microglobulin concentration is an index of the extent of the disease and of the prognosis. Occasionally, raised plasma concentrations may occur in a number of haematological malignancies. Beta$_2$-microglobulin is a surrogate marker for the overall body tumour burden.

Myelomatosis (multiple myeloma; plasma-cell myeloma)

Myelomatosis is caused by the malignant proliferation of plasma cells throughout the bone marrow. The condition becomes increasingly frequent after the age of 50; it can occur before the age of 30, but is rare. The sex incidence is about equal. The clinical features are due to malignant proliferation of plasma cells and disordered immunoglobulin synthesis and/or secretion from the cell.

Malignant proliferation of plasma cells

Bone pain may be severe and is due to pressure from the proliferating cells. X-rays may show discrete punched-out areas of radio-translucency, most frequently in the skull, vertebrae, ribs and pelvis. There may be generalized osteoporosis. Pathological fractures may occur. Histologically there is little osteoblastic activity around the lesion, which arises in the marrow rather than in the bone itself; consequently, the plasma alkaline phosphatase activity is normal unless there is liver involvement, in which case the raised level is of hepatic, not bony, origin. A normal plasma alkaline phosphatase activity, in cases with bone lesions, suggests myelomatosis rather than bony metastases. Hypercalcaemia may occur and also renal failure. The latter may occur as a result of Bence-Jones proteinuria as well as the hypercalcaemia. Amyloidosis is also associated.

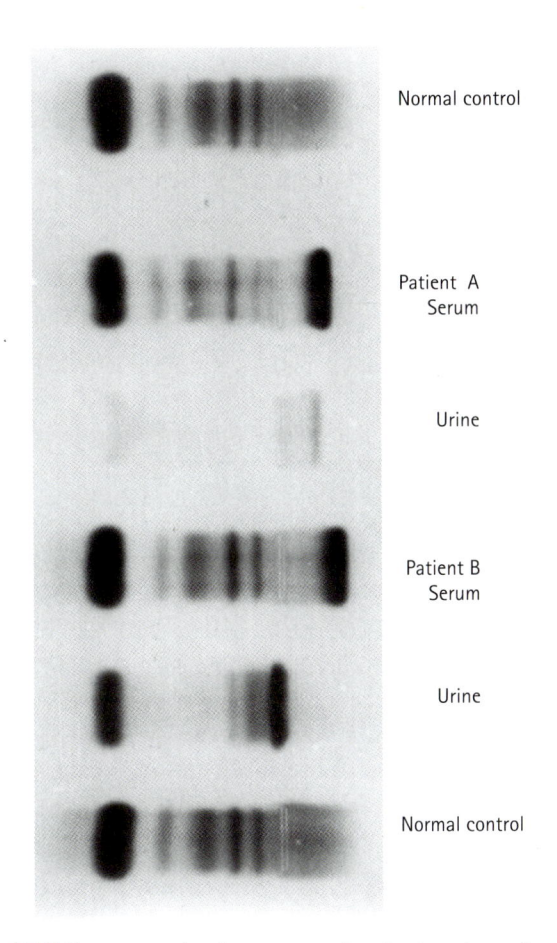

Fig. 19.7 Serum and urinary protein electrophoretic patterns in myelomatosis. Patient A with paraprotein and immune paresis in serum and Bence-Jones protein (BJP) band in urine. Patient B with paraprotein and immune paresis in serum and with heavy BJP on the right and leakage of albumin and other low molecular-weight proteins (glomerular permeability) in urine.

of malignant disease. It consists of free monoclonal L chains, or fragments of them, which have been synthesized much in excess of H chains, implying a degree of dedifferentiation. Due to its relatively low molecular weight (20–40 kDa), the protein is filtered at glomeruli and only accumulates in plasma if there is glomerular impairment or if it polymerizes. It may damage renal tubular cells and form large casts, producing the 'myeloma kidney'. It may also be a precursor for amyloid deposition in tissues.

- Amyloidosis can also occur (see later).

Immune paresis

The synthesis of immunoglobulins from other clones of cells may be suppressed by the proliferation of a single clone. In such cases the band, other than the narrow

> ## CASE 1
>
> A 72-year-old male presented to his general practitioner with back pain and weakness. The following are the results of some of his laboratory tests.
>
> *Plasma*
> Sodium 136 mmol/L (135–145)
> Potassium 4.9 mmol/L (3.5–5.0)
> Urea 13.7 mmol/L (2.5–7.0)
> Creatinine 160 µmol/L (70–110)
> Corrected calcium 3.20 mmol/L (2.15–2.55)
> Total protein 98 g/L (60–75)
> Albumin 34 g/L (35–45)
>
> ### DISCUSSION
> Note the impaired renal function, hypercalcaemia and raised total plasma protein concentration. The patient was also found to be anaemic, with a haemoglobin concentration of 9.3 g/dL. Dipstick urine testing showed proteinuria. Serum and urinary protein electrophoresis showed an IgG kappa paraprotein with immune paresis and Bence-Jones proteinuria. Skeletal bone survey showed lytic bone lesions, and bone marrow biopsy supported the diagnosis of multiple myeloma.

Disordered immunoglobulin synthesis and immune paresis

The immunoglobulin most frequently increased is IgG, and, less commonly, IgA (about 2.5:1). Occasionally, IgM, IgD or IgE is found, the last two being very rare. Bence-Jones protein may sometimes be present in plasma if renal failure is present. In about 20 per cent of cases, no paraprotein is detected in the plasma but BJP is detected in urine. Rarely, neither a paraprotein nor BJP can be found. In either case there is usually immune paresis. In IgD myelomatosis an increase in γ-globulin concentration may not be detectable by routine electrophoresis. The paraprotein should be typed and the plasma concentration monitored to follow progress. The serum free light chain ratio (kappa to lambda) may also be abnormal.

Bone marrow appearance

The proportion of plasma cells in the bone marrow is increased and many of these cells are atypical ('myeloma cells'). *Examination of a bone marrow aspirate must be carried out before myelomatosis is diagnosed or excluded.*

Soft tissue plasmacytoma

Rarely, myeloma involves soft tissues, without marrow changes (extramedullary plasmacytoma). Although the protein abnormalities of myelomatosis are often found, the behaviour and prognosis of the two conditions are different. Spread of soft-tissue plasmacytoma is slow and tends to be local. Local excision of the solitary tumour may be effective.

Waldenström's macroglobulinaemia

Waldenström's macroglobulinaemia is caused by a malignancy of B-cells, with increased synthesis of IgM; the cells resemble lymphocytes rather than plasma cells. There is generalized lymphadenopathy. Like myelomatosis, macroglobulinaemia usually occurs in older patients, over the age of 60, but, unlike myelomatosis, it is commoner in men than in women. Symptoms of the 'hyperviscosity syndrome' are commoner than in myelomatosis, probably because of the large size of the IgM molecule; skeletal manifestations are rarer.

The laboratory findings and diagnosis include the following.

- IgM monoclonal paraprotein in the γ-region on protein electrophoresis. The plasma IgA concentration is usually reduced, but that of IgG may be raised.
- The bone marrow aspirate or lymph node biopsy contains atypical lymphocytoid cells.

Heavy-chain disease

The heavy-chain diseases are a rare group of disorders characterized by the presence of an abnormal protein in plasma or urine, identifiable as part of the H chain (α, γ or µ). The clinical picture is that of:

- *intestinal lymphomatous lesions*, with severe malabsorption (α-chain disease); the condition usually affects young adults of Mediterranean origin;
- *generalized lymphadenopathy* with recurrent infections in the elderly (γ-chain disease);
- *chronic lymphatic leukaemia* (µ-chain disease).

In some of these conditions a paraprotein may be detectable.

Cryoglobulinaemia

Cryoglobulins are proteins that precipitate when cooled below body temperature. They may be associated with diseases known to produce paraproteins. About half of them can be shown to consist of a monoclonal immunoglobulin (usually IgM or IgG). The patient usually presents with other symptoms of the underlying disease and the cryoglobulin is found during investigation. Occasionally, intravascular precipitation may occur at temperatures above 22 °C and, if the concentration of protein is high, presenting symptoms and signs may be skin lesions such as purpura and Raynaud's phenomenon. In some cases the protein is polyclonal and includes complement; these cases may be associated with immune-complex disease. Occasionally no underlying abnormality can be found (essential cryoglobulinaemia).

To determine cryoglobulinaemia, the blood should be collected in prewarmed tubes at 37 °C and transported quickly to the laboratory. Aliquots can be taken, one at room temperature (22 °C) and the other at 37 °C. The cryoglobulin protein can be quantitated by subtracting the difference between the 37 °C sample and the supernatant of the 22 °C sample, as at 22 °C the protein/gel would be expected to precipitate, as lower than body temperature.

'Benign' paraproteinaemia

If a paraprotein is found on electrophoresis, investigation for one of the diseases discussed above should be initiated. In up to 30 per cent of hospital cases, and probably more in the 'well population', no cause can be found. The condition, which may be transient, has been called 'benign' or 'essential' paraproteinaemia or monoclonal gammopathy of undetermined significance (MGUS). The diagnosis should be made provisionally and the patients followed up; they may later develop myelomatosis or macroglobulinaemia. This condition is commoner in the elderly; BJP is not usually present and plasma paraprotein is often less than 5 g/L with no immune paresis.

Amyloid

Amyloid diseases are secondary protein structure diseases in which insoluble protein fibrils accumulate extracellularly. At least 20 different types of fibrils have been described in human amyloidosis, each with a different clinical picture. All types of tissue amyloid consist of a major fibrillar protein that defines their type. All amyloid types show certain features.

- Soluble in water and in buffers of low ionic strength.
- Amorphous eosinophilic appearance on light microscopy after haematoxylin and eosin staining.
- Green fluorescence seen under polarized light after Congo red staining.
- Regular fibrillar structure as observed by electron microscopy.
- X-ray diffraction shows β-pleated sheet structure.

Amyloidosis is usually classified biochemically. The amyloidoses are referred to with a capital A (for amyloid) followed by an abbreviation for the fibril protein. For example, in cases formerly termed primary amyloidosis and in myeloma-associated amyloidosis, the fibril protein is an immunoglobulin light chain or light-chain fragment (abbreviated L); thus, patients with these amyloidoses are now said to have light chain amyloidosis (AL). In instances previously termed senile cardiac amyloidosis and in cases formerly called familial amyloid polyneuropathy, the fibrils consist of the transport protein transthyretin (TTR); these diseases are now termed ATTR. (See Chapter 11.)

PROTEINS IN URINE

The loss of most plasma proteins through the glomeruli is restricted by the size of the pores in, and by a negative charge on, the basement membrane that repel negatively charged protein molecules. Alteration of either of these factors by glomerular disease may allow albumin and larger proteins to enter the filtrate. Low-molecular-weight proteins are filtered even under normal conditions; most are absorbed and metabolized by tubular cells. Normal subjects excrete up to 0.08 g of protein a day in the urine, amounts undetectable by usual screening tests. Proteinuria of more than 0.15 g a day almost always indicates disease.

Significant proteinuria may be due to renal disease or, more rarely, may occur because large amounts of low-molecular-weight proteins are circulating and therefore being filtered. Blood and pus in the urine and also urinary infection give positive tests for protein. (See also Chapter 3.)

Renal proteinuria

Glomerular proteinuria

Glomerular proteinuria is due to increased glomerular permeability, as in the nephrotic syndrome. Albumin is usually the predominant protein in the urine.

Transient proteinuria

Transient proteinuria may be associated with physical exertion, trauma, cardiac failure, fever and other acute illness.

'Orthostatic' ('postural') proteinuria

Proteinuria is usually more severe in the upright than in the prone position. The term 'orthostatic' or 'postural' has been applied to proteinuria, often severe, which disappears at night. Overnight urine collection shows normal albumin excretion (i.e. less than 50 mg during the 8-hour period). It appears to be glomerular in origin and is commonest in adolescents and young adults, typically those who are tall and thin. It may be associated with severe lordosis. Renal function is normal and proteinuria is usually less than 1 g/day. Although it is often harmless, evidence of renal disease may occur after some years.

Microalbuminuria

Sensitive immunological assays have shown the normal daily excretion of albumin to be less than 0.05 g. Patients with diabetes mellitus who excrete more than this, but whose total urinary protein excretion is 'normal', are said to have microalbuminuria and to be at greater risk of developing progressive renal disease than those whose albumin excretion is normal. This can be assessed from the urinary albumin:creatinine ratio or by timed urinary albumin collection. The incidence of this complication may be reduced by optimization of glycaemic control and also blood pressure using angiotensin-converting enzyme (ACE) inhibitors (see Chapter 12). Microalbuminuria can also occur in other diseases, such as inflammatory bowel disease or rheumatoid arthritis.

Tubular proteinuria

Tubular proteinuria may be due to renal tubular damage from any cause, especially pyelonephritis. If glomerular permeability is normal, proteinuria is usually less than 1 g/day and consists mainly of low-molecular-weight globulins and not albumin. Low-molecular-weight α-globulins and β-globulins are sensitive markers of renal tubular damage. Tubular proteinuria can be diagnosed by measuring certain low-molecular-weight proteins in urine, such as retinol-binding protein (RBP), N-acetyl-β-D-glucosaminidase or α_1-microglobulin.

However, because the β_2-microglobulins in urine are unstable, other proteins, such as RBP, may be better indicators of tubular damage. Tubular proteinuria is associated with Fanconi syndrome with glycosuria, amino-aciduria, hyperphosphaturia (hypophosphataemia) and renal tubular acidosis. This can be primary or secondary, for example to heavy metals and drugs such as cis-platinum.

Overflow proteinuria

This occurs when proteins of low molecular weight are filtered normally by the glomerulus and reabsorbed at the proximal tubule but are produced in amounts greater than the reabsorptive capacity of the proximal tubule.

Overflow proteinuria can be due to the production of BJP, to severe haemolysis with haemoglobinuria, or to severe muscle damage (rhabdomyolysis) with myoglobinuria. In the last two cases, the urine may be red or brown in colour.

Bence-Jones proteinuria can be inferred by comparison of urinary and serum electrophoretic patterns and by immunochemical assays. Bence-Jones protein is the only protein of a molecular weight lower than albumin that is likely to be found in significant amounts in unconcentrated urine in the absence of haemoglobinuria or myoglobinuria. The presence of a band in urine that is denser than that of albumin, especially if not present in the serum, is suggestive of BJP.

CASE 2

A 65-year-old patient with type 2 diabetes mellitus had an HbA1c of 10.3 per cent and random blood glucose concentration of 23.8 mmol/L in the diabetes clinic. He was taking metformin 500 mg twice a day. His blood pressure was 180/100 mmHg. A urinary albumin:creatinine ratio (ACR) was 9.9 g/mol. A year prior to this, his urinary ACR was normal, at less than 2.5 g/mol.

DISCUSSION

The patient has microalbuminuria, which was confirmed on repeat urine sampling. This can progress to proteinuria and eventually chronic renal failure. The aim of the clinician should be to try to optimize glycaemic control. In this case, the patient's HbA1c was high, reflecting poor control, and was improved by increasing his metformin and adding the sulphonylurea gliclazide, which brought his HbA1c to 7 per cent. He is hypertensive, which also needs treating, and he was started on an ACE inhibitor.

Apparent proteinuria

Apparent proteinuria has occasionally been found because the patient, or someone else, has added egg white or animal blood to their urine.

Nephrotic syndrome

An established case of the nephrotic syndrome is characterized by proteinuria, hypoalbuminaemia, oedema and hyperlipidaemia. The clinical condition is caused by increased glomerular permeability, resulting in a daily urinary protein loss of, by definition, more than 3 g (although some definitions state different values). There may be hypertension and evidence of other impaired renal function. Some of the causes are shown in Box 19.2.

Laboratory findings of nephrotic syndrome

Protein abnormalities

Proteinuria in the nephrotic syndrome usually ranges from 3 g or more a day. The relative proportion of different proteins lost is an index of the severity of the glomerular lesion. In mild cases, albumin (molecular weight 65 kDa) and transferrin (molecular weight 80 kDa) are the predominant urinary proteins, but α_1-antitrypsin (molecular weight 50 kDa) is also present. With increasing glomerular permeability, larger proteins such as IgG (molecular weight 160 kDa) appear.

The serum electrophoretic picture depends on the severity of the renal lesion. In early cases a low serum albumin concentration may be the only abnormality, but the typical pattern includes reduced albumin, α_1- and γ-globulin bands, with an increase in α_2-globulin because of an increase in the high-molecular-weight α_2-macroglobulin (Fig. 19.8). The γ-globulin concentration may be normal or raised. Urinary electrophoresis gives some idea of the severity of the glomerular lesion.

The differential protein clearance is a more precise measure of the selectivity of the lesion. The clearance of a low-molecular-weight protein, such as transferrin or albumin,

---

Box 19.2 Some causes of the nephrotic syndrome

Primary renal disease

Most types of glomerulonephritis, usually due to deposition of circulating immune complexes in the glomeruli in about 80% of cases

In children, 'minimal change' glomerulonephritis is the most common cause

Secondary renal disease

Diabetes mellitus
Myelomatosis
Hypertension
Cryoglobulinaemia
Amyloidosis
Systemic lupus erythematosus (due to deposition of immune complexes)
Malaria from Plasmodium malariae (due to immune complexes)
Inferior vena caval or renal vein thrombosis
Drugs and toxins, e.g.:
  gold
  penicillamine
  cis-platinium

CASE 3

A 47-year-old male attended the medical out-patients' department because of bilateral ankle oedema and hyperlipidaemia. A number of investigations were requested, with the following results.

Plasma (fasting)
Sodium 136 mmol/L (135–145)
Potassium 4.3 mmol/L (3.5–5.0)
Urea 8.7 mmol/L (2.5–7.0)
Creatinine 111 μmol/L (70–110)
Total protein 55 g/L (60–75)
Albumin 28 g/L (35–45)
Cholesterol 9.4 mmol/L (3.0–5.0)
Triglyceride 5.3 mmol/L (0.50–1.50)

A 24-hour urinary total protein determination was 7.8 g.

DISCUSSION

The patient had nephrotic syndrome presenting with peripheral oedema, hypoproteinaemia, hypoalbuminaemia and severe hyperlipidaemia. Note that the plasma creatinine and urea concentrations may not be too abnormal unless chronic renal failure ensues. A renal biopsy showed that the patient had focal segmental glomerulonephritis.

298 PROTEINS IN PLASMA AND URINE

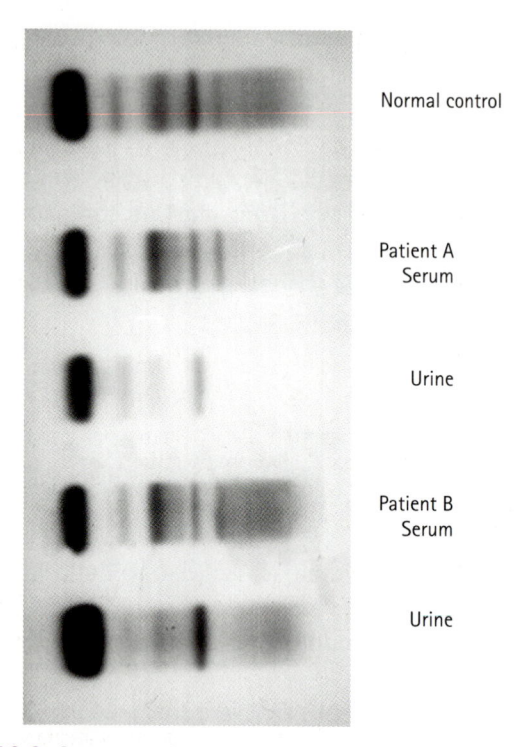

Fig. 19.8 Serum and urinary protein electrophoretic patterns from patients with the nephrotic syndrome. Patient A has selective glomerular proteinuria, and patient B has non-selective proteinuria.

is compared with that of a larger one, such as IgG. The result is usually expressed as a ratio, obviating the need for timed urine collections. A ratio of IgG to transferrin or albumin clearance of less than 0.2 indicates high selectivity (predominant loss of small molecules) and has a more favourable prognosis than a higher ratio; such cases usually respond well to steroid or cyclophosphamide therapy.

The consequences of the protein abnormalities are oedema caused by a fall in the intravascular colloid osmotic pressure, due to hypoalbuminaemia (see Chapter 2), and reduction in the concentration of protein-bound substances due to loss of carrier proteins; it is important not to misinterpret low plasma total concentrations of calcium, thyroxine, cortisol and iron.

In mild cases, plasma LDL concentrations increase, with consequent hypercholesterolaemia probably due to the increased rate of protein synthesis, including that of apolipoprotein B (apoB) lipoprotein, in the liver (see Chapter 17). In more severe cases, a rise in plasma very low-density lipoprotein (VLDL) (triglycerides) concentration may cause plasma turbidity. Fatty casts may be detectable in the urine.

In the early stages, glomerular permeability is high and the plasma urea and creatinine concentrations are normal, although uraemia may develop. At this stage, protein loss is reduced and plasma concentrations of protein and lipid may revert to normal, but this does not indicate recovery. Secondary hyperaldosteronism may also occur (see Chapters 2 and 3).

Testing for urinary protein

Several rapid screening tests are in routine use. It is essential that the sample is fresh. There are limitations of screening tests, such as the following.

- The tests were mainly developed to detect albumin and may be negative in the presence of other proteins, such as BJP.
- Because the tests depend on protein concentrations, very dilute urine may give negative results despite significant proteinuria.

One example of a urinary protein screening tests is Albustix. The test area of the reagent strip is impregnated with an indicator (tetrabromphenol blue) buffered to pH 3. At this pH it is yellow in the absence of protein. Protein forms a complex with the dye, stabilizing it in the blue form; it is green or bluish-green if protein is present. The colour after testing is compared with the colours on the chart provided, which indicate the approximate protein concentration. The strips should be kept in the screw-top bottles, in a cool place and the instructions should be followed carefully.

False-positive results occur:

- if the specimen is contaminated with vaginal or urethral secretions, including haematuria, semen or menstrual fluid;
- in strongly alkaline (infected or stale) urine, when buffering capacity is exceeded; a green colour in this case is a reflection of the alkaline pH;
- if the urine container is contaminated with disinfectants such as chlorhexidine.

False-negative results occur if acid has been added to the urine as a preservative (for example for the estimation of urinary calcium).

Investigation of proteinuria (Fig. 19.9)

- Normally urinary total protein is about 50–150 mg/day. Rather than a 24-hour urinary protein collection, it may be more convenient to use a random urinary protein:creatinine ratio. Normally this is less than 15.

- Consider orthostatic or postural proteinuria when an early-morning urine sample is negative for protein but pre-bed samples show proteinuria.
- A 24-hour protein measurement and/or random urinary protein:creatinine (P:C) ratio are then necessary to measure the proteinuria. A high degree of proteinuria (for example more than 3 g/day or P:C more than 300) is indicative of nephrotic syndrome. A selectivity index can then be calculated for the proteinuria to see whether or not it is non-selective.
- If proteinuria is confirmed, urinary protein electrophoresis may be useful to determine the pattern of proteinuria, i.e. whether there is glomerular or tubular pathology. Overflow proteinuria may also be revealed, such as Bence-Jones proteinuria, myoglobinuria or haemoglobinuria.
- Does the patient have diabetes mellitus and what is the degree of proteinuria. Diabetic nephropathy is also associated with diabetic retinopathy, i.e. representing increased microvascular permeability.
- Other tests may be indicated, such as autoantibodies, including anti-glomerular membrane antibodies, streptococcal antibodies and also complement C3 and C4. In addition, renal imaging, for example ultrasound, and renal biopsy may be required.

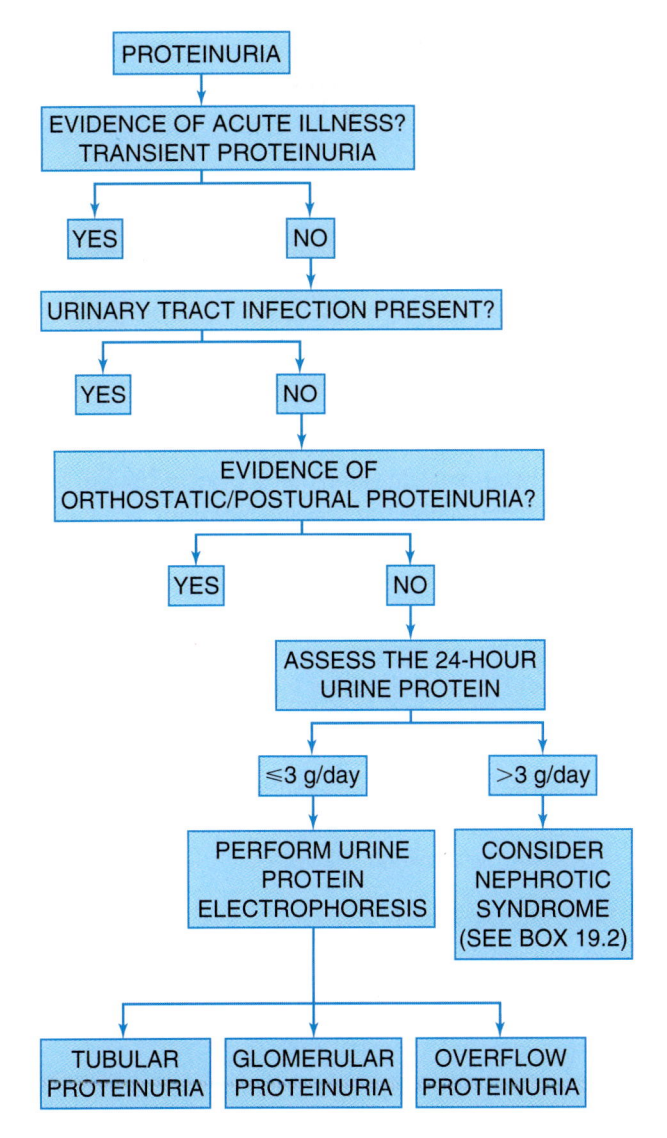

Fig. 19.9 Algorithm for the investigation of proteinuria.

Remember that urine dipstick tests can give false-positive results (see above).
- Exclude urinary tract infection; a midstream urine test may be useful.
- Is the proteinuria transient? Confirm on at least two or three occasions.
- Renal function tests, i.e. plasma urea and creatinine, should be performed and it is also important to check plasma albumin and protein for hypoalbuminaemia and hypoproteinaemia.
- Take a drug history for renal toxic agents, for example gold or penicillamine.
- Clinical history and examination may reveal systemic illnesses that can cause proteinuria (see above). Check plasma prostate-specific antigen in men to help assess for prostatic disease.

BLOOD SAMPLING FOR PROTEIN ESTIMATIONS

This chapter ends with the clinical indications for measuring serum or plasma protein and albumin.

Blood for protein estimations, including for immunoglobulins, should be taken with *a minimum of venous stasis*, otherwise falsely high results may be obtained.

Protein electrophoresis should be performed on serum from clotted blood, rather than on plasma, because the presence of fibrinogen may mask, or be interpreted as, an abnormal band or protein.

Samples for complement estimations must be taken and processed so as to minimize in-vitro activation.

Blood for cryoglobulin measurement should be collected in a syringe warmed to 37 °C, and should be maintained at this temperature until it has been tested. Failure to observe this precaution may result in false-negative findings, because the cryoprecipitate is incorporated into the blood clot on cooling. *It is important to contact your laboratory for advice before taking the blood.*

Indications for plasma or plasma total protein and albumin estimations

The following are the more common indications for plasma protein and albumin estimations.

- *To investigate oedema.* Very low plasma albumin and total protein concentrations in the presence of oedema indicate that hypoalbuminaemia may be the cause. Conditions causing severe hypoalbuminaemia include the nephrotic syndrome and hepatic cirrhosis, both of which have typical serum electrophoretic patterns. The diagnosis of nephritic syndrome depends on finding gross proteinuria.
- *To assess changes in hydration.* Changes in plasma total protein or albumin concentrations over short periods of time are almost certainly due to changes in hydration, or to changes in capillary permeability (see Chapter 2). Dehydration may evoke raised plasma albumin and protein concentrations, whereas the converse is true in over-hydration.
- *To help assess nutritional status.* Plasma albumin concentrations are sometimes used to help assess nutritional status. However, low albumin concentrations, although associated with malnutrition, are not specific as they can be low for other reasons (see Chapter 14).
- *To investigate suspected myelomatosis or macroglobulinaemia.* The difference between the total plasma protein and albumin concentration is called the 'globulin' concentration. This is raised in clinical situations when the globulin concentration is raised, such as in myelomatosis.

Protein electrophoresis should be carried out on serum to detect a paraprotein and, importantly, also on urine to detect BJP. The diagnosis of myelomatosis should be confirmed by microscopic inspection of a bone marrow aspirate or biopsy and usually also a skeletal survey. Plasma immunoglobulin concentrations should be measured to assess the degree of immune paresis.

- *To evaluate apparently abnormal concentrations* or changes in concentrations of a protein-bound substance. Estimation of plasma albumin estimation should always accompany that of total plasma calcium. If changes in this or other protein-bound substances parallel those of albumin, they are probably due to changes in protein concentrations.
- *As part of the investigation of hypogammaglobulinaemia.* A low total plasma protein concentration, if not due to hypoalbuminaemia, may be due to hypogammaglobulinaemia. Plasma immunoglobulin concentrations can be measured as part of the assessment of the adequacy of the immune system.

Note that these tests assess only *humoral* immunity: T cell abnormalities and their investigations are outside the scope of this book.

CONCLUSIONS

- Abnormalities of plasma and urinary proteins are relatively common in clinical practice and therefore knowledge of protein biochemistry is necessary for a full understanding of these conditions.
- Diagnostically, certain proteins can be specifically assayed or protein electrophoresis of serum and/or urine can be performed to show pattern changes.
- The acute-phase response and inflammation are essential mechanisms to protect the body. B-cells are concerned primarily with immunoglobulin synthesis and humoral immunity, whereas T-cells are involved in cellular immunity.
- Multiple myeloma is a plasma-cell malignancy associated with paraproteinaemia, Bence-Jones proteinuria, osteolytic bone lesions and hypercalcaemia.
- Proteinuria can be due to either glomerular or tubular disorders. The nephrotic syndrome is associated with peripheral oedema, hypoalbuminaemia and hypoproteinaemia.

20 PURINE AND URATE METABOLISM

Purines	301	Causes of low plasma urate concentrations	
Hyperuricaemia	303	(hypouricaemia)	307
Pseudogout	306		

Abnormalities of purine metabolism are often found in clinical practice, notably hyperuricaemia and gout. After exploring purine metabolic pathways, this chapter discusses the various disorders of purine metabolism, including their clinical features, diagnosis and treatment.

PURINES

Normal purine metabolism

Urate is the end-product of purine metabolism in humans. In most other mammals, it is further metabolized to the more water-soluble allantoin. Humans lack uricase and thus their uric acid levels are higher. It is because of the poor solubility of urate that humans are prone to the clinical effects of hyperuricaemia, such as gout and renal damage. The purines adenine and guanine are constituents of nucleic acid from DNA and RNA. The purines used by the body for nucleic acid synthesis may be derived from the breakdown of ingested nucleic acid, mostly from cell-rich meat, or they may be synthesized de novo from small molecules. About two-thirds of the body's urate (3–4 mmol/day) is produced endogenously, with one-third coming from exogenous dietary purines (1–2 mmol/day).

Synthesis of purines

The purine synthetic pathway involves the incorporation of many small molecules into the relatively complex purine ring. The upper part of Fig. 20.1 summarizes some of the more important synthetic steps. The following stages, especially, should be noted.

The first step in purine synthesis is condensation of pyrophosphate with phosphoribose to form phosphoribose diphosphate (phosphoribosyl pyrophosphate, PRPP).

The amino group of glutamine is incorporated into the ribose phosphate molecule and pyrophosphate is released. Amidophosphoribosyl transferase catalyses this rate-limiting or controlling step. The enzyme is subject to feed-back inhibition by increasing concentrations of purine nucleotides; thus the rate of synthesis is slowed when its products increase. The control of this rate-limiting step may be impaired in primary gout.

Glycine is added to phosphoribosylamine. The rate of purine synthesis is increased in primary gout. In Fig. 20.1, the atoms in the glycine molecule have been numbered to correspond with those in the purine and urate molecules, and the heavy lines further indicate the final position of the amino acid in these molecules.

Via a series of metabolic steps, purine ribonucleotides (purine ribose phosphates) are formed, which control the second step in the synthetic pathway – the formation of phosphoribosylamine. Ribose phosphate is cleaved off, thereby releasing the purines. Some cytotoxic drugs inhibit various stages of the pathway, thus preventing DNA formation and cell growth.

Fate of purines

Purines synthesized in the body, those derived from the diet and those liberated by endogenous catabolism of nucleic acids may be oxidized to urate or re-used for nucleic acid synthesis.

Purines oxidized to urate. Some adenine is oxidized to hypoxanthine, which is further oxidized to xanthine. Guanine can also form xanthine. Xanthine, in turn, is oxidized to form urate. The oxidation of both hypoxanthine and xanthine is catalysed by xanthine oxidase in the liver. Thus the formation of urate from purines depends on xanthine oxidase activity: gout may be treated using an inhibitor of this enzyme (allopurinol).

Purines re-used for nucleic acid synthesis. Some xanthine, hypoxanthine and guanine can be resynthesized to purine nucleotides by pathways involving, among other enzymes, hypoxanthine–guanine phosphoribosyl transferase (HGPRT) and adenine phosphoribosyl transferase (APRT).

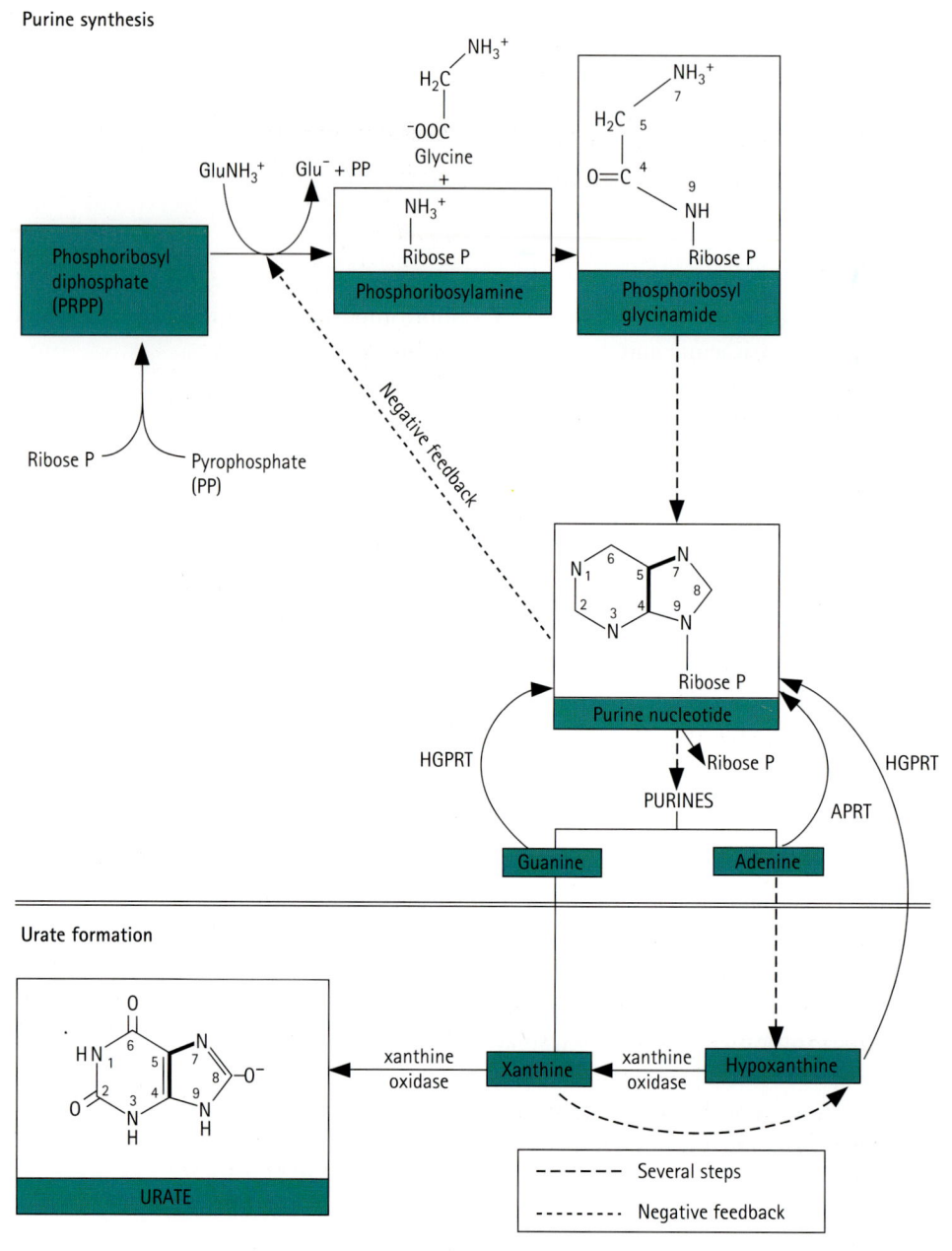

Fig. 20.1 Summary of purine synthesis and breakdown, showing the steps of clinical importance. ($GluNH_3^+$ = glutamine; Glu^- = glutamate; HGPRT = hypoxanthine–guanine phosphoribosyl transferase; APRT = adenine phosphoribosyl transferase.)

Excretion of urate

Urate is filtered through the glomeruli and most is reabsorbed in the proximal tubules. More than 80 per cent of that formed in urine is derived from more distal tubular secretion. Urinary excretion is slightly lower in males than in females, which may contribute to the higher incidence of hyperuricaemia in men.

Renal secretion may be enhanced by uricosuric drugs (e.g. probenecid or sulfinpyrazone), which block tubular urate reabsorption. Tubular secretion of urates is inhibited by organic acids, such as lactic and oxo-acids, and by ketones and thiazide diuretics. Seventy-five per cent of urate leaving the body is in urine. The remaining 25 per cent passes into the intestinal lumen, where it is broken down by intestinal bacteria, the process being known as uricolysis.

HYPERURICAEMIA

Causes of hyperuricaemia

Generally speaking, hyperuricaemia can occur by two main mechanisms: increased production (over-producers) and/or decreased excretion (under-excretors).

The factors that may contribute to hyperuricaemia (summarized in Fig. 20.2) are:

- increased synthesis of purines (step 1),
- increased intake of purines (step 2),
- increased turnover of nucleic acids (step 3),
- increased rate of urate formation (step 4),
- reduced rate of excretion (step 5).

Increased synthesis, due to impaired feedback control, is probably the most important mechanism causing primary hyperuricaemia, whereas abnormalities of the other steps are causes of secondary hyperuricaemia.

Consequences of hyperuricaemia

Urate is poorly soluble in plasma. At plasma pH, most urate is ionized at position 8 of the purine ring (see Fig. 20.1). This anionic group is associated with the predominant extracellular cation, sodium. Ionization of uric acid decreases as the pH falls, and it therefore becomes less soluble; at a urinary pH below about 6, uric acid may form renal calculi.

Crystallization in joints, especially those of the feet, produces the classic picture of gout. Urate precipitation at these sites causes an inflammatory response with leucocytic infiltration and it is thought that lactic acid production

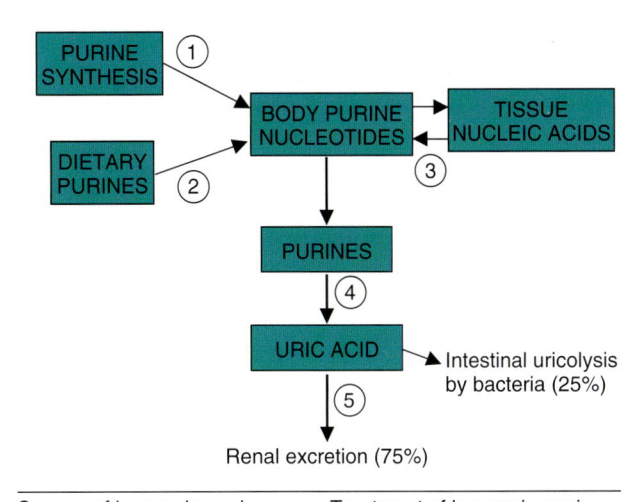

Causes of hyperuricaemia
1. Increased in primary hyperuricaemia
2. Affected by diet
3. Increased in malignancy, infection, cytotoxic therapy, psoriasis etc.
5. Decreased in renal failure, thiazide diuretic therapy, some cases of primary hyperuricaemia and acidosis

Treatment of hyperuricaemia
4. Reduced by xanthine oxidase inhibitors (e.g. allopurinol)
5. Increased by uricosuric drugs (e.g. probenecid)

Fig. 20.2 Urate metabolism in normal subjects.

by these cells causes a local fall in pH: this converts urate to uric acid, which is less soluble than urate, and a vicious circle is set up in which further precipitation, and therefore further inflammation, occurs. In acute attacks of gouty arthritis, local factors are more important than the plasma urate concentration, which is usually normal during the attack.

Precipitation may occur in subcutaneous tissues, especially of the ears, and in the olecranon and patellar bursae and tendons. Such deposits are called gouty tophi. A potentially serious effect of hyperuricaemia is precipitation of urate in the kidneys and renal calculi, causing progressive renal damage. For this reason it has been recommended that even asymptomatic cases should probably be treated if the plasma urate concentration is consistently higher than 0.6 mmol/L.

Hyperuricaemia can be primary or secondary.

Primary hyperuricaemia and gout

Familial incidence

In some cases a hereditary component is present, probably involving abnormalities of urate metabolic pathways.

Sex and age incidence

Primary hyperuricaemia and gout are very rare in children and unusual in women of child-bearing age. Plasma urate concentrations are low in children and rise in both sexes at puberty, more so in males than in females. Women become more prone to hyperuricaemia and gout in the post-menopausal period.

Precipitating factors

- A high meat diet contains a relatively high proportion of purines.
- Alcohol has been shown to decrease renal excretion of urate. This may be because it increases lactic acid production, which inhibits urate secretion.

Neither of these factors is likely to precipitate gout in a normal person, but, like thiazide diuretics, may do so in a subject with a hyperuricaemic tendency.

Biochemical defects in primary hyperuricaemia

Purine synthesis is increased in about 25 per cent of cases of primary hyperuricaemia due to over-activity of amidophosphoribosyl transferase, which controls the formation of phosphoribosylamine.

Reduced renal tubular secretion of urate has also been demonstrated in other cases of primary hyperuricaemia. Many subjects may have both increased synthesis and decreased excretion.

Familial juvenile gouty nephropathy is a rare autosomal dominant condition leading to progressive renal failure.

Rare causes of juvenile hyperuricaemia

Lesch–Nyhan syndrome is an *exceedingly* rare X-linked, recessively inherited disorder of urate metabolism caused by a reduced activity of HGPRT. Severe hyperuricaemia occurs in young male children. Hypoxanthine and other purines cannot be recycled to form purine nucleotides, and probably produce more urate. The syndrome is associated with mental deficiency, a tendency to self-mutilation, aggressive behaviour, athetosis and spastic paraplegia. Partial deficiency of HGPRT is called Kelley–Seegmiller syndrome. Hyperuricaemia can also occur with increased 5-PRPP synthase activity.

Secondary hyperuricaemia

High plasma urate concentrations may be secondary to the following.

Increased turnover of nucleic acids

- *In rapidly growing malignant tissue*, especially in leukaemias, lymphomas and polycythaemia rubra vera.
- *In psoriasis*, when turnover of skin cells is increased.
- *Following increased tissue breakdown*.
  - After the treatment of large malignant tumours by radiotherapy or cytotoxic drugs (tumour lysis syndrome). This can cause massive sudden release of urate, which may crystallize in and block renal tubules causing acute oliguric renal dysfunction. During such treatment, allopurinol should be given and, if glomerular function is not impaired, fluid intake kept high.
  - Due to trauma, including that of surgery; endogenous urate release is increased.
  - During starvation or prolonged fasting: the patient's own tissues may be used as an energy source, with increased urate release. Starvation may be associated with mild ketoacidosis, and protein catabolism releases acidic amino acid residues. The acidosis, by inhibiting the secretion of urate, may aggravate the hyperuricaemia. During complete fasting, plasma urate concentrations may exceed 0.9 mmol/L.

Reduced excretion of urate

This may be due to the following.

- *Thiazide diuretics*. Although hyperuricaemia is relatively common during diuretic treatment, clinical gout is a rare complication. It may, however, be precipitated in those patients with a gouty tendency.
- *Other drugs*, including low doses of salicylates, ciclosporin, nicotinic acid, methoxyflurane, levodopa, ethambutol and pyrazinamide.
- *Renal glomerular dysfunction*. Before the diagnosis of primary hyperuricaemia is made, the plasma concentration of urea and/or creatinine should be assayed on the same specimen as urate, to exclude renal dysfunction as a cause. It may be difficult to decide which abnormality is the primary one because hyperuricaemia can cause renal dysfunction. The urate:creatinine concentration ratio in a spot urine sample may help distinguish hyperuricaemia due to reduced renal excretion from renal impairment secondary to hyperuricaemia. A ratio less than 0.7 implies that renal impairment is responsible for the hyperuricaemia. A ratio greater than 0.7 suggests urate nephropathy. Clinical gout is rare in the secondary hyperuricaemia of renal disease.

> **CASE 1**
>
> A 62-year-old male was treated with chemotherapy by the oncologists for non-Hodgkin's lymphoma. His biochemistry results post-chemotherapy were as follows.
>
> *Plasma*
> Sodium 137 mmol/L (135–145)
> Potassium 5.6 mmol/L (3.5–5.0)
> Urea 11.5 mmol/L (2.5–7.5)
> Creatinine 138 µmol/L (60–120)
> 'Corrected' calcium 2.19 mmol/L (2.15–2.55)
> Phosphate 3.17 mmol/L (0.80–1.35)
> Urate 0.74 mmol/L (0.20–0.43)
>
> **DISCUSSION**
> Where there is rapid growth of dividing tumour cells and consequent elevated nucleic acid turnover, increased purine metabolism and hyperuricaemia can occur. This is a case of tumour lysis syndrome, which can occur after chemotherapy where there is rapid cell destruction and release of purine metabolites and intracellular ions such as potassium and phosphate, resulting in hyperkalaemia and hyperphosphataemia.

- *Prolonged metabolic acidosis* (see Chapters 3 and 4).
- *Chronic lead intoxication* (see Chapter 21).

Combined (both increased production and reduced excretion) causes

- *High alchol intake*.
- *Prolonged and severe exercise*.
- *Dyslipidaemia* and impaired glucose tolerance or type 2 diabetes mellitus. Hyperuricaemia is associated with insulin resistance and the metabolic syndrome.
- *Glucose-6-phosphatase deficiency* or von Gierke's disease (see Chapter 27). The tendency to hyperuricaemia in these patients may be directly related to the inability to convert glucose-6-phosphate (G-6-P) to glucose. More G-6-P is available for metabolism through intracellular pathways, including:
  - the pentose-phosphate pathway, thus increasing ribose phosphate (phosphoribose) synthesis; this may accelerate the first step in purine synthesis, with consequent urate over-production;
  - glycolysis, thus increasing lactic acid production; lactic acid may reduce renal urate excretion.

Principles of treatment of hyperuricaemia

- *Reducing dietary purine intake*, for example red meats. This treatment is rarely effective by itself.
- An acute attack of *gout* can be treated with a *non-steroidal anti-inflammatory drug* (NSAID).
- *Colchicine*, which has an anti-inflammatory effect and inhibits neutrophil activation, can be used in acute gouty arthritis but does not affect urate metabolism. It is sometimes used if NSAIDs are contraindicated.

- *Reducing urate production* by using drugs that inhibit xanthine oxidase activity, such as allopurinol (hydroxypyrazolopyrimidine), which is structurally similar to hypoxanthine, so acting as a competitive inhibitor of the enzyme. De-novo synthesis may also be decreased by this drug. However, allopurinol may worsen an acute gout attack. Initiation of allopurinol should be made a few weeks after the acute attack under the cover of an NSAID.
- *Increasing the renal excretion of urate with uricosuric drugs*, such as probenecid or sulfinpyrazone. These drugs may be effective if renal function is normal, but are less so if there is renal glomerular dysfunction. Fluid intake is usually kept high. Low doses of most uricosuric drugs reduce urate secretion; they are rarely used unless allopurinol is contraindicated.

Investigation of hyperuricaemia (Fig. 20.3)

- A careful drug history is important, as various drugs (Box 20.1) can evoke hyperuricaemia, such as thiazide diuretics as well as high alcohol intake.
- A family history may reveal a primary hereditary form of gout or hyperuricaemia.
- Check renal function with plasma urea and creatinine, as renal impairment is a common cause of hyperuricaemia. A spot urinary urate:creatinine concentration ratio may help distinguish hyperuricaemia due to reduced renal excretion from renal impairment secondary to hyperuricaemia.
- Consider secondary conditions with high cell turnover, such as tumours, psoriasis and polycythaemia (see Box 20.1).

```
                    HYPERURICAEMIA
                           │
                           ▼
           PATIENT ON URATE-RAISING AGENTS
                     │         │
                    NO         YES
                     │
                     ▼
                 MEASURE
            URINE URATE EXCRETION
                  │       │
                 LOW    NORMAL/HIGH
                  │         │
         IMPAIRED RENAL    EVIDENCE OF CONDITIONS
         FUNCTION?         WITH HIGH CELL TURNOVER?
           │    │              │       │
          NO   YES             NO     YES
           │                    │
      EVIDENCE OF          CONSIDER RARE ENZYME
      METABOLIC ACIDOSIS   DEFECTS OF PURINE METABOLISM
                           (SEE BOX 20.1)
```

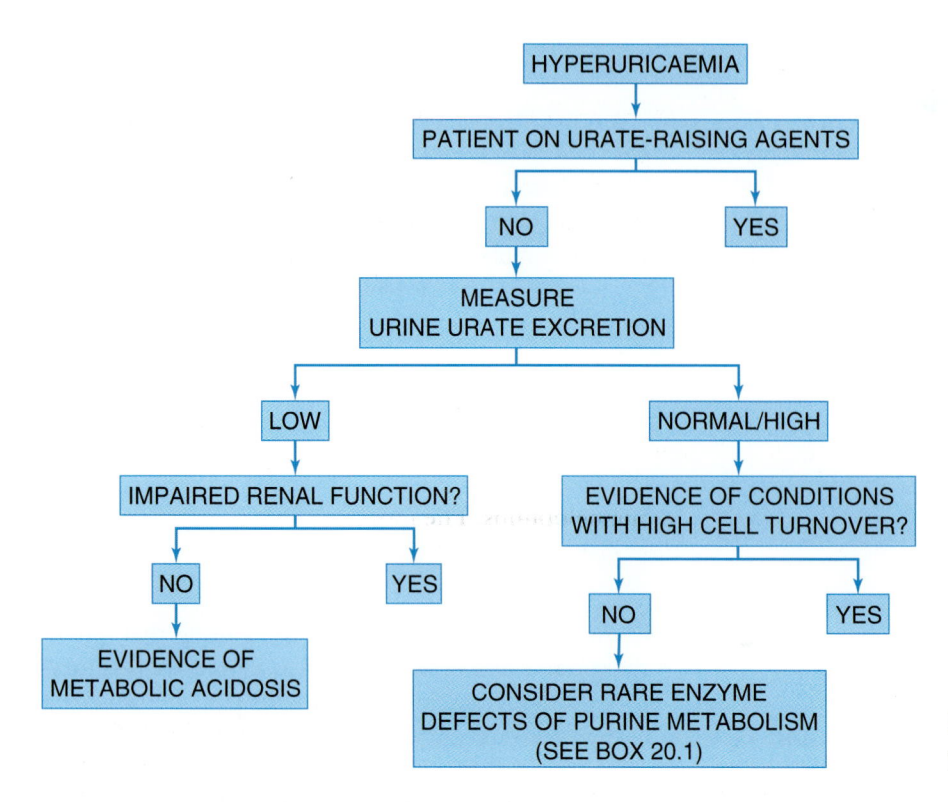

Fig. 20.3 Algorithm for the investigation of hyperuricaemia.

- Hyperuricaemia can also be seen in a metabolic acidosis due to reduced renal urate excretion (see Chapter 4).
- There is an association between hyperuricaemia and the metabolic syndrome with hypertriglyceridaemia, obesity and insulin resistance.
- A 24-hour urine analysis for urate excretion on and off a low purine diet may give an indication of whether the patient is an over-producer or under-excretor of urate.
- Do not forget the rare causes of hyperuricaemia, for example Lesch–Nyman syndrome or von Gierke's disease.

PSEUDOGOUT

Pseudogout is not a disorder of purine metabolism although the clinical presentation is similar to that of gout. Calcium pyrophosphate precipitates in joint cavities, and calcification of cartilages is demonstrable radiologically. The plasma urate concentration is normal. The crystals of calcium pyrophosphate may be identified in joint fluid using a polarizing microscope, when positive bifringence is observed. Patients may present with acute pseudogout arthopathy or chronic chondrocalcinosis. Pseudogout is associated with hyperparathyroidism, hypothyroidism, haemochromatosis and acromegaly.

> **Box 20.1 Some causes of hyperuricaemia**
>
> Drugs: thiazides, nicotinic acid, warfarin, cyclosporin, pyrazinamide, didanosine and ethambutol
> Poisoning by other agents, such as alcohol and lead
> Metabolic syndrome associated with insulin resistance and hypertriglyceridaemia, obesity and hypertension
> Impaired urate excretion:
>   acute or chronic renal failure
>   metabolic acidosis
> High cell turnover:
>   haemolytic anaemia
>   myeloproliferative disease
>   malignancies
>   psoriasis
>   tumour lysis syndrome
> Hereditary or genetic conditions:
>   glucose-6-phosphatase deficiency (von Gierke's disease)
>   Lesch–Nyman syndrome
>   Down's syndrome

CAUSES OF LOW PLASMA URATE CONCENTRATIONS (HYPOURICAEMIA)

This is rare unless it is the result of the treatment of hyperuricaemia with, for example, allopurinol or probenecid. It is associated with proximal renal tubular damage, in which the reabsorption of urate is reduced, and can be seen in Fanconi's syndrome. Hypouricaemia is also a finding in some patients receiving parenteral nutrition and in pregnancy, the syndrome of inappropriate antidiuretic hormone (SIADH, see Chapter 2) and type 1 diabetes mellitus.

Xanthinuria

This is a very rare inborn error of purine metabolism, inherited as an autosomal recessive disorder, in which there is a deficiency of xanthine oxidase in the liver. Purine breakdown stops at the xanthine–hypoxanthine stage, and plasma and urinary urate concentrations are very low. Increased xanthine excretion may lead to the formation of xanthine stones; this does not occur during the treatment of gout with xanthine oxidase inhibitors, perhaps because the drugs also inhibit purine synthesis.

CONCLUSIONS

- Urate is formed as a product of purine metabolism and is renally excreted.
- Raised plasma urate concentrations (hyperuricaemia) are associated with gout.
- Gout can be primary or secondary, and the clinical features include acute arthritis leading to chronic arthropathy, gouty tophi, renal calculi and obstructive uropathy.
- Allopurinol, a xanthine oxidase inhibitor, can be used clinically to lower plasma uric acid concentrations.
- Hypouricaemia is usually not of major clinical significance in itself, although factors associated with it include SIADH, pregnancy, Fanconi's syndrome and xanthinuria.

21 DISORDERS OF HAEM METABOLISM: IRON AND THE PORPHYRIAS

Haem metabolism	308	Iron therapy	313
Iron metabolism	310	Iron overload	314
Ferritin	313	Disorders of haem synthesis: the porphyrias	317
The soluble transferrin receptor	313		

Abnormalities of haem metabolism are important clinically. They include the porphyrias, which are rare, and disorders involving haem iron, such as iron deficiency, which are common in clinical practice.

HAEM METABOLISM

Most body tissues synthesize haem. In bone marrow it is incorporated into haemoglobin, an iron-containing pigment that carries oxygen from the lungs to tissues, and in muscle into myoglobin, which also binds oxygen. In other cells it is used for the synthesis of cytochromes and related compounds. The former are components of the electron transport chain, which is involved in oxidative phosphorylation. Quantitatively the liver is the major non-erythropoietic haem-producing organ. All haem pigments contain iron; the oxygen-carrying ability of the haem molecule depends on the presence of ferrous iron (Fe^{2+}), the form normally present in both haemoglobin and oxyhaemoglobin.

Red blood cells are broken down by the reticuloendothelial system, predominantly in the spleen. Released haemoglobin is split into the peptide chain, globin, which enters the general protein pool, and haem. The haem ring is split, a process catalysed by haem oxidase, to form a linear molecule, biliverdin. Released iron is reused and biliverdin is reduced to lipid-soluble bilirubin. The metabolism of bilirubin is discussed in Chapter 17 in the context of jaundice.

Biosynthesis of haem and haemoglobin

The main steps in the synthesis of haem are outlined below and in Figure 21.1.

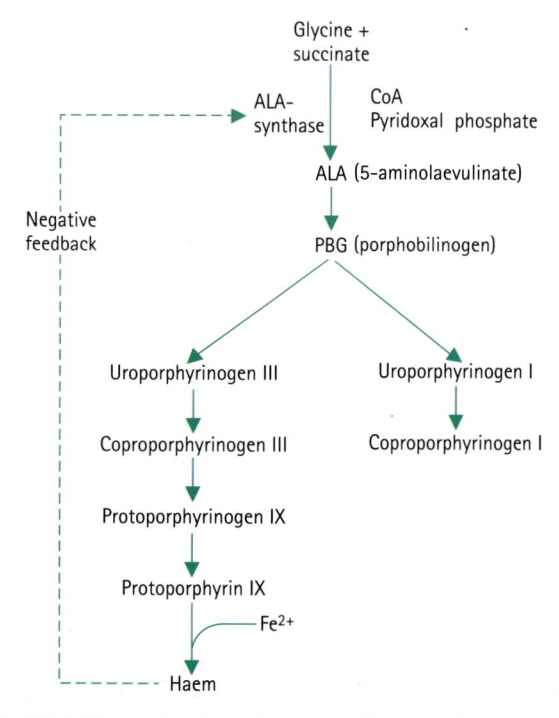

Fig. 21.1 Biosynthesis pathways of haem. (CoA = coenzyme A.)

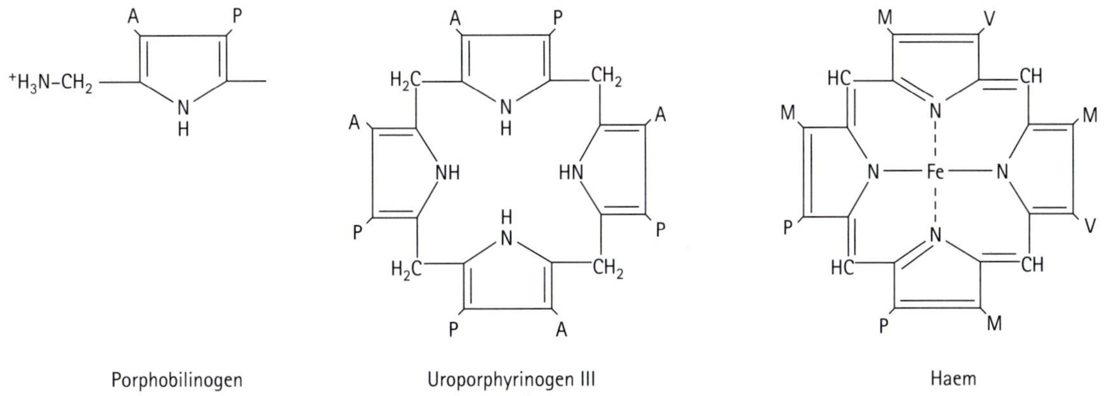

Fig. 21.2 Porphobilinogen, the tetrapyrrole uroporphyrinogen III, which incorporates four porphobilinogen units and haemoglobin. Uroporphyrinogen I differs only in the order of the side chains on one of the rings. (Side chains: A = acetate; M = methyl; P = propionate; V = vinyl.)

- 5-Aminolaevulinic acid (ALA) is formed by condensation of glycine and succinate. The reaction requires pyridoxal phosphate and is catalysed by ALA synthase. This is the rate-limiting step in the synthetic pathway and is regulated by feedback inhibition by haem.
- Two molecules of ALA condense to form a monopyrrole, porphobilinogen (PBG).
- Four molecules of PBG combine to form a tetrapyrrole ring, uroporphyrinogen (Fig. 21.2). Two isomers are formed, I and III. The major pathway involves the III isomer.
- Haem is formed by the successive production of coproporphyrinogen and protoporphyrin, followed by incorporation of Fe^{2+} into the centre of the ring.
- Haemoglobin consists of four haem molecules, covalently linked to four (two pairs of) polypeptide chains.

Excretion of haem precursors

Excess intermediates on the haem pathway are excreted in either urine or faeces.

The porphyrin precursors ALA, PBG and uroporphyrinogen are water soluble and appear in the urine. They are colourless, but PBG may spontaneously oxidize to form uroporphyrin when exposed to air and light. Porphyrinogens also oxidize spontaneously to the corresponding porphyrins, which are dark red and fluoresce in ultraviolet light. A urine specimen containing large amounts of porphyrinogens or their precursors will gradually darken if left standing.

Protoporphyrin is excreted in bile and appears in the faeces, whereas coproporphyrin(ogen) may be excreted by either route.

Haemoglobin and related compounds

When oxygen is incorporated into haemoglobin to form oxyhaemoglobin, the spatial arrangement of the haem complexes is altered in such a way as to facilitate further oxygen uptake. Other compounds related to haemoglobin may sometimes be formed and some of these may hinder the oxygen-carrying capacity.

Carboxyhaemoglobin

Carboxyhaemoglobin is cherry-red in colour and is formed when carbon monoxide binds to haemoglobin or displaces oxygen from oxyhaemoglobin; haemoglobin has a greater affinity for carbon monoxide than for oxygen. This occurs in carbon monoxide poisoning, which can be lethal. Once carbon monoxide is removed from inspired air, oxyhaemoglobin is reformed. Consciousness is not lost until the carboxy form has replaced about half the oxyhaemoglobin.

Myoglobin

Myoglobin, the single haem–polypeptide complex, is normally present in muscle. Plasma concentrations may rise if skeletal or myocardial muscle cells are damaged. Being of low molecular weight, it is rapidly cleared by the kidneys.

Methaemoglobin

Methaemoglobin is haemoglobin in which iron is in the ferric (Fe^{3+}) form (haemin); therefore, it cannot carry oxygen. It is brown and is normally present in very low plasma concentrations; drugs such as sulphonamides may increase methaemoglobin. The symptoms of methaemoglobinaemia are due to hypoxia, which causes cyanosis and an increased respiratory rate.

Methaemalbumin

Methaemalbumin is also brown. It is formed when haem combines with plasma albumin in conditions such as severe intravascular haemolysis or acute haemorrhagic pancreatitis when haemoglobin has been converted to haemin in the abdominal cavity and absorbed. Methaemalbumin occurs when the haemoglobin-binding capacity of haptoglobin has been exceeded.

Sulphaemoglobin

Sulphaemoglobin is similar to methaemoglobin but contains sulphur; unlike methaemoglobin, it cannot be reconverted to haemoglobin in vivo. It remains in intact red blood cells. Methaemoglobinaemia-producing drugs cause sulphaemoglobinaemia if hydrogen sulphide is present, usually in the gut.

IRON METABOLISM

Distribution of iron in the body

About 50–70 mmol (3–4 g) of iron are distributed amongst body compartments. There is considerable interchange of iron between stores and plasma.

Free iron is toxic. In normal subjects it is all protein bound: in plasma it is bound to transferrin, in the storage pools to protein in ferritin and haemosiderin, and in erythrocytes it is incorporated into haemoglobin.

About 70 per cent of the total iron is circulating, largely in erythrocyte haemoglobin. However, there are smaller amounts in muscle myoglobin and iron-containing enzymes and cytochromes.

Up to 25 per cent of the body iron is stored in the reticuloendothelial system, in the liver, spleen and bone marrow; bone marrow iron is drawn on for haemoglobin synthesis. Iron in stored as protein complexes, ferritin and haemosiderin. Ferritin iron is more easily released from protein than that in haemosiderin. Haemosiderin can be seen by light microscopy in unstained tissue preparations. Ferritin and haemosiderin, but not haem iron, stain with potassium ferrocyanide (Prussian blue reaction) and this staining characteristic may be used to assess the size of iron stores.

Iron deficiency only becomes haematologically evident when no stainable iron is detectable in the reticuloendothelial cells in bone marrow films.

Iron overload is likely when, because reticuloendothelial storage capacity is exceeded, stainable iron is demonstrable in parenchymal cells in liver biopsy specimens. This is the storage pool.

Only about 50–70 mmol (3–4 mg), or about 0.1 per cent of the total body iron, are circulating in plasma, all bound to transferrin; this fraction is measured in plasma iron assays. This is the transit pool.

Iron can only cross cell membranes by active transport in the Fe^{2+} form; it is in this reduced state in both oxyhaemoglobin and 'reduced' haemoglobin. It is in the Fe^{3+} form in ferritin and haemosiderin and when bound to transferrin.

Iron absorption

Body iron content control depends on absorption by an active process in the upper small intestine. Within the intestinal cell, some of the iron combines with the protein apoferritin to form ferritin.

Normally, about 18 μmol (1 mg) of iron is absorbed each day and this just replaces loss. This amounts to about 10 per cent of the iron ingested in the diet, although the proportion depends to some extent on the type of food. Once in the body, iron is in a virtually closed system (Fig. 21.3).

Iron absorption seems to be influenced by any or all of the following factors:

- oxygen tension in the intestinal cells,
- marrow erythropoietic activity,
- the size of the body iron stores.

Iron absorption is also increased in many non-iron deficiency anaemias.

Most normal women taking an adequate diet probably absorb slightly more iron than men and so replace their higher losses in menstrual blood and during pregnancy.

Iron requirements for growth during childhood and adolescence are similar to, or slightly higher than, those of menstruating women and can be met by increased absorption from a normal diet.

Iron excretion

This is poorly controlled, as loss from the body may depend on the ferritin iron content of cells lost by desquamation, mostly into the intestinal tract and from the skin. The total daily loss by these routes is about 18 μmol (1 mg). Urinary excretion is minimal, as circulating iron is protein bound and not water soluble.

Normal iron loss is so small, and normal iron stores are so large, that it would take about 3 years to become iron

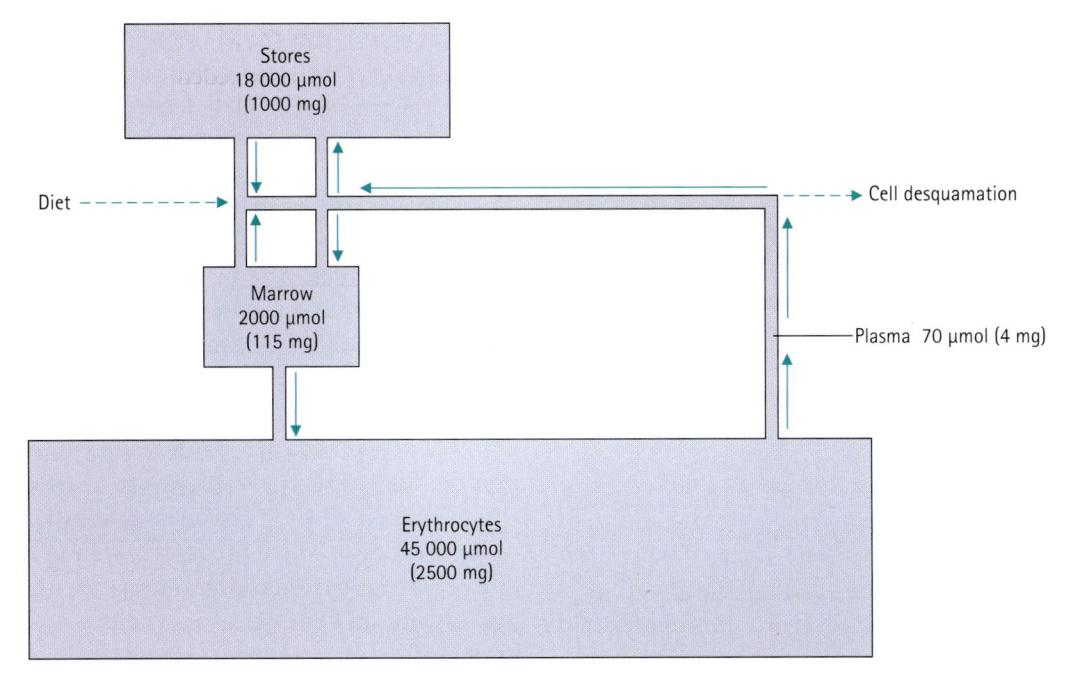

Fig. 21.3 Body iron compartments.

deficient on a completely iron-free diet. Of course, this period is much shorter if there is any blood loss, such as menstruation.

Iron transport in plasma

Iron is transported in the plasma in the ferric form, attached to the specific binding protein transferrin at a concentration of about 18 μmol/L. Transferrin is normally capable of binding about 54 μmol/L of iron and is therefore about a third saturated. Transferrin-bound iron is carried to stores and to bone marrow cells and in the latter some iron passes directly into developing erythrocytes to form haemoglobin.

Factors affecting plasma iron concentration

The plasma iron concentration is likely to be a poor index of the total body content because only a very small proportion is in this compartment; it has no function, except as a protein-bound transport fraction. Plasma iron concentration is very variable, even under physiological conditions.

Physiological factors

The causes of physiological changes in plasma iron concentrations are not well understood, but alterations can be very rapid and almost certainly represent shifts between plasma and stores, not changes in total body iron. The following factors are known to affect plasma concentrations within a population.

- *Sex and age differences.* Plasma iron concentrations, like those of haemoglobin and the erythrocyte count, are higher in men than in women, probably for hormonal reasons. The difference is first evident at puberty, before significant menstrual loss has occurred, and disappears at the menopause. Androgens tend to increase the plasma iron concentration and oestrogens to lower it.
- *Pregnancy and oral contraceptives.* In the first few weeks of pregnancy, the plasma iron may rise to concentrations similar to those found in men. A similar rise occurs in women taking some oral contraceptives.

Iron concentrations can vary within an individual by up to 100 per cent or more. This can be due to the following.

- *Random variations.* Day-to-day variations may be as much as three-fold and usually overshadow cyclical changes. They may be associated with physical or mental stress or diet, but usually no cause can be found.
- *Circadian (diurnal) rhythm.* The plasma iron concentration is higher in the morning than in the evening. If subjects are kept awake at night, this difference is less marked; it is reversed in night workers.
- *Monthly variations in women.* The plasma iron may reach very low concentrations just before or during the menstrual period. The reduction is probably due to hormonal factors rather than blood loss.

Pathological factors

Iron deficiency and iron overload usually cause low and high plasma iron concentrations respectively.

Iron deficiency is associated with a hypochromic, microcytic anaemia and with reduced amounts of stainable bone marrow iron. Plasma ferritin concentrations are usually, but not always, low.

Iron overload is associated with increased amounts of stainable iron in liver biopsy specimens, and plasma ferritin concentrations are high.

Other pathological factors that may affect plasma iron concentrations include the following.

- *Any acute or chronic illness* (even a bad cold) *causing a fall in plasma iron concentration*. Chronic conditions such as malignancy, renal disease, rheumatoid arthritis and chronic infections are often associated with normochromic, normocytic anaemia. Iron stores and plasma ferritin concentrations are normal or even increased; the anaemia does not respond to iron therapy. Iron deficiency may be superimposed on the anaemia of chronic illness, especially if drugs are being taken that cause gastrointestinal bleeding; plasma ferritin concentrations are then variable. The finding of hypochromic erythrocytes is the most sensitive index of this complication. Low plasma iron concentrations occur whether or not there is any iron deficiency.
- *Disorders in which the marrow cannot use iron*, either because it is hypoplastic or because some other essential erythropoietic factor, such as vitamin B_{12} or folate, is deficient; plasma iron concentrations are often high. Blood and marrow films may show a typical picture, but, for example in pyridoxine-responsive anaemia and in thalassaemia, the findings in the blood film may resemble those of iron deficiency; in the last two conditions the presence of stainable marrow iron stores excludes the diagnosis of iron deficiency.
- *Haemolytic anaemia*. The plasma iron concentration may be high during a haemolytic episode, as iron, liberated from the destroyed erythrocytes, enters the plasma; it is usually normal during the quiescent periods when the iron enters the reticuloendothelial system. Marrow iron stores and plasma ferritin concentrations are usually increased in chronic haemolytic conditions.
- *Acute liver disease*. Disruption of hepatocytes may release ferritin iron into the bloodstream and cause a transient rise in the plasma iron concentration. Cirrhosis may be associated with a similar finding, perhaps due to increased iron absorption and intake.

Transferrin and total iron-binding capacity

Plasma iron concentrations alone rarely give information about the state of iron stores. In rare situations in which doubt remains after haematological investigation, diagnostic precision may sometimes be improved by measuring both the plasma transferrin and iron concentrations.

Plasma transferrin can be directly assayed or measured indirectly by adding an excess of inorganic iron to the plasma, any not bound to protein being removed, usually with an exchange resin. The concentration of iron remaining is assayed and the result expressed as the total iron-binding capacity (TIBC). This is usually a valid approximation of the transferrin concentration. In rare circumstances, of which the most common is severe liver disease, plasma ferritin concentrations are high enough to bind significant amounts of iron and the results of iron-binding capacity measurements are then misleading as an assessment of the transferrin concentration.

Physiological changes in the plasma transferrin concentration

The plasma transferrin concentration is less labile than that of iron. However, it rises:

- after about the 28th week of pregnancy even if iron stores are normal,
- in women taking some oral contraceptive preparations,
- in any patient treated with oestrogens.

Pathological changes in the plasma transferrin concentration

Plasma transferrin concentration and TIBC:

- rise in iron deficiency and fall in iron overload,
- fall in those chronic illnesses associated with low plasma iron concentrations,
- may be unchanged in acute illness,
- may be very low in the nephrotic syndrome, associated with a low plasma iron concentration, because the relatively low-molecular-weight transferrin is lost in the urine together with iron.

Thus the low plasma iron concentration of uncomplicated iron deficiency is associated with a high transferrin concentration and TIBC; that of non-iron deficiency is associated with low concentrations.

Table 21.1 Biochemical findings associated with plasma iron abnormalities

	Plasma concentrations				Marrow iron stores
	Iron	Transferrin	Ferritin	TfR	
Low iron concentration					
Iron deficiency	↓	↑	Usually ↓	↑	↓
Acute illness	↓	–	– or ↑	–	–
Chronic illness	↓	↓	– or ↑	–	Usually ↑
High iron concentration					
Early pregnancy	↑	–	–	–	–
Late pregnancy or oral contraceptives	Variable	↑	–	↑	–
Iron overload	↑	↓	↑	↓	↑
Liver disease	↑	↓	↑	– or ↑	May be ↑
Haemolysis	↑	– or ↓	↑	↑	↑

TfR = transferrin receptor; ↑ = up; – = normal; ↓ = down.

If iron deficiency coexists with the anaemia of chronic illness, the opposing effects of the two conditions on the transferrin concentration make it difficult to interpret transferrin, as well as plasma iron, concentrations.

FERRITIN

Circulating ferritin is usually in equilibrium with that in stores. However, it is an 'acute-phase' protein and its synthesis is increased in many inflammatory conditions.

The normal plasma ferritin concentration is about 100 µg/L. A plasma ferritin concentration below about 10 µg/L suggests iron deficiency. Results can be misleading if there is coexistent inflammatory disease, since accelerated synthesis may lead to normal or even high plasma concentrations despite very low iron stores. In this situation, the results of plasma iron and transferrin assays are also difficult to interpret; haematological parameters remain the most reliable diagnostic indicators of iron deficiency, and possibly also assay of the soluble transferrin receptor (see later).

High concentrations of plasma ferritin always occur in significant iron overload, but may also be due to:

- inflammatory conditions,
- malignant disease,
- liver disease,
- haemolysis,
- high alcohol intake.

Thus the finding of a normal or low plasma ferritin concentration almost certainly excludes the diagnosis of iron overload, but a high one does not necessarily confirm it.

The laboratory findings in conditions that may affect plasma iron concentrations are summarized in Table 21.1.

THE SOLUBLE TRANSFERRIN RECEPTOR

Cells express transferrin receptors (TfRs) on their surface. Plasma or so-called soluble transferrin binds to TfR, preferring the diferric transferrin form. The TfR–transferrin complex is internalized into endosomes, where the iron is released into the cytosol. The transferrin bound to the TfR returns to the cell surface, where the apo–transferrin dissociates and another diferric transferrin can bind. It can therefore be seen that iron uptake into cells is dependent on the number of cell surface TfRs and the concentration and percentage saturation of transferrin.

Plasma TfR concentrations reflect total cellular TfR levels, which are increased in iron deficiency as TfR is up regulated due to the cell's requirements for iron, but, unlike ferritin, are not increased as a result of the acute-phase response of inflammation. Plasma TfR concentrations are also directly related to the rate of erythropoiesis and to increased erythrocyte turnover, such as occurs in haemolytic anaemia.

IRON THERAPY

As the body iron content is determined by control of absorption, rather than excretion, parenteral iron therapy (which bypasses absorption) and repeated transfusions of blood (which contains about 4.5 mmol (250 mg) of iron per unit) may cause iron overload. In anaemias other than those due to iron deficiency, stores are normal or even increased. Proven iron deficiency usually requires iron therapy and *the oral route is preferable, as anaphylaxis may occur with parenteral administration*. Repeated blood transfusions may be needed to correct severe non-iron deficiency anaemia, for example if the marrow is hypoplastic, but the danger of overload should be remembered.

Iron absorption is stimulated by anaemia even if iron stores are increased. The treatment of non-iron deficiency anaemia with oral iron supplements is not only ineffective, but can also lead to iron overload; this is especially likely in haemolytic anaemia, in which the iron released from destroyed erythrocytes remains in the body.

IRON OVERLOAD

The only route of iron loss is cell desquamation. Iron absorbed from the gastrointestinal tract or administered parenterally in excess of daily loss accumulates in body stores. If such 'positive balance' is maintained over long periods, iron stores may exceed 350 mmol (20 g), i.e. about five times the normal amount.

Causes of iron overload

- *Increased intestinal absorption*:
  - hereditary or primary haemochromatosis,
  - anaemia with increased, but ineffective, erythropoiesis,
  - liver disease (rare cause),
  - dietary excess,
  - inappropriate oral iron therapy.
- *Parenteral administration*:
  - multiple blood transfusions,
  - inappropriate parenteral iron therapy.

A very rare cause of iron overload is an inherited deficiency of transferrin.

Consequences of iron overload

The effect of the accumulated iron depends on its distribution in the body. This, in turn, is influenced partly by the route of entry. Two main patterns are seen at postmortem or in biopsy specimens.

Parenchymal iron overload occurs in haemochromatosis and in patients with ineffective erythropoiesis. Iron accumulates in the parenchymal cells of the liver, pancreas, heart and other organs. There is usually associated functional disturbance or tissue damage.

Reticuloendothelial iron overload is seen after excessive parenteral administration of iron or multiple blood transfusions. The iron accumulates initially in the reticuloendothelial cells of the liver, spleen and bone marrow.

In dietary iron overload, both hepatic reticuloendothelial and parenchymal overload may occur, associated with scurvy and osteoporosis. Whatever the cause of massive iron overload, there may be parenchymal accumulation and tissue damage.

Haemosiderosis is a histological definition. An increase in iron stores as haemosiderin can be seen. It does not necessarily mean that there is an increase in total body iron; for example, in many types of anaemia there is reduced haemoglobin iron but increased storage iron. *Haemochromatosis* describes the clinical disorder due to parenchymal iron-induced damage.

Syndromes of iron overload

Hereditary or primary haemochromatosis

Hereditary haemochromatosis has an autosomal recessive mode of inheritance and a defect of the haemochromatosis gene (*HFE*). Approximately 1 in 10 of people in Western societies are carriers and about 1 in 1000 are homozygous. The gene for this disorder is closely associated with the HLA gene locus on chromosome 6. Those members of a family with an HLA haplotype identical with that of the patient are likely to develop the disease. Factors such as alcohol abuse may hasten the accumulation of iron and the development of liver damage. Males are more likely to manifest the condition, as menstruation in females lowers tissue iron stores.

There is increased intestinal absorption of iron over many years, which produces large iron stores in the tissues, such as the liver, pancreas, joints, heart and gonads. It presents, usually in middle age, as cirrhosis of the liver, sometimes with diabetes mellitus, joint pains, cardiomyopathy, hypogonadism and greyish skin pigmentation due to melanin, not iron. It has been referred to as 'bronzed diabetes', although such skin features tend to occur late.

Examination of liver biopsy specimens may be useful, giving an idea of disease severity and showing increased iron content when stained by Perl's blue staining. There is an association with hepatocellular carcinoma, which can be screened for by assay of plasma α-fetoprotein.

The diagnosis may be made on the basis of the measurement of plasma ferritin, which is often greater than 1000 µg/L. Also plasma iron concentration and TIBC

> ## CASE 1
>
> A 46-year-old male was investigated in the hepatology clinic because of abnormal liver function tests. He was known to have type 2 diabetes mellitus. The results of some of his biochemistry tests prior to liver biopsy were as follows.
>
> *Plasma*
> Bilirubin 13 μmol/L (<20)
> Alanine transaminase 192 U/L (<42)
> Alkaline phosphatase 206 U/L (<250)
> Albumin 44 g/L (35–45)
> Gamma glutamyltransferase 224 U/L (<55)
> Ferritin 2343 μg/L (15–300)
> Iron 40 μmol/L (11–30)
> Total iron-binding capacity 42 μmol/L (54–80)
> Iron saturation 95% (plasma iron/TIBC × 100%)
>
> ### DISCUSSION
> The patient was found to have haemochromatosis. This was confirmed by studies of the *HFE* gene, which showed him to be homozygous for the C282Y mutation, and iron staining on liver biopsy. His diabetes mellitus may also have been secondary to this, as were the abnormal liver function tests. Elevated plasma ferritin concentrations can be seen in liver disease, haemolysis, alcohol excess and conditions in which there is an acute-phase response. However, the high iron saturation of more than 50 per cent suggests haemochromatosis.

with a saturation of greater than 50 per cent are indicative of haemochromatosis and may increase before plasma ferritin concentration does.

The relatives of patients with proven hereditary haemochromatosis should be investigated. Genetic tests are now available, with a majority of cases of haemochromatosis being due to the *C282Y* or *H63D HFE* gene mutations.

Treatment is often by venesection, aiming to reduce the plasma ferritin to less than 100 μg/L. Each 500 mL unit of blood removes about 250 mg of iron from the body.

Secondary iron overload

Anaemia and iron overload

Several types of anaemia may be associated with iron overload. In some, such as hypoplastic anaemia and the anaemia of chronic renal failure, the cause is multiple blood transfusions; the iron initially accumulates in the reticuloendothelial system. If overload is massive (often over 100 units of blood), deposition may occur in parenchymal cells, with the development of secondary haemochromatosis.

In anaemias characterized by erythroid marrow hyperplasia but with ineffective erythropoiesis, such as thalassaemia major and sideroblastic anaemia, there is, in addition, increased absorption of iron. Secondary haemochromatosis develops at a lower transfusion load than in hypoplastic anaemia.

Treatment of iron overload of anaemia

This can obviously not be treated by venesection. The tendency for transfusion to aggravate iron overload further can be minimized by giving the iron-chelating agent desferrioxamine each time; this can be excreted in the urine with any non-haemoglobin iron.

Dietary iron overload

Increased iron absorption due to excessive intake is rare. One well-described form is, however, relatively common in the rural black population of southern Africa. The source is beer brewed in iron containers. Usually, the excess is confined to the reticuloendothelial system and the liver (both portal tracts and parenchymal cells), and there is no tissue damage. In a small number of cases, deposition in the parenchymal cells of other organs occurs and the clinical picture may resemble that of primary haemochromatosis; it may be distinguished by the high concentration of iron in the reticuloendothelial system seen in the bone marrow.

Scurvy and osteoporosis may occur in this form of iron overload. The ascorbate deficiency may be due to its irreversible oxidation in the presence of excessive amounts of iron, and osteoporosis sometimes accompanies scurvy. Ascorbate deficiency also interferes with normal mobilization of iron from the reticuloendothelial cells; plasma iron concentrations may be low and the response to chelating agents poor, despite iron overload.

Investigation of disorders of iron metabolism

Investigation of iron deficiency of anaemia

There are many causes of anaemia, which may be due either to iron deficiency or to a variety of other conditions, sometimes associated with high iron stores. The subject of the diagnosis of anaemia, such as haemolytic or pernicious anaemia, is covered more fully in textbooks of haematology. Blood haemoglobin reflects the major metabolic pool of iron, ferritin the storage pool and transferrin the transit pool.

The clinical impression of anaemia should be confirmed by blood haemoglobin estimation. Iron deficiency can, however, exist with haemoglobin concentrations within the reference range.

The mean corpuscular volume (MCV) and mean corpuscular haemoglobin (MCH) should be checked and often a blood film examined. Iron deficiency anaemia is microcytic and hypochromic in type, and these findings may be evident before the haemoglobin concentration has fallen below the reference range. Normochromic, normocytic anaemia is a non-specific finding, usually associated with other chronic disease; it is associated with iron deficiency only if there has been very recent blood loss.

In most cases of anaemia, consideration of these findings together with the clinical picture may elucidate the cause. Anaemias such as those due to sickle cell disease, thalassaemia or of the sideroblastic type, although rarer, are most likely to confuse the picture, since they too are hypochromic but are not due to iron deficiency.

A low plasma ferritin concentration (less than 10 µg/L) is indicative of iron deficiency due to low iron stores.

One major diagnostic dilemma is to separate iron deficiency anaemia from anaemia of chronic disorders, for example carcinoma or inflammatory disease. In the latter there is often an acute-phase response, which can raise plasma ferritin concentrations, which are influenced by inflammation. This can, therefore, 'mask' a low plasma ferritin concentration due to iron deficiency. A plasma ferritin concentration more than 200 µg/L under these circumstances probably rules out iron deficiency anaemia, but values more than 10 µg/L but less than 200 µg/L are equivocal and do not distinguish between iron deficiency anaemia and anaemia of chronic disorders. Under these circumstances, plasma soluble TfR assay may be useful; this should be raised in iron deficiency but not in anaemia of chronic disorders.

An unequivocally low plasma ferritin concentration confirms iron deficiency, but a normal or high one should not be assumed to exclude it. A bone marrow film for iron staining may be needed to confirm the diagnosis of iron deficiency in ambiguous cases.

If a diagnosis of iron deficiency is made, it is essential to rule out blood loss and its source. Particularly important is to exclude gastrointestinal malignancy and also gynaecological pathology. Faecal occult blood samples may show the presence of gastrointestinal blood loss, which may necessitate prompt endoscopic investigation (see Chapter 16).

A patient with proven iron deficiency who shows no response to oral iron treatment within a few weeks may not be taking the tablets. If iron has been taken, malabsorption (usually as part of a general absorption defect) is a possible explanation of a poor response.

Investigation of suspected iron overload

Initial tests

Plasma iron, percentage saturation of transferrin, plasma ferritin

All of these should be measured. The plasma iron concentration is almost invariably high in primary haemochromatosis,

CASE 2

A 64-year-old female saw her general practitioner because of weight loss, tiredness and change in bowel habit (the recent development of loose stools). The following relevant laboratory results were returned.

Haemoglobin 9.0 g/dL (12–17)
White cells 5.1 × 10^9/L (3–10)
Platelets 430 × 10^9/L (150–450)
MCV 70 fL (80–95)
MCH 23 pg (28–34)

Plasma iron study results:
Ferritin 7 µg/L (15–300)

Iron 6 µmol/L (11–30)
Total iron-binding capacity 60 µmol/L (54–80)

Three faecal occult blood samples were all positive for blood.

DISCUSSION

The hypochromic, microcytic anaemia (suggested by the low MCH and MCV respectively) and also low plasma ferritin and iron concentrations all point to an iron deficiency. The patient was later shown by colonoscopy to have a carcinoma of her descending colon. Iron deficiency should prompt investigation as to why this is present, and bleeding needs to be excluded.

often more than 36 μmol/L. This is associated with a reduced plasma transferrin concentration and TIBC, and the percentage saturation is usually greater than 50 per cent, and may be nearer 100 per cent. In the presence of infection or malignancy, however, the plasma iron concentration and percentage saturation may be lower than expected; the plasma transferrin concentration remains low.

Plasma ferritin concentrations are high in most patients with iron overload (whether reticuloendothelial or parenchymal). It is rare in hereditary haemochromatosis to have a normal plasma ferritin concentration, although this may occur in the early stages, when the iron saturation may be more useful diagnostically. Remember that plasma ferritin can be elevated in hepatic disease and high alcohol intake. There is also a rare familial hyperferritinaemia due to a defect in ferritin synthesis that should not be misdiagnosed as haemochromatosis.

If all these values are normal, it is unlikely that the patient has iron overload. If there is doubt, particularly in the face of a positive family history, genetic studies of the *HFE* gene may be indicated.

Demonstration of increased iron stores

The diagnosis of iron overload usually needs demonstration of increased iron stores.

Liver biopsy

Liver biopsy specimens contain large amounts of stainable iron, which may be mainly in parenchymal or mainly in reticuloendothelial cells. If haemochromatosis is confirmed, liver function tests are necessary, as is exclusion of diabetes mellitus or impaired glucose regulation and other clinical features of iron overload such as pituitary or gonadal involvement. Cirrhosis may progress to hepatocellular carcinoma, which should be looked out for.

Bone marrow iron content

This is usually normal in haemochromatosis, in which overload is predominantly parenchymal, but may be greatly increased in reticuloendothelial overload. A similar loading of the reticuloendothelial cells is found when there is deficient use of marrow iron for haemoglobin synthesis, as in many haematological, neoplastic and chronic inflammatory diseases.

Family studies

The blood relatives of patients found to have haemochromatosis should be investigated. Estimations of plasma iron and percentage saturation of transferrin are the most sensitive tests and may change before ferritin levels rise if iron stores are not significantly increased. Genetic studies looking at *HFE* gene mutations are now being used.

DISORDERS OF HAEM SYNTHESIS: THE PORPHYRIAS

The porphyrias are a rare group of disorders of haem synthesis, resulting from a deficiency of one of the enzymes on the haem synthetic pathway (Fig. 21.4). Haem production is impaired, but reduced feedback inhibition of ALA synthase (the rate-limiting step) may maintain adequate haem levels at the expense of overproduction of porphyrins or their precursors.

Porphyrias can be classified into those that present with acute porphyric attacks and those with dermatological lesions (cutaneous) but not acute porphyric attacks.

The main porphyrias are as follows.

- The *acute porphyrias*:
  - PBG synthase deficiency,
  - acute intermittent porphyria,
  - hereditary coproporphyria,
  - variegate porphyria.
- The *cutaneous non-acute porphyrias*:
  - porphyria cutanea tarda,
      genetic predisposition,
      acquired,
  - congenital erythropoietic porphyria,
  - protoporphyria.

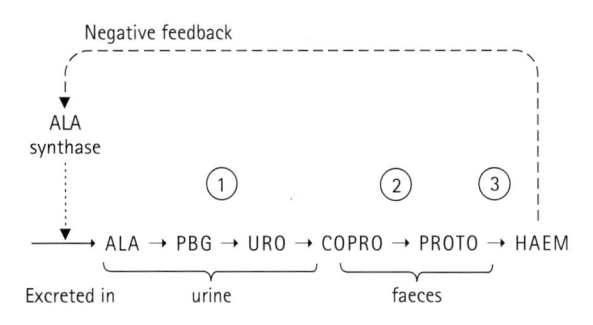

Fig. 21.4 Sites of enzyme deficiencies in (1) acute intermittent porphyria, (2) hereditary coproporphyria, (3) variegate porphyria. (ALA = 5-aminolaevulinic acid; PBG = porphobilinogen; URO = uroporphyrinogen; COPRO = coproporphyrinogen; PROTO = protoporphyrinogen.

Table 21.2 The major clinical features of the porphyrias

Clinical features	Acute porphyrias						Cutaneous porphyrias		
	AIP		VP		HC		PCT	CEP	PP
	Acute	Latent	Acute	Latent	Acute	Latent	Non acute		
Abdominal and neurological symptoms	+	−	+	−	+	−	−	−	−
Skin lesions	−	−	+	+	Rare	Rare	+	+	+

AIP = acute intermittent porphyria; VP = variegate porphyria; HC = hereditary coproporphyria; PCT = porphyria cutanea tarda; CEP = congenital erythropoietic porphyria; PP = protoporphyria.

CASE 3

A 17-year-old female was admitted under the care of the general surgeons because of abdominal pain, which she had been experiencing with varying severity over the preceding year. She underwent a laparotomy, although no abdominal abnormality was found. However, postoperatively her blood pressure rose from 128/70 mmHg to 170/120 mmHg. An acute porphyria was considered and the following porphyria screening results were obtained.

Urinary PBG 213 μmol/L (0–10)
Urinary total porphyrins 6400 nmol/L (20–330)
Faecal porphyrins 110 nmol/g dry weight (10–210)

DISCUSSION

Abdominal pain and hypertension can be presenting features of an acute porphyria. Further investigation, including family studies and genetic tests, confirmed the diagnosis of acute intermittent porphyria. Note that the anaesthetic agents given for the operation worsened the acute attack. Indeed, certain anaesthetic drugs, such as thiopental, can induce ALA synthase activity, thereby increasing flux through the porphyrin pathways. The lack of skin manifestations and normal faecal porphyrins support the diagnosis of acute intermittent porphyria.

The last two are also called the erythropoietic porphyrias.

The major clinical and biochemical features are outlined in Table 21.2 and discussed briefly below and correlate well with the biochemical abnormalities.

The acute porphyrias

Porphobilinogen synthase deficiency is an autosomal recessive condition; PBG concentration is not raised, although that of ALA is, and the condition is very rare. The other three acute porphyrias listed above are *autosomal dominantly* inherited disorders and have latent and acute phases. The symptoms and biochemical abnormalities of the latent phases differ and reflect the nature of the enzyme defect. In the acute phases, however, the biochemical and clinical pictures characteristic of excessive ALA and PBG production associated with neurological and abdominal symptoms develop. The similarities and differences are best explained by referring to a simplified scheme of the haem synthetic pathway (see Fig. 21.1).

Latent phase

The enzyme defect tends to reduce haem levels, which in turn increase ALA synthase activity by a decrease in negative feedback inhibition. Increased ALA synthase activity has been demonstrated in all the porphyrias. Haem levels are maintained at the expense of the accumulation and excretion of the substance immediately before the block.

In *acute intermittent porphyria* there is increased urinary ALA and PBG excretion, although it may not be detectable in all patients; the latent phase is usually asymptomatic. It is due to PBG deaminase deficiency.

In *hereditary coproporphyria* there is increased faecal coproporphyrin excretion; the increase in the concentration of porphyrins may produce skin lesions, but less commonly than in variegate porphyria. It is due to coproporphyrinogen oxidase deficiency.

In *variegate porphyria* there is increased faecal protoporphyrin excretion; the increase in the concentration of porphyrins may produce skin lesions. There is no increase in erythrocyte porphyrins; however, plasma emission fluorescence shows a peak of 624–626 nm when stimulated at 405 nm, whilst the other acute porphyrias show peaks at 615 nm. It is due to protoporphyrinogen oxidase deficiency.

Diagnosis of latent porphyria

It is essential to investigate the close blood relatives of any patient with porphyria. Screening tests for excess urinary PBG and ALA are inadequate to diagnose latent acute intermittent porphyria, and even quantitative estimation may fail to detect all carriers. The activity of the relevant enzymes can be measured in erythrocytes, and genetic tests may be useful.

Acute phase

Acute disturbances such as peripheral neuropathy or abdominal pain may occur in an acute attack, in which the precursors ALA and PBG are produced in excess. These features may be due to a direct toxic effect of ALA or PBG. Convulsions may occur in acute attacks, sometimes associated with hyponatraemia; this may be due to the syndrome of inappropriate antidiuretic hormone (see Chapter 2).

5-Aminolaevulinate synthase activity may be further increased by a number of drugs, particularly barbiturates, oestrogens, sulphonamides, phenytoin, halothane and griseofulvin. Also important are alcohol and smoking and acute illness such as infection (this may be a direct effect or may be due to an increased demand for haem).

Acute attacks occur only in a small proportion of patients exposed to the provoking agents. They are more common in premenstrual or pregnant women, and in women rather than in men, and usually only occur after puberty. Colicky abdominal pain, due to involvement of the autonomic nervous system, and neurological symptoms ranging from peripheral neuropathy to quadriplegia are usually the presenting features. Death may result from respiratory paralysis.

The acute attack closely resembles serious acute intra-abdominal conditions and, if the diagnosis is not made, the patient may be subjected to surgery with the use of a barbiturate anaesthetic; this and the stress of operation may aggravate the condition.

The acute attack is marked by an increase in ALA and PBG production. In acute intermittent porphyria, this increase is due to the block imposed by an inherited deficiency of PBG deaminase; in hepatic coproporphyria and variegate porphyria, this enzyme becomes rate limiting and is unable to respond normally to the increased demand. *The increase in urinary ALA and PBG concentrations is the hallmark of the acute porphyric attack* and, in hereditary coproporphyria and variegate porphyria, is superimposed on all the other biochemical abnormalities. The accelerated activity of the pathway and the spontaneous conversion of the precursors to porphyrin lead to increased urinary porphyrin excretion.

About 1 per cent of acute attacks are fatal. It is important to stop precipitating drugs and not to use medications that could evoke an attack. Convulsions may be treated with gabapentin or vigabatrin. Haem arginate given by slow intravenous infusion can result in a reduction in ALA and PBG concentrations and thus reduce some of the features of the acute attack, but not usually the neuropathy.

Cutaneous porphyrias (non-acute)

The cutaneous porphyrias include porphyria cutanea tarda, congenital erythropoietic porphyria and protoporphyria.

Porphyria cutanea tarda

This is the most common porphyria. In patients with porphyria cutanea tarda, the skin is unduly sensitive to minor trauma, particularly in sun-exposed areas; the commonest presenting feature is blistering on the backs of the hands. Less commonly, the lesions appear on the face. Increased facial hair and hyperpigmentation occur in chronic cases. Acute attacks do not occur, but this type of porphyria is associated with hepatic damage.

The basic defect is an inability to convert uroporphyrinogen to coproporphyrinogen due to a deficiency of uroporphyrinogen decarboxylase. There are two types of porphyria cutanea tarda.

- It may be an *autosomal dominantly inherited disorder*. The familial form is rare, although environmental factors are also important.
- Most cases are acquired. Factors that produce clinical disease, possibly by aggravating an underlying genetic deficiency, include alcohol abuse, iron overload or high-dose oestrogen therapy. Symptoms improve when the offending substance is withdrawn. Some liver toxins such as hexachlorobenzene directly inhibit the activity of the enzyme. There is an association with hepatitis C. Iron overload can also be present and haemochromatosis needs to be excluded.

The impaired conversion leads to an accumulation of uroporphyrinogen and porphyrins intermediate between it and coproporphyrinogen. These deposit in the skin and are excreted in the urine in increased amounts. Faecal porphyrins are not increased but the abnormal pattern of intermediate porphyrins may be detected by chromatography; this finding is of diagnostic value. It is important not to confuse this disorder with the coproporphyrinuria of liver disease (see below).

Erythropoietic porphyrias

Two rare inherited disorders are associated with the accumulation of porphyrins in erythrocytes. Acute porphyric attacks do not occur and ALA and PBG excretion are normal.

Congenital erythropoietic porphyria

Congenital erythropoietic porphyria is inherited as an *autosomal recessive* characteristic due to uroporphrinogen III synthase deficiency. Usually, blood erythrocyte and plasma uroporphyrin I concentrations are very high from infancy onwards and there is severe photosensitivity. Porphyrins are also deposited in bones and teeth, which fluoresce in ultraviolet light; the teeth may be brownish-pink in colour. Hirsutism, especially of the face, also occurs and there is haemolytic anaemia. Urinary porphyrin concentrations are grossly increased, although faecal porphyrin levels are less so.

Protoporphyria

This is an *autosomal dominantly* inherited disorder due to ferrochelatase deficiency in which protoporphyrin concentrations are increased in erythrocytes and faeces. There is mild photosensitivity, and hepatocellular damage may lead to liver failure.

These two conditions tend to give rise to photosensitivity, whereas there is increased skin fragility in the other porphyrias that involve the skin. The erythropoietic porphyrias can be treated by sunlight avoidance, for example by using skin sunblocks. In porphyria cutanea tarda, venesection may be used to reduce iron stores and oral chloroquine to increase the excretion of porphyrins. Carotene treatment may be useful in erythropoietic porphyria.

Other causes of excessive porphyrin excretion

Porphyria is not the only cause of disordered porphyrin metabolism, and positive screening tests *must be confirmed* by quantitative analysis, with identification of the porphyrin. Other causes must be considered.

Lead poisoning

Lead poisoning inhibits several of the enzymes involved in haem synthesis, including PBG synthase and ferrochelatase, and eventually causes anaemia. The urine contains increased amounts of ALA (an early and sensitive test), and coproporphyrin. Some of the symptoms of lead poisoning, such as abdominal pain and peripheral neuropathy, are similar to those of the acute porphyric attack, and may cause difficulty in diagnosis. However, the excretion of PBG is not usually increased. Zinc protoporphyrin concentration rises with increased lead exposure, although the method of choice for assessing exposure to inorganic lead is blood lead concentration. Other features of lead poisoning include lead staining of the teeth and basophilic stippling of red blood cells.

Liver disease

This may increase urinary coproporphyrin levels, possibly because of decreased biliary excretion. It is probably the commonest cause of porphyrinuria. Occasionally there is mild photosensitivity (in porphyria cutanea tarda, the more severe skin lesions are due to uroporphyrin excess).

Bleeding lesions of upper gastrointestinal tract

These lesions may produce raised levels of faecal porphyrin by degradation of haemoglobin. If there is bleeding from the lower part of the tract, the blood reaches the rectum before there is time for conversion; this may be of help in locating the approximate site of bleeding.

Iron deficiency and sideroblastic anaemia

This may also result in increased concentrations of erythrocyte porphyrins.

Investigation of suspected porphyria

The laboratory should be notified and a check made of which type of samples is required. Porphyrins are relatively stable, but samples must be protected from light. Porphobilinogen rapidly polymerizes to uroporphyrins and consequently a random fresh urine sample is more suitable than a 24-hour collection. All samples should be analysed as soon as possible after collection. Samples should not be sent simply requesting a 'porphyrin screen'; an indication should be given of which type of porphyria is suspected, giving the relevant clinical details, so that the laboratory can select the appropriate tests.

Generally, urine, faeces and blood (both plasma and erythrocytes) are needed for complete analysis. The technique of plasma fluorescence has recently proved useful to distinguish some of the porphyrias (Table 21.3). Specialist laboratories can carry out enzyme assays and genetic tests.

Table 21.3 Major biochemical features of the porphyrias

Porphyria	Urine		Faeces	Red blood cells	Plasma fluorescence (nm)[a]
	PBG	POR			
AIP	+	Copro III	—	—	615
HC	+	Copro III	Copro III	—	615
VP	+	Copro III	Proto IX	—	624–626
PCT	—	Urohepta	Isocopro	—	615
CEP	—	Uro I Copro I	Copro I	Zn-Proto	615
PP	—	—	Proto	Proto	632

PBG = porphobilinogen; POR = porphyrin; AIP = acute intermittent porphyria; HC = hereditary coproporphyria; VP = variegate porphyria; PCT = porphyria cutanea tarda; CEP = congenital erythropoietic porphyria; PP = protoporphyria; Copro = coproporphyrinogen I or III; Proto = protoporphyrinogen; Zn = zinc; Urohepta = uroheptaporphyrinogen; Uro = uroporphyrinogen; Isocopro = isocoproporphyrinogen; + = PBG present; − = PBG absent; [a] plasma fluorescence emission wavelength peak when stimulated at 405 nm.

Suspected acute porphyria

Fresh urine should be tested immediately for PBG using Ehrlich's reagent. If PBG is not present, it is highly unlikely that the patient is suffering from an acute porphyric attack unless he or she has the rare PBG synthase deficiency, in which case ALA concentration would be expected to be raised. A patient with a history of repeated attacks of abdominal pain or neurological symptoms may have acute intermittent porphyria, variegate porphyria or hereditary coproporphyria.

If an acute porphyria is confirmed, the concentration of porphyrins in urine and in a random sample of faeces should be measured. Raised values suggest variegate porphyria (protoporphyrin and coproporphyrin) or hereditary coproporphyria (coproporphyrin). Acute intermittent porphyria does not normally show abnormal faecal porphyrins. The following should be remembered.

Patients with acute intermittent porphyria who have once had an acute attack may continue to excrete increased amounts of PBG for many months. This condition does not show skin lesions, unlike the other acute porphyrias.

Plasma fluorescence may reveal different emission peaks when stimulated at 405 nm, e.g. variegate porphyria may show a peak at 625 nm when stimulated at 405 nm, whereas the other acute porphyrias show a peak at 615 nm.

It is possible to assay enzymes of haem metabolism in red blood cells. For example, decreased PBG deaminase is found in patients with acute intermittent porphyria. There is often overlap in levels between affected and normal people but, within a family, carriers can be shown to have levels about half those of unaffected members. This test may also detect affected children. However, the enzyme activity is related to the mean age of the red blood cells; this assay is not suitable for children under the age of about 9 months or for individuals with haemolytic disorders.

Negative urine and faeces porphyrin tests do not exclude the diagnosis of latent porphyria, and in these cases enzyme and genetic tests may be useful.

Suspected porphyria with skin lesions

Skin lesions may occur in any type of porphyria other than acute intermittent porphyria. Blood, urine and faeces should be sent for testing.

Increased concentrations of erythrocyte porphyrins suggest protoporphyria or congenital erythropoietic porphyria (very rare). High concentrations may also occur in iron deficiency anaemia and lead poisoning.

Increased concentrations of urinary porphyrins suggest porphyria cutanea tarda or congenital erythropoietic porphyria. The increased uroporphyrin excretion in these conditions must be distinguished from the coproporphyrinuria of liver disease.

Increased concentrations of faecal porphyrins occur in protoporphyria, variegate porphyria and hereditary coproporphyria. These may be distinguished by chromatographic separation of porphyrins; this will also demonstrate the abnormal pattern of porphyria cutanea tarda.

Protoporphyria shows a unique plasma fluorescence emission peak of 632 nm when stimulated at 405 nm.

Enzyme and genetic tests may be useful.

Investigation of family members

If one of the porphyrias is diagnosed, it is essential to investigate blood relatives. Those found to have the condition must be counselled regarding the medications that may precipitate an attack.

Carriers of variegate porphyria and hereditary coproporphyria may be identified after puberty by the demonstration of clearly increased faecal porphyrin excretion. Normal excretion before puberty does not exclude the diagnosis.

Some of the porphyrias may be diagnosed by enzyme determination, for example acute intermittent porphyria is detected by measuring red cell PBG deaminase activity.

Genetic studies are now possible by specialist laboratories to investigate the porphyrias.

CONCLUSIONS

- Haemoglobin contains most (70 per cent) of the body's iron. Iron is mandatory for normal haemopoiesis.
- Ferritin is an intracellular iron-binding protein. Iron is also absorbed in the small intestine and bound to transferrin within the circulation. It is stored bound to ferritin.
- Iron deficiency is common and blood loss needs to be excluded. A low plasma ferritin concentration suggests iron deficiency.
- Unbound iron is toxic to the body. Haemochromatosis is a genetic condition of chronic iron overload. This is associated with liver disease, diabetes mellitus, skin pigmentation, cardiac and endocrine problems.
- The haem moiety of haemoglobin contains tetrapyrrole rings synthesized from porphyrinogen precursors. Disorders of the haem synthetic pathways can lead to porphyria. Most of the porphyrias are autosomal dominant.
- The porphyrias can be divided into (a) the acute group, which can present with acute abdomen, neuropsychiatric symptoms and hypertension, and (b) cutaneous (non-acute) forms that may present with skin symptoms.

22 CARDIOVASCULAR DISEASE

Myocardial infarction	323	D-dimers and deep vein thrombosis	326
Cardiac failure and natriuretic peptides	326	Cardiovascular risk factors	326

The clinical biochemistry laboratory often plays a central role in the diagnosis and management of acute myocardial infarction. A number of cardiovascular risk factors have been described, some of which can be assayed in the biochemistry laboratory, and these are discussed in this chapter.

MYOCARDIAL INFARCTION

One of the largest killers in Western urbanized societies is acute myocardial infarction. Its diagnosis is usually made on the clinical presentation and electrocardiographic findings and confirmed by the characteristic changes in plasma enzyme activities or troponin levels. The American College of Cardiology and the European Society of Cardiology have defined acute myocardial infarction as a typical rise and fall of biochemical marker, for example plasma creatine kinase isoenzyme MB (CK-MB) or troponin, with at least one of the following: ischaemic symptoms, new pathological Q waves on electrocardiogram (ECG), ischaemic ECG changes (ST depression or elevation) and coronary artery intervention. This classification also recognizes that patients previously classified as having unstable angina or minor myocardial injury are now reclassified as having non-ST segment elevation myocardial infarction (NSTEMI).

It is useful to note that acute myocardial infarction and NSTEMI have a common pathophysiological pathway, namely acute coronary artery plaque rupture followed by a series of events resulting in thrombosis formation. The outcome is dependent on the state of the collateral circulation and the severity of artery occlusion. In other words, clinically we no longer think in terms of the presence or absence of an acute myocardial infarction, but instead of a spectrum of disease ranging from angina pectoris through to acute myocardial infarction; this stratification is based upon cardiac markers reflecting ischaemic damage.

It is also particularly important to diagnose acute myocardial infarction promptly, as thrombolytic therapy may be indicated to try to dissolve the thrombus in situ. The earlier this therapy is given, the better the prognosis, as 'minutes are myocardium'. Thus, biochemical markers need to be specific, sensitive and change rapidly to optimize the diagnosis and treatment of acute myocardial infarction.

Cardiac enzymes

The plasma enzyme estimation of greatest value is that of CK (see Chapter 18), although this has been largely superseded by the assay of cardiac troponins. At one time, the enzymes lactate dehydrogenase (LDH) or hydroxybutyrate dehydrogenase (HBD) and aspartate aminotransferase (AST) were used diagnostically, although they are now rarely assayed in the diagnosis of acute myocardial infarction or NSTEMI.

An approximate guide to the sequence of changes after acute myocardial infarction is given in Table 22.1 (see also Fig. 22.1).

All plasma enzyme activities (including that of CK-MB) may be normal until at least 4 hours after the onset of chest pain due to a myocardial infarction; *blood should not be taken for enzyme assay until this time has elapsed*. If the initial plasma CK activity is normal, a second sample should be taken about 4–6 hours later. A rise in the plasma CK activity supports the diagnosis of an infarction. The simultaneous measurement of plasma CK-MB activity, which is

Table 22.1 The time sequence of changes in plasma cardiac markers after acute myocardial infarction

Cardiac marker	Starts to rise (hours)	Time after infarction for peak rise (hours)	Duration of rise (days)
CK (total)	4–6	24–48	3–5
AST	6–8	24–48	4–6
LDH/HBD	12–24	48–72	7–12
Myoglobin	2–4	12–24	2–4
Troponin	4–6	12–24	7–10

CK = creatine kinase; AST = aspartate transaminase; LDH = lactate dehydrogenase; HBD = hydroxybutyrate dehydrogenase.

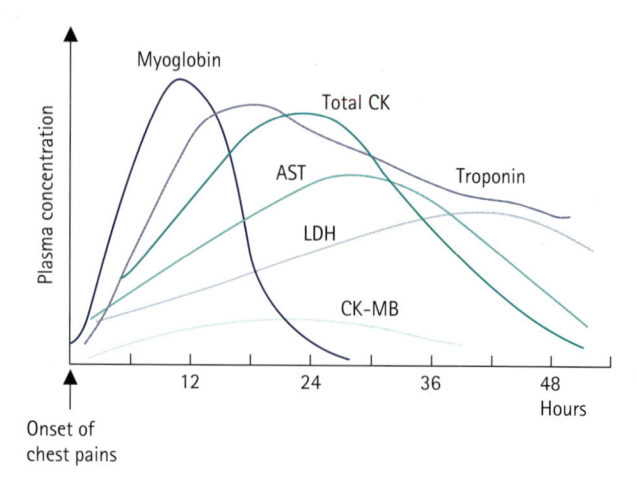

Fig. 22.1 Plasma cardiac markers post-acute myocardial infarction. (CK = creatine kinase; AST = aspartate transaminase; LDH = lactate dehydrogenase.) (Reproduced with kind permission from Candlish JK and Crook M, *Notes on Clinical Biochemistry*, Singapore: World Scientific Publishing, 1993.)

shown to exceed about 5 per cent of the total CK activity, may occasionally help in early diagnosis; a raised plasma CK-MB activity or concentration alone is not diagnostic of an infarction.

Most of the CK released after a myocardial infarction is, in fact, the MM isoenzyme (CK-MM), which is found in both skeletal and myocardial muscle and has a longer half-life than the MB fraction. After about 24 hours, the finding of a high MM and undetectable MB does not exclude myocardial damage as a cause of high total CK activities; by this time the plasma HBD activity is usually raised.

A raised plasma total CK activity, due entirely to CK-MM, may follow recent intramuscular injection, exercise or surgery. Plasma enzyme activities are raised in about 95 per cent of cases of myocardial infarction and are sometimes very high. The degree of rise is a crude indicator of the size of the myocardial infarct, but is of limited prognostic value. The prognosis often depends more on the site than on the size of the infarct. A second rise of plasma enzyme activities after their return to normal may indicate extension of the damage. A prolonged rise in plasma CK may suggest a cardiac ventricular aneurysm. These plasma enzyme activities do not usually rise significantly after an episode of angina pectoris without infarction, but troponins may do.

The sequence of changes in plasma AST activity after myocardial infarction are similar to those of CK (see Table

---

CASE 1

A 46-year-old male was admitted late at night (23.30 hours) to casualty by ambulance because of a tight central chest pain that had started at 03.00 hours the morning before. He had delayed calling for medical assistance because he thought it was only indigestion. In the ambulance, the paramedics gave him an intramuscular injection of diamorphine for pain relief. The ECG was normal.

Plasma
- Creatine kinase 565 U/L (<250)
- Troponin T 0.01 μg/L (<0.1)

DISCUSSION

The normal plasma troponin T makes a diagnosis of acute myocardial infarction unlikely, as this would be expected to be elevated in view of when the chest pain started. The elevated plasma CK concentration is not specific for cardiac damage and may have been raised as a result of muscle damage secondary to the intramuscular injection: beware of interpreting elevated plasma CK concentrations in the presence of intramuscular injections. A CK-MB concentration would be less likely than total CK concentration to be elevated in skeletal muscle damage, as CK-MB is predominantly cardiac in origin.

22.1), although it rises significantly less with respect to the upper reference limit. Even a small myocardial infarct does cause some hepatic congestion due to right-sided heart dysfunction, and this may contribute to the rise of plasma AST activity. This is rarely a diagnostic problem because the increase in plasma AST activity following an infarction is usually much greater. If there is primary hepatic dysfunction, congestive cardiac failure without infarction or pulmonary embolism (which, by impairing pulmonary blood flow, usually causes some hepatic congestion), plasma AST rises whereas LDH1 (HBD), but not total LDH, activity usually remains normal.

Many laboratory assays rely on measuring the enzyme activity of CK. However, it has been suggested that greater diagnostic accuracy may be obtained by measuring CK-MB mass by immunological assays instead of assaying the activity of the enzyme, although these assays may be more expensive and may be less readily available than activity measurements.

Creatine kinase-MB also exists as two isoforms, namely CK-MB1 and CK-MB2. The latter is predominantly released from the myocardium. Creatine kinase-MB that is routinely assayed reflects the sum of the two isoforms. Normally CK-MB1 predominates in plasma, but after an acute myocardial infarction this is reversed. The assay for CK-MB isoforms is, however, complicated and requires specialized technology.

Myoglobin

As mentioned in Chapter 21, myoglobin is a low-molecular-weight haem-containing protein found in both skeletal and cardiac muscle. Due to its low molecular weight, it is rapidly released from the myocardium upon damage, and a typical rise occurs within 2–4 hours after the onset of acute myocardial infarction. This is useful for the early diagnosis of acute myocardial infarction, as this rise is generally earlier than that of the other presently used cardiac markers. Unfortunately, myoglobin is not cardiac specific, being also found in skeletal muscle, and thus is less useful in the diagnosis of acute myocardial infarction unless used in conjunction with other markers.

Troponins

Troponins are muscle-regulatory proteins present in skeletal and cardiac muscle. Three troponins have been reported, namely troponin C (TnC), troponin I (TnI) and troponin T (TnT). There are no structural differences between cardiac and skeletal muscle TnC. However, the cardiac and skeletal forms of TnI and TnT are structurally different and can be distinguished by immunological assays.

Troponin I and TnT appear in the plasma 4–8 hours after symptoms of acute myocardial infarction, and are best measured 12 hours after the start of chest pain. They are therefore not early markers of acute myocardial infarction, but they do stay elevated for about 7–10 days in plasma, which makes them useful in the late presentation of chest pain.

Troponin T may be elevated in patients with chronic renal failure and thus may not be so cardio-specific. However, TnI can be extensively modified by proteolysis after release into the plasma. This means that measurements may give varying results as different antigenic epitopes are revealed, depending upon the commercial supplier of the assay. At present, there is no universal agreement as to which troponin assay, i.e. TnI or TnT, is best.

An increased TnI or TnT concentration is a sensitive marker of occult myocardial damage even in non-ischaemic conditions. Plasma troponin concentrations are increased in subarachnoid haemorrhage (due to vasoactive peptide release affecting the myocardium), hypertension, tachy-arrhythmias, cardiac surgery, sepsis, congestive cardiac failure, pulmonary embolism and hypothyroidism.

Research has shown that troponins allow a subset of patients with rest-unstable angina to be classified despite normal plasma CK-MB concentrations. Those with raised plasma cardiac troponin concentrations were more likely to have an acute myocardial infarction or die within 6 months of the event. In other words, troponins allow risk stratification of patients with acute coronary syndrome. In another study it was found that, unlike CK-MB, cardiac troponins have prognostic value after coronary thrombolysis therapy, with troponin concentrations on admission correlating with 6-week mortality. Low-molecular-weight heparin or platelet-receptor blockers (glycoprotein GIIB/IIIA inhibitors) reduce cardiac events in non-Q-wave coronary syndromes with raised concentrations of cardiac troponins compared with those without troponin concentration elevation.

In view of these findings, cardiac troponins have been recommended as the biochemical cardiac marker of choice. However, sometimes a panel of cardiac markers may be useful in making the diagnosis of acute myocardial infarction, for example myoglobin rises early, thus alerting the clinician to possible cardiac problems, whilst the later rise of troponin allows greater specificity. A new marker, ischaemia-modified albumin, is raised in the presence of myocardial ischaemia and may be used in the future in conjunction with conventional cardiac markers.

> ## CASE 2
>
> A 66-year-old male was sent by his GP to casualty because of tight chest pain that had occurred 3 days previously. The pain had largely resolved after 6 hours, but he was left feeling weak and breathless, which worsened over a few days, causing him eventually to seek medical attention. The following laboratory test results were found.
>
> *Plasma*
> - Creatine kinase 235 U/L (<250)
> - Troponin T 0.13 μg/L (<0.1)
>
> An ECG showed changes suggestive of a myocardial infarction in the lateral leads V4–V6.
>
> ### DISCUSSION
> The plasma CK activity has returned to normal because of the time delay since myocardial infarction, whilst the plasma troponin T concentration still remains elevated. Plasma CK usually starts to rise 4–6 hours after a myocardial infarction and to normalize at about 3–5 days. Conversely, plasma troponin T starts to rise at 4–6 hours post-infarct and remains elevated for as long as about 10 days. Troponins are thus useful cardiac markers in both the early hours and a few days later.

CARDIAC FAILURE AND NATRIURETIC PEPTIDES

Chronic heart failure can be defined as a clinical condition associated with symptoms and signs of left or right ventricular dysfunction. The diagnosis is often made clinically on the basis of the presence of dyspnoea, fatigue, signs of fluid overload, for example pulmonary crepitations, peripheral oedema and raised jugular venous pressure. However, sometimes the diagnosis can be difficult, and further investigations are necessary. Echocardiography requires experienced personnel and can measure cardiac ejection fraction, which may be reduced in chronic heart failure.

There are three major natriuretic peptides (NPs), namely atrial natriuretic peptide (ANP), brain natriuretic peptide (BNP) and C-type natriuretic peptide (CNP). Atrial natriuretic peptide is produced in the atria and is released upon increased atrial wall tension, such as occurs with increased intravascular volume. Brain natriuretic peptide is found in brain and cardiac ventricles and its concentration is increased in the plasma in cardiac failure and ventricular hypertrophy. C-type natriuretic peptide exists in a number of tissues, including the brain, kidney and endothelial cells. There are also NP receptors: the A-type receptors bind ANP and BNP; the B type binds CNP; and the C receptor binds all NPs and is involved in their clearance. Both ANP and BNP produce natriuresis (see Chapter 2) and increase venous capacitance as well as reducing extracellular fluid volume; CNP is a potent vasodilator and probably has a more local tissue action rather than working as a cardiac hormone.

It has been suggested that plasma BNP may be a useful marker of cardiac failure, as a normal plasma concentration virtually rules out the condition. Also, plasma BNP has prognostic value in patients with cardiac failure, with those with the highest levels having a greater mortality and morbidity. Plasma BNP is a marker of both right and left ventricular dysfunction.

D-DIMERS AND DEEP VEIN THROMBOSIS

The diagnosis of deep vein thrombosis (DVT), for example in leg or pelvic veins, can be difficult clinically, but it is important not to miss this condition as it may lead to a fatal pulmonary embolus. D-dimers are released into the plasma upon thrombosis formation when fibrinogen is converted to fibrin. A raised plasma fibrinogen concentration is a risk factor for cardiovascular disease. Raised plasma D-dimer concentration is, therefore, a useful marker of the presence of a thrombus and a useful tool in the diagnosis of a DVT. A raised plasma D-dimer concentration may lead the clinician to request ultrasound or other imaging techniques to look for a DVT or pulmonary embolus.

CARDIOVASCULAR RISK FACTORS
(Table 22.2)

Cardiovascular disease, including coronary heart disease and myocardial infarction, is responsible for the major

Table 22.2 Some major cardiovascular risk factors

Non-modifiable	Modifiable
Age	Hypercholesterolaemia
Sex	Hypertriglyceridaemia
Family history	Low plasma HDL cholesterol
Ethnicity	Smoking
	Hypertension
	Obesity
	Diabetes mellitus
	Insulin resistance
	Raised plasma fibrinogen
	Plasma lipoprotein (a)
	Plasma homocysteine
	Plasma hs-CRP

HDL = high-density lipoprotein; hs-CRP = high-sensitivity C-reactive protein.

burden of mortality in urbanized societies and is commoner in males, the elderly and those with a positive family history of premature coronary heart disease (for example below the age of 60 years). In addition, certain ethnic groups are more at risk of coronary heart disease, such as some South Asian groups.

There are probably at least 200 cardiovascular risk factors, although the major ones are abnormal lipids (high plasma cholesterol and triglycerides and low high-density lipoprotein [HDL] cholesterol), hypertension, smoking, diabetes mellitus, obesity and a family history of cardiovascular disease. These constitute the so-called 'classic' risk factors.

Homocysteine

Various recent studies have shown other cardiovascular risk factors, one of which is homocysteine, a sulphur-containing amino acid. It has been known for a while now that patients with homocystinuria, who have a deficiency of cystathionine β-synthase (an autosomal recessive condition with an incidence of 1:200 000), have a thrombotic tendency (see Chapters 15 and 27). This has led researchers to look at the part homocysteine may play in cardiovascular disease. There is an association between raised plasma homocysteine concentrations and cardiovascular disease, in that individuals with concentrations in the upper part of the reference range have an increased cardiovascular risk.

Homocysteine is derived from methionine by demethylation. It can also be metabolized to cysteine by transulphuration, or remethylated using betaine or methyltetrahydrofolate. Thus elevated plasma homocysteine can be due to deficiencies of vitamin B_{12}, folate or vitamin B_6. There is also evidence that a mutation of the methylene tetrahydrofolate reductase (*MTHFR*) gene (single base-pair substitution C677T) results in elevated plasma homocysteine levels (see Chapter 15).

Plasma homocysteine concentrations above 10 μmol/L confer increased cardiovascular risk. Concentrations of homocysteine increase with age, impaired renal function, hypothyroidism, psoriasis and certain drugs such as methotrexate, theophylline and L-dopa.

Treatment with folate and/or vitamin B_{12} and B_6 can lower plasma homocysteine levels and thus may reduce cardiovascular risk.

C-reactive protein

Research has shown that atherosclerosis involves inflammatory processes. Macrophages, monocytes and T lymphocytes are found in the atheromatous plaques, as are raised concentrations of cytokines with acute-phase reactants. Cytokines such as interleukin-6 (IL-6) increase the hepatic synthesis of acute-phase proteins, including C-reactive protein (CRP, see Chapter 19).

Plasma CRP concentration may reflect the likelihood of the atheromatous plaque rupturing. High-sensitivity CRP assays (hs-CRP) have recently been developed, and a positive association between future coronary events and plasma hs-CRP concentration has been found. Plasma hs-CRP may also have prognostic value in patients with acute coronary syndrome, with those with an hs-CRP of more than 3 mg/L at onset being more likely to suffer acute myocardial infarction or cardiovascular death. Desirable values are less than 1 mg/L, with those at intermediate cardiovascular risk having values 1–3 mg/L. In terms of cardiovascular risk event prediction, plasma hs-CRP may be stronger than the plasma total cholesterol:HDL ratio.

Hypertension

Hypertension can be defined as sustained systolic blood pressure of more than 140 mmHg and/or diastolic blood pressure more than 90 mmHg. It is a major risk factor for coronary heart disease and stroke. In most cases the cause is unknown and it is called essential hypertension. There are many causes of hypertension, including obesity, steroid use, insulin resistance and high alcohol intake. Rarer secondary causes include renal disease such as polycystic disease, scleroderma, pyelonephritis and renal artery stenosis (Table 22.3). Endocrine causes include phaeochromocytoma, Cushing's syndrome, Conn's syndrome, acromegaly

Table 22.3 Some secondary causes of hypertension and initial biochemical investigations that may be useful

Cause	Initial biochemical investigation
Diabetes mellitus/insulin resistance	Plasma glucose
Renal disease	Plasma urea or creatinine; urine for protein, blood and casts
Primary hyperaldosteronism	Plasma potassium and aldosterone:renin ratio, urine potassium
Cushing's syndrome	24-hour urinary free cortisol, dexamathasone suppression test
Primary hyperparathyroidism	Plasma 'corrected' calcium, phosphate and PTH
Acromegaly	Plasma IGF-1, oral glucose tolerance test (GH suppression)
Phaeochromocytoma	24-hour urinary catecholamines or HMMA (VMA)
Renal artery stenosis	Plasma urea, creatinine, potassium and aldosterone and renin
Liddle's or Gordon's syndrome	Plasma urea, creatinine, potassium and aldosterone and renin

PTH = parathyroid hormone; IGF = insulin-like growth factor; GH = growth hormone; HMMA = 4-hydroxy-3-methoxymandelic acid; VMA = vanillyl mandelic acid.

and hyperparathyroidism. Also consider aortic coarctation and, if the patient is pregnant, pre-eclampsia.

Clinical biochemistry tests have an important part to play in the management of hypertension. First, they have a role in diagnosis. The biochemical investigation of hyperparathyroidism, acromegaly, Cushing's syndrome, primary hyperaldosteronism (Conn's syndrome) and phaeochromocytoma, and of other rare conditions such as Liddle's syndrome and Gordon's syndrome, which may present with hypokalaemia or hyperkalaemia respectively, are covered in other chapters of this book.

Biochemical testing also has a role in assessing renal function (see Chapter 3) and in monitoring anti-hypertensive therapy. Hypokalaemia can develop in patients treated with thiazide diuretics (non-potassium sparing), as can hyperuricaemia, hypercalcaemia, hyperglycaemia and hyponatraemia.

Angiotensin-converting enzyme inhibitors and angiotensin receptor antagonists (ARAs) are also used to treat hypertension and may cause hyperkalemia and a rise in plasma creatinine, particularly in patients with renal artery stenosis. In renal artery stenosis, glomerular filtration is maintained by angiotensin II and these drugs can thus reduce the glomerular filtration rate, with a concomitant impairment in renal function, for example a 10–20 per cent rise in plasma creatinine may occur. It is for this reason that renal function should be closely monitored within days of initiating an angiotensin-converting enzyme inhibitor or ARA and after an increase in dose. Plasma renin concentration is usually raised in renal artery stenosis.

CONCLUSIONS

- Cardiovascular disease is one of the world's biggest killers. It has many risk factors, which can be divided into those that are modifiable and those that are not. Of the former, the major contributors are smoking, diabetes mellitus, abnormal lipids, hypertension and obesity.
- The diagnosis of acute myocardial infarction can be difficult, but it is important to make a prompt diagnosis, as thrombolysis needs to be given early. Biochemical tests have an important role in this respect. Plasma CK can be used, and exists as three major isoenzymes (BB, MB and MM). Total plasma CK lacks cardiac specificity and the CK-MB isoenzyme is more specific and either its activity or its mass amount can be assayed.
- The troponins are more specific cardiac markers than CK. Also, plasma troponin stays elevated for longer than CK after an infarct. Troponins are therefore useful for the late diagnosis of myocardial infarction.
- Plasma myoglobin becomes elevated within about 2–4 hours of myocardial infarction but is not specific for cardiac damage, as it is also found in skeletal muscle.
- Plasma natriuretic peptides may be elevated in ventricular dysfunction and are therefore useful in the diagnosis of cardiac failure.
- Biochemistry investigations may be useful in the management and investigation of hypertension.

23 CEREBROSPINAL AND PLEURAL FLUID

| Cerebrospinal fluid | 329 | Pleural fluid | 333 |

This chapter looks at two important biological fluids, namely cerebrospinal fluid (CSF) and pleural fluid, and how their biochemical analysis can be useful clinically.

CEREBROSPINAL FLUID

In adults, the total volume of CSF is about 135 mL, produced at a rate of 500 mL/day. This is predominantly formed by plasma ultrafiltration through the capillary walls of the choroid plexuses in the brain's lateral ventricles. These plexuses also actively secrete small amounts of substances such as chloride.

The fluid passes from the lateral, through the third and fourth ventricles, into the subarachnoid space between the pia and subarachnoid mater, from where much is reabsorbed into the circulation by arachnoid villi. The remaining fluid flows through the subarachnoid space, completely surrounding the brain and spinal cord; thus it supports and protects these structures against injury. Like lymph, CSF removes waste products of metabolism.

Cerebrospinal fluid circulates very slowly, allowing contact with cells of the central nervous system (CNS). The uptake of glucose by these cells probably results in lower concentrations relative to plasma. Concentrations of analytes in the CSF should always be compared with those in plasma because alterations in the latter are reflected in the CSF even when CNS metabolism is normal.

Flow is slowest, and therefore contact is longest, in the lower lumbar region, where the subarachnoid space comes to an end; therefore, the composition of CSF from lumbar puncture is different from that of cisternal or ventricular puncture.

Examination of the cerebrospinal fluid

Although biochemical investigation of the CSF is important, so is microbiological and cytological examination. Textbooks of microbiology and cytology should be consulted for further diagnostic details if required.

Sample collection

Cerebrospinal fluid is usually collected by lumbar puncture. This procedure may be dangerous if the intracranial pressure is raised, and the clinician should therefore check that there is no papilloedema before proceeding; sometimes brain imaging, for example computerized tomography (CT) scanning, may be indicated. Small-bore needles may reduce the risk of post-lumbar puncture headache.

Usually a total of about 5 mL of CSF should be collected as 1–2 mL aliquots into sterile containers and sent first for microbiological examinations; if necessary, any remaining specimen can then be used for biochemical analysis. If a CSF glucose concentration is indicated, 0.5 mL should be collected into a fluoride tube and promptly sent to the laboratory with a blood sample taken at the same time. The CSF is potentially highly infectious and must be handled and transported with care.

Appearance

Normal CSF is completely clear and colourless; slight turbidity is most easily detected by visual comparison with water.

> ### CASE 1
>
> A 17-year-old female student was admitted to hospital with fever, neck stiffness, headache, photophobia and a purpuric rash. She had the following CSF laboratory results.
>
> CSF glucose 2.0 mmol/L (concomitant plasma glucose 5.6 mmol/L)
> CSF protein 0.98 g/L (<0.4 g/L)
>
> Cerebrospinal fluid microscopy showed elevated leucocytes, and Gram staining showed Gram-negative *Meningococcus*.
>
> #### DISCUSSION
>
> A lumbar puncture to obtain CSF is potentially a dangerous, invasive investigation. It carries the risk of cerebral herniation, bleeding and infection. In this case, meningitis was suspected, which was confirmed by the CSF results. Note the raised protein and low glucose concentrations relative to plasma due to bacteria. The presence of bacteria is confirmed by microscopy. *Meningococcus* can rapidly cause death and is associated with massive haemorrhagic adrenal destruction, as in Waterhouse–Friderichsen syndrome.

Spontaneous clotting

Clotting occurs when there is excess fibrinogen in the specimen, usually associated with a very high protein concentration. This finding occurs with tuberculous meningitis or with tumours of the CNS.

Colour

A *bright red colour* may result from damage to a blood vessel during lumbar puncture (traumatic tap) or a recent haemorrhage into the subarachnoid space.

If CSF is collected as three separate aliquots, blood staining will be progressively less in the aliquots if bleeding is due to the lumbar puncture itself, whereas all aliquots would be expected to be bloody if there was a subarachnoid bleed.

Xanthochromia is defined as a *yellow* coloration of the CSF and results from altered haemoglobin, the colour appearing several days after a subarachnoid haemorrhage and, depending on the extent of the bleeding, lasting for up to a week or more or jaundice (which will be clinically obvious and may impart a yellow colour to the CSF).

Visual appraisal of CSF is not sufficiently sensitive to detect subtle degrees of xanthochromia for the diagnosis of subarachnoid haemorrhage. In such cases spectrophotometric examination of CSF is important. Spectrophotometric analysis may reveal an oxyhaemoglobin absorption peak of 413–415 nm; bilirubin shows an additional peak at 450–460 nm. This test is particularly useful in patients with subarachnoid haemorrhage who have a negative brain CT scan. The presence of methaemoglobin or bilirubin is strongly suggestive of a subarachnoid haemorrhage, as oxyhaemoglobin alone is not necessarily confirmatory because it may simply reflect a 'bloody' CSF tap.

Turbidity

Turbidity is usually due to infection or high CSF protein content. It may also occur after haemorrhage.

Biochemical estimations

The following are the most commonly requested CSF biochemical tests.

Glucose

The CSF glucose concentration is slightly lower than that in plasma and, under normal circumstances, is rarely less than 50 per cent of the plasma concentration. Provided that CSF for glucose assay has been preserved with fluoride, an abnormally low glucose concentration occurs in the following.

- *Hypoglycaemia*: the CSF glucose concentration parallels that of plasma, although there is a delay before changes in plasma glucose concentrations are reflected in the CSF. Hypoglycaemia may cause coma and low CSF glucose concentrations in the absence of any primary cerebral abnormality (see Chapter 12). *Both plasma and CSF concentrations must be measured.*
- *Infection*: if there is an increased polymorphonuclear leucocyte count or a bacterial infection, the CSF glucose concentration may be very low because of increased metabolism of glucose. The CSF glucose concentration may be particularly low in pyogenic meningitis and tuberculous meningitis; in viral meningitis, it is often normal. The estimation of CSF glucose does not reliably distinguish between different forms of infective meningitis because the result may be normal in any form.

- *Widespread malignant infiltration of the meninges* may also be associated with low CSF glucose concentrations.

Protein

The CSF protein concentration in the lumbar spine is up to three times higher than that in the ventricles; the normal lumbar concentration is below 0.4 g/L. In newborn infants, because of the relatively high vascular permeability, the CSF protein concentration is about three times that of the adult.

Changes in concentration of, for example, immunoglobulin G (IgG) do not necessarily indicate cerebral disease, but may simply reflect changes in plasma (normally 80 per cent of total CSF protein has transferred across from the plasma). Therefore the results of assays can only be interpreted if those of the two fluids are compared.

Cerebral disease may change the total concentration of CSF protein and the proportions of its constituents, for two reasons.

- The vascular and meningeal permeabilities can increase, allowing more protein to enter the CSF.
- Proteins (immunoglobulins) may be synthesized within the cerebrospinal canal by inflammatory or other invading cells.

Measurement of total CSF protein concentration

Measurement of CSF total protein is a relatively insensitive test for the diagnosis of cerebral disease, because early changes in the concentration of a specific protein do not always cause a detectable rise in the total protein concentration.

The CSF total protein concentration may be increased in the following situations.

- *In the presence of blood*, due to haemoglobin and plasma proteins.
- *In the presence of pus*, due to cell protein and to exudation from inflamed surfaces.
- *In non-purulent inflammation of cerebral tissue*, when there may be a definite rise in total protein concentration despite the absence of detectable cells in the CSF. Cells may also be undetectable in some cases of bacterial meningitis, particularly in children, in immunocompromised patients, or if antibiotics have been given before lumbar puncture.
- *If there is blockage of the spinal canal* which, by impairing the flow of CSF distal to the block, allows longer for equilibrium with the circulation and so brings the composition of CSF slightly nearer to that of plasma (Froin's syndrome). Increased pressure in the CSF may also increase protein. Such blockage may be caused by:
  - spinal tumours,
  - vertebral fractures,
  - spinal tuberculosis.
- *Where there is local synthesis of immunoglobulins* by plasma cells within the CSF.

Measurement of individual CSF protein concentrations

In the presence of blood or pus, tests for individual CSF proteins are not useful and may even be misleading. They may, however, detect abnormalities when the total protein concentration is equivocally raised or normal, and may help to elucidate the cause of a high concentration.

Increased capillary permeability, with a similar increase in the permeability of the blood–brain barrier, may be demonstrated by finding relatively high-molecular-weight proteins not normally present in CSF. This non-specific pattern is associated with a large number of inflammatory conditions, but may sometimes facilitate diagnosis. Such a pattern may be due to:

- infections,
- cerebral tumours,
- acute idiopathic polyneuropathy (Guillain–Barré syndrome), in which acute-phase proteins and immunoglobulins may also be synthesized locally.

Abnormal CSF protein synthesis

The identification of immunoglobulins synthesized within the CSF, particularly IgG and IgA, may help with the diagnosis of multiple sclerosis or other demyelinating disorders. Abnormal immunoglobulin synthesis may be detected by the following.

- The finding of a characteristic electrophoretic pattern with multiple ('oligoclonal') bands in the γ-globulin region. *Oligoclonal bands only signify cerebral disease if they are found in the CSF and not in the serum.* Although such bands can be detected in more than 90 per cent of patients with multiple sclerosis, the finding is not specific for this condition. Occasionally, intrathecal malignant B lymphocytes produce a local monoclonal band.
- Comparison of the IgG and albumin CSF:plasma ratio. Albumin has a lower molecular weight than IgG and its concentration increases disproportionately in CSF if increased vascular permeability due to

inflammation is the cause of the high protein concentration. In this case the CSF:plasma ratio of IgG to albumin will be low or, if permeability is so increased that the two proteins diffuse at almost the same rate, normal. In conditions such as multiple sclerosis in which IgG has been synthesized within the CSF, the ratio is high. This method is less sensitive than the detection of oligoclonal bands (see Chapter 19).

Increased CSF immunoglobulin synthesis, with oligoclonal bands, may be found in:

- multiple sclerosis (the most important indication for the test),
- viral infections:
  - meningitis,
  - encephalitis,
  - subacute sclerosing panencephalitis,
- prion disease, for example Creutzfeldt–Jakob disease,
- bacterial meningitis,
- tuberculosis,
- neurosyphilis,
- acute idiopathic polyneuropathy (Guillain–Barré syndrome),
- systemic lupus erythematosus,
- cerebral sarcoidosis,
- cerebral tumours (rarely).

Tau protein

As in any ultrafiltrate, the concentration of high-molecular-weight CSF proteins is very much lower than in plasma. Also, electrophoresis shows that the proportions of individual proteins are slightly different in CSF compared with those in serum. For example, in the CSF, the concentration of prealbumin is higher and of γ-globulin lower relative to other proteins than in plasma. The tau protein, detectable in the β–γ region in CSF, is a variant of transferrin (asialotransferrin), which cannot be absorbed as the ultrafiltrate passes through the choroid plexus; this modified form cannot be reabsorbed into the circulation and therefore is not found in plasma.

In plasma, the asialotransferrin concentration is very low, as desialylated glycoproteins are rapidly removed from the circulation by the hepatic asialoglycoprotein receptor. A nasal secretion (rhinorrhoea) containing tau protein is suggestive of the source being CSF, as normal nasal secretions do not contain tau protein.

Other CSF analytes

C-reactive protein and lactate have also been used in certain circumstances to indicate bacterial infection. However, these tests are not specific, as both can be elevated in other conditions. Microbiological tests are often more useful if infection is suspected.

Procedure for examination of the CSF

Consider the following.

- Heavily bloodstained (assuming a non-traumatic lumbar puncture) in three consecutive specimens: there has probably been a cerebral haemorrhage.
- Send for microbiological examination and for estimation for glucose and protein concentrations.
- Xanthochromic: in addition to the above tests, send the specimen for spectrophotometric examination.
- If indicated, intrathecal immunoglobulin synthesis may be confirmed, either using the CSF:plasma ratio of IgG to albumin or by the detection of multiple (oligoclonal) bands in the CSF.

CASE 2

A 43-year-old male attended the ear, nose and throat (ENT) department because of a nasal discharge. He had had surgery 3 years previously following a head injury. Although he had initially been treated as having allergic rhinitis, the ENT consultant sent some of the nasal fluid to the clinical biochemistry laboratory for tau protein analysis. The results returned showed the presence of tau protein in his nasal fluid.

DISCUSSION
Nasal fluid should not normally contain tau (or desialylated transferrin) protein, as this is usually found in CSF. Therefore the findings suggest that the nasal discharge contained CSF. The previous head injury had resulted in a dura tear, allowing CSF to leak from the nose.

PLEURAL FLUID

This is a plasma ultrafiltrate; there is usually less than 10 mL of this fluid in each pleural cavity. If the rate of removal is less than the rate of formation, pleural fluid will accumulate. Decreased removal may be due to decreased pleural space pressure (for example bronchial obstruction) or impaired lymphatic drainage (for example neoplasms). Pleural fluid production is increased if there is decreased colloid osmotic pressure (for example hypoproteinaemia), increased capillary vessel permeability (for example infection) or hydrostatic pressure elevation (as in cardiac failure).

Pleural effusion fluid can be divided into exudates and transudates (Box 23.1).

Pleural fluid is often 'tapped' with a needle (thoracentesis) and samples sent to the laboratory for analysis. A pleural fluid protein concentration of greater than 30 g/L is suggestive of an exudate. Raised lactate dehydrogenase (LDH) activity in pleural fluid is indicative of a malignancy or inflammatory process and is more in keeping with an exudate.

Light and colleagues used these observations to devise Light's criteria for the identification of exudates, for which both pleural and plasma analyses for protein and LDH are needed.

A pleural fluid is defined as an exudate if any one of the following three conditions is satisfied:

- pleural fluid LDH more than 200 U/L,
- pleural fluid:plasma protein ratio more than 0.5,
- pleural fluid:plasma LDH ratio more than 0.6.

Other biochemical tests (in addition to microbiological tests and cytology) on pleural fluid may include the following.

- Amylase concentration may be raised in pleural effusions secondary to acute pancreatitis, although other causes include some malignant effusions and oesophageal rupture.
- A raised pleural triglyceride concentration, in comparison to plasma, particularly if greater than 1.5 mmol/L, is suggestive of chylothorax. This occurs when lymph or chyle leaks from the thoracic duct into the pleural space.
- A low pleural fluid glucose concentration, below 1.2 mmol/L, may be found in effusions due to rheumatoid arthritis, although this may also be seen with bacterial infections.
- Tumour markers such as CEA, CA-125, CA-15-3 and CA-19-9 may sometimes be used to help diagnose malignant pleural effusions. However, cytological examination may be more useful.
- Adenosine deaminase is released from activated lymphocytes. A raised pleural fluid adenosine deaminase activity is suggestive of tuberculosis. This test is useful if organisms cannot be cultured.

Box 23.1 Some causes of a pleural effusion

Exudates

Infective inflammatory, e.g. pneumonia or tuberculosis
Non-infective inflammatory, e.g. pulmonary embolism, rheumatoid arthritis, drugs such as amiodarone
Neoplasm, e.g. primary lung or secondaries
Miscellaneous, e.g. trauma, chylothorax

Transudates

Congestive cardiac failure
Nephrotic syndrome
Cirrhosis
Hypothyroidism

CASE 3

A 69-year-old male smoker presented to the chest clinic with shortness of breath, haemoptysis, cough and weight loss. A chest X-ray revealed a left-sided pleural effusion and upper-zone 'shadow'. The effusion was 'tapped' and the following results were obtained.

Pleural fluid LDH 566 U/L (<200)
Pleural fluid protein 114 g/L, with concomitant plasma protein 60 g/L

DISCUSSION

These biochemical tests suggest a pleural exudate. Note the raised pleural fluid LDH and considerably raised pleural fluid protein (more than 30 g/L) concentrations. The cytology showed malignant cells. A lung carcinoma was found on bronchoscopy. Exudate pleural fluid is associated with malignant lung disease.

CONCLUSIONS

- In adults, the total volume of CSF is about 135 mL, produced at a rate of 500 mL/day. This is predominantly formed by plasma ultrafiltration through the capillary walls of the choroid plexuses in the brain's lateral ventricles.
- Laboratory analysis of CSF can be useful in the diagnosis of various diseases, including meningitis and subarachnoid haemorrhage.
- Pleural fluid can also be analysed in the laboratory and divided into transudates (protein less than 30 g/L) and exudates (protein more than 30 g/L). This may be useful when searching for the cause of the effusion.

24 METABOLIC EFFECTS OF TUMOURS

The diffuse endocrine system	335	Multiple endocrine neoplasia	338
Catecholamines	335	Ectopic hormone production	339
The carcinoid syndrome	337	Tumour markers	340

This chapter looks at how clinical biochemistry tests can be used to diagnose and monitor patients with malignant disease. Malignant disease is one of the world's major 'killers' and it is therefore important to know the basic principles of biochemical diagnosis and monitoring in such patients.

Neoplastic cells of differentiated tissues sometimes synthesize enough compounds not normally thought of as coming from that tissue to be detectable in body fluids. These substances fall into two principal groups:

- those that alter metabolism and thus may produce clinical effects, some of which are hormonal syndromes;
- those that, although biologically inactive, may be analytically detectable in body fluids; these are sometimes used as tumour markers.

THE DIFFUSE ENDOCRINE SYSTEM

Certain rare syndromes with endocrine or neurotransmitter properties are associated with neoplasia. These cells may share common cytological characteristics, originating in the embryonic ectoblast. Staining techniques have shown their ability for **a**mine **p**recursor **u**ptake and **d**ecarboxylation (APUD) with the production of amines. Tumours of these cells have therefore been called APUDomas (although this older classification has been challenged). Some secrete physiologically active amines, whereas others, such as the pituitary and parathyroid glands and the calcitonin-producing C-cells of the thyroid, secrete peptide hormones. Many occur in the gastrointestinal tract and pancreas. Secreting tumours of tissues of the sympathetic nervous system and the amine-secreting carcinoid tumours are discussed in this chapter.

CATECHOLAMINES

The sympathetic nervous tissue comprising the adrenal medulla and sympathetic ganglia is derived from the embryonic neural crest and is composed of two types of cells, the chromaffin cells and the nerve cells, both of which can synthesize active catecholamines (dihydroxylated phenolic amines). Adrenaline (epinephrine) is almost exclusively a product of the adrenal medulla, whereas noradrenaline (norepinephrine) is predominantly formed at sympathetic nerve endings.

Metabolism of catecholamines

Adrenaline and noradrenaline (epinephrine and norepinephrine) are formed from the amine precursor tyrosine via dihydroxyphenylalanine and dihydroxyphenylethylamine (dopamine). Adrenaline and noradrenaline are both metabolized to the inactive 4-hydroxy-3-methoxymandelic acid (HMMA), incorrectly called vanillyl mandelic acid (VMA), by similar pathways in which metadrenaline and normetadrenaline, respectively, are intermediates (Fig. 24.1). Adrenaline, noradrenaline and their metabolites can be measured in urine.

Action of catecholamines

Noradrenaline causes generalized vasoconstriction, with hypertension and pallor. Adrenaline dilates blood vessels

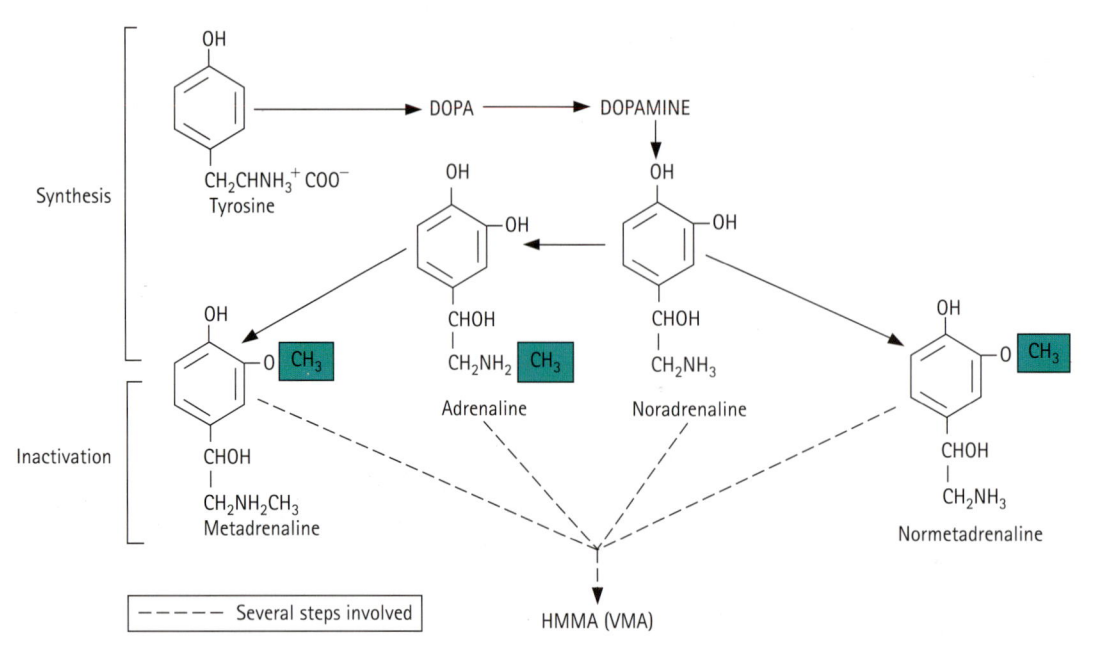

Fig. 24.1 Synthesis and metabolism of catecholamines. (HMMA = 4-hydroxy-3-methoxymandelic acid; VMA = vanillyl mandelic acid; DOPA = dihydroxyphenylalanine.)

in muscles, with variable effects on blood pressure and pulse rate. Adrenaline may also cause hyperglycaemia due to stimulation of glycogenolysis and other anti-insulin effects.

Catecholamine-secreting tumours

Phaeochromocytomas

Phaeochromocytomas present mainly in adults and occur in chromaffin tissue. About 10% are outside the adrenal medulla, 10% are bilateral and 10% are malignant. They are associated with the multiple endocrine neoplasia (MEN) syndrome. The symptoms and signs can be related to very high plasma concentrations of catecholamines.

The hypertension associated with phaeochromocytoma is potentially curable by surgery. Its presence should be excluded, particularly if a young adult presents with paroxysmal or persistent hypertension for no apparent reason or a patient presents with refractory hypertension or shows the classic triad of sweating, headaches and tachycardia associated with hypertension. Hyperglycaemia and, if the

---

CASE 1

A 34-year-old male was referred to the hypertension clinic because of uncontrolled hypertension. His blood pressure in the clinic was 186/104 mmHg, despite treatment with bendroflumethiazide, enalapril and felodipine. Some biochemistry tests were requested, which gave the following results.

Plasma
Sodium 138 mmol/L (135–145)
Potassium 4.2 mmol/L (3.5–5.0)
Urea 5.7 mmol/L (2.5–7.0)
Creatinine 90 μmol/L (70–110)

24-hour urinary HMMA 476 μmol/day (<25)

DISCUSSION
Phaeochromocytoma is the likely diagnosis, given the raised urinary HMMA concentration. This was confirmed by further tests, including a radioisotope metaiodobenzylguanidine (MIBG) scan and an adrenal MRI scan. The MEN syndrome needs to be excluded, given the known association with phaeochromocytoma. It is often wise to seek a secondary cause of hypertension in young individuals with hypertension, particularly those refractory to treatment.

plasma glucose concentration is high enough, glycosuria, may occur during the attack.

Diagnosis of phaechromocytomas

The biochemical diagnosis of these tumours can usually be made by measuring the daily urinary excretion of catecholamines (adrenaline, noradrenaline and dopamine) or HMMA, the major catabolic product of catecholamines. Metanephrines (which are also metabolites of catecholamines) can also be measured in urine and their concentration may be raised in some phaeochromocytomas when urinary HMMA is normal. A slightly increased excretion of urinary catecholamines can be found in cases of essential hypertension. Various dietary components and drugs affect some of the analytical methods, and therefore *it is important to consult your laboratory before starting a urine collection.* Labetalol, α-methyldopa and Sinemet (combined levodopa and carbidopa) may interfere with some of these assays.

In some cases, particularly if the tumours are small or hypertension is paroxysmal, metabolite excretion in a 24-hour urine collection may be misleading. If there is a high index of suspicion, it may be useful to repeat this estimation on three consecutive days. Raised plasma metanephrine concentrations have about 100 per cent sensitivity for the diagnosis of phaeochromocytoma and may be helpful if the patient is unable to give a reliable urine sample. However, the concentration of plasma metanephrines may also be raised in renal failure.

The clonidine or pentolinium suppression tests may have a place in the investigation if urinary catecholamines are positive or equivocal and imaging studies are negative. In normal individuals, concentration of urinary and plasma catecholamines should decrease after the administration of the suppressing agent, unlike the situation in a phaeochromocytoma, in which there is autonomous catecholamine secretion.

Imaging studies include abdominal computerized tomography, magnetic resonance imaging (MRI) and MIBG uptake scan. The MIBG is taken up specifically by the phaeochromocytoma tissue. The estimation of plasma catecholamine concentrations in samples obtained by selective venous catheterization may help to localize the tumour before surgery.

Neuroblastomas

Neuroblastomas are very malignant tumours of the sympathetic nervous tissue and usually occur in children. About 40 per cent occur in the adrenal medulla, and about 60 per cent are extra-adrenal.

The plasma catecholamine concentrations may be as high as, or higher than, those in patients with phaeochromocytomas. Some neuroblastomas secrete dopamine and its metabolite homovanillic acid whose concentration is raised in the urine and may be used as a tumour marker.

THE CARCINOID SYNDROME

Normal metabolism of 5-hydroxytryptamine

Some cells are called argentaffin because they reduce, and therefore stain with, silver salts. These are normally found in tissues derived from the embryonic gut and are most abundant in the ileum and appendix, but they are also found in the pancreas, stomach and rectum. They synthesize the biologically active amine 5-hydroxytryptamine (5-HT; serotonin) from the amine precursor tryptophan, the intermediate product being 5-hydroxytryptophan (5-HTP). 5-Hydroxytryptophan is inactivated by deamination and oxidation by monoamine oxidases to 5-hydroxyindole acetic acid (5-HIAA) (Fig. 24.2). The oxidases and aromatic amino acid decarboxylases are present in other tissues as well as in argentaffin cells; 5-HIAA is usually the main urinary excretion product of argentaffin cells.

Argentaffin cells may also excrete the peptide substance P, an excess of which causes flushing, tachycardia, increased bowel motility and hypotension.

Tryptophan →(Tryptophan-5-hydroxylase)→ 5-HTP (5-Hydroxytryptophan) →(Aromatic amino acid decarboxylase)→ 5-HT (5-Hydroxytryptamine: serotonin) →(Monoamine oxidase)→ 5-HIAA 5-Hydroxyindole acetic acid

Tryptophan ⇢ Nicotinamide

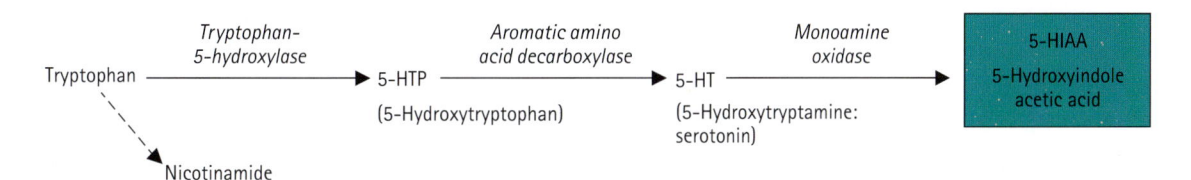

Fig. 24.2 Metabolism of tryptophan.

> **CASE 2**
>
> A 56-year-old male attended the gastroenterology department because of profuse diarrhoea. He also mentioned that he had felt increasingly breathless, and he looked flushed. A number of investigations were requested, but it was a 24-hour urinary 5-HIAA concentration of 544 μmol/day (less than 25) that suggested the diagnosis.
>
> **DISCUSSION**
> The patient had considerably raised urinary 5-HIAA concentration and symptoms suggestive of carcinoid syndrome. Note the flushing and diarrhoea as well as the breathlessness, probably due to bronchospasm induced by vasoactive and bronchoactive amines. The patient was subsequently found to have carcinoid syndrome involving a tumour of the ileum that had metastasized to the liver.

Causes of the carcinoid syndrome

The carcinoid syndrome is usually associated with abnormally high concentrations of plasma 5-HT. Ileal and appendiceal tumours only produce the typical clinical syndrome when they have metastasized, usually to the liver. The products of intestinal tumours are inactivated in the liver, but those from other sites, such as the bronchus, are released directly into the systemic circulation in an active form and may therefore cause symptoms.

Only one enzyme, tryptophan-5-hydroxylase, is needed to convert tryptophan to 5-HTP (see Fig. 24.2), and its derepression in malignant syndromes leads to excessive synthesis of 5-HTP. The decarboxylase and monoamine oxidases are present in normal non-argentaffin tissues, so 5-HTP accumulates. In the carcinoid syndrome associated with carcinoma of the bronchus, the urinary excretion of 5-HTP and 5-HT, compared with that of true carcinoid tumours, is proportionally higher than that of 5-HIAA.

The symptoms and signs of the carcinoid syndrome include:

- diarrhoea, which may be severe enough to cause the malabsorption syndrome,
- flushing,
- bronchospasm and right-sided fibrotic lesions of the heart, such as tricuspid incompetence and pulmonary stenosis; the heart lesions do not occur if the primary tumour is in the bronchus.

The symptoms and signs are more likely to be due to the presence of substance P than of 5-HT. Histamine has also been suggested as a cause of the flushing. A pellagra-type syndrome may occasionally develop, because tryptophan is diverted from nicotinamide to 5-HT synthesis. A carcinoid crisis occurs when the tumour releases large amounts of vasoactive substances into the circulation.

Diagnosis of the carcinoid syndrome

Urinary 5-HIAA secretion is usually very high in the carcinoid syndrome. A daily excretion of more than 25 μmol is elevated and greater than 100 μmol indicates carcinoid syndrome if walnuts and bananas (which are high in hydroxyindoles) have been excluded from the diet for about 24 hours before the urinary collection is started. Elevated urinary 5-HIAA has also been reported in association with small bowel disease and intestinal obstruction, e.g coeliac disease and sprue but usually concentrations are not as high as in carcinoid syndrome.

In very rare cases, usually of bronchial or gastric tumours, the argentaffin cells lack aromatic amino acid decarboxylase. In such cases, despite increased secretion of 5-HTP, urinary 5-HIAA excretion may not be increased to diagnostic levels. If there is a strong clinical suspicion of the carcinoid syndrome despite the finding of normal 5-HIAA excretion, estimation of total 5-hydroxyindole (5-HTP, 5-HT and 5-HIAA) excretion may be indicated. In some cases, if urine is not available, plasma 5-HT or its metabolites may be measured.

Carcinoid tumours may also secrete adrenocorticotrophic hormone (ACTH), which can result in Cushing's syndrome as well as being associated with MEN 1 syndrome. Octreotide, a somatostatin analogue, can be used to antagonize some of the effects of the released mediators in carcinoid syndrome.

MULTIPLE ENDOCRINE NEOPLASIA

In the rare syndromes of MEN (pluriglandular syndrome), two or more endocrine glands secrete inappropriately high amounts of hormones, usually from adenomas. There are two main groups of syndromes.

MEN 1 may involve two or more of the following endocrine tissues; the glands involved are listed in order of decreasing incidence of involvement:

- *parathyroid gland* (hyperplasia or adenoma),
- pancreatic islet cells:
  - gastrinomas
  - insulinomas
  - glucagonomas
  - vasoactive intestinal polypeptide-producing tumour (VIPoma)
  - pancreatic polypeptide-producing tumour (PPoma),
- *anterior pituitary gland*,
- adrenal cortex.

Remember the three Ps: parathyroids, pancreas and pituitary.

MEN 2 includes:

- medullary carcinoma of the thyroid gland,
- phaeochromocytoma,
- adenoma or carcinoma of the parathyroid gland.

MEN 2 can be subdivided into 2A (Sipple's syndrome) and 2B, the latter also being associated with marfanoid habitus, mucosal neuromas and abnormal corneal nerve fibres.

Both types of MEN are usually familial, inherited as a Mendelian dominant trait with variable penetrance. MEN 1 is due to a mutation in the *MENIN* gene, a tumour-suppressor gene; MEN 2 is the result of a proto-oncogene mutation called *RET*. Genetic tests can be used to screen families.

Calcitonin (see Chapter 6) is secreted by the thyroid parafollicular 'C' cells. Plasma calcitonin concentration can be raised in medullary carcinoma of the thyroid associated with MEN 2 syndrome. It can thus be used as a tumour marker for medullary thyroid carcinoma. Plasma calcitonin concentration can be used for screening for familial thyroid medullary carcinoma. In some cases, basal plasma calcitonin levels are not significantly raised but may become so after intravenous pentagastrin stimulation.

ECTOPIC HORMONE PRODUCTION

Mechanism of production

All cells have the potential to produce any peptide or protein coded for in the fertilized ovum. Malignant cells may produce ectopic hormones or other peptides if they partly revert to their early embryonic, pluripotential state. This may cause the histological changes associated with neoplasia, which are sometimes associated with the synthesis of significant amounts of a peptide not normally detectable in the fully differentiated tissue. There are two possible hypotheses, both of which include derepression:

- of part of the genome of the tissue cell that codes for the peptides, which are then synthesized in excess,
- of specialized neuroendocrine cells, which are scattered through many tissues.

Some substances are secreted more often by one type of tumour than by others, whereas some types of tumour secrete more than one 'foreign' substance.

Hormonal syndromes

Hormones produced at ectopic sites, such as those secreted by pathological over-activity of endocrine glands, are not under normal feedback control, and secretion continues under conditions in which it should be suppressed; such secretion is therefore inappropriate. Ectopic production is most clinically obvious if the peptide has hormone-like effects. Many of the syndromes associated with such hormonal syndromes are discussed in the relevant chapters of this book.

The following may be due to hormone secretion by the tumour.

Hyponatraemia due to antidiuretic hormone secretion

Although ectopic antidiuretic hormone (ADH) production is most commonly associated with the relatively rare oat-cell carcinoma of the bronchus, the syndrome of inappropriate ADH secretion has been reported in a wide variety of tumours. This syndrome, which is not confined to malignant disease, is discussed in Chapter 2.

Hypokalaemia due to adrenocorticotrophic hormone secretion

Ectopic ACTH secretion stimulates the secretion of all adrenocortical hormones except aldosterone; the clinical presentation often resembles that of primary hyperaldosteronism. The condition is usually associated with an oat-cell carcinoma of the bronchus but has occasionally been described in association with a variety of other malignant lesions, especially pulmonary carcinoid tumours. The patient may present with severe hypokalaemic alkalosis. (See Chapters 4 and 5.)

Hypercalcaemia due to secretion of parathyroid-hormone-related protein

Hypercalcaemia due to the secretion of parathyroid-hormone-related protein (PTHRP) is one of the commonest of these syndromes. It is associated with many types of malignant disease, including squamous cell carcinoma of the bronchus. Parathyroid-hormone-related protein is structurally similar to PTH and may have important actions in mineral metabolism in the fetus. The onset of hypercalcaemia can be very rapid, in contrast with that of primary hyperparathyroidism. (See Chapter 6.)

Polycythaemia due to erythropoietin secretion

Polycythaemia due to the secretion of erythropoietin or an erythropoietin-like molecule is a well-recognized complication of renal carcinoma; erythropoietin stimulates bone marrow erythropoiesis. Because erythropoietin is a normal product of the kidney, this is not an example of ectopic hormone secretion; however, the syndrome has been reported in association with other tumours, especially hepatocellular carcinoma (primary hepatoma).

Hypoglycaemia due to insulin or an insulin-like growth factor

Although rare, hypoglycaemia due to insulin or an insulin-like growth factor (IGF) has been reported in association with various tumours. Severe hypoglycaemia, with appropriately low plasma immunoreactive insulin and C-peptide concentrations and raised IGF-2 concentration, has been found in association with very large retroperitoneal or thoracic mesenchymal tumours resembling fibrosarcomas, or with hepatocellular carcinoma. (See Chapter 12.)

Gynaecomastia due to chorionic gonadotrophin secretion

This has been reported in association with various tumours, including carcinoma of the bronchus, breast and liver, due to raised circulating concentrations of chorionic gonadotrophin. In children with hepatoblastoma this may also cause precocious puberty.

Galactorrhoea

Galactorrhoea may also occur due to the ectopic secretion of prolactin or prolactin-like molecules. (See Chapter 7.)

Hyperthyroidism due to thyroid-stimulating hormone secretion

Some tumours of trophoblastic cells, such as choriocarcinoma, hydatidiform mole and testicular teratoma, have been shown to secrete a thyroid-stimulating hormone-like substance similar to human chorionic gonadotrophin (hCG). Clinical hyperthyroidism is unusual, even when plasma hormone concentrations are high. (See Chapter 11.)

TUMOUR MARKERS

For the measurement of a tumour marker to be clinically useful, the result should clearly separate those patients with from those without a tumour. Therefore (although in practice this is not the case), a tumour marker should ideally be:

- 100 per cent *sensitive*: levels should be raised if the tumour is present;
- 100 per cent *specific*: levels should *not* be raised if the tumour is *not* present.

Tumour markers may be used for the following.

- *To screen for disease*: very few markers are sufficiently sensitive or specific to be used to screen for the presence of a tumour (see Chapter 1).
- *To diagnose a tumour*: if a patient presents with clinical signs or symptoms, the measurement of a marker in plasma or urine may very occasionally be used to confirm a diagnosis.
- *To determine the prognosis*: in some cases the concentration of a specific marker is related to the mass or spread of the tumour.
- *To monitor the response to treatment*: if a tumour marker is present, the rate of its decrease in concentration may be used to assess the response to treatment such as surgery, chemotherapy or radiotherapy.
- *To identify the recurrence of a tumour*: if the concentration of the marker was previously raised, intermittent measurement during remission may sometimes be used to identify recurrence. Occasionally, however, tumours may dedifferentiate and fail to express the marker despite continued growth and spread.

Some examples of tumour markers

Prostate-specific antigen

Prostate-specific antigen (PSA) is a marker for prostatic carcinoma, a common male tumour, and is a 33 kDa protein and is homologous with the protease kallikrein family; it has a plasma half-life of about 3 days. One of its probable functions is to help liquidize semen. Its level is raised in benign prostatic hyperplasia (BPH) and prostatic carcinoma but also in prostate infection, for example prostatitis, and after rectal examination.

Levels of PSA increase with age, which is mainly due to the increase in the volume of the prostate that occurs. Therefore age-adjusted reference ranges should be used. There may also be a place for expressing plasma PSA in terms of prostate volume as found on ultrasound examination.

One diagnostic limitation is that the values of PSA overlap in BPH and prostatic carcinoma. After a radical prostatectomy, plasma PSA levels become undetectable at 2–3 weeks. Finasteride, a 5-α-reductase inhibitor that is sometimes used to treat BPH, decreases plasma PSA by up to 50 per cent.

The PSA is bound in the plasma to either α_1-antichymotrypsin or α_2-macroglobulin. The concentration of bound or complexed PSA is higher in prostate carcinoma, whereas that of free PSA is higher in BPH. The ratio of free to total PSA is lower in men with prostatic carcinoma. The PSA index is expressed as the percentage of the total plasma PSA that is free; an index above about 17 per cent is suggestive of BPH and one of less than 17 per cent of prostate carcinoma.

Plasma PSA concentrations greater than 10 μg/L are strongly suggestive of carcinoma, although carcinoma may be present even if values fall within the reference range. A PSA above 20 μg/L is suggestive of prostatic carcinoma that has spread beyond the prostate gland.

Plasma PSA assays in conjunction with digital rectal examination may be used as part of a screening programme for prostatic carcinoma in at-risk males. There is, however, no universally agreed screening protocol for prostatic

CASE 3

A 68-year-old, non-smoking female was under the care of the general surgeons because of colonic carcinoma, for which she had had a left hemi-cholectomy 10 months previously. Her plasma carcinoembryonic antigen (CEA) was 43 μg/L (normally less than 2.5 in non-smokers) prior to the operation. At the time she left hospital for surgery, her plasma CEA had reduced to less than 4.0 μg/L. Three months after her surgery, her plasma CEA was less than 2.5 μg/L.

The results from a recent outpatient follow-up clinic showed a plasma CEA of 19 μg/L.

DISCUSSION

The postoperative results indicate that her tumour had been largely resected, as the plasma CEA concentrations were reduced to near 'normal' levels. Tumour remission seemed likely at 3 months post-operation, as the plasma CEA concentrations remained low. Unfortunately, tumour recurrence had occurred at the time of her recent outpatient follow-up visit, as evidenced by the considerable rise in plasma CEA concentration. Tumour markers are usually less useful for diagnosing a malignancy than for following the progression of a tumour by observing the changes in their concentration.

CASE 4

A 67-year-old male attended the urology outpatients' clinic because of urinary hesitancy, lower back pain and nocturia. Rectal examination revealed a large, firm and craggy prostate gland. Some of his biochemistry results were as follows.

Plasma
Prostate-specific antigen 28 μg/L (<4)
'Corrected' calcium 2.98 mmol/L (2.15–2.55)
Phosphate 0.92 mmol/L (0.80–1.35)

DISCUSSION

The grossly elevated plasma PSA concentration is suggestive of malignant prostate disease. A bone scan showed osteosclerotic bony secondaries in his lumbar spine. Further investigations, including prostatic biopsy, confirmed metastatic prostatic carcinoma. This would also be a likely explanation for his hypercalcaemia.

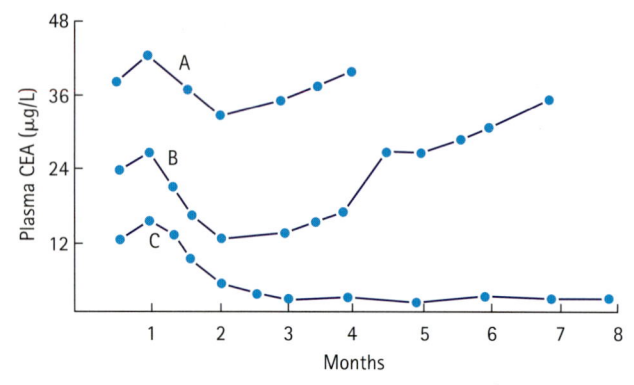

Fig. 24.3 The use of the tumour marker carcinoembryonic antigen (CEA) in monitoring disease progression. Patient A had an advanced gastrointestinal tumour and after initial chemotherapy died. Patient B had initial remission as a result of surgery but died after tumour relapse. Patient C had successful surgery with CEA essentially normalizing. (Reproduced with kind permission from Candlish JK and Crook M, *Notes on Clinical Biochemistry*, Singapore: World Scientific Publishing, 1993.)

carcinoma in the general population. Prostate biopsy is usually necessary if the PSA concentration is above 10 µg/L; however, the decision regarding biopsy is more difficult if PSA levels are 4–10 µg/L, although the PSA index may help.

Carcinoembryonic antigen

Carcinoembryonic antigen may be produced by some malignant tumours, especially colorectal carcinomas. If the initial plasma concentration is raised, serial plasma CEA estimations may sometimes help to monitor the effectiveness of, or recurrence after, treatment (Fig. 24.3). Plasma concentrations correlate poorly with tumour mass, but a very high concentration usually indicates a bad prognosis. Plasma concentrations may also rise in non-malignant disease of the gastrointestinal tract and in smokers.

Alpha-fetoprotein

Alpha-fetoprotein (AFP) is an oncofetal protein, the synthesis of which is suppressed as the fetus matures. Concentrations may be very high in the plasma of patients with certain tumours such as hepatocellular carcinoma (primary hepatomas and hepatoblastomas) and teratoma. Moderately raised concentrations may be due to non-malignant liver disease.

Human chorionic gonadotrophin

Human chorionic gonadotrophin is normally produced by the placenta, but also by trophoblastic cells of gonadal and extragonadal germ cell tumours. Ectopic secretion has been observed in some bronchial carcinomas. The measurement of hCG can be used to screen for choriocarcinoma in women who have had a hydatidiform mole (see Chapter 10). Plasma concentrations may be raised in patients with malignancy of the gonads such as seminomas, and hCG may be used to monitor the response to treatment and tumour recurrence.

Carbohydrate antigens

Carbohydrate antigens (CAs) are a group of tumour markers, raised plasma concentrations of which may be used to monitor the response to treatment and the recurrence of certain tumours.

- *CA 125* concentration may be raised in the plasma of patients with ovarian carcinoma. It can also be raised in endometriosis and pelvic inflammatory disease. Its use in conjunction with transvaginal ultrasonography has been proposed as a means of screening for ovarian carcinoma.
- *CA 15-3* concentration may be raised in the plasma of some patients with advanced breast carcinoma, although it can also be raised in cirrhosis, and with ovarian cysts.
- *CA 19-9* concentration may be raised in the plasma of patients with pancreatic or colorectal carcinoma and those with obstructive liver disease.

None of the CA tumour markers fulfils the criteria of an ideal marker, as none is sufficiently sensitive or specific to be used to screen for early disease. Furthermore, some advanced tumours dedifferentiate and fail to produce a marker despite continued growth and spread. These tumour markers may, however, be useful in the monitoring of patients with tumours and in the assessment of therapy. High levels are associated with tumour spread and relapse, and low levels are suggestive of tumour remission.

Other tumour markers

- *Serum paraprotein and urinary Bence-Jones protein* (discussed in Chapter 19 for multiple myeloma).
- *Plasma lactate dehydrogenase* (LDH): the concentration can be raised in certain haematological tumours such as lymphomas.

- *Placental alkaline phosphatase*: true placental alkaline phosphatase and placental-like isoenzyme concentrations are raised in seminoma and dysgerminoma. Levels are not usually raised in teratomata. In conjunction with AFP and hCG, it is useful in the diagnosis and monitoring of extragonadal and gonadal germ cell tumours. However, plasma concentrations are also elevated in smokers. (See Chapter 18.)
- *Thyroglobulin*: this high-molecular-weight protein is produced in the follicular cells of the thyroid. Its concentration is raised in follicular or papillary carcinoma of the thyroid. Spuriously low levels may be found in the presence of thyroglobulin antibodies, which interfere with the assay.
- *Neuronal-specific enolase*: plasma levels may be raised in small-cell lung carcinoma and neuroblastoma; it is derived from neurodectal tissue.
- *Inhibin*: this is secreted by the granulosa cells of the ovary and by the Sertoli cells of the testis. It can be used as a plasma tumour marker of ovarian granulosa cell tumours and testicular Sertoli cell tumours.
- *Squamous cell carcinoma antigen*: this is a recently described plasma tumour marker of potential use in squamous cell carcinoma of the cervix.

New tumour markers are likely to be revealed in the future and this chapter is not all-inclusive. Genetic tests are also being developed that may be useful to predict those individuals at risk of developing various carcinomas, for example *BRCA* gene mutations for breast carcinoma. Tumour-modified DNA, RNA and nucleic acids also circulate in the blood and may be useful in the diagnosis of certain cancers.

CONCLUSIONS

- Laboratory biochemical tests can be useful in the investigation and management of certain malignant disorders.
- Tumours alter metabolism and thus may produce clinical effects, some of which are hormonal syndromes. In addition, tumours may release compounds that, although biologically inactive, may be analytically detectable in body fluids. These are sometimes used as tumour markers.
- In the rare syndromes of MEN (pluriglandular syndrome), two or more endocrine glands secrete inappropriately high amounts of hormones, usually from adenomas.
- The diagnosis of phaeochromocytomas may be facilitated by the assay of urinary catecholamines or metanephrines.
- Similarly, raised urinary 5-HIAA concentration may be useful in the diagnosis of carcinoid syndrome.
- For the measurement of a tumour marker to be clinically useful, the result should clearly separate those patients with a tumour from those without. Therefore a tumour marker should ideally be sensitive (concentrations should be raised if the tumour is present) and specific (levels should not be raised if the tumour is not present).
- Tumour markers are generally best used for monitoring the progression of tumours with therapy (remission or relapse).

25 THERAPEUTIC DRUG MONITORING AND POISONING

Monitoring drug treatment	344	Biochemical monitoring of possible side-effects of drug treatment	351
Factors affecting drug plasma concentrations	345	Diagnosis of drug or substance overdose of unknown cause	351
When to measure individual drug concentrations to monitor treatment	347		
Pharmacogenetics	350		

Drug overdose and the consequences of drug side-effects are common causes of hospital medical admissions. This chapter also looks at therapeutic monitoring of particular drugs and how the clinical biochemistry laboratory can be involved in the management of various drug overdoses.

The blood (usually plasma or serum) concentrations of many drugs can be measured or, more rarely, those of other body fluids, although in only a few situations is this of proven benefit.

Pharmacokinetics is the study of the fate of drugs after administration and is concerned with their absorption, distribution in body compartments, metabolism and excretion. Absorption depends on whether the drug is taken orally, by intravenous or intramuscular injection, sublingually or rectally.

Possible indications for measuring drug concentrations in various body fluids are to:

- check that the patient is taking the drug as prescribed (compliance);
- ensure that the dose is sufficient to produce the required effect but not so high as to be likely to cause toxic effects;
- help diagnose drug side-effects and drug interactions;
- determine the type of drug or drugs taken in cases of suspected overdose and to assess the need for treatment.

MONITORING DRUG TREATMENT

One can assess whether the dose of a drug is optimal either clinically or by laboratory assays. An example of the former would be monitoring the action of antihypertensive drugs by measuring the blood pressure. Examples of laboratory biochemical effects, which are discussed in the relevant chapters, include the following:

- plasma potassium concentrations during potassium supplementation (Chapter 5);
- thyroid-stimulating hormone concentrations whilst on thyroxine therapy (Chapter 11);
- plasma calcium concentration and alkaline phosphatase activity during vitamin D treatment for hypocalcaemia or osteomalacia (Chapter 6);
- plasma cholesterol after hydroxy-malonyl-glutaryl coenzyme A reductase inhibitor therapy (Chapter 13);
- clotting status as judged by prothrombin time and International Normalized Ratio (INR) for determining warfarin dosage.

The drug or metabolite concentrations can also be measured in biological fluids, although these may not parallel cellular effects. However, the measurement of plasma concentrations may be indicated in the following situations.

- If the desired result cannot be measured precisely: for example, the incidence of epileptic fits is a poor indicator of the optimal dosage of anticonvulsants.
- If the range of plasma levels that is most effective in producing the desired result without toxic side-effects (the therapeutic range) has been defined: this is particularly true if there is a narrow margin between therapeutic and toxic drug concentrations, such as in the case of digoxin or lithium.
- If the prescribed drug is the main active compound and is not metabolized significantly to an active metabolite: otherwise the active metabolite may be measured, for example phenobarbital in primidone treatment.

FACTORS AFFECTING DRUG PLASMA CONCENTRATIONS

The total amount of drug in the extracellular fluid depends on the balance between that entering and that leaving the compartment; the plasma concentration depends on the volume of fluid through which the retained drug is distributed.

Timing of the sample

Blood samples must be taken at a standard time after ingestion of the drug, the exact time varying with the known differences in the rate of absorption, metabolism and excretion of different drugs (Table 25.1).

The following factors may affect the blood concentration of some drugs.

Patient compliance

It has been shown that not all in-patients take a drug exactly as prescribed; compliance with instructions is likely to be even worse outside hospital. The patient may not take the drug at all, take more than the prescribed dose, take the drug intermittently or become confused about the timing and dose, particularly if taking more than one drug.

Clinicians should realize that poor compliance might cause a poor clinical response or toxicity. A regular review of therapy and careful explanation to the patient are important. Assay of plasma concentrations is only a crude method of assessing compliance and only tests the situation at the time when blood was taken.

Table 25.1 Therapeutic drug monitoring in adults[a]

Drug	Sampling time	Major route of elimination	Comments
Carbamazepine	Trough	Liver	May cause hyponatraemia
Ciclosporin	Trough	Liver	Monitor renal and liver function
Digoxin	6–8 hours post-dose	Liver Renal (60–80%)	Check plasma potassium concentration
Gentamicin	Trough Peak: 30 min post-i.v., 60 min post-i.m.	Renal	Monitor renal function.
Lithium	12 hours post-dose	Renal	May cause hypothyroidism
Phenobarbital	Trough	Liver	
Phenytoin	Trough	Liver	Undergoes saturable metabolism
Primidone	Trough	Liver	Partially metabolized to phenobarbital
Tacrolimus	Trough	Liver	Monitor renal and liver function
Theophylline		Liver	
Oral	2 hours post-dose		
Slow release	4–6 hours		
Intravenous infusion	6–8 hours		
Valproate	Trough	Liver	Only useful to assess compliance or confirm toxicity

[a]Therapeutic ranges are less reliable for patients taking a number of drugs. Sampling times are only a general guide. In some cases, samples taken at other times may be appropriate. i.v. = intravenous; i.m. = intramuscular.

Entry of the drug into, and distribution through, the extracellular fluid

Absorption

Lipid-soluble drugs can pass through cell membranes more readily, and are therefore absorbed more rapidly, than water-soluble ones; they reach the highest plasma concentrations at between 30 and 60 minutes after ingestion. The rate of absorption in an individual patient may be affected by:

- the timing of ingestion in relation to meals;
- the rate of gastric emptying: this must be allowed for, for example during treatment with drugs affecting gut motility or after gastric surgery;
- vomiting, diarrhoea or malabsorption syndromes;
- the administration of other compounds, such as the bile acid sequestrants which may also bind certain drugs within the intestinal lumen.

Volume of distribution

The final plasma concentration of a drug reached after a standard amount has been absorbed depends on the volume through which it has been distributed. For example, it may be difficult to predict the appropriate dose in oedematous or obese patients who, because they have a larger than normal volume of distribution, may have unexpectedly low plasma concentrations. By contrast, in small children, with a low volume of distribution, there is a danger of overdosage. The patient's weight or surface area may need to be allowed for when the dose is calculated.

Binding to plasma albumin

Many drugs, like many endogenous substances, are partly inactivated by protein binding, usually albumin. Most drug assays estimate the total concentration of the free plus the protein-bound drug. Biological feedback mechanisms do not control free drug concentrations as they do those of plasma calcium and hormones; therefore, the method of interpretation to allow for altered protein binding is different. Measured plasma concentrations fall little due to a reduction in protein binding; a larger proportion of the measured drug will be in the unbound, free, active form, so that metabolism and excretion will increase. Unless this is realized, dangerously high plasma free concentrations may be interpreted as being within, or even below, the therapeutic range if the plasma albumin concentration is very low.

The bound proportion varies with differing plasma albumin concentrations and there is no valid correction factor that allows for protein abnormalities. About 90 per cent of phenytoin, 70 per cent of salicylic acid, 50 per cent of phenobarbital and 20 per cent of digoxin is protein bound. However, binding may be affected by the following.

- *Abnormalities in plasma albumin concentration*: blood should be taken without stasis to minimize a possible rise in plasma albumin, and albumin-bound drug, concentrations. Low concentrations, such as those often found in hepatic cirrhosis or the nephrotic syndrome, may reduce the proportion of protein-bound drugs.
- *Competition for binding sites on protein*: many drugs, unconjugated bilirubin and hydrogen ions compete with each other for binding sites.

Metabolism and excretion of drugs

The blood concentrations of a drug depend on normal hepatic and renal function as well as on acid–base and electrolyte balance.

The time taken for the plasma drug concentration to fall to half its original concentration is called its effective half-life. To maintain a reasonably steady plasma concentration, drugs with a short half-life should be taken more frequently than those with a long one. After starting treatment, a steady state is usually reached after about five times its half-life has elapsed; the first specimen of blood for monitoring should not be taken earlier than this.

The rate at which the plasma drug concentration falls after it has reached peak concentration depends on the rate of distribution through the extracellular fluid (see above), the rate of entry into cells and the rate at which it is metabolized and excreted, whether in urine or bile.

The rate of elimination of most drugs depends on their plasma concentration. A small increase in the dose of some, such as phenytoin, may exceed the capacity of the metabolic or excretory pathways and so cause a disproportionate increase in plasma levels; the plasma concentrations of these drugs should be monitored carefully. The rate at which this occurs is termed saturation kinetics.

Metabolic conversion to active or inactive metabolites

Some drugs are only active after metabolic conversion; others are inactivated, usually by conjugation in the liver.

Ideally, a drug assay should measure all the active forms, whether the parent compound or its active metabolite, and none of the inactive forms.

Drug–drug interactions

If a number of different drugs are being prescribed, one may affect the plasma concentration of another by altering its binding to plasma proteins, rate of metabolism or excretion. For example, sodium valproate displaces phenytoin from its protein-binding sites and reduces its rate of metabolism.

Tolerance

Some drugs (for example phenytoin) may induce the synthesis of enzymes that inactivate them and consequently higher doses than usual may be needed to produce the desired effect. In other cases, reduced receptor sensitivity may require higher doses than normal in order to increase the plasma concentration and to achieve the desired effect.

Patient variations

The rate of metabolism of some drugs depends on the age of the patient.

- *Premature infants*, with immature detoxifying mechanisms, metabolize and excrete some drugs more slowly than adults.
- *Children*, who have a higher metabolic rate than adults, may eliminate some drugs more rapidly than adults.
- *The elderly* may metabolize drugs slowly; they are particularly sensitive to digoxin.

The rate of metabolism of some drugs may be affected by genetic or racial factors (see 'Pharmacogenetics' below) as well as by metabolic causes, for example increased sensitivity to digoxin evoked by hypokalaemia or hypercalcaemia.

WHEN TO MEASURE INDIVIDUAL DRUG CONCENTRATIONS TO MONITOR TREATMENT

Only a few drug assays are of proven clinical value. The clinical picture must be taken into account and all the above factors must be allowed for when interpreting the results. The following are some of the drug measurements that have been claimed to be useful for therapeutic monitoring.

Cardiac anti-arrhythmic drugs

Digoxin

This drug is used in congestive cardiac failure and atrial fibrillation. Estimation of plasma digoxin concentrations may be useful in the following situations.

- To assess compliance: the elderly, for whom digoxin is frequently prescribed, are often taking several different drugs and are liable to be confused about which tablets to take and at what time.
- In patients, such as the elderly, who are likely to have a low threshold for toxicity, and in premature infants, who have an increased elimination half-life.
- If it is difficult to calculate the appropriate dose because of an abnormal volume of distribution due to obesity or oedema, or in infants.
- If excretion is impaired, perhaps due to renal dysfunction.
- If the patient is taking another drug, such as amiodarone, which possibly reduces its rate of excretion.

Plasma digoxin concentrations, even within the therapeutic range, are very difficult to interpret in the presence of conditions that may alter receptor sensitivity, such as:

- hypokalaemia, hypercalcaemia or hypomagnesaemia,
- hypoxia or acidosis,
- hypothyroidism.

Blood should be taken at least 6 hours after the last dose, when absorption and distribution are usually complete (see Table 25.1). It is also important to check plasma potassium levels and renal function, as digoxin is renally excreted. The assay of digoxin can be problematic, as the antibodies used in certain immunoassays may cross-react with endogenous compounds – so-called digoxin-like immunoreactive substances. The latter can occur in pregnancy. Sometimes digoxin overdose/toxicity can be treated by the administration of inactivating digoxin antibodies (Digibind).

Amiodarone

This is used to treat various cardiac arrhythmias, including ventricular tachycardias and atrial fibrillation. The drug is highly protein bound and has a long half-life, up to 10–40 days after a single dose and up to 100 days on chronic therapy.

> ### CASE 1
>
> A 69-year-old male was on once-daily digoxin 250 µg, once-daily bendroflumethiazide 2.5 mg, and once-daily warfarin 4 mg for atrial fibrillation and hypertension. He attended his anticoagulant clinic to have his blood warfarin levels checked. The following results were returned.
>
> *Plasma*
> Sodium 140 mmol/L (135–145)
> Potassium 3.8 mmol/L (3.5–5.0)
> Urea 6.7 mmol/L (2.5–7.5)
> Creatinine 102 µmol/L (60–120)
> International Normalized Ratio 2.7 (2–3)
> Digoxin 3.3 µg/L (0.8–2.2)
>
> **DISCUSSION**
> The attending doctor was worried about digoxin toxicity given the raised plasma concentrations. However, after discussion with the laboratory and phlebotomy, it transpired that the blood samples had been taken within an hour of the patient taking his digoxin tablet. Repeat testing 7 hours after taking the digoxin showed a plasma concentration of 1.2 µg/L, within the therapeutic range. This case illustrates the importance of the correct timing of blood sampling for therapeutic drug monitoring (in the case of digoxin, this is optimally about 6–8 hours post-dose).

It is not excreted in the urine, but is predominantly metabolized in the liver. The metabolite desethylamiodarone is also active. Amiodarone is potentially very toxic, sometimes causing photosensitivity reactions, pulmonary fibrosis and corneal micro-deposits. Additionally, it blocks free thyroxine to free tri-iodothyronine conversion and can evoke hypothyroidism. Conversely, as it contains iodine, it can also cause thyrotoxicosis (see Chapter 11).

Flecainide

This is another anti-arrhythmic drug for which therapeutic drug monitoring may be beneficial.

Anticonvulsants

Once the dose that gives stable plasma concentrations within the therapeutic range has been determined, monitoring is probably only necessary in the following cases:

- to assess compliance,
- if the frequency of fits increases in a previously well-controlled patient,
- if the clinical picture suggests toxicity,
- if another drug is prescribed that may affect the plasma concentrations.

Plasma concentrations in children and in pregnant women should be monitored more frequently, as these groups are more likely to develop toxicity.

Phenytoin

Phenytoin is used in the treatment of partial and generalized tonic–clonic seizures by inhibiting voltage-gated sodium channels.

Measurement of plasma phenytoin may be useful, because it exhibits saturation kinetics. Thus a small increase in dose of phenytoin may result in a large increase in plasma concentration and be associated with toxicity. Sodium valproate displaces phenytoin from its binding sites and reduces its rate of metabolism; free plasma phenytoin may then cause toxicity despite apparently appropriate total plasma concentrations. Phenytoin is a potent enzyme-inducing drug (as, indeed, are phenobarbital and carbamazepine) and may enhance the metabolism of other drugs as well as causing an elevation in plasma gamma-glutamyl transferase, which does not necessarily mean abnormal hepatic toxicity. (See Chapter 17.)

Carbamazepine

Like phenytoin, carbamazepine can be used in the treatment of partial and generalized tonic–clonic seizures by inhibiting voltage-gated sodium channels. Additionally, it can be used in the treatment of trigeminal neuralgia and diabetic neuropathy and also for prophylaxis of bipolar disorders. It has an active metabolite formed in the liver called carbamazepine 10,11-epoxide. Carbamazepine induces its own metabolism and thus plasma concentrations may fall at the end of the first month of therapy, which results in the need for a dose increase.

Valproate

This is used to treat myoclonic seizures, generalized absence seizures and partial and generalized tonic–clonic seizures. It is also finding a place in the treatment of bipolar affective disorders.

Plasma concentrations of sodium valproate correlate poorly with the dose prescribed, the clinical response and toxicity, probably because of the presence of active metabolites. Consequently, the main justification for measuring plasma concentrations is to assess compliance. However, valproate is hepatotoxic and it is therefore important to check liver function tests.

Phenobarbital, primidone and ethosuximide are less used today in the treatment of epilepsy, although therapeutic drug monitoring may be useful.

There are several new anti-epileptic drugs now available, for which the need to monitor plasma concentrations is under evaluation. Vigabatrin, an inhibitor of γ-aminobutyric acid metabolism, has a long action because it binds avidly to receptors; therefore, plasma concentrations are unlikely to predict therapeutic response or toxicity. Other new anti-epileptic drugs include lamotrigine, which inhibits excitatory neurotransmitter release, and gabapentin, but it remains to be seen how useful therapeutic drug monitoring will be in patient management.

Lithium

The margin between therapeutic and toxic concentrations of lithium at high dosage is narrow and therefore plasma concentrations should be monitored regularly.

Lithium may be given to psychiatric patients for bipolar affective disorders. It is not protein bound, and interpretation of the results of assays is not complicated by protein abnormalities. Plasma concentrations should be measured on a specimen taken 12 hours after the evening dose.

Lithium usage is associated with hypothyroidism (see Chapter 11), and plasma concentrations above about 1.4 mmol/L can be nephrotoxic. Oliguria and acute renal failure, which can be precipitated by reduced salt intake or diuretic usage, can reduce lithium clearance. It is important, therefore, to monitor thyroid and renal function tests in such patients. Plasma lithium levels above 2.5 mmol/L are associated with significant mortality and may necessitate dialysis.

Theophylline

Theophylline assays may be useful, especially in acute asthmatic attacks that are not responding clinically; the results may help to ensure that the poor response is not due to under-dosage and, if it is not, that increasing the dosage will not lead to toxic plasma levels.

Theophylline and its active metabolite caffeine are used in the management of recurrent apnoea in the newborn; at this age, their clearance is slow and theophylline is partially metabolized to caffeine. Both plasma theophylline and caffeine concentrations may need to be assayed if theophylline has been given, in order to assess therapeutic or toxic effects.

Samples for theophylline assays should be taken at between 2 and 4 hours after the last dose. The half-life of theophylline is shortened in smokers.

CASE 2

A 40-year-old female was admitted to casualty because of confusion. She was known to be on lithium therapy for a bipolar disorder. The following blood results were obtained.

Plasma
Sodium 150 mmol/L (135–145)
Potassium 5.0 mmol/L (3.5–5.0)
Urea 7.8 mmol/L (2.5–7.5)
Creatinine 134 μmol/L (60–120)
Thyroid-stimulating hormone 18.7 mU/L (0.20–5.0)
Free thyroxine 6.8 pmol/L (12–25)
Lithium 2.8 mmol/L (therapeutic range 0.5–1.0)

DISCUSSION

The elevated plasma lithium concentration indicates a potential risk of toxicity. The level should be checked to ensure correct sample timing, as incorrect timing, i.e. not trough levels, is a common cause of elevated drug levels.

The hypernatraemia can be explained by the polyuria and nephrogenic diabetes insipidus secondary to lithium toxicity upon the kidney. Hypothyroidism can also be secondary to lithium toxicity.

Antibiotics

Aminoglycosides, such as gentamicin, are given intramuscularly or intravenously and, in contrast to many other antibiotics, the margin between the therapeutic range and toxic levels is narrow. Toxic levels may cause ototoxicity and nephrotoxicity.

Measurement is particularly indicated if there is serious infection or the treatment is so prolonged that the risk of toxicity is increased or renal function is impaired.

Aminoglycoside concentrations are often measured twice. The first specimen should be taken immediately before injection, when the 'trough level' is expected, to ensure that concentrations are not already high and that further administration is not likely to cause toxicity, or that they are not so low as to be ineffective. The second should be taken about an hour after injection, at the time of the anticipated 'peak level', to ensure that an adequate concentration has been achieved for antibacterial action.

Two new glycopeptide antibiotics, namely vancomycin and teicoplanin, are used to treat aerobic and anaerobic Gram-positive bacteria. Like gentamicin, they may cause nephrotoxicity and ototoxicty, a risk increased by concomitant aminoglycoside usage. Therapeutic drug monitoring also has a role in the use of these drugs.

Methotrexate

Methotrexate is used as a cytotoxic agent and, to achieve this, plasma concentrations should exceed 1 μmol/L for at least 36 hours. It is a folate antagonist, which inhibits DNA synthesis at lower concentrations. It is also used as an immunosuppressant in psoriasis and rheumatoid arthritis.

When used as a cytotoxin, plasma levels above 5–10 μmol/L at 24 hours, 0.5–1.0 μmol/L at 48 hours and 0.1 μmol/L at 72 hours post-dose are associated with an increased risk of marrow suppression.

Methotrexate excretion is predominantly renal and is facilitated by a good urine flow and an alkaline pH greater than 6.5. After high-dose methotrexate, 'rescue therapy' with folinic acid is given to reduce toxicity by providing cells with folate co-factors for DNA synthesis.

Immunosuppressants

Ciclosporin

This is an immunosuppressant that inhibits T-lymphocyte activation by binding to calcineurin phosphatase and is used to prevent the rejection of transplanted organs, for example kidney. Ciclosporin is a cyclic peptide derived from the fungus *Tolypocladium inflatum Gams*. It is also used (usually at lower dose) in the treatment of inflammatory bowel disease, rheumatoid arthritis and psoriasis.

The dosage may be difficult to assess because there is considerable variation amongst individuals in the rate of absorption and clearance; there is also a relatively narrow margin between therapeutic and toxic drug concentrations. The main toxic action is on the kidney, although hepatic dysfunction can also occur. During the first 6 months, when the risks of rejection are highest, plasma concentrations should be measured regularly.

Peak ciclosporin concentrations occur 1–4 hours after oral dosage and require adequate bile flow. Over half of the drug binds to red blood cells and then redistributes in plasma, where a majority is found bound to lipoproteins, as ciclosporin is strongly lipophilic. EDTA is necessary for assay. Ciclosporin levels should be determined on trough samples, i.e. 12 hours after the previous dose on a twice-daily regimen. Daily monitoring is usual after transplantation; in the first few months, levels of 100–400 μg/L are usual, decreasing to about 100–200 μg/L afterwards.

Tacrolimus

This is a macrolide lactone and, like ciclosporin, inhibits calcineurin phosphatase, thereby inhibiting T-lymphocyte activation.

Although useful as an immunosuppressant, it is nephrotoxic and cardiomyopathy may occur. It has an advantage over ciclosporin in having a greater potency, and impaired biliary function is less likely to alter its absorption. Therapeutic drug monitoring seems to be of value, and levels over 25 μg/L are associated with increased toxicity.

PHARMACOGENETICS

Various enzymes are responsible for the metabolism of drugs. For example, the inactivation of isoniazid by acetylation depends on whether the patient is genetically capable of carrying out this process at a normal rate; toxicity is likely at lower plasma concentrations in 'slow acetylators' than in 'fast acetylators'.

Thiopurine methyltransferase (TPMT) is involved in the metabolism of azathioprine, which is used as a cytotoxic and also as an immunosuppressant agent. The enzyme TPMT shows pharmocogenetic variation and about 90 per cent of the UK population have high enzyme levels. However, about 10 per cent are heterozygotic for TPMT deficiency and about 0.3 per cent are homozygotic for no functional activity. The latter two groups are more susceptible to azathioprine toxicity. Determination of red cell TPMT activity prior to azathioprine administration may give a guide as to who should have therapy and what dose should be given.

Similarly, debrisoquine hydroxylase activity can be used as a guide to cytochrome P450 phenotype. The cytochrome family is involved in the metabolism of various drugs. Debrisoquine hydroxylase activity reflects cytochrome (CY) 2D6 status, which is involved in the metabolism of a number of drugs, including certain anti-arrhythmics and antidepressants.

BIOCHEMICAL MONITORING OF POSSIBLE SIDE-EFFECTS OF DRUG TREATMENT

Some drugs have harmful side-effects. For example, the plasma urea, creatinine, sodium and potassium concentrations should be checked for patients on diuretic therapy or taking angiotensin-converting enzyme inhibitors. The assessment of liver damage (for example plasma transaminase activities) or of renal function may be indicated during treatment with potentially hepatotoxic (for example valproate) or nephrotoxic (for example ciclosporin) drugs, respectively. The statins may sometimes cause muscle damage or rhabdomyolysis, which can be detected by measuring the plasma concentration of creatine kinase (CK).

DIAGNOSIS OF DRUG OR SUBSTANCE OVERDOSE OF UNKNOWN CAUSE

Drug overdosage must always be excluded as a cause of coma of unknown origin. Unexplained clinical or laboratory findings may suggest effects due to drug or alcohol ingestion despite denial by the patient. Hypokalaemia, for example, may be due to purgative abuse, and hypoglycaemia may be a presenting finding associated with alcohol ingestion. Raised plasma transaminase activities, thought to be due to alcoholic liver disease, may be investigated by measuring random plasma alcohol concentrations. A raised plasma CK concentration may be indicative of 'Ecstasy' or cocaine abuse. Measurement of blood gases is useful to determine whether there is an acid–base disturbance, for example a metabolic acidosis may be seen in paracetamol overdose. As discussed above, some drugs, such as digoxin and lithium, may cause renal impairment.

About half the patients attempting suicide take several drugs, sometimes with alcohol. Qualitative screening of plasma, urine or gastric aspirate may be needed to help identify the drugs.

The measurement of plasma drug concentrations (and also sometimes of other biological fluids such as vomit or gastric contents) may be supplemented by screening the urine for drugs or their metabolites. Sometimes specialized toxicological laboratories may need to be consulted. The careful labelling and identification of samples that may have associated medico-legal issues is essential.

It is often unnecessary to measure the plasma concentrations of drugs that the patient is known to have taken in overdose. The need for gastric lavage and measures to increase the urinary excretion of the drug and to maintain adequate respiration and circulation are not usually affected by knowledge of drug concentrations. The treatment of many drug overdoses is often supportive, with close monitoring of the patient and clinical intervention when necessary. However, in some cases specific antidotes are indicated.

Drugs or poisons for which there is a specific antidote

Paracetamol (acetaminophen)

It is *essential* to measure plasma drug concentrations in suspected paracetamol poisoning, for the following reasons.

- A metabolite of paracetamol is hepatotoxic: its metabolism is saturable and is detoxified by conjugation with glutathione. Depletion of glutathione is implicated in the liver damage. The patient may die of liver failure despite recovery from the immediate effects.
- A specific antidote to the hepatotoxic effect is available.
- The antidote is only useful if given within a defined period of time and if defined plasma concentrations are reached.
- The likelihood of hepatotoxicity cannot be predicted from the clinical picture at presentation (Fig. 25.1).

N-acetylcysteine and methionine are both relatively effective antidotes, because they enable paracetamol to be converted to non-toxic metabolites. Methionine is given orally but may cause vomiting. N-acetylcysteine is most often used and is given intravenously. It is only effective

Case 3

A 23-year-old male took a paracetamol overdose. The following results were obtained 2 days after treatment with intravenous N-acetylcysteine.

Plasma
Bilirubin 33 μmol/L (<20)
Alanine aminotransferase 881 U/L (<42)
Alkaline phosphatase 127 U/L (<250)
Albumin 42 g/L (35–45)
Gamma-glutamyl transferase 266 U/L (<55)
International Normalized Ratio 3.1 (2–3)

DISCUSSION

The results show severely abnormal liver function tests secondary to paracetamol overdose. The raised alanine aminotransferase concentration suggests hepatocyte damage evoked by the paracetamol. Paracetamol overdose can induce a number of biochemical disturbances, including a metabolic acidosis, raised plasma anion and osmolal gap. The raised INR is concerning and suggests severe paracetamol toxicity and the risk of life-threatening hepatic damage, in some cases necessitating liver transplant.

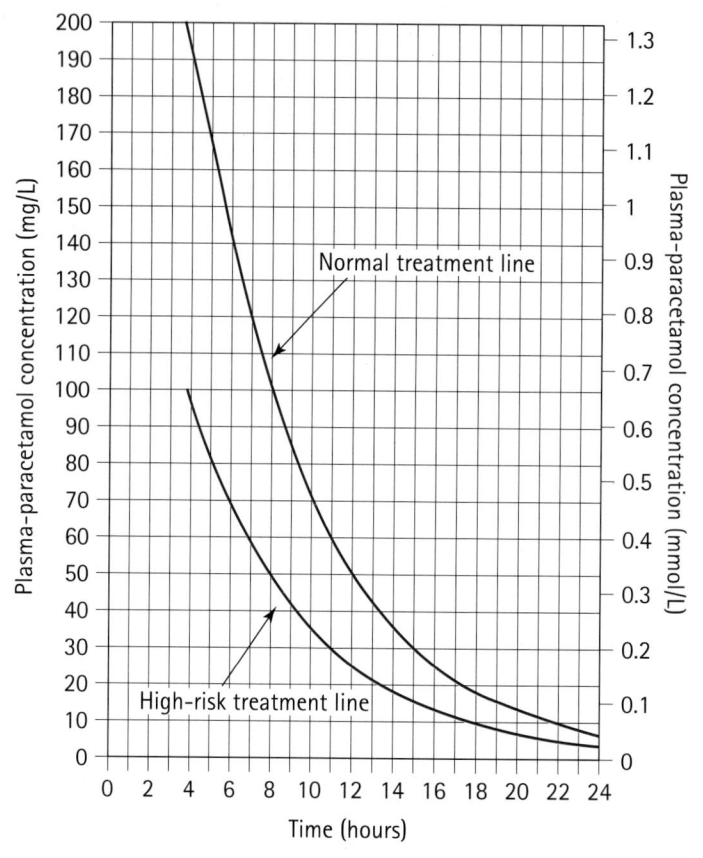

Fig. 25.1 Patients whose plasma-paracetamol concentrations are above the *normal treatment line* should be treated with acetylcysteine by intravenous infusion (or, if acetylcysteine cannot be used, with methionine by mouth provided the overdose has been taken *within 10–12 hours* and the patient is not vomiting). Patients on enzyme-inducing drugs (e.g. carbamazepine, phenobarbital, phenytoin, primidone, rifampicin, alcohol and St John's wort) or who are malnourished (e.g. in anorexia, in alcoholism, or those who are HIV-positive) should be treated if their plasma-paracetamol concentrations are above the *high-risk treatment line*. The prognostic accuracy after 15 hours is uncertain but a plasma-paracetamol concentration above the relevant treatment line should be regarded as carrying a serious risk of liver damage. (Graph reproduced courtesy of University of Wales College of Medicine Therapeutics and Toxicology Centre.)

in clearly defined circumstances and should only be given after the following factors have been taken into account.

Plasma concentrations of paracetamol cannot be interpreted and should not be measured until absorption and distribution are nearly complete, at about 4 hours after ingestion. If treatment is to be effective, it should be started as soon as possible following ingestion. Concentrations should be measured on specimens taken as early as possible, ideally between 4 and 20 hours after ingestion.

Patients taking enzyme-inducing agents such as phenytoin, rifampicin, carbamazepine or alcohol or those who are malnourished, for example because of anorexia or infection with human immunodeficiency virus, are more at risk of paracetamol toxicity. Take serial measurements of plasma transaminase activities (which may rise to 10 000 U/L or more), renal function (as renal failure can develop) and prothrombin time or INR. Prothrombin time or INR is probably the best marker of the severity of liver failure.

Iron overdosage

This is more likely in children, who may mistake the tablets for sweets. Desferrioxamine chelates iron and the chelate is excreted in the urine. Concentrations above 90 µmol/L in young children and above 150 µmol/L in adults are said to be indications for treatment.

Other drugs and substances

The following are some of the other drug and chemical poisonings for which there are specific antidotes.

Benzodiazepines

Respiratory depression, leading to a respiratory acidosis, can occur and measurement of blood gases may therefore be useful. Flumazenil may reverse some of their actions.

Ethylene glycol (antifreeze)

This may cause a metabolic acidosis, renal and hepatic dysfunction and also hypocalcaemia (due to oxalate conversion and calcium chelation as calcium oxalate). Therapeutic ethanol administration may reduce the conversion of this to toxic metabolites by competition with alcohol dehydrogenase.

Cyanide

This can result in lactic acidosis, and measurement of arterial blood gases may be useful. Antidotes include dicobalt edetate, sodium nitrite and sodium thiosulphate, which may protect the blocking of cyanide on the electron transport system in the mitochondria.

Methanol

Renal failure, hypoglycaemia, metabolic acidosis and rhabdomyolysis may occur, as can raised plasma amylase concentration. Ethanol infusion inhibits alcohol dehydrogenase, which converts methanol to toxic formic acid.

Opiates

These can cause respiratory depression leading to a respiratory acidosis. Naloxone may reverse some of the effects of opiates such as morphine or heroin.

Carbon monoxide

Carbon monoxide can cause hypoxia without cyanosis. Carboxyhaemoglobin above 60 per cent can cause respiratory failure and death. Arterial blood gases are important, and a metabolic acidosis may ensue. Oxygen therapy, sometimes hyperbaric, may increase the washout of carboxyhaemoglobin.

Organophosphorous insecticides

Antidotes include cholinesterase inhibitors such as atropine or pralidoxime, with the treatment being monitored using acetyl-cholinesterase activity.

Drugs or poisons for which there is no specific antidote

There are no specific antidotes for the majority of drug overdoses. Salicylate overdose is worth considering in further detail, as it is probably one of the commonest overdoses encountered. Forced diuresis may increase the excretion of salicylate in severe overdose (induction of alkalosis often further increases the excretion rate of acidic drugs), but neither forced diuresis nor induction of alkalosis is without risk. If an alkaline diuresis is induced, plasma potassium concentrations, as well as blood pH, must be monitored because of the danger of acute hypokalaemia.

In adults, a respiratory alkalosis occurs initially, followed by a metabolic acidosis (possibly due to uncoupling of oxidative phosphorylation). Children seem less likely to develop the respiratory alkalosis. Hypokalaemia and either hyperglycaemia or hypoglycaemia may also occur.

Where there is no specific drug antidote, treatment is supportive, although biochemical tests for electrolytes, acid–base balance, renal and hepatic function and blood gases are often useful.

Case 4

A 24-year-old female took an aspirin overdose of about forty 300 mg tablets that she had purchased from the local chemist. The following biochemical results were obtained in the casualty department 8 hours after ingestion.

Plasma
Sodium 140 mmol/L (135–145)
Potassium 5.0 mmol/L (3.5–5.0)
Chloride 100 mmol/L (95–105)
Bicarbonate 20 mmol/L (24–32)
Urea 3.8 mmol/L (2.5–7.5)
Creatinine 104 μmol/L (60–120)
Arterial blood pH 7.55 (7.35–7.45)
$PaCO_2$ 4.0 kPa (4.6–6.0)
PaO_2 12.0 kPa (9.3–13.3)

DISCUSSION
The patient displays a respiratory alkalosis due to the aspirin (salicylate) overdose as it can stimulate the respiratory centre. Aspirin can, however, also result in a metabolic acidosis, particularly in children, which can present with an increased plasma anion gap. Other biochemical changes that may be seen with aspirin overdose are hypoglycaemia or hyperglycaemia and disturbances in liver function tests and electrolytes.

CONCLUSIONS

- The biochemical laboratory plays an important role in the monitoring of the concentrations of some drugs, usually those for which there is a narrow therapeutic window. The common drugs for which this may be useful are the anti-epileptic drugs and some of the cardiac anti-arrhythmic agents, as well as certain antibiotics, lithium and chemotherapy drugs.
- Therapeutic drug monitoring may be useful for detecting patient drug compliance and for observing changes in drug levels if used in combination with other drugs to help avoid drug interaction. Therapeutic drug monitoring can be used to 'tailor' drug dosage to patient needs.
- Drug or substance overdoses are a common cause of hospital admissions, and measuring drug concentrations and biochemical monitoring, for example of renal, liver and acid–base status, can be useful.

26 CLINICAL BIOCHEMISTRY AT THE EXTREMES OF AGE

| Neonates | 355 | Elderly | 366 |

This chapter looks at clinical biochemistry at the extremes of age, i.e. neonates and the elderly.

NEONATES

Some preliminary definitions are useful. A premature or preterm baby is one born before 37 completed weeks' gestation. A neonate is a live baby within 1 month of birth. A low-birth-weight baby is one less than 2.5 kg and a very low-birth-weight baby is one less than 1.5 kg.

One of the most significant advances in recent medical care has been the survival rate of very small premature infants, which has increased because of improved specialized medical and nursing techniques for treating the newborn. However, these infants can experience a number of abnormal biochemical conditions, which are briefly summarized in this chapter.

Diseases occurring during the neonatal period can be divided into two main groups: those of infants born before term, in whom immaturity contributes to the severity of the disease, and those of full-term infants.

The commonest disorders in both groups are perinatal asphyxia, the respiratory distress syndrome (RDS), infection and inborn errors.

Compared with about 5 L in a 70-kg adult, the blood volume of a premature infant weighing 1 kg is only about 90 mL. Therefore only a small amount of blood can be taken without causing volume depletion or anaemia. Sometimes capillary samples are used as an alternative to venous (or arterial) samples, although the former may be more prone to contamination from the interstitial and cellular fluids. Prior to requesting tests on small samples, the clinician should contact the laboratory to discuss the best strategy for obtaining test samples. The interpretation of test results may be influenced by the different reference ranges at different ages, which can be difficult to define.

Renal function

The kidneys usually have a full complement of nephrons by about the 36th week of gestation, but renal function is not fully developed until the age of about 2 years. Glomerular function develops more rapidly than that of the tubules. Fetal urine is produced from about the ninth week.

The glomerular filtration rate (GFR) doubles during the first 2 weeks of life because of an increase in renal blood flow. The GFR (which is related to surface area) reaches adult values by about 6 months of age.

The plasma urea concentration is low in newborn infants compared with that in adults, despite the relatively low GFR; the high anabolic rate results in more nitrogen being incorporated into protein rather than into urea than in adults. Plasma urea concentrations fluctuate markedly with varying nutritional states, metabolic rates and states of hydration.

The plasma creatinine concentration (which is inversely related to GFR) at birth is similar to the mother's. It decreases rapidly at first, averaging about 35 μmol/L, the fall being slower in preterm infants, and then rises before reaching adult values (allowing for the surface area) by about 6 months.

Renal function in newborn infants can maintain basic homeostasis but may not be able to respond adequately to illness or other stresses. It is often difficult to determine if there is renal impairment because of the unsatisfactory nature of renal function tests at this age. A plasma urea concentration above about 8 mmol/L suggests retention due to glomerular impairment, whether parenchymal or pre-renal in origin, especially if the urinary output can be shown to be low. Management depends to a large extent on clinical criteria. In the neonate, neither the plasma urea nor the creatinine concentration is a very sensitive indicator of renal function.

Renal dysfunction in neonates can be due to factors such as hypotension, birth asphyxia, renal toxic drugs, renal agenesis, septicaemia or dehydration or can occur post-surgery.

The daily excretion of urine is about 15–60 mL in full-term newborns, increasing to about 500–600 mL/day at about 1 year (see Chapter 3).

Water

About 80 per cent of the weight of a neonate consists of water, compared with about 60 per cent of that of an adult; the relative amount of water is related more to the proportion of fat to lean tissue than to total body weight. Proportionally, there is probably more water in the extracellular than in the intracellular compartment at birth. During the first week of life, the extracellular fluid compartment contracts; urinary loss may account for the relatively high total amount of sodium excreted by preterm infants and does not necessarily indicate a disturbance in sodium homeostasis.

Renal concentrating capacity is lower in the newborn than in the adult and increases during the first 2 years; the maximum urinary osmolality that can be achieved in response to water deprivation, even if stimulated by exogenous antidiuretic hormone (ADH), is between 500 and 700 mmol/kg. The countercurrent mechanism is relatively inefficient, partly because the loops of Henle do not penetrate as deeply into the renal medulla as in the adult and partly due to the relatively low rate of urea production and therefore excretion. Because reabsorption of urea from the collecting ducts contributes to the interstitial medullary osmolality, so facilitating water reabsorption in response to ADH, renal concentrating ability may rise if urea production is increased when a high-protein diet is given.

'Insensible' water loss is proportionately much higher in infants than in adults because the ratio of surface area to body volume is high, more fluid is lost through the skin because the epidermis is not fully developed before about the 28th week of gestation, there is very little subcutaneous fat, and metabolic and respiratory rates are high.

Insensible transepidermal water loss can increase by up to 50 per cent due to phototherapy or overhead baby warmers – hence the importance of maintaining high ambient humidity.

Daily fluid requirements are therefore up to five times higher per kilogram of body weight than in adults. It is important to pay close attention to this, as high insensible losses can occur, leading to renal and circulatory failure and haemoconcentration and hypernatraemia. The average basal water loss in a neonate is about 20 mL/kg per day (see Chapter 2).

Sodium

The total body sodium content of a newborn infant of 1 kg is less than 100 mmol, compared with about 3000 mmol in the adult. A premature infant may need up to 6 mmol/kg of sodium a day because of the high losses, and a normal full-term infant about 2–4 mmol/kg, compared with about 1.5 mmol/kg in an adult. In preterm infants, plasma renin, aldosterone and angiotensin II concentrations are high.

Renal conservation of sodium is inefficient in premature infants, despite relatively high plasma renin activities and aldosterone concentrations compared with adults, because of immature renal tubular function. Excretion of a sodium load is impaired, perhaps because of the low GFR. Sodium balance should be carefully controlled, bearing in mind the very low total body sodium content at this age.

The total body sodium and the plasma sodium concentrations (and therefore osmolality) may fluctuate because renal function is immature. Sodium excretion declines after birth. Preterm babies may have a failure of sodium tubular reabsorption leading to sodium deficit, particularly if there is low sodium input. The newborn infant, unlike fully conscious children and adults, is unable to make its need for water clear and it may be difficult to assess the requirements accurately. Rapid changes in extracellular osmolality due to inappropriate intake of water cause significant shifts of water between the intracellular and extracellular compartments; signs varying from listlessness to convulsions, or even coma, may be caused by changes in cerebral hydration. The plasma sodium concentration should be monitored to ensure that the proportion of sodium to water is correct.

Hyponatraemia

The following are some of the causes of hyponatraemia.

- *Prolonged maternal infusion of oxytocin* (Syntocinon) or other hypo-osmolal fluid, e.g 5 per cent dextrose, during labour. Oxytocin has an antidiuretic action similar to that of ADH and may cause dilutional hyponatraemia in both mother and infant.
- *Inappropriate ADH secretion*: following postpartum intracranial haemorrhage or meningitis in severe pulmonary disease, such as RDS (hyaline membrane disease) or pneumonia.

- *Infusion of water in excess of sodium to the baby*, either as 5 per cent dextrose or as hypo-osmolal sodium solutions.
- *Acute renal disease*, including acute tubular necrosis, especially if hypo-osmolal fluid is given to a child with glomerular dysfunction.
- *Diuretic treatment*, particularly in premature infants.

Congenital adrenal hyperplasia, adrenal insufficiency, hypothyroidism and cystic fibrosis should always be considered as a possible cause of hyponatraemia at this age.

Clinical signs of hyponatraemia may be associated with hypotension, drowsiness and convulsions.

Hypernatraemia

Hypernatraemia develops if water loss exceeds that of sodium, or if excess of sodium relative to water is infused or fed.

If replacement is inadequate, the high 'insensible' water loss, aggravated by impaired urinary water retention, may cause rapid extracellular fluid depletion with hypotension and, if water depletion is predominant, hypernatraemia. This is particularly likely if 'insensible' loss is increased through the:

- skin – for example due to sweating caused by pyrexia or overhead heaters or to phototherapy for jaundice,
- lungs – if the patient is hyperventilating, for example because of pneumonia,
- intestine – if there is vomiting or diarrhoea.

Iatrogenic causes in infants include giving sodium bicarbonate or excess salt. Neonates are more susceptible than adults to developing hypernatraemia because the addition of a given amount of extra sodium increases the very low extracellular sodium content proportionally more than if it were diluted in a larger pool, as it is in adults; this tendency is aggravated by impaired renal excretion.

Nephrogenic diabetes insipidus is a rare cause of neonatal hypernatraemia.

Potassium

The total body potassium of a newborn infant of 1 kg is less than 100 mmol, compared with about 3000 mmol in an adult. A normal full-term infant requires about 2–4 mmol/kg of potassium a day (compared with about 1 mmol/kg in an adult) to replace losses.

As in the adult, artefactual causes of abnormal plasma potassium concentrations must be excluded. Pseudohyperkalaemia is especially likely if capillary samples are used, because tissue cells may be damaged if the skin is squeezed as in a heel prick. It may also be due to in-vitro haemolysis, or to withdrawal of blood from a cannula through which a potassium solution is being infused. Conversely, pseudohypokalaemia may result if the infused fluid is potassium free.

Hypokalaemia

Hypokalaemia may be caused by increased gastrointestinal loss due to diarrhoea or an alkalosis, e.g pyloric stenosis. In this age group also consider renal tubular acidosis (type I or II). Iatrogenic causes include diuretic use.

Hyperkalaemia

Iatrogenic causes include excess potassium treatment. Other common causes include acute renal failure, exchange transfusion and tissue damage resulting from hypoxia or birth trauma, for example severe bruising or haematoma. Consider also congenital adrenal hyperplasia or adrenal insufficiency (see Chapter 5).

Pulmonary function

Perinatal asphyxia

Renal complications and disturbances of electrolyte balance are more likely to develop in infants with perinatal asphyxia.

Cerebral oedema or haemorrhage may stimulate ADH secretion, causing oliguria and a dilutional hyponatraemia with hypo-osmolality, accompanied by a high urinary sodium concentration due to plasma volume expansion.

The hypotension occurring during asphyxia may reduce renal blood flow enough to cause acute oliguric renal failure (acute tubular necrosis). In addition to the oliguria and hyponatraemia, there may be uraemia and hyperkalaemia, with proteinuria. Hypoglycaemia and hypocalcaemia may also occur.

Fetal pH can be measured during delivery, usually from a capillary sample from the baby's scalp. This may be indicated if changes in cardiotocograph or fetal heart rate indicate fetal distress. A pH value below 7.2 indicates the need for urgent delivery.

Hypoxaemia

Fetal lung fluid production ceases at birth, probably as a result of increases in adrenaline concentration during delivery. Labour squeezes liquid from the mouth, and absorption takes place into the pulmonary lymphatics and capillaries. Type 2 pneumocytes produce surfactant, which serves to reduce lung surface tension, thus facilitating lung expansion. Deficiency of surfactant as in prematurity can cause RDS.

Normal term neonatal arterial P_{O_2} breathing air is about 8–11 kPa. Oxygen therapy can cause toxicity, including bronchopulmonary dysplasia and stiff lungs, and should be closely monitored, for example by transcutaneous gas analysis. Retinopathy of prematurity (previously known as retrolental fibroplasia) may lead to blindness.

Acid–base homeostasis

The plasma bicarbonate concentration is normally about 3 mmol/L lower in newborn infants than in adults. This is due partly to renal immaturity and partly to the low concentration of urinary buffers; both these factors impair bicarbonate 'reabsorption' and regeneration. However, the plasma concentrations must be interpreted with caution, as they are likely to be artefactually low in very small samples. The neonate is more vulnerable to acid–base disturbances (for further discussion see Chapter 4). The specific conditions that affect neonates are discussed here.

Metabolic acidosis

The causes of metabolic acidosis include the following.

- Renal dysfunction.
- Lactic acidosis due to:
  - tissue hypoxia resulting from poor tissue perfusion caused by hypotension and the low P_{O_2} accompanying asphyxia or sepsis,
  - some inborn errors of metabolism, such as glucose-6-phosphatase deficiency.
- Inborn errors of amino acid or organic acid metabolism (see Chapter 27).

Also consider:

- congenital heart disease and patent ductus arteriosus,
- acute blood loss.

Metabolic alkalosis

This can result from pyloric stenosis, with which projectile vomiting can occur. This is associated with hypokalaemic alkalosis.

Respiratory acidosis

Respiratory distress may be caused by pulmonary disorders such as RDS, pneumonia and meconium aspiration during birth.

The commonest cause in the preterm infant is the RDS, the incidence of which is inversely related to the gestational age of the infant at birth. Respiratory distress syndrome is due to immaturity of the enzymes responsible for the intrauterine synthesis of pulmonary surfactant, which maintains the patency of the alveoli. Surfactant synthesis begins at about the 20th week of gestation and increases rapidly after about the 34th week following maturation of the alveolar cells. Surfactant deficiency is commoner in male infants, those of diabetic mothers and those with asphyxia and hypothermia.

The condition presents with pulmonary collapse (atelectasis), with secondary lung infections being common. The blood P_{CO_2} is high, causing respiratory acidosis. The low blood P_{O_2} and reduced blood flow due to hypotension cause tissue hypoxia with lactic acidosis; renal dysfunction may aggravate the metabolic acidosis. The combination of respiratory and metabolic components may cause severe acidosis.

An infant with respiratory distress syndrome may benefit from the administration of surfactant, given through an endotracheal tube, and from positive-pressure ventilation, which help to expand the lungs and correct blood gas abnormalities. If these treatments are successful, the improved general condition increases tissue perfusion, correcting the lactic acidosis and improving renal function.

The P_{O_2} and P_{CO_2} of cutaneous capillary blood can be monitored continuously using electrodes placed on the skin. The electrodes bring the capillary P_{O_2} and P_{CO_2} to near arterial levels by heating the skin to about 44 °C, thus increasing cutaneous blood flow. The electrodes must be repositioned every 4 hours to prevent local burns and need to be recalibrated frequently. *Transcutaneous blood gas monitoring supplements, but does not replace, arterial blood gas analysis* (see Chapter 4).

Respiratory alkalosis

The conditions associated with a respiratory alkalosis that occur in neonates include septicaemia, meningitis, hyperammoniaemia and hepatic failure.

Gastrointestinal tract

The fetal gastrointestinal tract has limited functional development before 26 weeks. This helps to explain why premature babies may have poor tolerance of enteral feeding. Lactose may be poorly absorbed within the first week of life.

Liver

The metabolism of the neonatal liver is initially slower than in adults. As will now be seen, this is important with regard to neonatal bilirubin metabolism, particularly that of conjugation.

Plasma transaminase activities are up to twice the upper limit of the adult reference range during the first 3 months of life and fall to adult levels by the age of about 1 year. The plasma total alkaline phosphatase activity is higher in infancy and during childhood because of the contribution from actively growing bone; it falls to adult levels after the pubertal growth spurt.

Bilirubin metabolism

Neonatal abnormalities of bilirubin metabolism are discussed here (see Chapter 17 for further details).

Unconjugated hyperbilirubinaemia

Proportionally more unconjugated bilirubin reaches the liver in the newborn infant than in the adult, for the following reasons.

- Delayed clamping of the umbilical cord may significantly increase red cell mass.
- Bruises may occur during birth, and resorption of haemoglobin breakdown products from these increases the plasma bilirubin concentration. A cephalo-haematoma can release large amounts of bilirubin.
- The red cell half-life is shorter; the blood haemoglobin concentration falls rapidly during the first week of life, even in normal infants.

The mature liver can conjugate very large amounts of bilirubin and, due to increased bilirubin production, jaundice is rarely severe in adults. In the newborn, even at term, the conjugating process is not fully developed.

Physiological jaundice (unconjugated hyperbilirubinaemia) is defined as mild jaundice which is not present at birth but which develops during the first few days and continues during the first 10 days of life, and for which there is no obvious pathological reason. Such jaundice is very common in normal newborn infants (about 50 per cent of normal babies develop this after 48 hours), the incidence being inversely related to the gestational age at birth. The plasma total bilirubin rarely exceeds 200 µmol/L, with the conjugated bilirubin unlikely to be greater than 40 µmol/L.

Physiological jaundice can be aggravated by prematurity, infections, dehydration, hypoxia and poor nutrition, to name but a few.

Plasma unconjugated bilirubin concentrations may be very high in premature infants because of hepatic immaturity. If the bilirubin concentration exceeds the albumin-binding capacity, the unbound, fat-soluble unconjugated bilirubin may cross cell membranes and be deposited in the brain, causing kernicterus. This is a serious complication, which may result in permanent brain damage or death.

The risk of kernicterus is increased:

- the more premature the infant;
- if the plasma unconjugated bilirubin concentration is rising rapidly, perhaps due to haemolysis;
- if the bilirubin-binding capacity is low, due to:
  - hypoalbuminaemia,
  - displacement of bilirubin from albumin by some drugs;
  - displacement of bilirubin from albumin by hydrogen ions in acidosis due to hypoxia or other serious illness.

CASE 1

A term infant was jaundiced and his plasma bilirubin concentration was 182 µmol/L 2 days after delivery. Further testing showed that this was predominantly unconjugated bilirubin (176 µmol/L). The baby was otherwise well, and within 5 days the plasma bilirubin concentration decreased to 36 µmol/L (<20).

DISCUSSION

The jaundice was attributed to physiological jaundice of the newborn. This is the most likely explanation given the only moderate elevation of bilirubin concentration that presented 2 days after delivery. The bilirubin was predominantly unconjugated due to 'immaturity' of the glucuronyltransferase system in some infants that is responsible for conjugation of bilirubin.

Jaundice during the first 24 hours of life is more likely to be pathological than physiological. It may have the following causes.

- Maternofetal rhesus or ABO blood group incompatibility: this is particularly likely in infants born to multiparous mothers, who may have developed antibodies during previous pregnancies.
- Inherited erythrocyte abnormalities associated with haemolysis, such as glucose-6-phosphate dehydrogenase deficiency, pyruvate kinase deficiency or hereditary spherocytosis. The first of these is X-linked and more common in people of Mediterranean or African origin.
- Intrauterine infections that affect the liver, such as syphilis, rubella or toxoplasmosis.

Bilirubin should be measured in blood taken from the umbilical cord of all infants known to be at risk for one of the above reasons; blood group typing and Coombs' testing for red cell antibodies can also be performed on cord blood.

Management

If the plasma bilirubin concentration is rising rapidly or exceeds about 340 μmol/L in full-term infants, exchange transfusion may be needed. This 'action level' may be significantly lower in the preterm infant. Biochemical complications of exchange transfusions are usually due to the anticoagulant used in the infused blood, and are transitory. They include hyperkalaemia, hypocalcaemia, metabolic acidosis and hypoglycaemia.

Bilirubin is destroyed by ultraviolet light and lesser degrees of unconjugated hyperbilirubinaemia may be treated by phototherapy. Water loss from the skin may be high and fluid balance must be carefully monitored. There are action charts available that help with treatment decisions based on hours after birth and the plasma bilirubin concentration.

Prolonged unconjugated hyperbilirubinaemia, i.e. persisting beyond 10 days in a term baby, not in itself requiring treatment, may accompany chronic infections, such as with cytomegalovirus, or hypothyroidism. It is more common in breast-fed infants than in those given formula, possibly because a factor(s) in maternal milk inhibit uridine-diphosphate-glucuronyltransferase activity. (See Chapter 17.)

Conjugated hyperbilirubinaemia

Impaired excretion of bilirubin that has been conjugated in hepatocytes may be due to the following.

- *Congenital biliary atresia* (Byler's disease): it is important to make this diagnosis early because some forms may be amenable to surgical treatment. The stools are usually pale and there is increased urinary bilirubin concentration with abnormal liver function tests. Biliary tree ultrasound and radioisotope scans together with liver biopsy can aid diagnosis. Early surgery by the Kasai hepato-portoenterostomy procedure may be life saving.
- *Biliary obstruction* caused by pressure on the bile ducts by, for example, extrabiliary tumours, although this is a rare cause in children. Alagille's syndrome is a very rare condition associated with decreased intrahepatic bile ducts, congenital cardiac defects and facial dysmorphism.

Neonatal hepatitis rarely presents clinically until after the first week of life. Its causes include intrauterine infection, such as syphilis, toxoplasmosis, cytomegalovirus infection, hepatitis A or B and rubella.

Metabolic causes of jaundice include galactosaemia and α_1-antitrypsin deficiency. It may also be associated with parenteral nutrition.

Other inherited abnormalities associated with jaundice include the Dubin–Johnson syndrome.

Investigation of jaundice in the newborn period

- Neonatal jaundice should be investigated if:
  - it is present on the first day of life,
  - it is prolonged beyond 10 days of age,
  - it is severe, for example plasma bilirubin greater than 300 μmol/L,
  - conjugated bilirubin concentration is raised (Table 26.1).

Table 26.1 Some causes of prolonged neonatal jaundice

Unconjugated	Conjugated
Breast-feeding	Biliary atresia
Infection	Total parenteral nutrition
Rhesus/ABO iso-immunization	Alagille syndrome
Crigler–Najjar syndrome	Alpha$_1$-antitrypsin deficiency
Hypothyroidism	Tyrosinaemia
Haemolysis, e.g. glucose-6-phosphatase deficiency	Galactosaemia deficiency
	Cystic fibrosis
	Zellweger's syndrome
	Hepatitis
	Dubin–Johnson syndrome

- Plasma bilirubin concentration should be quantitated and separated into unconjugated and conjugated fractions. Liver function tests, urinary bilirubin and stool colour should be checked.
- Consideration should also be given to any medications that might be implicated in the jaundice or whether the neonate is on parenteral nutrition.
- Neonatal infection and congenital hypothyroidism should be excluded as causes of the jaundice.
- If unconjugated bilirubin predominates, the blood film and reticulocytes should be checked and a Coombs' test performed; these are useful to exclude haemolysis.
- Remember also that unconjugated hyperbilirubinaemia can be seen in breast-milk jaundice.
- In cases of severe unconjugated bilirubinaemia, the Crigler–Najjar syndrome should be considered.
- If conjugated bilirubin predominates, it is important to exclude liver disease, including hepatitis.
- Depending on the clinical findings, if liver function is found to be abnormal, various biochemical tests may be indicated in an inborn error of metabolism such as plasma α_1-antitrypsin deficiency, plasma and urinary amino acids. Exclude galactosaemia (see Chapter 27). Liver ultrasound may also be useful.
- It is important that biliary atresia is excluded, for example with imaging techniques.
- In the presence of conjugated hyperbilirubinaemia and normal liver function tests, the Dubin–Johnson or Rotor syndrome should be considered.

Glucose metabolism and hypoglycaemia

The newborn

Causes of hypoglycaemia in the newborn period (and, for completeness, also in childhood) are shown in Box 26.1. Hepatic glycogen stores increase about threefold and adipose tissue (another source of energy) is laid down during the last 10 weeks of pregnancy. Very premature infants therefore have little liver glycogen and adipose tissue and are especially prone to hypoglycaemia. Full-term infants may become hypoglycaemic if initially adequate stores are drawn on more rapidly than normal, for example during perinatal asphyxia. Infants at greater risk of hypoglycaemia include those with infections, asphyxia, Rhesus haemolytic disease and exchange transfusion, those that are small for dates and those born to diabetic mothers.

Plasma glucose concentrations as low as 1.7 mmol/L during the first 72 hours of life in the premature infant,

> **Box 26.1 Some causes of neonatal and childhood hypoglycaemia**
>
> *Reduced production of glucose*
> 'Small for dates' baby
> Prematurity
> Birth asphyxia
> Sepsis
> Poor nutrition
> Hypothermia
> Congenital heart disease
>
> *Inborn errors of metabolism*
> Glycogen storage disease, e.g. type 1
> Organic acidurias
> Disorders of fat oxidation, e.g. medium chain acyl coenzyme a dehydrogenase deficiency
> Disorders of gluconeogenesis, e.g. pyruvate carboxylase deficiency
> Galactosaemia and hereditary fructose intolerance
> Carnitine deficiency
> Amino acid disorders, e.g. tyrosinaemia
> Ketotic hypoglycaemia of infancy
> Leucine sensitivity
>
> *Hyperinsulinaemia*
> Maternal diabetes
> Nesidioblastosis
> Beckwith–Wiedemann syndrome
> Insulinoma
> Erythroblastosis fetalis
>
> *Hormone deficiencies*
> Hypothyroidism
> Hypopituitarism
> Adrenal insufficiency
> Congenital adrenal hyperplasia

or 2.0 mmol/L during the later neonatal period, may not be associated with any clinical signs. When clinical features do occur they include tremors, apnoeic attacks and convulsions. However, impaired neurological development has been reported in full-term infants in whom the plasma glucose concentration repeatedly fell to below 2.0 mmol/L despite the absence of clinical signs. It has been recommended that the plasma glucose concentration be maintained above 2.0 mmol/L in at-risk patients.

If a baby has hypoglycaemia and is asymptomatic, milk feeds are usually given until blood glucose levels are above 2.0 mmol/L. However, in the presence of symptoms of hypoglycaemia, intravenous 10 per cent dextrose (glucose) may need to be given. Nesidioblastosis is due to overgrowth of insulin-producing beta cells in the pancreas and presents with severe hypoglycaemia and hyperinsulinaemia. Beckwith–Wiedemann syndrome is due to a short-arm deletion of chromosome 11 and is associated with hypoglycaemia, visceromegaly, exomphalos and mental retardation.

Hypoglycaemia determined by near-patient glucose tests *must* be confirmed by proper laboratory testing in a fluoride sample. Lack of ketonuria in the presence of hypoglycaemia implies hyperinsulinaemia or a defect of fat oxidation.

The babies of diabetic mothers tend to be large, jaundiced and hypocalcaemic and to have lung immaturity and congenital defects. Neonatal hypoglycaemia is related to the degree of maternal glycaemic control.

Early infancy

Soon after birth, or the introduction of milk to the diet, hypoglycaemia may be due to one of the following causes.

Glycogenoses or glycogen storage disorders

A deficiency of one of the enzymes involved in glycogenesis or glycogenolysis results in the accumulation of normal or abnormal glycogen with hepatomegaly. In von Gierke's disease, the least rare glycogen storage disorder, there is a deficiency of glucose-6-phosphatase. Fasting hypoglycaemia occurs because the enzyme is essential for the conversion of glucose-6-phosphate (G-6-P) to glucose. There may also be ketosis and endogenous hypertriglyceridaemia due to excessive lipolysis caused by low insulin activity, lactic acidosis due to excessive anaerobic glycolysis, and hyperuricaemia.

The diagnosis is made either directly, by demonstrating the absence of the enzyme in a liver biopsy specimen, or indirectly, by demonstrating failure of plasma glucose concentrations to rise after giving glucagon to stimulate glycogenolysis. Infusion of galactose or fructose, which are normally converted to glucose via G-6-P, also fails to increase plasma glucose concentrations because G-6-P cannot be converted to glucose.

Treatment involves giving frequent meals to maintain normal plasma glucose levels and so prevent cerebral damage.

Hereditary fructose intolerance

This is a rare cause of hypoglycaemia. It is due to deficiency of fructose-1-phosphate aldolase. The accumulation of fructose-1-phosphate in several tissues causes many of the clinical features; hypoglycaemia may be due to the inhibition of glycogenolysis and gluconeogenesis. Symptoms only present after sucrose-containing (fructose and glucose) and fructose-containing fruit or fruit drinks have been introduced into the diet. Hypoglycaemia, with nausea, vomiting and abdominal pain, and fructosuria follow about 30 minutes after fructose ingestion or intravenous infusion; this can be used as a diagnostic test. The infant fails to thrive. Liver accumulation of fructose-1-phosphate causes hepatomegaly with jaundice; this may progress to cirrhosis with ascites.

Later infancy

Idiopathic hypoglycaemia of infancy

The diagnosis of this condition is made by excluding other causes of hypoglycaemia. Symptoms usually develop after fasting or a febrile illness. Brain damage is a risk. In some cases there is excessive insulin secretion and it may not be possible to differentiate this condition from an insulinoma. Islet cell hyperplasia (nesidioblastosis or endogenous-persistent hyperinsulinaemic hypoglycaemia of infancy) is a difficult diagnosis to make and is an uncommon cause of hypoglycaemia occurring before the age of 3 years.

During the second year of life, hypoglycaemia associated with ketosis may also develop after fasting or a febrile illness (ketotic hypoglycaemia). These children were usually 'small for dates' at birth.

Adult causes of hypoglycaemia, including insulinoma, must always be considered in the differential diagnosis.

Leucine sensitivity

There is often a familial incidence of leucine sensitivity. During the first 6 months of life, casein (present in milk) may cause severe hypoglycaemia due to its high leucine content. Leucine sensitivity is probably due to the stimulation of insulin secretion by the amino acid. The condition appears to be self-limiting and does not usually persist beyond the age of 6 years. The diagnosis is confirmed by demonstrating hypoglycaemia within 30 minutes after an oral dose of leucine or casein. Normal subjects do not respond to leucine with a significant fall in plasma glucose concentration, but a number of patients with insulinoma are leucine sensitive.

Treatment involves giving a diet low in leucine-containing food.

Other causes of hypoglycaemia in childhood are shown in Box 26.1 and discussed in Chapter 12.

Calcium, phosphate and magnesium metabolism

Calcium metabolism in adults is discussed in Chapter 6.

Calcium and phosphate are actively transported across the placenta; total and free ionized calcium concentrations are higher in fetal than in maternal plasma. 25-hydroxycholecalciferol, but not its active metabolite 1,25-dihydroxycholecalciferol or parathyroid hormone (PTH), can pass placental membranes. Calcium and phosphate accumulate rapidly only between the 30th and 36th week of fetal life; therefore, a very premature infant may become calcium and phosphate deficient when feeds are not supplemented.

During intrauterine life, the relatively high maternally derived fetal plasma free ionized calcium concentration suppresses PTH release from the fetus's own parathyroid glands. Fetal plasma calcium concentration is usually higher than in the mother due to active calcium transport across the placenta. The glands may take time to recover after birth and there may be transient hypoparathyroidism. Plasma total and free ionized calcium concentrations fall by up to 30 per cent immediately after birth, but, in the normal infant, spontaneously regain adult concentrations within about 3 days; this fall rarely needs to be treated.

The reference range for plasma total calcium concentration in the newborn period is wider than that for adults. Plasma phosphate concentrations are higher in actively growing infants and in children compared with adults, as is the concentration of plasma alkaline phosphatase.

Neonatal hypocalcaemia

Hypocalcaemia during the first 2 weeks of life can be divided into two groups (Box 26.2).

Hypocalcaemia of early onset occurs during the first 3 days of life and is commonest:

- in low-birth-weight, preterm infants, for the reasons given above,
- following perinatal asphyxia,
- in the infants of diabetic mothers.

It may also occur if the mother was hypercalcaemic during pregnancy, for example due to primary hyperparathyroidism; the maternal hypercalcaemia is reflected in the fetus, and the suppressed fetal parathyroid glands may take some time to recover. This condition is a more severe form of the 'physiological' condition described above.

Box 26.2 Some causes of neonatal hypocalcaemia

Physiological
Birth asphyxia
Diabetic mother
Prematurity
Small birth weight

Non-physiological
Low calcium or high phosphate intake
Exchange transfusion
Vitamin D deficiency
Renal or hepatic disease
Hypoparathyroidism
Pseudohypoparathyroidism
Hypomagnesaemia
Organic acidurias
Maternal hyperparathyroidism or vitamin D deficiency

CASE 2

A preterm baby was born at 28 weeks weighing only 900 g. The following biochemical results were obtained.

Plasma
Sodium 137 mmol/L (135–145)
Potassium 5.0 mmol/L (3.5–5.0)
Urea 1.7 mmol/L (2.5–7.0)
Creatinine 60 μmol/L (70–110)
Albumin 35 g/L (35–45)
'Corrected' calcium 1.80 mmol/L (2.15–2.55)
Phosphate 1.6 mmol/L (0.80–1.35)
Bilirubin 159 μmol/L (<20)
Glucose 1.6 mmol/L (3.5–5.5)

DISCUSSION
The results show hypocalcaemia and hypoglycaemia, which are sometimes seen in severe prematurity, although other causes may need to be excluded. Premature neonates may also show renal, liver and acid–base abnormalities. The baby here was also jaundiced (note the raised plasma bilirubin concentration).

Prolonged hypocalcaemia persisting beyond 3 days needs investigating.

Hypocalcaemia of late onset is less common. It usually followed the use of high-phosphate-containing feeds, such as unmodified cows' milk formulas, which are less used nowadays.

Primary hypoparathyroidism in neonates is rare but can be inherited, including an X-linked form. Maternal hyperparathyroidism may suppress neonatal PTH, evoking hypocalcaemia. There is also a rare transient form of hypoparathyroidism presenting up to a year of age. Di George's syndrome is a disorder in which hypoparathyroidism is associated with cardiac defects, thymic aplasia and immunodeficiency.

Rickets of prematurity

Bone demineralization (osteopenia) is common in small preterm infants and often resolves spontaneously before obvious clinical features of rickets develop. The plasma alkaline phosphatase activity may rise to more than six times the upper adult reference limit; the plasma calcium concentrations are usually low-normal and those of phosphate are low.

Rickets of prematurity usually becomes clinically evident between the fourth and 12th weeks of life, and occurs more commonly in very premature, low-birth-weight infants than in infants of older gestational age at birth. Longitudinal growth slows, and the decalcification of the bones predisposes to pathological fractures; in severe cases, respiration is impaired by the soft ribs.

X-ray changes may be minimal or absent in early cases. In more advanced disease, the classical radiological changes appear at the ends of long bones.

Rickets of prematurity may be due to the following.

- *Calcium and phosphate depletion*: if an infant is born prematurely, unsupplemented breast-milk may not contain enough of these minerals to replace that which should have accumulated in utero during the last 10 weeks of gestation.

  Phosphate depletion is probably the commonest cause and is indicated by a very low plasma phosphate concentration, compared with the appropriate reference range, and low urinary phosphate excretion.
- *Maternal vitamin D deficiency during pregnancy or in the infant after birth*: in very premature infants, such deficiency may be due to low activity of the renal 1α-hydroxylase needed to convert 25-hydroxyvitamin D to the active 1,25-dihydroxyvitamin D.
- *Drugs*, such as furosemide, which increase urinary calcium loss.
- *Renal tubular disorders of phosphate reabsorption*, which may cause phosphate depletion: in such cases the plasma calcium concentration is usually normal, but may even be high because the calcium cannot be deposited in bone without phosphate.

Treatment

Vitamin D and calcium and phosphate supplementation may be monitored by measuring serial plasma alkaline phosphatase activities. Despite successful treatment, these may continue to rise for several weeks, when bone is being actively laid down, before falling once the bone is adequately calcified.

Hypercalcaemia in the newborn period

Hypercalcaemia is less common than hypocalcaemia at this age. It may be associated with phosphate depletion and hypophosphataemia because calcium cannot be deposited in bone without phosphate and because hypophosphataemia enhances 1α-hydroxylase activity and therefore the formation of the active vitamin D metabolite. After treatment with phosphorus, the plasma calcium concentration may fall rapidly enough to cause clinical symptoms.

Idiopathic hypercalcaemia may occur in full-term infants receiving inappropriately high-dose vitamin D prophylaxis. Other conditions include vitamin D excess, familial hypocalciuric hypercalcaemia and Williams' syndrome. The last-mentioned is associated with mental retardation, 'elfin' facies and cardiac defects.

Magnesium

Hypomagnesaemia often accompanies hypocalcaemia and may be caused by dietary deficiency or by increased intestinal or urinary loss. Low plasma magnesium concentrations may impair the release and action of PTH and so delay correction of plasma calcium concentrations. Hypomagnesaemia should be considered if the infant has convulsions despite normocalcaemia.

Plasma proteins

At birth, the relative concentrations of individual plasma proteins differ from those found in adults. The concentration of total protein is about 12 g/L lower than in adults, but that of albumin is only slightly lower; as always, the latter may fall during illness. The acute-phase proteins (reflected in the α-globulins and β-globulins in the electrophoretic pattern) reach adult concentrations by about 6 months, but are affected by illness, again as they are in adults.

The immunoglobulin pattern differs significantly from that of adults. During normal pregnancy, placental transfer of maternal immunoglobulin G (IgG) leads to a gradual increase in fetal plasma concentrations of this immunoglobulin. After birth, maternally derived IgG is degraded and endogenous immunoglobulin synthesis starts. Adult concentrations of plasma IgM are reached by about 9 months, of IgG by between 3 and 5 years, and of IgA by the age of 15.

Measurement of plasma immunoglobulin concentrations may be indicated if an immune-deficiency state, whether primary, secondary or transient, is suspected. It may also help to detect infection, whether it occurred during the intrauterine period or has developed after birth. Results must be compared with age-matched reference ranges, allowance being made for both the time since conception (gestational age) and age since birth (postnatal age).

A high plasma IgM concentration in blood obtained from the umbilical cord, or within the first 4 weeks of life, may indicate intrauterine or neonatal infections such as syphilis, rubella, toxoplasmosis or cytomegalovirus infection. Allowance must be made for the normal rise in plasma IgM that starts after about 6 weeks of postnatal age.

Specific inborn errors, such as α_1-antitrypsin deficiency, may be diagnosed by measuring the appropriate plasma protein.

Hyperammonaemia

In term neonates and infants, plasma ammonia should be less than 100 μmol/L, and less than 200 μmol/L in preterm neonates. Clinical features of hyperammonaemia include seizures, coma, lethargy and respiratory alkalosis. Plasma ammonia should be assayed in fresh samples collected in heparin.

Sepsis (including urinary tract infections), cardiac failure and certain tumours can result in hyperammonaemia, as can valproate treatment. Acute hepatic failure or chronic liver disease can also evoke hyperammonaemia, as the liver is an important deaminating organ; Reye's syndrome is also associated. This is thought to be due to a mitochondrial disorder leading to fatty liver degeneration and acute encepalopathy.

The urea cycle disorders may also present with severe hyperammonaemia and, if urinary organic acid concentrations are raised, this is suggestive of an organic aciduria (see Chapter 27). The plasma amino acid pattern may give clues as to the amino acid disorder causing the hyperammonaemia, such as arginaemia, citrullinaemia, 3H syndrome and arginosuccinic aciduria. Inborn errors of metabolism are covered in more detail in Chapter 27.

Thyroid function

Immediately after birth, plasma thyroid-stimulating hormone (TSH) concentrations rise rapidly, probably in response to the stress of birth, to about 15 times the upper adult reference limit. They reach a peak within the first hour, before falling, rapidly at first, during the next week. Plasma total thyroxine concentrations peak within the first 24–48 hours and then fall gradually (Fig. 26.1).

Most laboratories in the UK screen with TSH alone, using a heel prick sample, although this may miss the even rarer cases of secondary hypothyroidism. Screening tests for neonatal congenital hypothyroidism should be delayed for about a week after birth to allow the plasma TSH concentration to stabilize. In premature babies TSH may not increase after birth and thus give false negative results; therefore, testing should be repeated when they are equivalent to 40 weeks.

About 1 in 3500 neonates have congenital hypothyroidism, with most cases being due to thyroid dysgenesis and about 10 per cent resulting from dyshormonogenesis. Thyroid function tests should be repeated in infants found to have a positive screening test at a week after birth; if the diagnosis is confirmed, thyroid replacement should be started immediately. Thyroid function should be reassessed, after the withdrawal of treatment, at the age of 1 year because neonatal hypothyroidism is sometimes transient.

Hypothyroidism may be suspected clinically, for example because of failure to thrive or persistent jaundice.

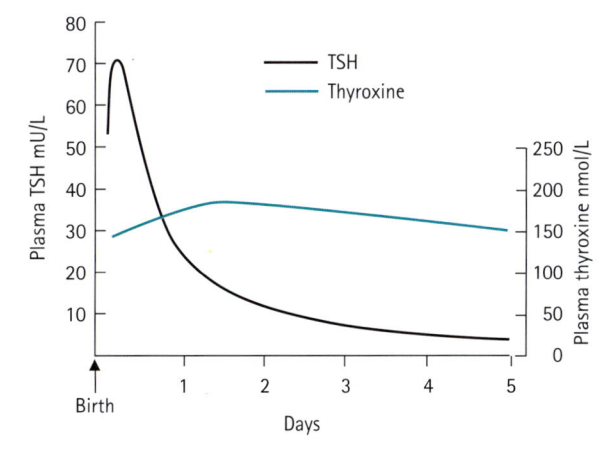

Fig. 26.1 Thyroid function in the newborn infant. (TSH = thyroid-stimulating hormone.)

(See also Chapter 11 for discussion of thyroid disease.) Neonatal screening is discussed further in Chapter 27.

ELDERLY

Within the next 50 years or so, about a quarter of the world's population will be over the age of 65 years.

Just as in the neonate, it is important to understand the biochemical changes that occur with age when it comes to interpreting chemical pathology results in the elderly.

First, it is pertinent to realize that multiple pathologies are sometimes present in the elderly. In addition, they may well be on numerous medications, and therefore drug interactions are more likely.

Some diseases are more common in the elderly, including type 2 diabetes mellitus, Paget's disease, osteoporosis, renal impairment, thyroid disease and certain tumours. Multiple myeloma is far more prevalent as age increases as in other malignant disease.

The increased morbidity and mortality of the elderly are not helped by the fact that nutritional disorders are also more common. Some elderly people, particularly if on low incomes, may have poor diets, and deficiency states have been described, including osteomalacia and scurvy.

Cardiovascular disease

Ischaemic heart disease and cerebrovascular disease constitute the major causes of death in the elderly and their risk increases with age. Plasma cholesterol concentration also increases with age, although there may be a decline in those over the age of 75 years.

Renal function

Renal function deteriorates with age, and over the age of 70 years, plasma creatinine concentration may be about 130 μmol/L and creatinine clearance 80–90 mL/min. This is important to remember when it comes to prescribing medications that are dependent on renal excretion (see Chapter 3).

Diabetes mellitus

This is more common in the elderly, in whom it is usually type 2. Generally, glucose intolerance increases with age (see Chapter 12).

Thyroid disease

Abnormalities of thyroid function also increase with age; both hyperthyroidism and hypothyroidism are more common in the elderly. The former is more likely to be associated with atrial fibrillation and the latter with hypothermia. Because of the increased likelihood of disease in the elderly, sick euthyroidism is also more common (see Chapter 11).

The pituitary gland diminishes in size in the elderly. Microadenomas are more likely, as is growth hormone deficiency.

CASE 3

An 83-year-old woman was seen by her general practitioner because of increasing confusion. She was known to have congestive cardiac failure, hypertension, diabetes mellitus, osteoporosis and diverticular disease. She was taking ten different medications. Some of her biochemical results were as follows.

Plasma
Sodium 135 mmol/L (135–145)
Potassium 5.1 mmol/L (3.5–5.0)
Urea 9.7 mmol/L (2.5–7.0)
Creatinine 136 μmol/L (70–110)
Albumin 36 g/L (35–45)
Corrected calcium 1.90 mmol/L (2.15–2.55)
Phosphate 0.68 mmol/L (0.80–1.35)

Glucose 12.6 mmol/L (3.5–5.5)
Thyroid-stimulating hormone 11.9 mU/L (0.2–5.0)
Free thyroxine 8.5 pmol/L (12–25)

DISCUSSION
The patient was subsequently shown to have had a cerebrovascular accident. Her biochemical tests suggest hypothyroidism, hypocalcaemia (found to be due to osteomalacia) and impaired renal function. The elderly may present with multiple pathologies. Renal function declines with age. Type 2 diabetes mellitus is also relatively common in the elderly. Another clinical problem is 'poly-pharmacy', with some elderly patients being treated with multiple drugs for multiple conditions and therefore running the risk of dangerous drug interactions.

Gonadal disorders

The female menopause occurs at about the age of 51 years and is associated with decreased plasma oestrogen and raised luteinizing hormone and follicle-stimulating hormone concentrations. The use of hormone replacement therapy is controversial. Gonadal decline is more variable in the male, as fertility may continue into the seventies and beyond, when plasma testosterone concentration may be reduced.

Bone disease

The most common bone disorder is osteoporosis (see Chapter 6). The reason is multifactorial, but includes decreasing endocrine function, including reduced oestrogen and testosterone, as well as nutritional factors. Paget's disease is also more prevalent and partly accounts for the higher plasma alkaline phosphatase activities found in this age group. Additionally, osteomalacia is increased due to vitamin D deficiency.

Dementia

About 10 per cent of people over the age of 65 years have dementia. This can be defined as a decline in global cognition in clear consciousness. It may be due to many factors, although the most common causes are vascular and Alzheimer's disease. It is essential to exclude treatable causes such as hypothyroidism, infection and nutritional deficiencies.

Potentially useful laboratory tests include full blood count, plasma folate and vitamin B_{12}, plasma glucose, thyroid function tests, liver and renal function tests, plasma calcium, syphilis screen and paraprotein screen.

CONCLUSIONS

- Neonates show a number of biochemical features that are different from those found in adults.
- Unconjugated hyperbilirubinaemia can be physiological in neonates, but severely raised plasma bilirubin concentration (more than 350 μmol/L approximately) can result in kernicterus associated with neurological damage.
- Premature neonates may present with hypocalcaemia, jaundice, hypoglycaemia and renal, hepatic and acid–base disorders.
- The elderly may present with multiple pathologies. Renal function declines with age. Type 2 diabetes mellitus is also relatively common in the elderly. Another clinical problem is 'poly-pharmacy', with many elderly people being treated with multiple drugs for multiple conditions, which runs the risk of drug interaction.

27 INBORN ERRORS OF METABOLISM

Some metabolic consequences of genetic defects	368	When to suspect an inborn error of metabolism	369
Clinical importance of inborn errors of metabolism	369	Principles of treatment of inborn errors of metabolism	370
Neonatal screening	369	Diseases due to inborn errors of metabolism	371
Prenatal screening	369		

The inherited characteristics of an individual are determined by about 50 000 gene pairs, arranged on 23 pairs of chromosomes, one of each pair coming from the father and one from the mother. Genotype diversity is introduced by random selection and recombination during meiosis, as well as by occasional mutation. These genetic variants may at one extreme be incompatible with life, or at the other produce biochemical differences detectable only by special techniques, if at all. Between the two extremes there are many variations that produce functional abnormalities or inborn errors of metabolism (IEM). Incidences of IEM range from about 1 in 100 to 1 in 200 000, depending on the disorder and the population involved. (See Chapter 28.)

SOME METABOLIC CONSEQUENCES OF GENETIC DEFECTS

Inherited inborn disorders may involve any peptide or protein, and are usually most obvious if there is an enzyme abnormality. Deficiency of a single enzyme in a metabolic pathway may produce its effects in several ways.

Suppose that substance A is acted on by enzyme X to produce substance B, and that substance C is on an alternative pathway (Fig. 27.1). A deficiency of X may cause:

- deficiency of the product (B) of the enzyme reaction, for example cortisol deficiency in congenital adrenal hyperplasia;

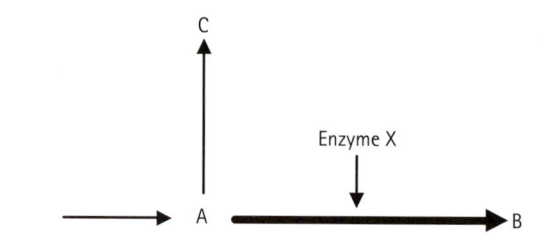

Fig. 27.1 Metabolic consequences of genetic defects.

- accumulation of the substance (A) acted on by the enzyme, for example phenylalanine in phenylketonuria (PKU);
- diversion through an alternative pathway: some product(s) of the latter (C) may accumulate and produce effects, for example congenital adrenal hyperplasia when accumulation of androgens causes virilization.

The effects of the last two types of abnormality will be aggravated if the whole metabolic pathway is controlled by negative feedback from the final product. For example, in congenital adrenal hyperplasia, cortisol deficiency reduces negative feedback, thereby increasing the rate of steroid synthesis and therefore the accumulation of androgens, causing virilization in the female (see Chapter 8).

The clinical effects of some IEM may be modified by, or depend entirely on, physiological or environmental factors. For example, iron loss occurs during menstruation and pregnancy; women with hereditary haemochromatosis accumulate iron less rapidly than men with the same condition and they rarely present with clinical features before the menopause (see Chapter 21). Patients with cholinesterase variants develop symptoms only if the muscle relaxant suxamethonium is given (see Chapter 18).

CLINICAL IMPORTANCE OF INBORN ERRORS OF METABOLISM

Some inborn errors are probably harmless. However, they are important because they produce effects that may lead to misdiagnosis, for example renal glycosuria and Gilbert's disease. In others, it is important to make a diagnosis, even though no effective treatment is yet available.

There is a group of diseases for which recognition in early infancy is of great importance because treatment may prevent irreversible clinical consequences or death. Some of the more important of these are PKU, galactosaemia and maple syrup urine disease.

NEONATAL SCREENING

Many countries have instituted programmes for screening all newborn infants for certain inherited metabolic disorders or congenital defects. The criteria should depend on the following characteristics of the disorder or of the test.

- The disease should not be clinically apparent at the time of screening and should have a relatively high incidence in the population screened.
- The disease should be treatable or early treatment should improve outcome.
- It must be possible to obtain the result of the screening test before irreversible damage is likely to have occurred.
- The screening test should be simple and reliable and the cost of the programme should, ideally, be at least partly offset by the cost savings resulting from early treatment. For example, such treatment may sometimes eliminate the need for prolonged institutional care.

Not all these criteria are necessarily fulfilled in all screening programmes.

In the UK, at between 5 and 8 days, babies are screened for certain conditions by taking a small capillary blood sample from a heel-prick stab. Blood is placed on a paper card (blood spots), which can be posted to the regional laboratory for assay.

In the UK, screening is generally carried out for neonatal hypothyroidism (see Chapters 11 and 26) and PKU. Other conditions that may be screened in certain regions include cystic fibrosis, sickle-cell disease or thalassaemia, glucose-6-phosphatase deficiency, galactosaemia and congenital adrenal hyperplasia. (These conditions are discussed elsewhere in this book.) The use of DNA technology and tandem mass spectroscopy in antenatal screening can be expected to increase in the future.

PRENATAL SCREENING

Prenatal screening, of high-risk groups only, may be performed for some disorders in order to plan the appropriate place and method of delivery for the well-being of the infant or to offer termination, if the diagnosis is made early enough and if it is acceptable.

Prenatal screening for inherited metabolic disorders most commonly involves demonstrating the metabolic defect in cultured fetal fibroblasts obtained by amniocentesis early in the second trimester, or by chorionic villus sampling during the first trimester. Examples of those groups in whom such screening may be indicated include women with a previously affected infant and ethnic groups thought to have a relatively high incidence of the carrier state, such as of Tay–Sachs disease in Ashkenazi Jews. In these high-risk populations, screening is often performed before conception, enabling genetic advice and prenatal diagnosis to be offered to couples who are carriers.

If, as in cystic fibrosis, the gene defect of the parent of an affected infant is known, there may be a case for selective screening of subsequent pregnancies using molecular biological techniques. Prenatal screening for congenital disorders, for example neural tube defects, or chromosomal abnormalities may also be performed.

WHEN TO SUSPECT AN INBORN ERROR OF METABOLISM

The possibility of an inherited metabolic defect should be considered if there are unusual, unexplained clinical features (Box 27.1) or abnormal laboratory findings in infancy or early childhood, especially if more than one infant in the family has been affected or there has been a consanguineous marriage.

Screening tests should be interpreted with caution and a suspected diagnosis confirmed by more specific techniques in a laboratory specializing in such disorders.

Inborn errors presenting acutely are usually due to an enzyme abnormality. This may be demonstrated *indirectly*,

> **Box 27.1 Some clinical findings suggestive of an inborn error of metabolism**
>
> *Early*
> Hypoglycaemia
> Metabolic acidosis
> Failure to thrive
> Vomiting
> Fits or spasticity
> Hepatosplenomegaly
> Prolonged jaundice
> A peculiar smell, or staining, of the nappies
> Death of child in family and positive family history
> Cataracts or retinitis pigmentosa
>
> *Late*
> Retarded mental development
> Refractory rickets
> Renal calculi
> Neuropathy
> Short stature
> Dysmorphic features

> **Box 27.2 Possible laboratory investigation of a suspected inborn error of metabolism[a]**
>
> Full blood count
> Serum electrolytes, bicarbonate and blood gases for acid–base status
> Renal function tests, including plasma urea and creatinine
> Liver function tests
> Plasma ammonia
> Blood glucose
> Urine ketones
> Serum cholesterol and triglyceride
> Plasma lactate
> Plasma uric acid
> Thyroid function tests
> Porphyrins
>
> *Further specialist tests*
> Plasma and urine amino acids
> Urine orotic acid
> Urine organic acidurias
> Plasma carnitine
> Metabolites in urine or plasma by tandem mass spectroscopy
> Specific enzyme assays
> DNA analysis of leucocytes or fibroblasts
> Histological studies of affected tissue
>
> [a] This is best carried out in conjunction with a specialist metabolic paediatric laboratory. Many patients present with at least one of the following: metabolic acidosis, hypoglycaemia or hyperammoniaemia. The laboratory tests may include those listed above.

by detecting a high concentration of the substance normally metabolized by the enzyme, or a low concentration of the product; or *directly*, by demonstrating a low enzyme activity in the appropriate tissue or blood cells; these assays may only be available at special centres. If possible, all cases should be confirmed in this way.

Examples of indirect screening methods include:

- estimation of plasma ammonia concentration to test for disorders of the urea cycle or organic acidurias, in which it accumulates;
- chromatography of plasma and urine for amino acids for the detection of disorders of amino acid metabolism;
- detection of organic acids in urine in disorders of branched-chain amino acid metabolism and organic acidurias.

If the clinical signs and symptoms are strongly suggestive of a particular disorder, specific measurements, such as those of urinary glycosaminoglycan excretion and white cell enzymes characteristic of mucopolysaccharidoses (MPS), may be used. The technique of tandem mass spectroscopy is proving useful in the investigation of various IEM.

Genetic tests are being used more frequently, and their use is likely to increase still further. Box 27.2 gives a suggested investigation plan.

PRINCIPLES OF TREATMENT OF INBORN ERRORS OF METABOLISM

Some inborn errors can be treated by:

- limiting the dietary intake of precursors in the affected metabolic pathway, such as phenylalanine in PKU or lactose in galactosaemia;
- supplying the missing metabolic product, such as cortisol in congenital adrenal hyperplasia;
- removing or reducing the accumulated product, such as ammonia in urea cycle disorders.

Experimental treatments may be tried for some disorders with particularly poor prognoses. One of these is enzyme replacement by bone marrow transplantation, but the results have sometimes been disappointing and it is not without its own complications. Insertion of the missing or defective gene is being attempted for disorders such as adenosine deaminase deficiency. However, for many disorders there is, at the time of writing, still no treatment unless they respond to one of the measures listed above.

DISEASES DUE TO INBORN ERRORS OF METABOLISM

Only a few of the known IEM are discussed here. Some of these conditions are mentioned briefly in the relevant chapters in this book.

For the sake of convenience, nine general categories of IEM are arbitrarily defined.

1. Urea cycle defects.
2. Disorders of amino acid metabolism, for example amino-acidurias.
3. Lysosomal storage defects.
4. Disorders of carbohydrate metabolism, for example glycogen storage disorders, gluconeogenesis and carbohydrate intolerance defects.
5. Lipid, fatty acid oxidation defects and organic acidurias.
6. Mitochondrial disorders.
7. Peroxisomal disorders.
8. Abnormalities of drug metabolism.
9. Miscellaneous causes.

1. Urea cycle disorders

Urea cycle defects are another cause of hyperammoniaemia and there may also be raised urinary orotic acid concentration, an intermediate metabolite of pyrimidine synthesis derived from carbamyl phosphate. The urea cycle defects can present not only with severe hyperammoniaemia, but also with a respiratory alkalosis and low plasma urea concentration (Fig. 27.2). Carbamyl phosphate

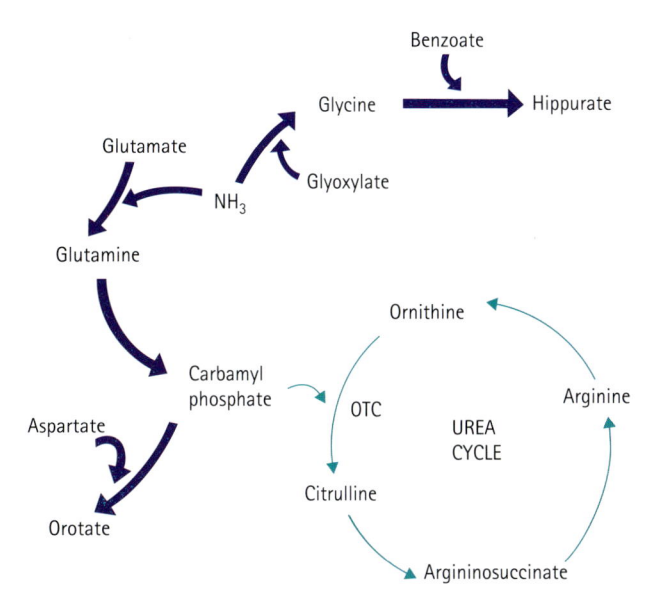

Fig. 27.2 Summary of the urea cycle. (OTC = ornithine transcarbamylase.) (Reproduced with kind permission from Candlish JK and Crook M, *Notes on Clinical Biochemistry*, Singapore: World Scientific Publishing, 1993.)

CASE 1

A 3-month-old male infant was seen in the paediatric out-patients' department because of failure to thrive and hypotonia. The family had previously lost a male child, who had died at the age of 9 months. Some of the presenting child's abnormal biochemistry results were as follows.

Plasma
Sodium 142 mmol/L (135–145)
Potassium 3.8 mmol/L (3.5–5.0)
Urea 0.5 mmol/L (2.5–7.5)
Creatinine 44 μmol/L (40–80)
Ammonia 654 μmol/L (<20)

Plasma amino acid analysis revealed elevated alanine, glutamine and orotic acid concentrations.

DISCUSSION
The diagnosis was established as ornithine transcarbamylase deficiency, one of the urea cycle defects, which is X-linked. Note that the child shows hyperammoniaemia and low plasma urea concentration and that he is male, in keeping with a sex-linked condition. There are relatively few causes of a low plasma urea concentration in neonates, and this combined with severe hyperammoniaemia supports a diagnosis of a urea cycle disorder. An inborn error of metabolism should be suspected on the death of a baby or when a child presents with failure to thrive.

synthetase deficiency (CPS deficiency) is a urea cycle disorder in which, unlike with other defects in this pathway, urinary orotic acid is not raised. Ornithine transcarbamylase deficiency is probably the commonest urea cycle defect and is sex linked.

2. Disorders of amino acid metabolism

Many disorders of amino acid metabolism are characterized by raised plasma concentrations of one or more amino acids, with overflow amino-aciduria.

The main metabolic pathway for aromatic amino acids is outlined in Fig. 27.3, which also indicates the known enzyme defects. Tyrosine, normally produced from phenylalanine, is the precursor of several important substances, inherited disorders of which are considered briefly.

Phenylketonuria

Phenylketonuria is an autosomal recessive disorder caused by an abnormality of the phenylalanine hydroxylase system. In the UK the incidence is about 1 in 10 000. This is the enzyme most commonly affected, but in about 3 per cent of cases the enzymes responsible for the synthesis of the cofactor tetrahydrobiopterin are abnormal. Therefore several different inherited deficiencies may have very similar biochemical and clinical consequences. Phenylalanine cannot be converted to tyrosine, and accumulates in plasma and is excreted in the urine with its metabolites, such as phenylpyruvic acid (a phenylketone).

The clinical features include:

- mental retardation developing at between 4 and 6 months, with psychomotor irritability;
- a tendency to reduced melanin formation because of reduced production of tyrosine; many patients are pale skinned, fair haired and blue eyed;
- irritability, feeding problems, vomiting and fits during the first few weeks of life;
- often generalized eczema.

Diagnosis may involve measuring the phenylalanine concentration in blood taken from a heel prick. The microbiological Guthrie test was used to assay phenylalanine, but now many laboratories use chromatography methods or tandem mass spectroscopy. In the newborn, and especially in premature infants, the enzyme system may not be fully developed and false-positive results are likely if the test is performed too early. If a positive result is found, the test should be repeated later, to allow time for development of the enzyme. The phenylalanine concentrations may be greater than 240 μmol/L.

Heterozygotes may be clinically normal, but can be detected by biochemical tests. A variant – persistent hyperphenylalaninaemia – without mental retardation has been described. Infants who are exposed in utero to the high phenylalanine concentrations of undiagnosed or poorly controlled phenylketonuric mothers may be mentally retarded, although they themselves do not have detectable PKU (maternal phenylketonuric syndrome).

The aim of treatment is to lower plasma phenylalanine concentrations by giving a low-phenylalanine diet. Such treatment should be monitored carefully, especially if the patient is planning to conceive or is pregnant. It is now generally recommended that in proven cases dietary restriction should be life long, with supervision by an expert dietician. Remember that the artificial sweetener aspartame is metabolized to phenylalanine.

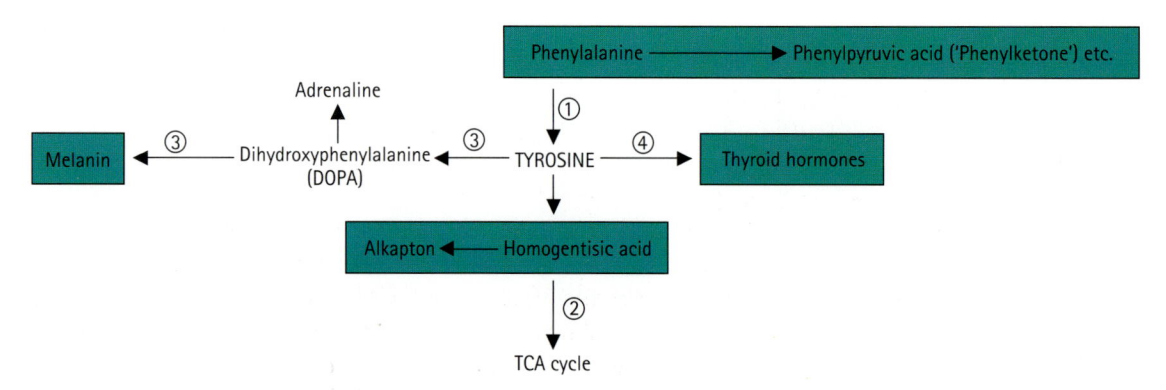

Fig. 27.3 Diagram showing the metabolism of tyrosine and some inborn errors of the aromatic amino acid pathway. Substances highlighted may be present in abnormal amounts in certain inborn errors of metabolism. (1) phenylalanine hydroxylase – phenylketonuria (PKU); (2) homogentisic acid oxidase – alkaptonuria; (3) tyrosinase – albinism; (4) thyroid enzymes – thyroid dyshormonogenesis. (TCA = tricarboxylic acid.)

Tyrosinaemia

Tyrosinaemia presents with renal tubular dysfunction, hypoglycaemia and severe liver disease with very raised plasma alkaline phosphatase concentration. The defect is due to abnormal fumarylacetoacetase leading to raised tyrosine, succinylacetone and hydroxyphenylpyruvate. Diagnosis is by showing raised urinary succinylacetone concentration and assay of fumarylacetoacetase in cultured leucocytes or fibroblasts. Treatment can be dietary, by liver transplantation or by nitro-trifluoromethylbenzoyl cyclohexanedione, which is thought to reduce the accumulation of some of the toxic metabolites.

Alkaptonuria

Alkaptonuria is an autosomal recessive disorder associated with a deficiency of homogentisic acid oxidase. Homogentisic acid accumulates in tissues and blood, and is passed in the urine. Oxidation and polymerization of homogentisic acid produce the pigment alkapton, in much the same way as polymerization of dihydroxyphenylalanine results in melanin. The deposition of alkapton in cartilages, with consequent darkening, is called ochronosis and results in visible darkening of the cartilages of the ears and often arthritis in later life. The conversion of homogentisic acid to alkapton is accelerated in alkaline conditions, and sometimes the most obvious abnormality in alkaptonuria is darkening of the urine as it becomes more alkaline on standing.

However, the condition is compatible with a normal life span, despite the tendency for patients to develop arthritis in later life. Homogentisic acid, a reducing substance, reacts with Clinitest tablets.

Albinism

A deficiency of tyrosinase in melanocytes causes one form of albinism; it is inherited as an autosomal recessive disorder. Pigmentation of the skin, hair and iris is reduced and the eyes may appear pink. Reduced pigmentation of the iris causes photosensitivity, and decreased skin pigmentation is associated with an increased incidence of certain skin cancers. The tyrosinase involved in catecholamine synthesis is a different isoenzyme, controlled by a different gene; consequently, adrenaline (epinephrine) metabolism is normal.

Homocystinuria

Homocystinuria is an autosomal recessive disorder due to deficiency of cystathionine synthase. These pathways involve sulphur-containing amino acids. Patients may show progressive central nervous system dysfunction, thrombotic disease, eye disease, including cataracts, and cardiovascular problems. The diagnosis of homocystinuria is based on the presence of raised urinary and plasma homocystinuria with low plasma methionine concentrations. The defective enzyme can be assayed in cultured skin fibroblasts.

Maple syrup urine disease

In maple syrup urine disease, which is inherited as an autosomal recessive condition, there is deficient decarboxylation of the oxoacids resulting from deamination of the three branched-chain amino acids, leucine, isoleucine and valine. These amino acids accumulate in the plasma and are excreted in the urine with their corresponding oxoacids. The sweet smell of the urine is like that of maple syrup, hence the condition's name.

The disease presents during the first week of life and if not treated, severe neurological lesions develop which cause death within a few weeks or months. If a diet low in branched-chain amino acids is given, normal development is possible.

The diagnosis of maple syrup urine disease is made by demonstrating raised concentrations of branched-chain amino acids in plasma and urine and low plasma alanine concentration. It may be confirmed by demonstrating the enzyme defect in leucocytes.

Histidinaemia

Histidinaemia is associated with deficiency of histidinase, an enzyme needed for normal histidine metabolism, and is probably inherited as an autosomal recessive trait. Some cases may have mental retardation and speech defects, but others may be normal.

The diagnosis is made by demonstrating raised plasma levels of histidine, and by finding histidine and the metabolite imidazole pyruvic acid in the urine.

Inherited disorders of amino acid transport mechanisms

Groups of chemically similar substances are often transported by shared or interrelated pathways. Such group-specific mechanisms usually affect transport across all cell membranes, and defects often involve both the renal tubules and intestinal mucosa. Inborn errors of the following amino acid group pathways have been identified:

- *the dibasic amino acids* (with two amino groups) cystine, ornithine, arginine and lysine (cystinuria) – COAL is a useful mnemonic;

- *many neutral amino acids* (with one amino and one carboxyl group) (Hartnup disease);
- *the imino acids* proline and hydroxyproline, which probably share a pathway with glycine (familial iminoglycinuria).

Amino-aciduria

Amino acids are usually filtered by the glomeruli, reach the proximal tubules at concentrations equal to those in plasma and are almost completely reabsorbed as they pass through this part of the nephron. Amino-aciduria may therefore be of two types.

- *Overflow amino-aciduria*: in which, because of raised plasma concentrations, amino acids reach the proximal tubules at concentrations higher than the reabsorptive capacity of the cells.
- *Renal amino-aciduria*: in which plasma concentrations are low because of urinary loss due to defective tubular reabsorption.

Amino-aciduria may also be subdivided according to the pattern of excreted amino acids.

- *Specific amino-aciduria* is due to increased excretion of either a single amino acid or a group of chemically related amino acids. It may be overflow or renal in type.
- *Non-specific amino-aciduria*, in which there is increased excretion of a number of unrelated amino acids, is almost always due to an acquired disorder. It may be overflow in type, as in severe hepatic disease when impaired deamination of amino acids causes raised plasma concentrations; more commonly, renal amino-aciduria results from non-specific proximal tubular damage, and other substances that are usually almost completely reabsorbed by the proximal tubule are also lost (phosphoglucoamino-aciduria; Fanconi syndrome). If it occurs due to an inborn error of metabolism, it is rarely a direct result of the genetic defect, but more commonly secondary to tubular damage caused by deposition of the substance not metabolized normally, such as copper in Wilson's disease.

Cystinuria

Cystinuria is the result of an autosomal recessive inherited abnormality of tubular reabsorption, with excessive urinary excretion, of the dibasic amino acids cystine, ornithine, arginine and lysine. A similar transport defect has been demonstrated in the intestinal mucosa, but although dibasic amino acid absorption is reduced, deficiencies do not occur because they can be synthesized in the body. Cystine is relatively insoluble and, because of the high urinary concentrations in homozygotes, may precipitate and form calculi in the renal tract. In heterozygotes, increased excretion can be demonstrated, but concentrations are rarely high enough to cause precipitation.

The diagnosis of cystinuria is made by demonstrating excessive urinary excretion of the characteristic amino acids. All these amino acids must be identified to distinguish this from cystinuria occurring as part of a generalized amino-aciduria.

The management of cystinuria aims to prevent calculi formation by reducing urinary concentration. The patient should drink plenty of fluid. Alkalinizing the urine increases the solubility of cystine. If these measures prove inadequate, D-penicillamine may be given; this forms a chelate, which is more soluble than cystine alone. (See Chapter 3 for a discussion of renal calculi.)

Cystinosis

This is a very rare but serious disorder of cystine metabolism, characterized by intracellular accumulation and storage of cystine in many tissues. It must be distinguished from cystinuria, a relatively harmless condition. Renal tubular damage by cystine causes the Fanconi syndrome. Amino-aciduria is non-specific and of renal origin. Affected individuals may die young.

Hartnup disease

Hartnup disease is a rare autosomal recessive disorder in which there are renal and intestinal transport defects involving neutral amino acids.

Many of the clinical manifestations can be ascribed to reduced intestinal absorption and increased urinary loss of tryptophan. This amino acid is normally partly converted to nicotinamide, the conversion being especially important if the dietary intake of nicotinamide is low.

The clinical features of Hartnup disease are intermittent and resemble those of pellagra, namely a red, scaly rash on exposed areas of skin; reversible cerebellar ataxia and mental confusion of variable degree.

Despite the generalized defect of amino acid absorption, there is no evidence of protein malnutrition; this may be because intact peptides can be absorbed by a different pathway.

Excessive amounts of indole compounds, originating from bacterial action on unabsorbed tryptophan, are absorbed from the gut and excreted in the urine.

The diagnosis of homozygotes is made by demonstrating the characteristic amino acid pattern in the urine.

Familial iminoglycinuria

Increased urinary excretion of the imino acids proline and hydroxyproline, and of glycine, despite normal plasma concentrations, is due to a transport defect for these three compounds. The condition is inherited as an autosomal recessive trait. It is apparently harmless, but must be differentiated from other more serious causes of iminoglycinuria, such as the defect of proline metabolism, hyperprolinaemia.

3. Lysosomal disorders

The mucopolysaccharidoses

The MPS are rare conditions caused by defects of any of the several enzymes that hydrolyse mucopolysaccharides (glycosaminoglycans), which therefore accumulate in tissues such as the liver, spleen, eyes, central nervous system, cartilage and bone.

Hurler's syndrome (MPS I H) is the least rare, and is inherited as an autosomal recessive disorder. Patients present in infancy or early childhood with the characteristic coarse features of 'gargoylism', short stature, mental retardation and clouding of the cornea. They usually die young of cardiorespiratory disease. Scheie's syndrome (MPS I S) is difficult to distinguish clinically from Hurler's syndrome at the time of diagnosis, but has a much better prognosis; there is little mental retardation.

Hunter's syndrome (MPS II), in contrast to all the other MPS, is inherited as a sex-linked recessive trait.

There are other mucopolysaccharide conditions, including Sanfilippo, which manifests severe central nervous system abnormalities, and Morquio, which is associated with short stature, barrel chest, knock knees and other skeletal abnormalities.

The MPS can initially be diagnosed biochemically by demonstrating increased urinary excretion of sulphated glycosaminoglycans, such as dermatan, heparan and keratan sulphates, the excretion pattern being characteristic of each syndrome. The diagnosis should be confirmed by direct enzyme assay and gene tests with family studies. There is, as yet, no proven effective treatment.

Lipid storage disorders

Here a deficiency of a lysosomal hydrolase is inherited, resulting in the accumulation of sphingolipid. The following are some examples.

- GM1 gangliosidosis defect of β-galactosidase.
- GM2 gangliosidosis such as Tay–Sachs disease, due to hexosaminidase deficiency.
- Gaucher's disease, due to a deficiency of β-glucosidase (glucocerebrosidase).
- Niemann–Pick disease, resulting from sphingomyelinase deficiency.
- Fabry's disease, resulting from α-galactosidase A deficiency.
- Metachromic leucodystrophy, resulting from arylsulphatase deficiency.

Clinical features of these conditions may include organomegaly, skeletal abnormalities, pulmonary infiltration and cherry-red macular spot on ophthalmologic examination.

4. Carbohydrate disorders

A variety of inborn disorders involve carbohydrate metabolism. Some are discussed in Chapter 26 in the context of neonatal hypoglycaemia.

Disorders of sugars

Galactosaemia is an autosomal recessive disorder due to galactose-1-phosphate uridyl transferase (Gal-1-PUT) deficiency (Fig. 27.4).

Galactose is necessary for the formation of cerebrosides, of some glycoproteins and, during lactation, of milk. Excess is rapidly converted into glucose. The symptoms of galactosaemia only become apparent if the infant is taking milk; the plasma galactose concentrations then rise. The main features include:

- vomiting and diarrhoea, with failure to thrive,
- prolonged prothrombin time,
- hepatosplenomegaly with jaundice and cirrhosis,
- cataract formation,
- mental retardation,
- renal tubular damage due to the deposition of galactose-1-phosphate in the tubular cells (Fanconi syndrome).

Galactose is a reducing substance. The urine may give a positive reaction with Clinitest tablets; this feature may be absent if the subject is not receiving milk and therefore galactose. Tubular damage may cause a generalized amino-aciduria.

The diagnosis is made by identifying galactose by thin-layer chromatography and by demonstrating a deficiency of Gal-1-PUT activity in erythrocytes. Urinary reducing substances are usually positive provided the infant is on a lactose-containing milk diet.

Treatment involves eliminating galactose in milk and milk-products from the diet. Sufficient galactose for the body's needs can be synthesized endogenously as uridyl disphosphate-galactose. This will reverse the acute symptoms but not some of the chronic long-term neurological complications.

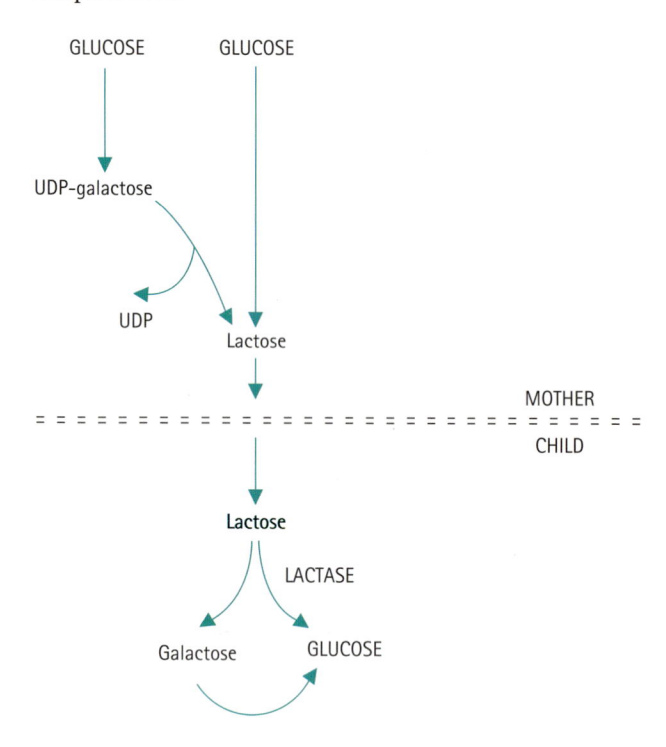

Fig. 27.4 Lactose and galactose cycle. (UDP = uridyl diphosphate.) (Reproduced with kind permission from Candlish JK and Crook M, *Notes on Clinical Biochemistry*, Singapore: World Scientific Publishing, 1993.)

The glycogen storage disorders

Glycogen storage disease type I

This is known as von Gierke's disease and is a deficiency of glucose-6-phosphatase (see Fig. 27.5 and Chapters 12 and 26). Patients may display a lactic acidosis, hypoglycaemia, hyperuricaemia and hypertriglyceridaemia.

Glycogen storage disease type II

Pompe's disease or maltase deficiency (α-1,4 glucosidase) is a lyosomal defect. It is associated with skeletal myopathy, including muscular hypotonia and cardiomyopathy.

Glycogen storage disease type III

This is a defect of debranching enzyme and is known as Forbes–Cori disease. Abnormal glycogen with short external branches accumulates in skeletal muscle, heart and liver. This can result in growth retardation, muscular weakness and cardiomyopathy.

Glycogen storage disease type IV

This is a defect of glycogen branching enzyme and is also called Andersen's disease. There is hepatosplenomegaly and also cardiac and skeletal muscle defects.

Glycogen storage disease type V

McArdle's disease is a deficiency of muscle phosphorylase. Muscle cramps and fatigue occur on heavy exertion. The urine may be burgundy-red in colour due to myoglobin from muscle breakdown.

CASE 2

A 4-year-old boy was seen in the paediatric out-patients' department because of hepatomegaly, metabolic acidosis and growth retardation. Some of his abnormal fasting blood results were as follows.

Plasma (fasting)
Glucose 2.0 mmol/L (3.0–5.5)
Urate 0.61 mmol/L (0.20–0.43)
Lactic acid 3.7 mmol/L (0.5–1.5)
Cholesterol 5.4 mmol/L (3.0–5.0)
Triglycerides 6.7 mmol/L (0.5–1.5)

DISCUSSION

The child has hyperlactataemia, hypoglycaemia, hyperuricaemia and hyperlipidaemia. He was later found to have von Gierke's disease (or type I glycogen storage disease) due to glucose-6-phosphatase deficiency. The glucose-6-phosphatase deficiency leads to abnormalities of glycolysis and gluconeogenesis, resulting in the hypoglycaemia and lactic acidosis. The raised plasma lactic acid concentration may interfere with uric acid renal excretion, leading to hyperuricaemia.

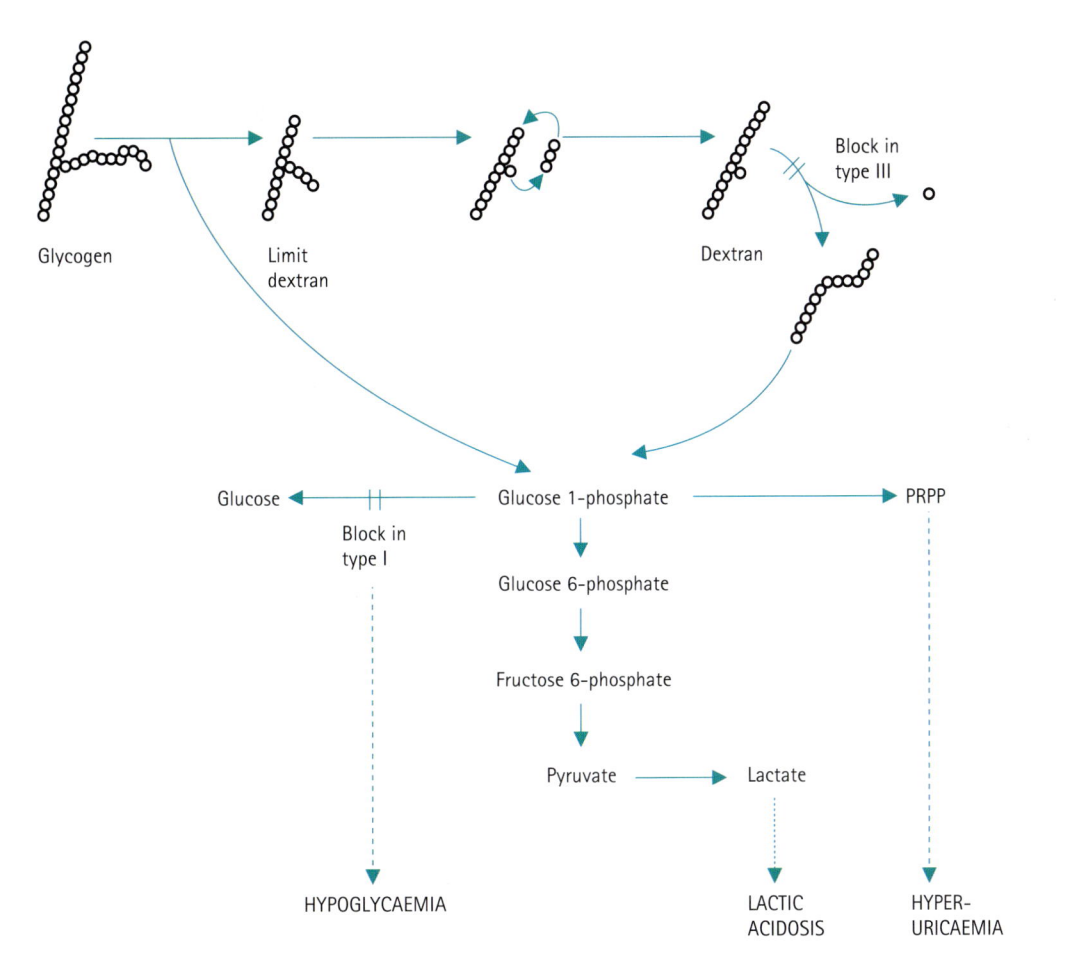

Fig. 27.5 Summary of glycogen metabolism in relation to glycogen storage disease types I and III. Glycogen is converted to limit dextran with four-unit stubs, after which a transferase removes a trisaccharide and attaches it to a free end, leaving a dextran with single 1,6-linked glucosyl units. If amylo-1,6-glucosidase is lacking, as in glycogen storage disease type III, the process stops at that point and hypoglycaemia results. In type I, where the glucose-6-phosphatase is lacking, formation of glucose for the maintenance of euglycaemia is blocked, and the enhanced alternative pathways tend to produce lactic acidosis and hyperuricaemia. (PRPP = 5-phosphoribosylpyrophosphate; o = glucose units in the dextrans.) (Reproduced with kind permission from Candlish JK and Crook M, *Notes on Clinical Biochemistry*, Singapore: World Scientific Publishing, 1993.)

Glycogen storage disease type VI

Hers' disease is due to hepatic phosphorylase deficiency. Symptoms may be mild, although growth retardation may occur.

Glycogen storage disease type VII

Tarui's disease is due to phosphofructokinase deficiency. The symptoms are similar to those of type V.

5. Lipid disorders and organic acidurias

Some inborn errors involving lipid disorders are discussed in Chapter 13.

Those organic acids derived from the metabolism of amino acids, carbohydrates and lipids are often detectable in the urine; others accumulate if there is an enzyme deficiency in a specific metabolic pathway. Examples include methylmalonic acidaemia, glutaric acidaemia, isovaleric acidaemia and proprionic acidaemia. These disorders, known as organic acidurias, are individually rare, but collectively have an incidence of about 1 in 12 000 births, similar to that of PKU. They may present in the neonatal period with life-threatening metabolic acidosis, vomiting and hypotonia, or in early infancy with failure to thrive, a Reye-like syndrome and convulsions associated with profound hypoglycaemia. They may also be a cause of sudden infant death.

> **CASE 3**
>
> A 5-month-old female infant had been referred to the teaching hospital paediatric department because of failure to thrive, lethargy and convulsions. Some of her biochemistry results were as follows.
>
> *Plasma*
> Sodium 136 mmol/L (135–145)
> Potassium 4.9 mmol/L (3.5–5.0)
> Urea 2.9 mmol/L (2.5–7.5)
> Creatinine 48 µmol/L (40–80)
> Bicarbonate 11 mmol/L (24–32)
> Glucose 4.5 mmol/L (3.0–5.5)
> Ammonia 721 µmol/L (<20)
>
> Plasma amino acid analysis showed increased glycine concentration, and the urine showed increased concentrations of ketones and methylmalonic acid.
>
> **DISCUSSION**
> The findings support the diagnosis of methylmalonic acidaemia, one of the organic acidurias. Note the severe hyperammoniaemia and raised methylmalonic acid concentration, which confirm the diagnosis. The child had a metabolic acidosis. Remember to consider IEM in children who fail to thrive.

The diagnosis is suggested by the clinical findings and supported by initial tests demonstrating a metabolic acidosis and sometimes hyperammoniaemia, with or without ketosis. It is confirmed by measuring urinary organic acid excretion and subsequent enzyme analysis, which should only be performed in specialized laboratories.

Medium-chain acyl coenzyme A dehydrogenase deficiency is autosomal recessive and is one of the most common fatty acid oxidation defects (about 1 in 10 000 live births). This potentially fatal condition may present with hypoketotic hypoglycaemia, encephalopathy, seizures and hepatomegaly following diarrhoea and vomiting (reduced food intake). Urinary dicarboxylic aciduria with glycine conjugates may occur, along with increased plasma octanoylcarnitine (an acylcarnitine).

6. Mitochondrial disorders

Mitochondrial DNA (mtDNA) is derived from the mother. This differs from nuclear DNA in that there are no introns and replication of mtDNA lacks proofreading, and the mutation rate is thus 10–100 times greater than that of nuclear DNA. Mitochondria lack an adequate DNA-repair mechanism. A number of clinical features may be present, including neuropathy, mental retardation, lactic acidosis, myopathy, ocular defects, diabetes mellitus, anaemia and hearing loss.

There are a number of mitochondrial disorders, including Leigh's syndrome, MELAS syndrome (**m**itochondrial **e**ncephalomyopathy, **l**actic **a**cidosis, **s**troke), Kearns–Sayre syndrome, NARP syndrome (**n**europathy, **a**taxia, **r**etinitis **p**igmentosa) and LHON syndrome (**L**eber's **h**ereditary **o**ptic **n**europathy).

The arterial or venous lactate:pyruvate ratio may be high (more than 50:1), which suggests a metabolic block in the respiratory chain system. There is often a high plasma lactate at rest. Plasma creatine kinase concentration may be raised and rhabdomyolysis can occur with myoglobinuria. Specialized muscle histology may be useful, and also genetic tests and family studies.

7. Peroxisomal disorders

In this group of disorders there is either a deficiency of a peroxisomal enzyme or a defect in forming intact peroxisomes.

There are probably about 20 of these disorders affecting about 1 in 30 000 individuals. Peroxisomes are involved in a number of metabolic processes. The following are some of the defects that have been described: defects of phytanic acid oxidation (Refsum's disease), dihydroxyacetone phosphate acyltransferase abnormality (Zellweger's syndrome), catalase defects (neonatal adrenoleucodystrophy), and abnormal plasmalogen biosynthesis (rhizomelic chondrodysplasia punctata).

These conditions may present with a variety of features, including dysmorphia, cataracts, liver disease, retinitis pigmentosa, adrenal insufficiency, peripheral neuropathy, deafness and ataxia.

8. Drugs and inherited metabolic disorders

The variation in individual response to drugs may partly be due to genetic variation. There are a number of well-defined inherited disorders that are aggravated by, or which only become apparent after, the administration of certain drugs. These disorders may be classified into two groups.

Disorders resulting in deficient metabolism of a drug

The muscle relaxant, suxamethonium (succinyl choline, or scoline) normally has a very brief action because it is rapidly broken down by plasma cholinesterase. In suxamethonium sensitivity (see Chapter 18), a cholinesterase variant of low biological activity impairs the breakdown of the drug, and prolonged postoperative respiratory paralysis may result ('scoline apnoea').

Two other inherited disorders are characterized by defective metabolism of the drugs isoniazid and phenytoin. In both, toxic effects occur more frequently, and at lower dosages, than in normal individuals. The genetic differences in the metabolism of azathioprine are discussed in Chapter 25.

Disorders resulting in an abnormal response to a drug

Deficiency of glucose-6-phosphate dehydrogenase (G-6-PD) may cause haemolytic anaemia, and is relatively common in ethnic groups such as those of Mediterranean origin. It is X-linked. This enzyme catalyses the first step in the hexose monophosphate pathway and is needed for the formation of nicotinamide adenine dinucleotide phosphate, which is probably essential for the maintenance of intact red cell membranes. Numerous variants of G-6-PD deficiency have been described. Haemolysis may be precipitated by certain antimalarial drugs, such as primaquine, and by sulphonamides.

In the inherited hepatic porphyrias (see Chapter 21), acute attacks may be precipitated by several drugs, particularly barbiturates. Some people react to general anaesthetics (most commonly halothane with suxamethonium) with a rapidly rising temperature, muscular rigidity and acidosis (malignant hyperpyrexia), which is associated with high mortality. Many, but not all, susceptible subjects in affected families have a high plasma creatine kinase activity.

9. Miscellaneous disorders

There are many other IEMs in addition to those mentioned above, including congenital adrenal hyperplasia (see Chapter 8), adenosine deaminase deficiency, electron transport chain defects and sulphite oxidase deficiency.

CONCLUSIONS

- The incidence of IEM ranges from about 1 in 100 to 1 in 200 000, depending on the disorder and the population involved.
- The presence of an inborn error should be considered in children with family histories of IEM, failure to thrive, convulsions and other metabolic abnormalities.
- Neonatal screening programmes based on the analysis of neonate blood spots are used to screen for certain metabolic disorders, including hypothyroidism and PKU.
- Neonatal screening laboratories use highly skilled biochemical and molecular biology techniques.
- Some inborn errors can be treated by:
  - limiting the dietary intake of precursors in the affected metabolic pathway, such as phenylalanine in PKU or lactose in galactosaemia;
  - supplying the missing metabolic product, such as cortisol in congenital adrenal hyperplasia;
  - removing or reducing the accumulated product, such as ammonia in urea cycle disorders.

28 GENETICS AND DNA-BASED TECHNOLOGY IN CLINICAL BIOCHEMISTRY

General principles	380	Genetic diagnosis	382
Patterns of inheritance	380		

Genetic disorders fall into three main categories.

- *Chromosomal disorders* due to the absence, or abnormal arrangement, of chromosomes affecting many genes and therefore many gene products. Examples include Down's syndrome (trisomy for chromosome 21), Turner's syndrome (45,XO) and Klinefelter's syndrome (47,XXY).
- *Monogenic disorders* due to an abnormality of a single gene, which is the primary determinant of the disorder and which is inherited in a predictable pattern, such as phenylketonuria.
- *Multifactorial or polygenic disorders* due to the interaction of multiple genes with environmental or other exogenous factors, such as diabetes mellitus.

GENERAL PRINCIPLES

Genes, located on chromosomes, comprise a sequence of bases on deoxyribonucleic acid (DNA) and code for the synthesis of proteins by ribonucleic acid (RNA) in its 'messenger' form (mRNA).

All nucleated cells contain an identical complement of genes, but only about 1 per cent is expressed.

A genotype is the actual genes present in an individual; phenotype is the physical expression of that genotype, usually via production of a polypeptide or protein.

Genes differ in length, sometimes containing many thousands of bases. However, only 10 per cent of the genome incorporates the protein-coding sequences (exons) of genes. Interspersed within many genes are intron sequences, which have no coding function. The rest of the genome consists of other non-coding regions (such as control sequences and intergenic regions).

Humans can synthesize about 100 000 varying polypeptides or proteins, which are usually composed of about 20 different kinds of amino acids. Genes contain specific sequences of three DNA bases (codons) instructing the cell's protein-synthesizing apparatus to add specific amino acids.

In disorders of single genes (monogenic), the abnormalities may be of:

- a *structural gene*, with production of an abnormal protein: in this case all the biochemical abnormalities can be explained by defective synthesis of a single peptide;
- a *controlling (enhancing) gene*, which, by altering the rate at which one or more structural genes function, affects the amounts of one or more structurally normal peptides.

The affected protein may be an enzyme, but in other conditions it may, for example, be a receptor, a transport or a structural protein, a peptide hormone, an immunoglobulin or a coagulation factor. With the Human Genome Project, more and more genes and their functions are being discovered.

PATTERNS OF INHERITANCE

Every inherited characteristic is governed by a pair of genes on homologous chromosomes, one gene being received from each parent. Different genes governing the same characteristic are called alleles. An individual with two identical alleles is homozygous for that gene or inherited characteristic; an individual with two different alleles is heterozygous. Genes may be carried on the autosomes (similar in both sexes) or on the sex chromosomes (X and Y); the patterns of inheritance differ.

Autosomal inheritance (Fig. 28.1)

If one parent (Parent 1 in the example in Fig. 28.1a) is heterozygous for an abnormal gene (A) and the other parent is homozygous for the normal gene (N), the possible combinations in the offspring are shown in the square in this figure.

On a statistical basis, half the offspring will be heterozygous (AN) for gene A, like Parent 1. None will be homozygous for the abnormal gene (AA).

If both parents are heterozygous (AN; Fig. 28.1b), a quarter of the offspring will be homozygous (AA) and half will be heterozygous (AN).

If one parent is homozygous (AA) and the other normal (NN), all the offspring will be heterozygous.

The metabolic consequences of an abnormal gene depend on the effectiveness of that gene compared with the normal one.

Autosomal dominant inheritance

Dominant abnormal genes affect both heterozygotes (AN) and homozygotes (AA), although homozygotes may be more severely affected. In the first example, Parent 1 (AN) and half the offspring will be affected, and in the second example both parents and three out of four of the offspring (AA and AN) will be affected. Characteristically, if there is autosomal dominant inheritance:

- every affected individual has at least one affected parent;
- offspring in successive generations are affected;
- clinically normal offspring are not carriers of the abnormal gene;
- statistically, three in four children are affected if both parents are heterozygous; if one parent is heterozygous, there is a one in two chance of an offspring being the same.

An example is familial hypercholesterolaemia (Chapter 13).

Autosomal recessive inheritance

Recessive abnormal genes only affect homozygous offspring (AA). In the first example, neither parent nor the

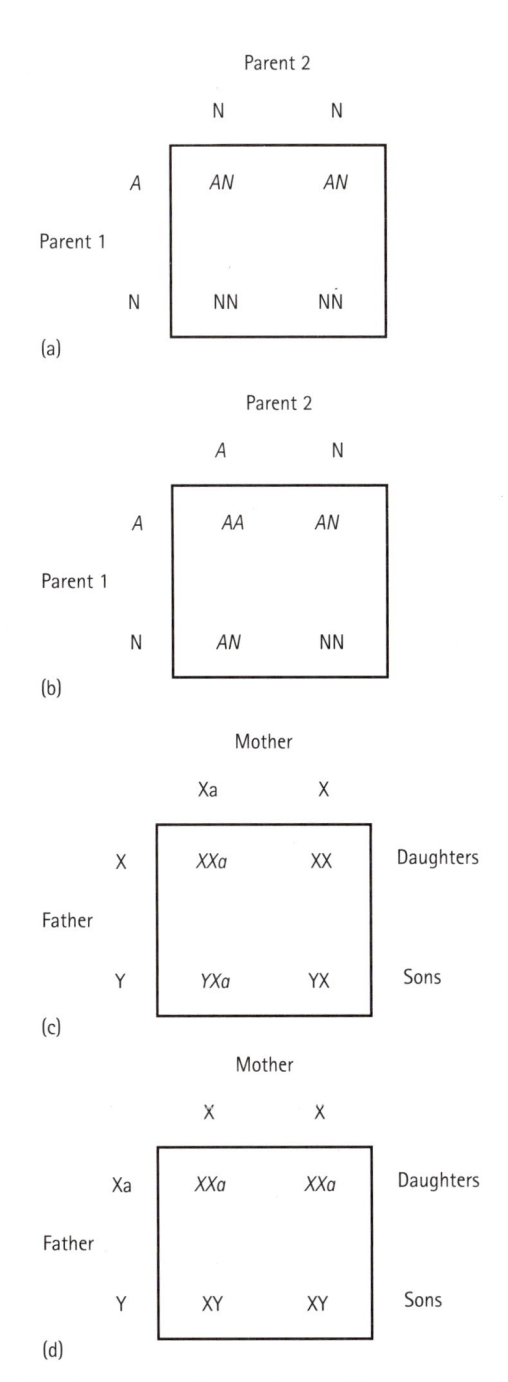

Fig. 28.1 Inheritance of genetic conditions.

offspring will be affected, and in the second example both parents will appear normal, but statistically one in four of the offspring will be affected. Therefore, in autosomal recessive inheritance:

- heterozygous parents are not usually clinically affected;
- clinical consequences may miss offspring in succeeding generations;
- clinically normal children may be heterozygous and therefore may be carriers of the abnormal gene;

- on average, one in four children of heterozygous parents are clinically affected.

Disorders inherited as a recessive trait have a lower expression frequency in affected families than dominant disorders, but tend to be more severe.

An example is cystic fibrosis (Chapter 16).

Sex-linked inheritance

Some abnormal genes are carried only on the sex (almost always the X) chromosomes.

X-linked recessive inheritance

Women have two X chromosomes and men have one X and one Y chromosome. In X-linked recessive inheritance, an abnormal X chromosome (Xa) is latent when combined with a normal X chromosome, but active when combined with a Y chromosome. If the mother carries Xa, she will appear to be normal, but statistically half her sons will be affected (XaY). Half her daughters will be carriers (XaX), but all her daughters will be clinically unaffected (Fig. 28.1c).

If the father is affected and the mother carries two normal genes, none of the sons will be affected, but all the daughters will be carriers (Fig. 28.1d).

Inherited disease manifesting in male offspring and carried by females is typical of X-linked inheritance. Females are only clinically affected in the extremely rare circumstance when they are homozygous for the abnormal gene. This will only occur if the female inherited the abnormal genes from an affected father and a carrier mother.

Haemophilia is the classic example of an X-linked recessive disorder.

X-linked dominant inheritance

In this type of inheritance, both XaX women and XaY men are affected. An example of this very rare type of disorder is familial hypophosphataemia.

Multiple alleles

Occasionally there may be several alleles governing the same characteristic. In such cases, different pair combinations may produce different disease patterns, for example some of the haemoglobinopathies, or the variant may only be detectable by biochemical testing, such as, for example, some of the plasma protein variants.

In rare cases, spontaneous new mutations may occur and may produce dominant disorders in unaffected families.

The terms 'dominant' and 'recessive' are relative. A dominant gene may fail to manifest itself (incomplete penetrance) and may therefore appear to skip a generation. A gene may vary in its degree of expression, and therefore in the degree of abnormality that it produces. A recessive gene, which produces disease only in homozygotes (*AA*), may be detectable by laboratory tests in clinically unaffected heterozygotes.

GENETIC DIAGNOSIS

In recent years there has been a huge growth in DNA technology and research, such that clinical diagnosis can now be made in certain conditions using small tissue samples. This chapter gives a brief outline of such technology; for a more detailed exposition, the reader is advised to refer to a specific molecular biology textbook.

Basics principles of molecular biology

Chromosomes consist of approximately equal parts of protein and DNA; chromosomal DNA contains an average of 100–200 million bases. DNA is a nucleoside polymer arranged in two strands as a double helix. There are four bases in DNA, namely adenine (A), cytosine (C), guanine (G) and thymine (T). These nucleotides consist of ester-linked phosphate residues at the $5'$-hydroxyl residue of a deoxyribose molecule that itself is linked to a purine or pyrimidine base by its $1'$-hydroxyl group.

Each of the DNA strands has polarity, namely $5'$ and $3'$ ends with the two opposite-running strands in opposite directions (anti-parallel).

The two strands are complementary, so that C on one strand pair bonds by hydrogen bonds with G on another strand and A pairs with T. These bases are always numbered from the $5'$ to the $3'$, with letters indicating the nucleotide bases.

Genetic material can copy itself (replication) during the S phase of the cell cycle. DNA polymerase needs a pre-existing DNA template and moves along the two strands and adds the appropriate nucleotides, following the base pairing rules, to the growing chain. Two new double strands of DNA are formed, identical to the original double strand. Every new double strand is half old and half new (semi-conservative).

The strands are anti-parallel. DNA polymerase always moves from $3'$ to $5'$ along the template strand, i.e. the reverse of the newly forming strand.

A gene is a unique sequence of nucleotides that codes for a particular protein or peptide and can be represented by one or more alleles.

The polypeptide or protein-coding instructions from the genes are transcribed indirectly through mRNA, i.e. transcription. The mRNA moves from the nucleus to the cellular cytoplasm, serving as the template for protein synthesis. The ribosomal system then translates the codons into an amino acid chain that will constitute the polypeptide or protein molecule for which it codes (translation). The genetic code is thus a series of codons that instruct which amino acids are needed to synthesize specific polypeptides or proteins.

DNA technologies

DNA can easily be prepared from very small amounts of biological samples, often blood. This essentially involves three steps: leucocyte lysis, chloroform/phenol extraction to remove contamination by proteins, followed by proteinase and RNAase treatment to remove remaining protein and RNA contamination.

Samples of DNA may be separated by electrophoresis due to its strong negative charge at neutral pH. By running the DNA through agarose gels, it can be separated into separate DNA molecules from 100–10 000 base pairs. Smaller DNA pieces can be separated by polyacrylamide gels, which are a tighter molecular sieve than agarose.

DNA probes can be a piece of DNA of variable length that can be inserted into the DNA of a plasmid. These circular pieces of double-stranded DNA can be artificially introduced into bacteria and incorporated into their DNA by a process called transformation. The bacteria are made permeable to DNA by divalent cations. At the same time, a selectable marker such as antibiotic resistance is also inserted, and only those bacteria containing this will grow in media containing the antibiotic. The probes can be labelled to locate them in DNA experiments, with either radio-labelled phosphorus-32 or non-radio-labelled using horseradish peroxidase-enhanced chemiluminescence or digoxigenin.

Hybridization

If DNA in solution is heated, the hydrogen bonds between the complementary strands become disorganized and dissociate (denaturing or melting). On lowering the temperature, the two strands are able to come together again – a process called renaturation or annealing.

It is possible to anneal nucleic acids from different sources in a process called hybridization. This is an essential principle of DNA technologies and allows a complementary sequence of bases (the target) to be annealed to a short piece of DNA (the probe). By adjusting the reaction conditions (increasing stringency), such as temperature and ionic strength, it is possible to ensure that the probe only hybridizes to a perfectly matching genomic DNA sequence.

The probes can either be complementary to lengths of the DNA within the gene under study (genomic probe) or complementary to exon regions of the gene under study that give rise to mRNA (cDNA probe).

Allele-specific oligonucleotide probes are short, single-stranded DNA probes that differ in composition by one single nucleotide and are thus able to detect single DNA point mutations.

DNA polymorphisms

DNA can be cut into smaller fragments by restriction endonucleases derived from bacteria. These are named by abbreviating the names of the originating bacteria. These endonucleases often work in a palindromic way, i.e. the sequence of bases on one DNA strand is repeated in reverse on the other. A restriction enzyme/restriction endonuclease is an enzyme that recognizes a specific nucleotide sequence (restriction site) and cuts (restricts) the nucleic acid at that particular site. An example of a restriction endonuclease is EcoRI made by *Escherichia coli*. EcoRI is specific for the sequence:

- 5′ … GAATTC … 3′
- 3′ … CTTAAG … 5′.

The base pairs on the DNA strands throughout the genome differ at particular locations in individuals. This is called polymorphism, and when the differences occur in introns (non-coding sequences of DNA), no overall change occurs in the final coded protein product. If the polymorphic location occurs at a particular restriction endonuclease site, either the site is not recognized by the enzyme or an alternative site may be created elsewhere in the DNA strand. This in turn leads to differences in the sizes of the DNA fragments produced – restriction fragment length polymorphisms (RFLPs). These RFLPs can, therefore, be used as markers of certain loci that may be implicated in disease states (Fig. 28.2).

Southern blotting

E.M. Southern devised a gel electrophoresis to allow specific DNA fragments to be separated. This method, called Southern blotting, is based on the re-association of DNA

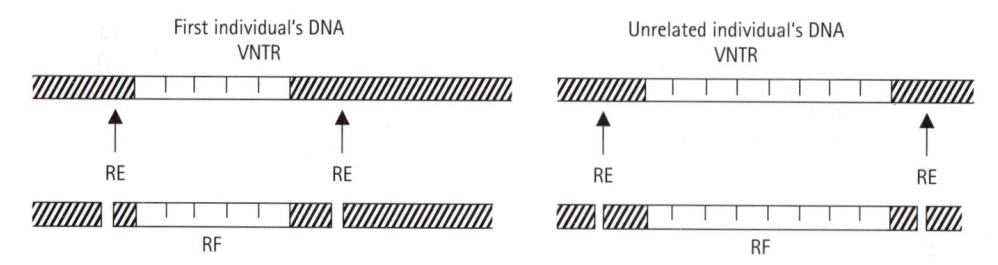

Fig. 28.2 Summary of DNA fingerprinting techniques. (VNTR = variable number of tandem repeats; RE = restriction endonuclease; RF = restriction fragment.) (Reproduced with kind permission from Candlish JK and Crook M, *Notes on Clinical Biochemistry*, Singapore: World Scientific Publishing, 1993.)

strands after denaturation and then detecting the fragments by a labelled probe.

The DNA fragments are separated after denaturation in alkaline solution. The DNA is transferred to a membrane by capillary action (blotting). It is then fixed to the membrane (either nitrocellulose or nylon) by baking or ultraviolet irradiation.

A probe is prepared which is either a DNA or RNA molecule that is complementary to the particular sequence under study. The probe is labelled, with radio-labelled phosphorus-32, fluorescent or immunological techniques. The labelled probe is incubated with the blotted membrane under conditions that favour re-association of the DNA strands – a process called hybridization.

If the conditions are set correctly, i.e. optimal stringency, the probe will only bind to areas of complementary DNA. The probe can then be located, thus locating the homologous DNA sequences.

Northern blotting

RNA molecules can be separated by electrophoresis and can be hybridized with an RNA or DNA probe. The mRNA from a particular gene can be identified and characterized. This is based on the principle that the mRNA will be abnormal either in amount or size if there is a corresponding gene mutation.

Northern blots can also be used to study the tissue-specific expression or development of particular genes, as well as identifying and characterizing mRNAs derived from genes of interest.

Micro-arrays

These are sometimes called DNA chips and are used to detect changes in gene expression in different cells. It is possible to place very small amounts of defined DNA molecules onto a membrane, which are then mixed with a sample to see if RNA molecules are present – somewhat like a reverse Northern blot.

Polymerase chain reaction

The essence of this technique is that a DNA segment is amplified by two primers using repeated cycles of denaturation, primer annealing and extension by DNA polymerase.

The reaction mixture consists of the original template DNA, the four nucleotides, and a large excess of oligonucleotide primers. The temperature is initially set to 95 °C to separate the DNA strands. It is then reduced to 50 °C so that the complementary primers bind and anneal, and then raised to 72 °C for about 1 minute – the optimal temperature for the DNA polymerase. The polymerase can usually incorporate 50–100 nucleotides per second. After this, the temperature is again raised to 95 °C to complete the cycle. There is thus a cycle of denaturation, primer annealing and primer-directed extension.

Taq polymerase is a heat-stable DNA polymerase derived from the organism *Thermus aquaticus*. Polymerase chain reaction (PCR) can amplify DNA up to a million-fold. It can be used in the diagnosis of known mutations of genomic DNA using amplification refractory mutation system. DNA cannot undergo PCR amplification if an oligonucleotide primer contains a 3′ nucleotide mismatch. In site-directed mutagenesis, a mutation or polymorphism destroys or creates a restriction endonuclease cutting site, which can be identified by PCR followed by endonuclease digestion (Fig. 28.3).

Examples of DNA diagnosis (Fig. 28.4)

Cystic fibrosis

Cystic fibrosis is often due to a 3 base-pair deletion in codon 508 of the cystic fibrosis chloride channel gene although

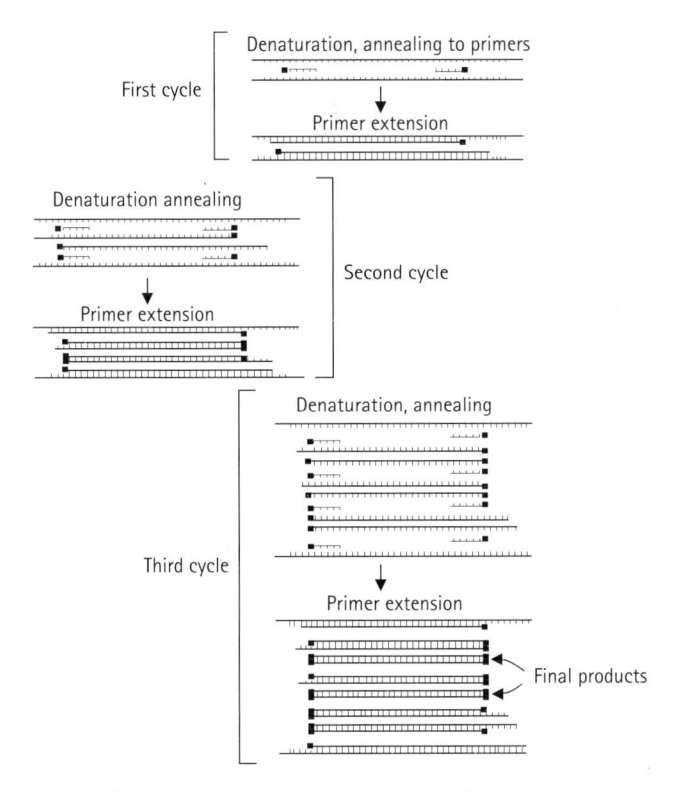

Fig. 28.3 Principles of the polymerase chain reaction. Basically, polymerization can be conducted in one vessel because the DNA polymerase can survive cycles of heating and cooling. Initially the genomic DNA double helix is separated into single strands (shown here as serrated lines) by heating, then cooled and allowed to anneal to DNA primers (the small serrated segments) complementary to the portion of the gene to be amplified. Then the enzyme and the added nucleotides form double-stranded DNA in the primer extension step. In the second cycle there is again denaturation by heating, annealing to primers in the cold, then primer extension. The first segments of DNA of the desired length are obtained, but annealed to strands of indeterminate length. It is only in the third cycle that the final products are obtained, but are thereafter multiplied exponentially. Note also that the base sequence of the gene, or part of it, has to be known for the design of the primers. (Reproduced with kind permission from Candlish JK and Crook M, *Notes on Clinical Biochemistry*, Singapore: World Scientific Publishing, 1993.)

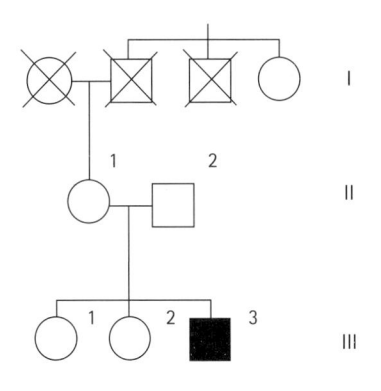

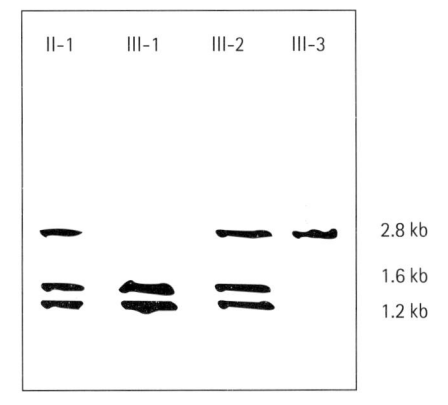

Fig. 28.4 A hypothetical case of the use of DNA probes to diagnose genetic conditions. Conventionally, squares represent males and circles females. The deceased are marked with crosses and the known male case is represented as a solid square. After electrophoresis of the fragments derived from the genomic DNA of the subjects, the 2.8 kb band in the affected male is found to be present in the mother, although in only one of the sisters, who is almost certainly a carrier if the mother is a carrier. (Reproduced with kind permission from Candlish JK and Crook M, *Notes on Clinical Biochemistry*, Singapore: World Scientific Publishing, 1993.)

Muscular dystrophies

Both Duchenne's and Becker's muscular dystrophies are due to deletions in the dystrophin gene on chromosome 21. The former is due to an absence of dystrophin, whereas the latter is due to partially functioning dystrophin.

Polymerase chain reaction techniques are being used to detect carriers and those affected (see Figs 28.3 and 28.4).

Alpha$_1$-antitrypsin deficiency

Alpha$_1$-antitrypsin deficiency can result in severe emphysema or cirrhosis. The gene is polymorphic, with more than 50 genetic variants. At one time the abnormalities

other mutations may also occur. The genetic defect can be detected using PCR and polyacrylamide gel, and this can be used to screen for carriers or affected pregnancies using chorionic villous sampling. (See Chapter 16.)

could be detected by protein isoelectric focusing, but this has now been superseded by the use of PCR to detect clinically important alleles. (See Chapter 19.)

Phenylketonuria

Phenylketonuria can be detected by measuring phenylalanine on neonatal blood spots. However, new PCR technology may allow affected pregnancies to be tested by chorionic sampling. (See Chapter 27.)

Genetics of lipid disorders

Familial hypercholesterolaemia is an autosomal dominant defect of the low-density lipoprotein receptor of chromosome 19. A variant is familial defective apolipoprotein B-100 (apoB-100), caused by a mutation of the apoB gene at the 3500 position. These conditions may be screened for by PCR technology. Apolipoprotein E shows polymorphism, with the apoE2 homozygote being associated with type III dyslipoproteinaemia and the apoE4 allele associated with Alzheimer's disease. Previously, apoE phenotyping was performed using isoelectric focusing, but this can give discordant results due to post-translational modifications of the apoE lipoprotein during its sojourn in the circulation. This method has now been superseded by PCR methods to characterize the apoE genotype. (See Chapter 13.)

Haemochromatosis

The diagnosis of haemochromatosis is now more commonly being made with DNA techniques. Genetic tests are now available, for example a majority of cases of haemochromatosis are due to the *C282Y* or *H63D HFE* mutation. (See Chapter 21.)

Sickle-cell anaemia

Sickle-cell anaemia is due to a single A to T substitution in the sixth codon of the β-globin gene. This can be detected during amniocentesis, for example by allele-specific hybridization.

Thalassaemia

Thalassaemia is characterized by the absence or size alteration of the globin mRNA. This can be detected by using Northern blotting techniques.

Infectious agents

Polymerase chain reaction can be used to verify the presence of specific pathogens. DNA primers are chosen that are specific to DNA sequences of the pathogen. Such pathogens include human immunodeficiency virus (HIV), hepatitis C and *Helicobacter pylori*.

Paternity testing and forensic diagnosis

DNA technology is now used to determine the genetic father in paternity disputes and also in forensic science to identify body tissues and fluids.

CONCLUSIONS

- Genetic disorders fall into three main categories:
  - chromosomal disorders,
  - monogenic disorders,
  - multifactorial or polygenic disorders.
- DNA technology will undoubtedly increase over the next few years and its use can be expected to increase in clinical biochemistry testing.
- The examples given in this chapter are only a selection of the DNA tests that may become available in the future. However, diseases such as cystic fibrosis and muscular dystrophy are already being diagnosed by DNA technology.
- The polymerase chain reaction is an important diagnostic molecular biology technique.

29 PATIENT SAMPLE COLLECTION AND USE OF THE LABORATORY

| Requesting patient samples | 388 | Collection of patient specimens | 388 |

Most clinical laboratories take stringent precautions to control the analytical accuracy and precision of results. Indeed, many laboratories undergo carefully regulated accreditation procedures.

Generally, laboratory users need only limited knowledge of the technical details of the laboratory tests. However, they should understand that the appropriate collection of patient specimens can affect results (Table 29.1), and they

Table 29.1 Some extra-laboratory factors leading to erroneous results

Cause of error	Some possible consequences
Patient not fasting	High plasma triglyceride and glucose
Keeping blood overnight before sending it to the laboratory or refrigerating blood sample	High plasma K^+, phosphate, LDH, AST
Haemolysis of blood	As above, lower plasma ALP
Prolonged venous stasis during venesection	High plasma protein, total Ca^{2+} and cholesterol
Taking blood from an arm with an infusion running into it	Electrolytes and glucose concentrations similar to dilution of everything else
Putting blood into wrong vial or tipping it from one vial into another	e.g. EDTA or oxalate cause low plasma Ca^{2+}
Blood for glucose not put into fluoride	Low blood or plasma glucose
Delay in analysing blood gases	Low bicarbonate concentration
Failure to keep sample cool or delay separating and freezing plasma	Low PTH, ACTH, insulin
Incorrect anticoagulant	e.g. gut peptide hormones falsely low if no protease inhibitor used
Palpation of prostate by rectal examination, passage of catheter, enema etc. in last few days	High tartrate-labile acid phosphatase and PSA
Inaccurately timed urine collection	Poorly timed 24-hour urinary excretion values Abnormal renal clearance values
Incorrect urine or no preservative	Falsely low result, e.g. urea or calcium
Loss of stools during faecal fat collection	Falsely low faecal fat results (test now rarely done)

LDH = lactate dehydrogenase; AST = aspartate transaminase; ALP = alkaline phosphatase; EDTA = ethylenediamine tetra-acetate; PTH = parathyroid hormone; ACTH = adrenocorticotrophic hormone; PSA = prostate-specific antigen.

should therefore work with the laboratory in its attempt to produce answers rapidly and accurately and identifiable with the relevant patient. To this end, one should understand the importance of:

- accurately completed request forms,
- the collection of specimens by the correct technique at the appropriate time,
- correctly labelled specimens,
- appropriate laboratory liaison,
- speedy delivery to the laboratory.

Remember that treatment based on technically correct results from a wrongly labelled or collected specimen may be as dangerous as a faulty surgical procedure. 'Unlikely' results are checked in most laboratories to make sure that they have not been transposed with the results for another patient.

All patient samples are potentially infection risks. Informed consent may be needed for acquired immunodeficiency syndrome testing and also certain genetic tests. All blood specimens should be sent in leak-proof, sealed plastic bags, with the request form in a different pocket in the bag. Failure to comply with these guidelines may put many people, including porters and laboratory staff, at unnecessary risk.

REQUESTING PATIENT SAMPLES

Patient identification

Accurate and legibly written information about the patient is essential, although electronic requesting systems are now available. This information includes the patient's:

- hospital case number,
- surname and first name(s), correctly and consistently spelt,
- date of birth, rather than age.

Any of these may be recorded inaccurately on the form and, unless there is complete agreement with previous details, results may be entered into the wrong patient's record either on a computer or in the patient's case notes, causing confusion and possible danger to the patient. In future, the National Health Service number will be used as a unique individual identifier in the UK.

Location of the patient and identification of the clinician

It should be obvious that if the ward or department is not stated, it may take time and effort to determine where the results should be sent. The requesting doctor must sign the form legibly, and also state how he or she can be notified rapidly, for example by 'bleep number', in case abnormal results requiring urgent action are found or advice needs to be sought about treatment. The doctor must check the completed request form to be sure that the information given is correct; it is also important to include their name and contact details.

Request forms designed by pathology and other departments ask only for information that is essential to ensure the most efficient possible service to the clinician and therefore to the patient. We are beginning to see the introduction of electronic test requesting, which should improve patient identification and speed up the process and may replace 'paper' requests.

COLLECTION OF PATIENT SPECIMENS

Collection of blood

If a clinically improbable result has been checked analytically and the second result is in close agreement with the first, a fresh specimen should be analysed. Although contamination at some stage of blood collection is an obvious possibility, this is relatively rare and should not be accepted until other, more common, causes have been excluded.

Effect on results of procedures before venepuncture

- *Some tests may require the patient to fast,* for example plasma glucose or triglyceride (see Chapters 12 and 13).
- *Oral medication*: some assays may be affected by oral medication.
  - Blood should be taken for drug assays at a standard time after the dose; misleadingly high plasma concentrations may occur at the time of peak absorption (see Chapter 25).
  - There may be significant hypokalaemia for a few hours after taking potassium-losing diuretics due to rapid clearance of potassium from the extracellular fluid. The plasma concentration returns to its 'true' level as equilibration occurs between cells and extracellular fluid (see Chapter 5).
  - Interfering substances: previous administration of a substance may affect a plasma analyte concentration for some time, for example certain antibiotics

Case 1

A 22-year-old male had the following postoperative biochemical results after an appendectomy.

Plasma
Sodium 165 mmol/L (135–145)
Potassium 1.9 mmol/L (3.5–5.0)
Urea 1.1 mmol/L (2.5–7.0)
Creatinine 38 µmol/L (70–110)
Glucose 43 mmol/L (3.5–6.0)

The clinical biochemistry laboratory suggested an immediate repeat blood sample, which gave the following results.

Plasma
Sodium 136 mmol/L (135–145)
Potassium 3.9 mmol/L (3.5–5.0)
Urea 5.4 mmol/L (2.5–7.0)
Creatinine 89 µmol/L (70–110)
Glucose 4.5 mmol/L (3.5–6.0)

DISCUSSION

The first sample seems to display profound hypernatraemia, hyperglycaemia and hypokalaemia. In addition, the plasma urea and creatinine concentrations are both low. The repeat sample values are completely different. It later transpired that the first sample had been taken out of the patient's drip arm, which had a dextrose–saline infusion going into it. This had resulted in dilution of the analytes and elevated sodium and glucose concentrations.

---

may interfere with chemical reactions used in creatinine assays (see Chapter 3).
- *Effect of posture:* for example the concentrations of plasma proteins and of substances bound to them are lower when the patient is supine compared with when standing up (see Chapter 19).
- *Intravenous infusion:* for example a spuriously low plasma sodium concentration may result if the sample is taken from a dextrose drip arm (see Chapter 2).
- *Clinical procedures:* for example palpation of the prostate by rectal examination may possibly release large amounts of acid phosphatase and prostate-specific antigen into the circulation; the spuriously elevated concentrations in blood may persist for several days (see Chapter 18).

Effects on results of the technique of venepuncture

Venous stasis

It is usual to apply a tourniquet proximal to the site of venepuncture to make it easier to enter the vein with the needle. If occlusion is maintained for more than a short time, the combined effect of raised intracapillary pressure and hypoxia of the vessel wall increases the rate of passage of water and small molecules from the lumen into the surrounding interstitial fluid. Large molecules, such as proteins, cannot pass through the capillary wall at the same rate; their plasma concentrations therefore rise.

Many plasma constituents are partly bound to protein. Prolonged venous stasis can raise the plasma total calcium concentration, sometimes to equivocal or slightly high levels. Therefore, ideally, blood samples for plasma calcium estimation should be taken without stasis, especially if high plasma concentrations have previously been found (see Chapter 6).

Prolonged stasis may also cause local hypoxia; consequent leakage of intracellular constituents, such as potassium and phosphate, may cause falsely high plasma concentrations. It is sometimes difficult to enter 'bad veins' without applying stasis. A tourniquet may be used and released as soon as the needle is in the vein; a suitable specimen may be obtained after waiting at least a further 15 seconds before withdrawing blood.

Site of venepuncture

If the patient is receiving an intravenous infusion, the administered fluid in the veins of the same limb, whether proximal or distal to the infusion site, has not mixed with the total plasma volume; local concentrations will therefore be unrepresentative of those circulating through the rest of the body. Blood taken from the opposite arm will give valid results. Note that glucose infusion may cause systemic hyperglycaemia and glycosuria. Only if the hyperglycaemia persists after infusion has stopped should the diagnosis of diabetes mellitus be considered (see Chapter 12).

Containers for blood

Most hospital laboratories issue a list of the types of container suitable for different assays; this list may vary from hospital to hospital. For example, most laboratories specify that:

- blood for glucose estimation should be put into a tube containing an inhibitor of erythrocyte glycolysis, such as fluoride;
- potassium should be estimated on plasma from heparinized blood rather than serum. Potassium is released from cells, especially platelets, during clotting. Serum potassium concentrations are usually higher than those of plasma by a variable amount; this difference can be clinically misleading. Marked differences may be found in patients with leukaemia, in whom the number of white blood cells is usually significantly increased.

Laboratories should only accept blood in the correct containers. Even with this precaution, serious errors can arise if blood is decanted from one container to another, although this is less likely to occur if a closed vacuum system is used for obtaining blood. The anticoagulant actions of oxalate and of sequestrene (ethylenediamine tetra-acetic acid; EDTA) depend on the precipitation or chelation of calcium, respectively, thus invalidating the results of calcium estimation. EDTA is usually in the form of its potassium salt; therefore, it renders the sample unsuitable for potassium analysis.

The use of sodium (instead of lithium) heparin may give a falsely high plasma sodium result. This anticoagulant is often used in specimens taken for 'blood gases'; apparent plasma sodium concentrations of 160–170 mmol/L can result from transferring an aliquot of sodium heparinized blood into a lithium heparin vial. The use of lithium heparin leads to a falsely high plasma lithium concentration and it should therefore not be used as an anticoagulant for lithium determination.

Effects of haemolysis and delayed separation of blood

Haemolysis

The concentration of many substances is very different in erythrocytes from that in the surrounding plasma. Haemolysis releases the cell contents into plasma and, consequently, if this occurs in vitro, the concentrations of some plasma constituents, such as potassium, phosphate and aspartate transaminase, may be falsely increased. The increase is variable and is not related to the intensity of the red colour of plasma due to haemoglobin. It is uncommon if haemolysis occurs in vivo because these constituents are distributed throughout the total extracellular, not just plasma, volume.

Haemoglobin may interfere with some chemical reactions, falsely increasing the apparent plasma bilirubin concentration and lowering alkaline phosphatase activity. The chance of haemolysis is minimized if the blood is treated gently and if a closed vacuum system is used.

CASE 2

A blood sample had been taken from a 44-year-old female on the medical ward and the results were as follows.

Plasma
Sodium 140 mmol/L (135–145)
Potassium >10 mmol/L (3.5–5.0)
Urea 4.1 mmol/L (2.5–7.0)
Creatinine 68 μmol/L (70–110)
'Corrected' calcium <0.5 mmol/L (2.15–2.55)
Phosphate 0.92 mmol/L (0.80–1.35)

Repeat blood sampling on the same day gave the following results.

Plasma
Sodium 139 mmol/L (135–145)
Potassium 3.6 mmol/L (3.5–5.0)
Urea 4.2 mmol/L (2.5–7.0)
Creatinine 68 μmol/L (70–110)
Corrected calcium 2.43 mmol/L (2.15–2.55)
Phosphate 0.90 mmol/L (0.80–1.35)

DISCUSSION

The first blood sample had been collected in a potassium-EDTA tube (this is normally used for certain haematology tests such as full blood count) by mistake and then the blood had been decanted by the doctor into the correct chemistry lithium heparin tube. Note in the first sample the raised plasma potassium and low calcium concentrations due to chelation by potassium-EDTA.

Delayed separation of blood

It is important to check the sample date. The differential concentrations of some analytes across cell membranes are maintained by energy, derived from glycolysis. In vitro, erythrocytes soon use up the available glucose and therefore the energy source; concentrations of these analytes in plasma will then tend to equalize with those in erythrocytes by passive diffusion across cell membranes. If plasma is not separated from blood cells within a few hours, the effect on plasma concentrations will be similar to that resulting from haemolysis. However, there are a few important differences.

- Because haemoglobin is not released, the plasma colour looks normal; the error is therefore easily overlooked.
- The plasma potassium concentration rises as the plasma glucose falls; initially, there may be a slight fall in the plasma potassium concentration as it moves into the erythrocytes.

Many plasma constituents, such as bilirubin, deteriorate even if the plasma is correctly separated and stored. Whenever possible, blood should reach the laboratory early in the working day, when most assays are being performed.

If the plasma sample is haemolysed or separation has been delayed, the plasma potassium concentration may still be clinically significant. For example, if the sample is visibly haemolysed and the plasma potassium concentration is only 2.8 mmol/L, this may indicate profound hypokalaemia; the laboratory staff should contact the requesting doctor directly to discuss the significance of the comment 'haemolysed specimen' on the report form.

Refrigeration

The refrigeration of whole blood has the effect of raising the plasma potassium concentration probably by reducing the activity of the ATPase pump. Transport of samples in cold weather may have a similar effect. Freezing will result in haemolysis. Therefore blood specimens must be centrifuged and the plasma separated from the cells before storing, for example overnight.

Collection of urine

Urine estimations performed on timed collections are expressed as units/time (for example mmol/24 hours); this figure is calculated by multiplying the concentration by the volume collected during the timed period. The accuracy of the final result depends largely on that of the urine collection. Sometimes, if the patient is a child or incontinent, accurate urine collection is particularly difficult.

For example, a 24-hour specimen may be collected between 09.00 hours on Sunday and 09.00 hours on Monday. The volume excreted by the kidneys during this period is the crucial one: urine already in the bladder at 09.00 hours on Sunday was secreted earlier and should not be included. Therefore the procedure is as follows.

- *09.00 hours on Sunday*: the bladder is emptied completely, whether or not the patient feels the need, and the specimen is discarded.

Case 3

A sample had been taken in the morning from a 43-year-old male and was then sent to the laboratory from the local health centre. The sample was analysed in the evening of the same day, as there had been a transport delay, and the following results were obtained.

Plasma
Sodium 143 mmol/L (135–145)
Potassium 6.0 mmol/L (3.5–5.0)
Urea 5.1 mmol/L (2.5–7.0)
Creatinine 88 μmol/L (70–110)

The laboratory contacted the patient's general practitioner and an urgent repeat sample showed the following results.

Plasma
Sodium 145 mmol/L (135–145)
Potassium 4.2 mmol/L (3.5–5.0)
Urea 5.2 mmol/L (2.5–7.0)
Creatinine 88 μmol/L (70–110)

DISCUSSION
The first patient sample shows hyperkalaemia, but repeat analysis on a 'fresh' sample shows a 'normal' potassium concentration. The spuriously raised potassium result in the first sample was due to delay in sample assay and leak of intracellular potassium ions out of cells, resulting in pseudohyperkalaemia. It is important to transport samples to the laboratory as quickly as possible to avoid storage artefacts.

- Collect all urine passed until *09.00 hours on Monday* when the bladder is completely emptied, whether or not the patient feels the need, and the specimen is added to the collection.

The shorter the period of collection, the greater the error if this procedure is not followed.

Before collection, a urine container should be obtained from the laboratory; this may contain a preservative to inhibit bacterial growth (which might destroy the substance being estimated) but that does not interfere with the relevant assay. The patient must be told not to discard the preservative in the container and that it might be toxic and harmful if spilt.

Collection of faeces

Rectal emptying is usually erratic and, unlike that of the bladder, can rarely be performed to order. Results of faecal estimations of, for example, fat may vary by several hundred per cent in consecutive 24-hour collections. If the collection period lasted for weeks, the *mean* 24-hourly output would be very close to the true daily loss from the body into the intestinal tract. To render collection more accurate, orally administered 'markers' are used in certain circumstances.

Faecal collections and estimations are time consuming and unpleasant for all concerned and are now rarely required. The administration of purgatives, enemas or barium before or during the collection period alters conditions and invalidates the result.

Labelling patient specimens

All specimens must be accurately labelled and the information should correspond with that on the accompanying request form in every detail, as error may cause a medico-legal disaster. The date, and preferably the time, of specimen collection should be included, and should be written at the time of collection.

Sending the specimen to the laboratory

Many estimations can be performed rapidly if the result is needed urgently. Non-urgent late blood samples can be separated from cells and stored overnight. In cases of true clinical emergency, the requesting clinician should notify the laboratory, preferably before the specimen is taken, indicating the reason for the urgency, so that the laboratory can be ready to deal with the specimen as soon as it arrives. It is the clinician's responsibility to indicate the degree of urgency. The words 'urgent, please phone' should only be used after contacting one of the senior laboratory staff to discuss the indication. The misuse of emergency services may delay truly urgent results.

CONCLUSIONS

- It is essential to liaise closely with the laboratory when collecting patient samples to help ensure correct sampling times and collection conditions.
- In-vitro haemolysis can lead to a spurious increase of predominantly intracellular ions in the plasma, such as potassium (pseudohyperkalaemia).
- Particular attention should be paid to avoiding blood samples being collected from the same arm as an intravenous infusion, leading to 'drip arm' results.
- It is also essential to ensure correct sample labelling and patient identification to avoid potentially life-threatening errors and medico-legal disasters.

30 POINT OF CARE TESTING

| Some major advantages of point of care testing | 393 | Some possible clinical settings for point of care testing devices | 394 |

Recently, laboratories have tended to become more specialized and centralized and may process millions of samples per year. High throughput, cost-effective automation (perhaps including the use of robotics), stringent quality assurance processes, computerization with data storage and retrieval systems, and highly skilled, monitored personnel are now common. In contrast, 'point of care testing' (POCT) has now developed, which enables clinicians or patients to perform tests without necessarily using the laboratory directly.

SOME MAJOR ADVANTAGES OF POINT OF CARE TESTING

Turnaround times

One of the main advantages of POCT over laboratory testing is the relative immediacy of results. This may enable prompt treatment, shortened patient waiting time and a reduced number of outpatient appointments and clinic visits for the patient.

Many POCT devices require minimal specimen preparation or collection (in some cases using a finger prick of blood). The machine is in the near-patient setting, thus reducing the delays associated with the transport of specimens and reports.

Technological advances and ease of use

The recent increase in POCT has partly been due to technological changes in the design of analysers. With the advent of micro-chips, computerization and miniaturization, it has become easier to bring analysis nearer to the patient and for it to be performed by personnel with minimal training or by the patients themselves. Some of the modern POCT devices incorporate biosensors, electrodes and dry and solid-phase chemistry reagents. These allow for small sample and reagent volumes, quick assay reaction times, ease of use and disposal of used reagents, more than one analyte to be measured simultaneously and probably less technical skill.

Transcutaneous biosensors allow continuous measurements to be made through the patient's skin without the need for blood collection. Near-infrared spectroscopy may allow continuous monitoring of more than one analyte as well as in-vivo glucose monitoring with implantable sensors in diabetic patients.

In choosing a POCT analyser system, remember that duplication may occur within the hospital at separate sites. Different analysers on the same site may result in the use of different reference ranges and thus difficulties in comparing patient results. Many of the new POCT analysers are relatively easy to maintain, but maintenance may need to be carried out by non-laboratory staff out of the laboratory setting. It is also likely that results will need to be interpreted and troubleshooting performed by non-laboratory personnel.

Costs

The reduction in turnaround time may result in a reduction in total costs if patient episodes are shorter and transport costs are reduced, for example courier costs. However, on a direct charge basis including capital costs, POCT may be more expensive than central laboratory testing. This can be due in part to duplication of tests overall and to economies of scale. The costs of reagents and machines, quality control

> **Box 30.1 Some possible advantages and disadvantages of point of care testing (POCT)**
>
> *Advantages*
>
> The methods may be less clinically invasive, e.g. finger prick of blood or biosensor
> There is usually a shorter result turnaround time and thus earlier treatment modification or initiation
> Patients can be more involved in their care
> There is a possibility of on-line monitoring of patients
> It may offer advantages in remote areas
> There is greater laboratory test selectivity, as there is less of a requirement to be restricted to analyser-dedicated 'profiles'
> There is the possibility of reduced on-call staff costs, but this is institution dependent
> It may save sample transport and reporting costs
>
> *Disadvantages*
>
> The ready availability of tests may cause increased inappropriate testing
> The tests may be performed by inexperienced, non-laboratory trained staff
> Reference ranges and results may differ from those of the laboratory, thus making comparison difficult
> Care is needed in machine maintenance and repairs
> Poor training may lead to inadequate quality control
> There may be a lack of back-up support should a device fail
> Duplication of equipment is possible in different hospital sites
> Without economies of scale, tests may become expensive

materials, maintenance, storage of report forms and results and training may all need to be taken into consideration when embarking on POCT. Labour costs are more difficult to assess in POCT, but may incorporate nursing staff; however, set against this are possible savings of on-call or out-of-hours costs for laboratory staff.

Depending on the structure and organization of the POCT setting, the overall costs could be less when the merits of rapid therapeutic responses and shorter hospital stays are taken into consideration (Box 30.1).

SOME POSSIBLE CLINICAL SETTINGS FOR POINT OF CARE TESTING DEVICES

A few examples of clinical situations in which POCT may be useful are given below.

Accident and emergency

One of the potential advantages of POCT is the possibility of fast result turnaround time, which is particularly important in the accident and emergency (A&E) department.

A significant number of A&E departments have blood gas machines, blood glucose meters and even small hand-held analysers for common biochemical tests. One area in A&E where POCT is very important is in the biochemical diagnosis of acute myocardial infarction using troponin T or I.

The introduction of thrombolytic therapy for myocardial infarction has been shown to improve survival, but ideally should be instigated as soon as possible, hence the interest in POCT.

CASE 1

A 13-year-old female with known type 1 diabetes mellitus was admitted to a casualty department because of drowsiness. A blood stix finger-prick test done in the casualty department showed blood glucose of 20 mmol/L. The medical senior house officer was going to give her some more insulin but decided, wisely, to confirm the result by sending a blood sample to the laboratory. The result was returned as 1.8 mmol/L!

DISCUSSION
It later transpired that the girl's fingers had been contaminated with vomit after she had been given some orange squash to drink, which led to a spuriously high blood glucose concentration result by POCT.

The moral of this case is to ensure proper sample collection and staff training. Check unexpected abnormal results with the laboratory.

In cases of drug overdose, it may take a few minutes for the results of POCT measurement of plasma paracetamol concentrations to be obtained.

Coagulation clinics

A number of devices are available which, using capillary or venous blood, can measure prothrombin or activated partial thrombin time. These can be used in coagulation clinics or by patients on warfarin to monitor their own treatment.

Drug addiction clinics

Measuring for drugs of abuse or ethanol is eliciting considerable interest in drug and alcohol addiction clinics. Various drugs can be assayed, including opiates, cocaine, cannabis, benzodiazepines, amphetamines and methadone. In the future it may also be possible for individuals to test their level of ethanol, which would be particularly useful in the context of drink-driving.

General practice, outpatient clinics and wards

Many outpatient clinics and wards as well as general practices use urine dipstick testing for screening patients, and various urine-testing strips are available. Some of these tests can be useful to screen for urinary tract infections.

There are also machines to determine cholesterol, triglyceride and high-density lipoprotein-cholesterol concentrations. Some desktop analysers allow other parameters to be assayed, for example creatinine, glucose, bilirubin and haemoglobin.

Special care baby units and adult intensive care

One blood test for which POCT is very relevant in the special care baby units is the determination of bilirubin using POCT bilirubinometers. In addition, blood gas machines and mini-analysers have been developed. One advantage is the need for only small blood samples.

Patient self-testing

Pregnancy testing is one of the most commonly used forms of POCT that patients can perform themselves.

The test of faecal occult blood as a diagnostic aid for colorectal carcinoma is another possibility for POCT by the patient.

Near-patient testing and diabetes mellitus

The patient management of diabetes mellitus is one area in medicine in which POCT or self-monitoring is frequently used. Broadly, this can be considered as involving urinary glucose concentration determinations, ketone urinary or plasma tests, blood glucose measurements, glycated haemoglobin assays and urinary microalbumin tests.

Box 30.1 gives some of the advantages and some of the disadvantages of POCT.

CONCLUSIONS

- The use of POCT is increasing in clinical medicine.
- POCT allows prompt patient result turn-around and thus the potential for speedy clinical management.
- POCT plays a large role in the management of diabetes mellitus, with some patients testing their own blood glucose levels and adjusting their diabetes therapy accordingly.
- However, POCT also has potential problems, and there should be close liaison with the hospital laboratory to ensure optimal usage. Good quality control is essential.

APPENDIX 1
UNITS IN CLINICAL CHEMISTRY

Results in clinical chemistry have been expressed in a variety of units. For example, the concentrations of electrolytes were formerly usually quoted in mEq/L, the concentration of protein in g/100 ml and that of cholesterol in mg/100 ml. The units used might vary from laboratory to laboratory: calcium concentrations might be expressed as mg/100 ml or mEq/L; in Britain plasma urea concentrations were expressed as mg/100 ml of urea, whereas in the United States it is usual to report mg/100 ml of urea nitrogen. This situation can be confusing and with patients moving, not only from one hospital to another, but from one country to another, dangerous misunderstandings have arisen.

SYSTÈME INTERNATIONAL D'UNITÉS (SI UNITS)

International standardization is obviously desirable, and such standardization has long existed in many branches of science and technology. The main recommendations for clinical chemistry are as follows:

- If the molecular weight (MW) of the substance being measured is known, the unit of quantity should be the mole or a subunit of a mole.

$$\text{Number of moles (mol)} = \frac{\text{weight in g}}{\text{MW}}$$

In clinical chemistry, in the UK, millimoles (mmol), micromoles (μmol) and nanomoles (nmol) are the most common units.

- The unit of volume should be the litre. Units of concentration are therefore mmol/L, μmol/L or nmol/L.

Examples

Results previously expressed as mEq/L

$$\text{Number of equivalents (Eq)} = \frac{\text{weight in g}}{\text{Equivalent weight}}$$

$$= \frac{\text{weight in g} \times \text{valency}}{\text{MW}}$$

- In the case of univalent ions, such as sodium and potassium, the units will be numerically the same. A sodium concentration of 140 mEq/L becomes 140 mmol/L.
- For polyvalent ions, such as calcium and magnesium (both divalent), the old units are divided by the valency. For example, a magnesium concentration of 2.0 mEq/L becomes 1.0 mmol/L.

Results previously expressed as mg/100 ml

If results were previously expressed in mg/100 ml the method of conversion to mmol/L is to divide by the molecular weight (to convert from mg to mmol) and to multiply by 10 (to convert from 100 ml to L). Thus effectively the previous units are divided by a tenth of the molecular weight. For example, the molecular weight of urea is 60, and of glucose 180. A urea concentration of 60 mg/100 ml and a glucose concentration of 180 mg/100 ml are both equivalent to 10 mmol/L. The factor of 10 is, of course, only used for concentrations. The total amount of urea excreted in 24 hours in mg is numerically 60 times that in mmol.

Exceptions

- *Units of pressure* (for example mmHg) are expressed as pascals (or kilopascals [kPa]). One kPa equals 7.5 mmHg, so that a P_{O_2} of 75 mmHg is 10 kPa. Pascals are SI units.
- *Proteins.* Body fluids contain a complex mixture of proteins of varying molecular weights. It is therefore recommended that the gram (g) be retained, but that the unit of volume be the litre (L). Thus a total protein of 7.0 g/100 ml becomes 70 g/L.
- 100 mL should be expressed as decilitre (dL).
- *Enzyme units* are not yet changed. Note that the definition of international units for enzymes does not state the conditions of the reaction.
- Some constituents, such as some hormones, are still expressed in 'international' or other special units.

APPENDIX 1: UNITS IN CLINICAL CHEMISTRY

A conversion table for some of the commoner results is listed in Table A.1. Note that:

1 mol = 1000 mmol (millimoles)
1 mmol (10^{-3} mol) = 1000 μmol (micromoles)
1 μmol (10^{-6} mol) = 1000 nmol (nanomoles)
1 nmol (10^{-9} mol) = 1000 pmol (picomoles)

Table A.1 Some approximate conversion factors for SI units

	From SI units		To SI units	
Bilirubin	μmol/L × 0.058	= mg/dL	mg/dL ÷ 0.058	= μmol/L
Calcium				
Plasma	mmol/L × 4	= mg/dL	mg/dl ÷ 4	= mmol/L
Urine	mmol/24 hours × 40	= mg/24 hours	mg/24 hours ÷ 40	= mmol/24 hours
Cholesterol	mmol/L × 39	= mg/dL	mg/dL ÷ 39	= mmol/L
Cortisol				
Plasma	nmol/L × 0.036	= μg/dL	μg/dL ÷ 0.036	= nmol/L
Urine	nmol/24 hours × 0.36	= μg/24 hours	μg/24 hours ÷ 0.36	= nmol/24 hours
Creatinine				
Plasma	μmol/L × 0.011	= mg/dL	mg/dL ÷ 0.011	= μmol/L
Urine	μmol/24 hours × 0.11	= mg/24 hours	mg/24 hours ÷ 0.11	= μmol/24 hours
P_{O_2}	kPa × 7.5	= mmHg	mmHg ÷ 7.5	= kPa
P_{CO_2}	kPa × 7.5	= mmHg	mmHg ÷ 7.5	= kPa
Glucose	mmol/L × 18	= mg/dL	mg/dL ÷ 18	= mmol/L
Iron	μmol/L × 5.6	= μg/dL	μg/dL ÷ 5.6	= μmol/L
TIBC	μmol/L × 5.6	= μg/dL	μg/dL ÷ 5.6	= μmol/L
Phosphate	mmol/L × 3	= mg/dL	mg/dL ÷ 3	= mmol/L
Proteins				
All serum	g/L ÷ 10	= g/dL	g/dL × 10	= g/L
Urine	g/L × 100	= mg/dL	mg/dL ÷ 100	= g/L
	g/24 hours		No change	
Triglyceride	mmol/L × 88	= mg/dL	mg/dL ÷ 88	= mmol/L
Urate	mmol/L × 17	= mg/dL	mg/dL ÷ 17	= mmol/L
Urea				
Plasma	mmol/L × 6	= mg/dL	mg/dL ÷ 6	= mmol/L
Urine	mmol/24 hours × 60	= mg/24 hours	mg/24 hours ÷ 60	= mmol/24 hours
5-HIAA	μmol/24 hours × 0.2	= mg/24 hours	mg/24 hours ÷ 0.2	= μmol/24 hours
HMMA	μmol/24 hours × 0.2	= mg/24 hours	mg/24 hours ÷ 0.2	= mmol/24 hours
Faecal 'fat'	mmol/24 hours × 0.3	= g/24 hours	g/24 hours ÷ 0.3	= mmol/24 hours

APPENDIX 2
ABBREVIATIONS USED IN THE TEXT

ABC1	adenosine triphosphate-binding cassette protein 1	**CAT**	computerized axial tomography
ACE	angiotensin-converting enzyme	**CBG**	cortisol-binding globulin (transcortin)
ACP	acid phosphatase	**CD**	carbonate dehydratase (carbonic anhydrase)
ACR	albumin:creatinine ratio	**CEA**	carcinoembryonic antigen
ACTH	adrenocorticotrophic hormone (corticotrophin)	**CETP**	cholesterol ester transfer protein
ADH	antidiuretic hormone (arginine vasopressin)	**CK**	creatine kinase
A&E	accident and emergency	**CNP**	C-type natriuretic peptide
AFP	alpha-fetoprotein	**CNS**	central nervous system
AIDS	acquired immunodeficiency syndrome	**COPD**	chronic obstructive pulmonary disease
AIS	autoimmune insulin syndrome	**CRH**	corticotrophin-releasing hormone
ALA	5-aminolaevulinic acid	**CRP**	C-reactive protein
ALP	alkaline phosphatase	**CSF**	cerebrospinal fluid
ALT	alanine aminotransferase (also known as glutamate pyruvate aminotransferase, GPT)	**CT**	computerized tomography
AMC	arm muscle circumference	**Cys C**	Cystatin C
ANP	atrial natriuretic peptide	**DDAVP**	1-desamino-8-D-arginine vasopressin (desmopressin acetate)
APA	aldosterone-producing adenomas	**DHEA**	dehydroepiandrosterone
Apo	apolipoprotein	**DHEAS**	dehydroepiandrosterone sulphate
APRT	adenine phosphoribosyl transferase	**DIT**	di-iodotyrosine
APUD	amine precursor uptake and decarboxylation	**DNA**	deoxyribonucleic acid
ARA	angiotensin receptor antagonist	**2,3-DPG**	2,3-diphosphoglycerate
AST	aspartate aminotransferase (also known as glutamate oxaloacetate aminotransferase, GOT)	**DVT**	deep vein thrombosis
ATP	adenosine triphosphate	**ECF**	extracellular fluid
BJP	Bence-Jones protein	**ECG**	electrocardiogram
BMD	bone mineral density	**EDTA**	ethylenediamine tetra-acetic acid
BMI	body mass index	**ENT**	ear, nose and throat
BMR	basal metabolic rate	**ERCP**	endoscopic retrograde cholangiopancreatography
BNP	brain natriuretic peptide	**ESR**	erythrocyte sedimentation rate
BPH	benign prostatic hyperplasia	**EUS**	endoscopic ultrasonography
CA	carbohydrate antigen	**FAD**	flavine adenine dinucleotide
CAE	calcium excreted per litre of glomerular filtrate	**FCH**	familial combined hyperlipidaemia
CAH	congenital adrenal hyperplasia	**FDH**	familial dysalbuminaemic hyperthyroxinaemia
cAMP	cyclic adenosine monophosphate	**FENa%**	fractional excretion of sodium
CaSR	calcium-sensing receptor	**FE**	fractional excretion
		FEPi%	fractional excretion of phosphate
		FMN	flavine mononucleotide
		FSH	follicle stimulating hormone

APPENDIX 2: ABBREVIATIONS USED IN THE TEXT

GAD	glutamic decarboxylase	MEN	multiple endocrine neoplasia
GDM	gestational diabetes mellitus	MIBG	meta-iodobenzylguanidine
GFR	glomerular filtration rate	MIT	mono-iodotyrosine
GGT	gamma-glutamyltransferase	MODY	maturity-onset diabetes of the young
GH	growth hormone	MPS	mucopolysaccharidosis
GHRH	growth hormone-releasing hormone	MRCP	magnetic resonance cholangiopancreatography
GnRH	gonadotrophin-releasing hormone		
G-6-P	glucose-6-phosphate	MRI	magnetic resonance imaging
G-6-PD	glucose-6-phosphate dehydrogenase	mRNA	messenger ribonucleic acid
GRA	glucocorticoid remediable aldosteronism	MSH	melanocyte-stimulating hormone
		mtDNA	mitochondrial DNA
HAV	Hepatitis A virus		
HBD	hydroxybutyrate dehydrogenase	NAD	nicotinamide adenine dinucleotide
HBV	Hepatitis B virus	NADP	nicotinamide adenine dinucleotide phosphate
hCG	human chorionic gonadotrophin		
HCV	Hepatitis C virus	NASH	non-alcoholic steatotic hepatitis
HDL	high-density lipoprotein	NEFA	non-esterified fatty acid
HELP	heparin extracorporeal low-density lipoprotein precipitation	NICTH	non-islet cell tumour hypoglycaemia
		NP	natriuretic peptide
HGPRT	hypoxanthine–guanine phosphoribosyl transferase	NSAID	non-steroidal anti-inflammatory drug
		NSTEMI	non-ST segment elevation myocardial infarction
5-HIAA	5-hydroxyindole acetic acid		
HIV	human immunodeficiency virus		
HMG-CoA	3-hydroxy-3-methyl glutaryl coenzyme A	OGTT	oral glucose tolerance test
HMMA	4-hydroxy-3-methoxymandelic acid	PABA	p-amino benzoic acid
HNF	hepatocyte nuclear factor	PBG	porphobilinogen
HONK	hyperosmolar non-ketotic	PCR	polymerase chain reaction
HRT	hormone replacement therapy	PH	primary hyperaldosteronism
hs-CRP	high-sensitivity C-reactive protein	PI	protease inhibitors
5-HT	hydroxytryptamine (serotonin)	PKU	phenylketonuria
5-HTP	hydroxytryptophan	PNI	prognostic nutritional index
HVA	homovanillic acid	POCT	point of care testing
		PPAR	peroxisome proliferator-activated receptors
IAH	idiopathic adrenal hyperplasia	PRPP	phosphoribosyl pyrophosphate
IDL	intermediate-density lipoprotein	PSA	prostate-specific antigen
IEM	inborn errors of metabolism	PTH	parathyroid hormone
IFG	impaired fasting glucose	PTHRP	parathyroid hormone-related protein
IFN	interferon		
Ig	immunoglobulin	RBP	retinol-binding protein
IGF	insulin-like growth factor	RDS	respiratory distress syndrome
IGT	impaired glucose tolerance	RFLP	restriction fragment length polymorphism
IL	interleukin		
INR	International Normalized Ratio	RNA	ribonucleic acid
		ROC	receiver operator curve
LCAT	lecithin-cholesterol acyltransferase		
LDH	lactate dehydrogenase	SCID	severe combined immunodeficiency
LDL	low-density lipoprotein	SHBG	sex-hormone-binding globulin
LH	luteinizing hormone	SIADH	syndrome of inappropriate antidiuretic hormone
MCH	mean corpuscular haemoglobin		
MCV	mean corpuscular volume	SLE	systemic lupus erythematosus

T_3	tri-iodothyronine	TSH	thyroid-stimulating hormone
T_4	thyroxine	TSI	thyroid-stimulating immunoglobulin
TBPA	thyroxine-binding pre-albumin	TTKG	transtubular potassium gradient
TBG	thyroxine-binding globulin		
TBW	total body water	UGT	uridine glucoronyl transferase
TCA	tricarboxylic acid	URL	upper reference limit
TfR	transferrin receptor		
TIBC	total iron-binding capacity	VIP	vasoactive intestinal polypeptide
TNF	tumour necrosis factor	VLCFA	very long-chain fatty acids
TPO	thyroperoxidase	VLDL	very low-density lipoprotein
TPMT	thiopurine methyltransferase		
TRH	thyrotrophin-releasing hormone	WHO	World Health Organization

INDEX

'vs' indicates the differentiation of various conditions.

abbreviations used 399–401
abdominal obesity in metabolic syndrome X 183
abdominal pain 248–9
absorption in GI tract 232, 234–8
　defects *see* malabsorption
　drug 346
accident and emergency, point of care testing 394
acetaminophen poisoning 351–3
acetazolamide 84, 89
　hyperchloraemic acidosis associated with 67
Acetest 196
acetyl CoA 175, 179
acetylation, isoniazid 350
acetylcholinesterase 277
　fetal 156
　red cell, reduced 278
N-acetylcysteine 351–2
acid
　bile 236
　gastric *see* stomach
acid–base balance 58–80
　definitions and terminology 58–9
　neonatal 358
　regulation 59–64
　see also pH
acid–base balance disturbances (=H$^+$ disturbances) 64–77
　arterial blood estimation in 79, 80
　summary of findings 76
　compensatory changes in 76–7
　investigations (other than blood gases) 80
　mixed 76–7
acid phosphatase 276–7
　prostatic 279
acidaemia 64
acidophils (pituitary) 116
acidosis
　metabolic 64, 65–71
　　causes 75
　　compensatory changes in 76
　　diabetic ketoacidosis *see* ketoacidosis
　　hyperchloraemic acidosis 67, 80
　　hypokalaemic acidosis 88–9
　　lactic acidosis 58, 67, 180–2
　　management 69–71
　　mixed respiratory acidosis and 76, 77
　　neonatal 358

renal tubular acidosis *see* tubules, renal
　tests determining cause 70
　potassium in 83, 91
　respiratory *see* respiratory acidosis
　severe, blood pH indicating 59
　urinary buffers in correction of 63
acromegaly 119–20
　glucose tolerance test 119, 120, 191
ACTH *see* adrenocorticotrophic hormone
acute-phase reactions and proteins 281–2, 284–6
　neonatal 364–5
acyl-CoA dehydrogenase deficiency, medium chain 378
addiction clinics, point of care testing 395
Addison's disease (hypoadrenocorticism; chronic adrenocortical insufficiency) 19, 129, 134–5, 136–7
　hyperkalaemia 91
　investigation in suspected disease 136–7
Addisonian crisis 136
adenine phosphoribosyl transferase (APRT) 302
adenomas
　adrenal 131, 140, 141
　　removal 141
　pituitary 123, 124–5
　　growth hormone-producing 119, 120
　　prolactin-producing 125, 146–7
adenosine deaminase 333
　gene therapy 371
ADH *see* antidiuretic hormone
adipose tissue *see* fat
adipsic hypernatraemia 21
adrenal cortex 127–43
　hyperfunction 130–4, 138–43
　hypofunction/insufficiency (hypoadrenalism) 131, 134–7
　　acute (Addisonian crisis) 136
　　chronic *see* Addison's disease
　　investigation 136–7, 142
　　secondary (ACTH deficiency) 118, 124, 136
adrenal hyperplasia
　adenoma vs 141, 142
　congenital (CAH) 128, 138–40, 153
　　diagnosis 139–40
　　treatment 140
　idiopathic 140

adrenal medulla 127
　phaeochromocytoma 336
adrenaline metabolism and actions 335–6
adrenocorticotrophic hormone (ACTH) 116, 130
　actions 116
　deficiency 118, 124, 136
　ectopic 338, 339
　　Cushing's syndrome 131, 134, 338
　　hypokalaemia in 86, 339
　excess 118, 124, 134
　measurements 133–4, 136
　secretion (and its regulation) 116, 127–8, 129
　　in stress 129
　see also tetracosactrin stimulation test
agammaglobulinaemia, infantile sex-linked 290
age 355–67
　drug metabolism and 347
　test results related to 3
　　plasma enzyme levels 270
　　plasma iron 311
　see also children; elderly; infants; neonates
air, expired, water loss 8
airways, small, obstruction 78
Alagille's syndrome 360
alanine aminotransferases (ALT) 253, 254, 266, 269, 270–1
　non-disease factors affecting 370
albinism 373
albumin 283–4
　CSF 331–2
　plasma 253, 254, 283–4
　　calcium binding to 94, 95
　　drug binding to 346
　　electrophoresis 281
　　haem binding to 310
　　indications for estimation 300
　　low levels *see* hypoalbuminaemia
　　in nutritional assessment 216
　　synthesis, abnormalities 283
　urinary, and its estimation 186, 296
albumin-corrected calcium 94–6
　raised 102
Albustix 298
alcohol abuse
　Cushing's syndrome vs 133
　hypoglycaemia in 194

alcohol abuse (*contd*)
  liver disease 257, 261, 266, 277
aldolase 273
aldosterone (mineralocorticoid) 9, 129
  actions 9, 42
  deficiency *see* hypoaldosteronism
  excess (aldosteronism;
      hyperaldosteronism;
      mineralocorticoid excess)
    hypokalaemia with 23, 24, 85
    metabolic alkalosis in 73, 74, 88
    primary *see* Conn's syndrome
    secondary 22–3, 85
  in low renal blood flow and GFR 42
  measurements 140–1, 141
  potassium loss in urine and 83
alfacalcidol administration 109
alkalaemia 64
alkaline phosphatase levels 254, 265, 274–6
  in bone disease 275, 276
    malignancy 101
  in cholestasis 255, 265
  isoenzymes 275–6
    Regan isoenzyme (=placental alkaline
      phosphatase) 275–6, 276, 279, 343
  in liver disease 265, 275
  in malignancy 279, 343
    of bone 101
  non-disease factors affecting 370
  in pregnancy 159
  raised 3
alkalosis 72–7
  metabolic 72–4
    causes 73
      compensatory changes in 76
      hypokalaemic alkalosis 24, 73, 87–8
      management 73–4
      neonatal 358
      of pyloric stenosis or chronic vomiting
        73, 75, 80
    potassium in 83, 84
    respiratory *see* respiratory alkalosis
    severe, blood pH indicating 59
alkaptonuria 196, 373
allele(s)
  inheritance patterns 381–2
  multiple 382
  oligonucleotide probes specific to 383
allergy and IgE 289
Allgrove's syndrome 135
allopurinol 302, 304, 305
alpha$_1$-antitrypsin 285
  deficiency 260, 266, 283, 291–2, 385–6
    genetic tests 385–6
  electrophoresis 283
  neonatal 365
alpha-fetoprotein
  neural tube defects 156
  tumours 342

alpha$_1$-globulins, electrophoresis 281
  in disease 282, 283
alpha$_2$-globulins, electrophoresis 281
  in disease 281, 282, 283
aluminium toxicity 232
alveoli and blood gas results 77–8
amenorrhoea 149–50, 159
amidophosphoribosyl transferase 301
  overactivity 304
amine precursor uptake and decarboxylation,
    tumours of cells involved 335
amino acids
  absorption 236
    defective 244
  hepatic deamination 251
    impaired 259–60
  metabolic/transport disorders 372–5
  parenteral 217
p-aminobutyric acid (PABA) test 239, 246
5-aminolaevulinic acid (ALA) 309
  raised levels 318, 319
5-aminolaevulinic acid (ALA) synthase 309
  increased activity 318, 319
aminotransferases 253, 265–6, 270–1, 279
amiodarone 347–8
  therapeutic monitoring 347–8
  thyroid function and 172, 348
ammonia
  neonatal 365
  urinary buffering 62, 63
ammonium chloride loading test 79
amniotic fluid measurements 156
amylase 235, 273–4
  isoenzymes 274
  measurements 238, 269, 273–4
    case study 274
    in diabetic ketoacidosis 188
    pleural fluid 333
amyloid 295
anaemia 315
  B-cell malignancy 293
  of chronic illness, iron concentrations in
    312, 313, 315, 316
  haemolytic 312
  iron-deficiency 315–16
  malabsorption as cause of 242–3, 244,
    245–6
  sickle-cell 386
  sideroblastic, porphyrinuria of 320
  vitamin A deficiency 223
  vitamin B$_6$ deficiency 227
  vitamin B$_{12}$ and folate deficiency 227, 228
  vitamin C deficiency 230
anaerobic carbohydrate metabolism 58, 180
anaesthetics, general, and malignant
    hyperpyrexia 379
analbuminaemia 283
analysers, point of care 393
Andersen's disease 376

androgens 127
  adrenal 129
    deficiency (hypoandrogenism) 135
      males 152
    excess (hyperandrogenism) 138
      in Cushing's disease 131
  gonadal 129
    female (ovarian) 145
    male (testicular) 145–6
androstenedione 145
anencephaly 156
angioneurotic oedema, hereditary 291
angiotensin I 9
angiotensin II 9
angiotensin II receptor blockers/antagonists
  diabetic nephropathy 186
  hyperkalaemia 90
  hypertension 328
angiotensin-converting enzyme 9, 278
angiotensin-converting enzyme inhibitors
  diabetic nephropathy 186
  hyperkalaemia 90
  hypertension 328
anion gap
  plasma 65
    high 65, 66–7
  urinary 66, 68–9
anorexia nervosa 220
anovulation *see* ovulation
antenatal tests *see* prenatal tests
antiarrhythmic drug monitoring 347–8
antibiotic monitoring 350
antibodies/immunoglobulins (in general)
    287–9
  in CSF, synthesis 331–2, 332
    by plasma cells 331
  deficient production 290
  in infection 288–9
    detection in viral hepatitis 256–7
  in liver disease, assays 266
  monoclonal, elevated levels *see*
    paraproteinaemia
  neonatal 365
  in plasma cell myeloma, disordered
    synthesis 294
  structure 287–8
antibodies/immunoglobulins in autoimmune
    disease
  in diabetes mellitus 182, 183
    to insulin 182, 194, 194
  in primary biliary cirrhosis 255
  to thyroid hormones 166, 167, 169
    interfering with assays 166
anticoagulants, blood samples 390
anticonvulsant monitoring 348–9
antidiuretic hormone (ADH; arginine
    vasopressin) 8–9
  actions 8–9
    countercurrent exchange 39

failure of homeostatic mechanisms
    involving 20–1
impaired renal tubular response to *see*
    nephrogenic diabetes insipidus
inappropriate secretion of (SIADH)
    24–5, 339
    case study 26
    hyponatraemia 25, 339, 356
    management 29
    neonatal 356
secretion (and its regulation) 8, 14, 18
    impaired *see* cranial diabetes
        insipidus
    with renal blood flow reduction 42
    sodium depletion and 19
see also DDAVP
antidiuretic hormone (ADH; arginine
    vasopressin) deficiency, consequences
    see diabetes insipidus
antidotes, specific
    drugs with 351–3
    drugs without 353
antiepileptic monitoring 348–9
antifreeze poisoning 353
antigens
    Ig binding site 288
    viral hepatitis 256–7
antihypertensive drugs 328
antipsychotic (neuroleptic) drugs 117
α_1-antitrypsin *see* alpha$_1$-antitrypsin
anuria, causes 45–6
apolipoproteins 201, 202, 204
    apoA$_1$ deficiency 210
    apoB
        ApoB$_{3500}$ mutation (=familial
            defective apolipoprotein B-100)
            207, 386
        metabolic defect 210
    apoC$_2$ deficiency 206
    apoE
        apoE$_2$ genotype/homozygosity/variants
            208, 209, 213
        phenotyping 386
APUDomas 335
argentaffin cells 337
arginine hydrochloride, growth hormone
    deficiency 123
arginine vasopressin *see* antidiuretic
    hormone
arm muscle circumference 215
arrhythmias
    hypercalcaemia 99
    hypokalaemia 87
    therapeutic drug monitoring 347–8
arterial blood *see* blood
arthritis, rheumatoid 333
arylsulphatase deficiency 375
ascites 259
ascorbate *see* vitamin C

aspartate aminotransferases (AST) 253, 254,
    266, 269, 270
    in myocardial infarction 269, 323, 324–5
asphyxia, perinatal 357
ATPase *see* sodium/potassium exchange
atrial natriuretic peptide 10, 326
autoimmune disease
    adrenal 134
    diabetes as 183
    hepatobiliary system 255–6, 266
    parathyroid 107
    thyroid 166–7
    see also antibodies
autosomal inheritance 381–2
azathioprine 350–1

B-cells/lymphocytes 284
    defects 290
    disorders 292
bacterial flora, intestinal,
    alterations/overgrowth 237, 243–4
    investigation/diagnosis 243, 245, 246
bacterial infection of CSF (and meningitis)
    330, 332
Bartter's syndrome 86, 87
basal metabolic rate (BMR)
    daily 216–17
    in starvation 215
basophils (pituitary) 116
Becker's muscular dystrophy, genetic tests 385
Bence-Jones proteins 292–3
    urinary 296, 342
benzodiazepine overdose 353
beriberi 225
beryllium poisoning 102
beta-cell (β-cell), pancreatic islet 175
    tumours *see* insulinoma
beta-globulins, electrophoresis 281
beta$_2$-microglobulin 293
bicarbonate (HCO_3^-)
    CO_2 conversion to 59
    fall/reduction leading to metabolic
        acidosis 64, 65
        in diabetes mellitus 187, 190
        with high anion gap 66–7
    generation/formation
        by erythrocytes 60–1
        in GI tract 63–4
        in kidney 61, 62
    in Henderson–Hasselbach equation 59
    in intravenous fluids 11
    measurement in blood/plasma 80
        in hyperkalaemia 92
    reclamation/reabsorption in kidney 61,
        61–2
    regulation of plasma bicarbonate 59
    rise/increase leading to metabolic alkalosis
        72, 72–3
    see also sodium bicarbonate

biguanides 185
bile 263
    formation 263
    obstructed flow *see* biliary tract
    stasis *see* cholestasis
bile acids 236, 263
    in obstetric cholestasis 255
    synthesis 236, 251, 263
bile salts 204, 236, 263
    deficiency 263
    sequestrants 210–11
biliary atresia, congenital 360
biliary cirrhosis, primary 255–6, 266
biliary tract 263–4
    calculi/stones 255, 263–4
    obstruction 243, 255, 264, 266
        neonatal 360
    sodium bicarbonate secretion 64
bilirubin 251–3
    CSF 330
    excretion 251–2
    formation 251–2
    measurements 254, 266
        in cholestasis 255
    metabolism 252
        neonatal 359–60
    retention in plasma 252–3
    urinary (bilirubinuria) 253, 254, 265
    see also hyperbilirubinaemia
biochemical effects of drugs 344
biopsy, liver 266
    iron overload 317
        primary haemochromatosis 314
biosensors in point of care testing 393
biotin 227, 229
bisalbuminaemias 283
bisphosphonates
    hypercalcaemia 103, 104
    osteoporosis 110
    Paget's disease of bone 110
bleeding *see* haemorrhage
blind loop (contaminated bowel) syndrome
    237, 242, 243
blood (arterial)
    gases 77–80
        factors affecting results 77–8
        indications for estimation 79–80
        specimen collection for estimations
            79
        see also carbon dioxide; oxygen
    in hydrogen ion disturbances, summary of
        findings 76
    pH
        abnormalities 59–60
        regulation/buffering 60–2
blood (CSF), presence 331
blood group incompatibility, fetomaternal
    157
    jaundice 360

blood pressure abnormalities *see* hypertension; hypotension
blood samples
  collection 388–91
    for blood gases 79
    for drug monitoring, timing 345
  containers 390
  delayed separation 391
  in diabetes 191
  in coma 190
  haemolysis 390
  neonatal screening for inborn errors of metabolism 369
  prenatal screening 369
  for protein estimations 299–300
  refrigeration 391
blood tests, faeces occult 247
body mass index, classification 220
Bohr effect 77
bone
  disorders 275, 276
    alkaline phosphatase *see* alkaline phosphatase
    elderly 367
    not normally affecting calcium levels 109–10
    in primary hyperparathyroidism 100
  growth *see* growth
  malignancy 275
    hypercalcaemia with metastatic deposits 101
    parathyroid hormone actions 96, 97
  in vitamin C deficiency 229
bone marrow
  iron use by, disorders affecting 312
  in plasma cell myeloma, appearance 294
bone mineral density estimation 110
bowel *see* intestine
brain-derived natriuretic peptide 326
branching enzyme deficiency 376
breast enlargement, males 153, 340
breastfeeding (lactation) 155
breath test 247
  hydrogen 244
  triolein 237, 243
broad β hyperlipidaemia 208–9
bromocriptine 117, 120, 147
  in amenorrhoea and infertility 161
Bruton's disease 290
buffering 58, 59, 60–4
  blood 60–2
  buffer pairs 59, 63
  urinary 62–3
burns, metabolic response 215

C-peptide (insulin) 175
  measurements 193, 194
C-reactive protein (CRP) 285–6, 327
  infections 285, 332

C-type natriuretic peptide 326
C1 esterase inhibitor defect/deficiency 291
C3 component of complement 286
CA 15-3 342
CA 19-9 342
CA 125 342
cabergoline 147
cadmium toxicity 232
caeruloplasmin 230, 231, 260
calciferol *see* vitamin D
calcitonin 97
  in hypercalcaemia 104
  in medullary carcinoma of thyroid 339
  see also procalcitonin
calcium 94–109
  absorption 238
  intake
    factors affecting 94
    reduced 105, 106
  in intravenous fluids 11
  loss/depletion
    factors affecting 94
    neonatal 364
  metabolism 94–8
    disorders *see* hypercalcaemia; hypercalciuria; hypocalcaemia
    neonatal 363–4
  plasma, regulation 94–8
  renal handling 38
  renal stones containing 55
calcium gluconate
  in hyperkalaemia 92
  in hypocalcaemia 109
calcium pyrophosphate deposition 306
Calcium Resonium 93
calcium-sensing receptor 98
calculi/stones
  biliary (gallstones) 255, 263–4
  renal 54–7
    in cystinuria 56, 57, 374
    in hypercalcaemia 55, 98, 100
    in hyperuricaemia 55, 203
cancer *see* malignancy
capillary membrane
  albumin redistribution due to increased permeability 283
  water distribution across 14
captopril test 141
carbamazepine monitoring 345, 348
carbamyl phosphate synthetase deficiency 371–2
carbenoxolone 86, 87
carbimazole 170
carbohydrate 174–97
  chemistry 174
  digestion/absorption 235
  malabsorption 243
  metabolism 174–97
    anaerobic 58, 180

growth hormone effects 119, 177
inborn errors 375–7
nutrition and 214
carbohydrate antigens 342
carbon dioxide
  bicarbonate generation in response to PCO_2 rise 60
  blood
    estimation of total plasma CO_2 80
    fall leading to respiratory alkalosis 74
    rise leading to respiratory acidosis 64, 71
    conversion to bicarbonate 59
  in lung, control 59–60
  see also hypercapnic respiratory failure
carbon monoxide poisoning 309, 353
  pulse oximetry in 79
carbonate dehydratase (CD; carbonic anhydrase) 60, 61, 62
  inhibitors 67, 84, 89
carbonic acid in Henderson–Hasselbach equation 59
carbonic anhydrase (carbonate dehydratase; CD) 60, 61, 62
carboxyhaemoglobin 79, 309, 353
carcinoembryonic antigen 341, 342
carcinoid syndrome 227, 241, 337–8
carcinoma
  adrenal 131
  cervical squamous cell 343
  colorectal *see* colorectal carcinoma
  gallbladder 264
  gastric 234
  hepatocellular 260, 266
  lung 333
  pancreatic 239
  prostate 279, 340–1
  thyroid 339, 343
cardiovascular disease 323–8
  in chronic renal failure 48
  in diabetes mellitus 184
  elderly 366
  HDL-cholesterol protective effect 205–6
  in hypercalcaemia 99
  in hypokalaemia 87
  pulse oximetry inaccuracies in 79
  risk factor assessment 212, 326–8
    C-reactive protein 286, 327
  see also heart
catecholamines 335–7
  hypokalaemia and 83, 86
  metabolism and actions 335–6
  tumours secreting 336–7
cations, plasma anion gap decreased by 66
cells
  damage and proliferation assessment 268–9
  in liver *see* hepatocytes
  electrolyte distribution between interstitial fluid and 11

fluid compartment within 11
membrane *see* membrane
cerebral tissue inflammation,
non-purulent 331
cerebrospinal fluid (CSF) 329–32
biochemical tests 330–2
examination 329–30
procedures for 332
sample collection 329
cervical squamous cell carcinoma 343
Child–Pugh classification of cirrhosis 259
childbirth
delivery 159
labour induction 35
children
alkaline phosphatase, raised activity 276
androgen excess 138
drug metabolism 347
growth retardation 122–3, 124
see also infants; neonates
chloride
estimation of plasma and urinary Cl⁻ 80
intestinal reabsorption 64
in intravenous fluids 11
see also hyperchloraemia; hypochloraemia
chloride shift 61
cholecalciferol (vitamin D_3) 97
cholecystitis 264
cholecystokinin 235, 238
cholestasis 255, 264, 277
causes 264
drug-induced 258
intrahepatic vs extrahepatic 255
obstetric 255
detection 254
cholesterol 200
inactivation/excretion by liver 251
steroids synthesis and 127
structure 198
synthesis 200, 204
transport/metabolism 204–6, 236
see also high-density lipoprotein-cholesterol; hypercholesterolaemia
cholesterol ester, structure 198
cholesterol ester transfer protein (CETP) 204
cholesterol stones 263
cholinesterase 277–8
causes of increased and decreased activity 277
suxamethonium sensitivity and 277–8, 379
variants 277, 278
choriocarcinoma 159
chorionic gonadotrophin *see* human chorionic gonadotrophin
chromaffin tissue tumour 336–7
chromium 231
chromium-51-labelled EDTA, GFR calculation 51
chromophobes 117

chromosomes 382
abnormalities/disorders 380
antenatal tests 157
sex, and sex determination 147
chronic illness/disease
anaemia of 312, 313, 315, 316
iron concentrations in 312
chylomicrons 200
elevated (in chylomicron syndrome) 206, 213
transport/metabolism 202–3
chylothorax 333
chymotrypsin, faecal 239
ciclosporin monitoring 345, 350
circadian/diurnal variations 3
cortisol levels 3, 129
iron levels in plasma 311
circulatory causes of lactic acidosis 67
cirrhosis 258–9, 266
in alpha₁-antitrypsin deficiency 292
plasma protein electrophoresis 282
primary biliary 255–6, 266
renal dysfunction and 261
clearance in glomerular filtration rate assessment 50–1
clinician identification in test requesting 388
Clinitest tablets 196
clonidine
growth hormone deficiency 123
suppression test 337
clotting *see* coagulation
coagulation (clotting)
CSF 330
point of care testing 395
vitamin K and 224
coagulation factors, hepatic synthesis 251
cobalamins *see* vitamin B_{12}
cobalt 232
Cockcroft–Gault equation 51
coefficient of variation 5
coeliac disease 240, 241
Cohen–Woods classification of lactic acidosis 67
colchicine 305
colic, biliary 264
colipase 236
colitis, ulcerative 245, 286
collagen in vitamin C deficiency 229
collecting ducts 37
colloid osmotic pressure 14
gradient decrease 22
colorectal carcinoma 247–8
carcinoembryonic antigen 341, 342
case study 260
colour, CSF 330
coma in diabetes 188, 188–90
hyperosmolal non-ketotic (HONK) 188, 189, 190

hypoglycaemic 186, 189–90
treatment 189–90
complement 286, 287
deficiency 291
compliance, patient 345
congenital adrenal hyperplasia *see* adrenal hyperplasia
congenital biliary atresia 360
congenital erythropoietic porphyria 320, 321
congenital hypothyroidism 167, 365–6
conjugation reactions in liver
bilirubin 251–2
see also hyperbilirubinaemia, conjugated
steroid hormones 129, 251
Conn's syndrome (primary hyperaldosteronism) 23, 23–4, 140–2
diagnosing cause 141
hypokalaemia 23, 24, 85
investigations 140–1
treatment 141–2
connective tissue disease, C-reactive protein in 285
containers
blood sample 390
urine 392
contaminated bowel (blind loop) syndrome 237, 242, 243
contraceptive pill *see* oral contraceptives
contraction alkalosis 73
copper 230–1
deficiency 230
metabolic defect (of Wilson's disease) 230–1, 260, 266
coproporphyria, hereditary 318
coproporphyrin(ogen) 309
Cori cycle 180, 181
Cori disease 376
coronary heart disease 211, 212
lipid-lowering in prevention of 211, 212
risk
assessment 326–8
in homozygous familial hypercholesterolaemia 207
corpus luteum 145
corticosteroids *see* glucocorticoids; mineralocorticoids; steroids
corticosterone 128
corticotroph 116
corticotrophin *see* adrenocorticotrophic hormone
corticotrophin-releasing hormone (CRH) 129
intravenous, test employing 134
cortisol (hydrocortisone) 127
actions 128
mineralocorticoid 129
circadian variations in secretion/plasma levels 3, 129

cortisol (hydrocortisone) (contd)
    deficiency/defective synthesis 127–8, 138–9
        acute 135
    excess 130
        investigation 131–3, 136–7
        see also Cushing's syndrome
    factors affecting plasma levels 130–1
    measurement 130–1, 131–3, 136, 136–7
    stress and 129
    synthesis (normal) 129
cortisol-binding globulin 128–9
cortisone 129
cost of point of care testing 393–4
countercurrent exchange 39
countercurrent multiplication 39
cranial diabetes insipidus 20–1
    causes 30
    investigations and management 30, 33, 34, 35
    polyuria in 30
creatine kinase 271–3
    in case studies 4, 324, 326
    causes of raised activities 272–3
        muscular dystrophy 278–9
    ethnic differences 3, 4, 270
    isoenzymes 271–2, 271–2, 323, 323–4, 325
    neonatal 355
creatinine
    plasma
        in diabetic ketoacidosis 188
        measurement 50
    urinary 299
        in hyperuricaemia 305
        in nutritional assessment 216
Crigler–Najjar syndrome 361
critical (intensive) care, point of care testing 395
Crohn's disease 247
    C-reactive protein in 286
cryoglobulins
    blood samples for measurement 299
    elevated (cryoglobulinaemia) 294–5
Cushing's disease 131
Cushing's syndrome 23, 24, 130–4
    causes 131, 133–4
        ectopic tumours 131, 134, 338
        pituitary 118, 124, 131, 133, 134
    hypertension 131, 328
    hypokalaemia 23, 24, 86
    investigations/diagnosis 125–6, 131–3
    mimicking conditions 133
cutaneous disorders see skin lesions
cyanide poisoning 353
cyanocobalamin 228
cystatin C 51–2
cystic fibrosis 238–9, 241–2, 384–5
    diagnosis 384–5
        prenatal testing 242, 369

cystine stones and cystinuria 56, 57, 373, 374
cytochrome P450 status and debrisoquine hydroxylase activity 351
cytokines 284, 285

D-dimers 326
daily variations see circadian variations
DDAVP test 34, 52
dead space, alveolar 78
deamination see amino acids
debranching enzyme deficiency 376
debrisoquine hydroxylase 351
decarboxylation, oxoacid, deficient 373
deep vein thrombosis 326
dehydration, definition 17
dehydroepiandrosterone (DHEA) and its sulphate 129, 150
delivery (in childbirth) 159
dementia
    elderly 367
    nicotinamide deficiency 226
depression vs Cushing's syndrome 133
dermatological lesions see eczema; skin lesions
1-desamino-8-D-arginine vasopressin (DDAVP) test 34, 52
desferrioxamine 353
detoxification in liver 251
dexamethasone suppression test
    high-dose 134
    low-dose 133
dextrose saline
    components 11
    sodium depletion due to incorrect use 18, 19
diabetes insipidus 20
    cranial see cranial diabetes insipidus
    investigations 33–5
    management 30
    nephrogenic 21
diabetes mellitus 182–92
    elderly 366
    idiopathic 182
    investigations 191–2
    ketoacidosis see ketoacidosis
    long-term effects 184–5
    management 185–92
    maternal see pregnancy
    point of care testing 394, 395
    risk factors 183
    type 1 182
    type 2 (non-insulin-dependent DM) 182, 183
    types other than 1 and 2 182–3
diagnostic value of test abnormalities 4
dialysis 53–4
diarrhoea
    disaccharide deficiency 243

nicotinamide deficiency 226
osmotic 247
secretory 247
dibasic amino acid transport disorders 373–4
DIDMOAD syndrome 21
diet see nutrition
diffuse endocrine system 335
DiGeorge's syndrome 107, 364
digestion 233–9
    enzymes involved see enzymes
digestive tract see gastrointestinal tract
digoxin monitoring 345, 347
    case study 348
dihydrotestosterone 146
1,25-dihydroxyvitamin D (1,25-dihydroxycholecalciferol) 97–8
    administration 107
    low concentrations 106
    receptor defect 106
    renal production 37, 97
dilution hypoalbuminaemia 283
dilutional hyponatraemia 18–19, 28
disaccharidases 235
    deficiency 243
disaccharides 174
    digestion/absorption 235
    see also sugars
distal tubules, function 36–7, 42
    acidosis due to defect in 68
    potassium handling 82
        hypokalaemia due to alterations in 85–6
    tests 52
distribution, drug 346
diuresis
    osmotic 9, 30, 33, 41–2
    water 41
diuretics
    neonatal, causing hyponatraemia 357
    potassium-losing see potassium-losing diuretics
    potassium-sparing 84
    thiazide see thiazide diuretics
diurnal variations see circadian variations
DNA 380, 382–3
    hybridization see hybridization
    mitochondrial, disorders related to 378
    polymorphisms 383
    structure 382
    synthesis/replication 382
    transcription 383
DNA chips 384
DNA technology 383–4
    see also genetic tests
dominant inheritance
    autosomal 381
    X-linked 382
dopamine
    drugs blocking actions (antagonists) 117

drugs stimulating actions (agonists) 117, 118, 147
  prolactin and 144
Down's syndrome 156–7
drugs 344–54
  addiction, point of care testing 395
  adverse/side-effects 351
    biochemical monitoring 351
    diabetes 182–3
    on glucose tolerance 192
    hypercalcaemia 99, 101
    hyperkalaemia 90, 91
    hyperprolactinaemia 147
    hyperuricaemia 304
    hypocalcaemia in pregnancy and neonates 364
    hypokalaemia 86, 89
    infertility 161
    osteoporosis 110
    thyroid hormones 171, 172
  albumin binding and consequences of hypoalbuminaemia 284
  blood (serum and plasma) levels 344–50
    factors affecting 345–7
    measurement/monitoring 347–50
  genetic factors influencing reactions to see pharmacogenetics
  interactions 347
  oral, assays affecting by 388–9
  overdose see toxins and drugs
  plasma enzyme levels raised by 269
  therapy with
    diabetes mellitus 185, 186
    hypercalcaemia 103, 104
    hyperlipidaemia see lipid-lowering drugs
    hypertension 328
    hyperthyroidism 170
    monitoring of drugs 344–51
    pituitary growth hormone-producing tumours 120
    pituitary prolactin-producing tumours 147
    respiratory acidosis 71–2
    thyroid function tests and effects of 165–6
Dubin–Johnson syndrome 262, 361
Duchenne muscular dystrophy 278–9
  genetic tests 385
dumping syndrome 234
duodenum
  enzyme measurements 239
  fluid loss, hyperchloraemia associated with 67
  ulcers 234
dwarfs, Laron 122
dysbetalipoproteinaemia 208–9
dyslipidaemias see hyperlipidaemias
dystrophin gene mutations, tests 385

eczema (dermatitis)
  IgE and 289
  nicotinamide deficiency 226
EDTA (ethylene diamine tetra-acetic acid; sequestrene)
  blood samples 390
  radiochromium-labelled, GFR calculation 51
efficiency of test 5
egg (oocyte) development 147
elastase, faecal 239, 241, 246
elderly 366–7
  drug metabolism 347
electrolytes
  distributions in fluid compartments 11
  i.v. administration 11
    in diabetic ketoacidosis 190
  measurement in polyuria 33
  in re-feeding syndrome (parenteral nutrition), abnormalities 219
  see also ions
electrophoresis 281–3, 299
  lipoproteins see lipoprotein
  nucleic acid on gels see gel electrophoresis
  plasma protein 266, 281–2, 300
    in disease 281–3
  urinary proteins 281–3
emesis see vomiting
encephalopathy, hepatic 259–60
  in hyperbilirubinaemia see kernicterus
endocrine function 115–73
  abnormalities/disorders 115–73
    diabetes due to 182
    diagnostic principles 115–16
    hypercalcaemia due to 99–101, 102
    hypoglycaemia due to 193
    kidney failure (chronic) due to 48
    osteoporosis due to 109
  kidney 37
  see also multiple endocrine neoplasia
endocrine system, diffuse 335
endoscopy, malabsorption 246
energy
  balance 214
  sources
    normal 214
    parenteral nutrition 217
enolase, neuronal-specific 343
enteral nutrition 217
enzymes
  cardiac 323–5
  digestive 233–4, 235, 236, 238–9
    duodenal measurements 239
    faecal measurements see faeces
    plasma measurements 238–9
  digestive, deficiency/impaired activity 241–2
    carbohydrate malabsorption due to 243–4

hepatic, measurement 253, 265, 266
induction 277
plasma 268–79
  normal levels 270–8
  in specific diseases 278–9
plasma, measurement 268–79
  factors affecting results 269–70
  units 397
epilepsy, therapeutic drug monitoring 348–9
epinephrine (adrenaline) metabolism and actions 335–6
ergocalciferol (vitamin D_2) 97
erythrocytes (red cells)
  acetylcholinesterase, reduced activity 278
  bicarbonate generation 60, 60–1
  inherited disorders, causing haemolysis 360
  porphyrins, increased concentrations 321
  transketolase activity 226
erythropoietic porphyrias 320, 321
erythropoietin
  secretion, polycythaemia due to 340
  use in chronic renal failure 53
ethnic/racial factors
  diabetes risk 183
  test results 3
    creatine kinase 3, 4, 270
ethylene diamine tetra-acetic acid see EDTA
ethylene glycol poisoning 353
euthyroid state
  goitre 171
  thyroxine levels 164
    elevated 171–2
  see also sick euthyroid syndrome
euvolaemic hypernatraemia 30
euvolaemic hyponatraemia 26, 28
excretion
  drug 346
  by liver 251
    assessment 254
  see also specific substances
exercise test, hypoglycaemia 195
exomphalos 156
expired air, water loss 8
extracellular fluid 11
  distribution
    aldosteronism due to redistribution 22
    control 280
    drug 346
  potassium in 83
    loss from ECF into intestinal secretions 87
  see also interstitial fluid; plasma
exudates, pleural 333
eye problems, vitamin A deficiency 223

F(ab)$_2$ 288
Fabry's disease 375

faeces/stools
  appearance in malabsorption 245
  calcium loss in 94
  collection 392
  enzyme assays 239
    in chronic pancreatitis 241
  fat estimation 237, 246
  occult blood test 247
  osmolality of faecal water, calculation 247
  porphyrins, increased levels 321
  see also diarrhoea; steatorrhoea
false positive or negative result 5
familial studies (incl. relatives)
  haemochromatosis 315, 317
  hyperuricaemia incidence 303
  porphyria 322
Fanconi's syndrome 52, 57, 68, 375
fasting 388
  in hypoglycaemia
    overnight 195
    prolonged 195
  impaired glucose 183
  see also starvation
fat (body fat; adipose tissue)
  assessment 215
  fatty acid metabolism 199
  glucose metabolism and ketosis 178–80
  see also lipid
fat-soluble vitamins 223–4
  absorption 237
    deficiency due to defects in 244
father, genetic, determination 386
fatty acids 199–200
  hepatic metabolism 178, 179
  intestinal absorption 237
  non-esterified/free (NEFA; FFA) 169, 199
  hormones affecting levels 176
  omega-3 211
fatty liver 261, 266
Fc receptors 288
females (women)
  androgens 145
    adrenal excess 138, 139
  daily basal metabolic rate 216
  GFR measurement 51
  infertility see infertility
  menopause 149, 367
  ovarian hormones see sex hormones
  pregnancy see pregnancy
  sexual development see sexual development
feminization 160
ferritin 266, 310, 313
  abnormal levels 313
    iron deficiency and 316
    measurements in iron overload 316–17
      primary haemochromatosis 314–15, 316–17

fertility
  elderly males 367
  problems see infertility
fetus
  abnormality detection see prenatal tests
  blood group incompatibility with mother see blood group incompatibility
  lung immaturity 157
  see also prenatal tests
fibrates 211
  alkaline phosphatase levels affected by 276
fibrin D-dimers 326
filtration, glomerular see glomerulus
fish oils 211
flecainide monitoring 348
fludrocortisone suppression test 141
fluid balance
  abnormalities/disturbances
    in hypoalbuminaemia 284
    in intestine 233
    in re-feeding syndrome 219
  monitoring 10
  neonatal 356
  see also water
fluid compartments 10–11
  electrolyte and water distribution 11
  see also specific compartments
fluid infusions, intravenous 18
  in diabetic ketoacidosis 190
  effects 18
  in hypercalcaemia 104
  in hypernatraemia 30
  incorrect, sodium depletion due to 18–19
  regimens/available forms 11
fluid intake, increased, causing polyuria 30
fluorescence, plasma, porphyrias 320, 321
folate 227–9
  administration lowering homocysteine levels 327
  deficiency 227, 229, 237–8
follicle-stimulating hormone (FSH) 116, 144
  excess/deficiency 118
  females
    in infertility investigations 160
    in menopause 149
    in menstrual cycle 148, 149
  males
    abnormalities 153
    in infertility investigations 160
    secretion and function 145, 146
  measurement 154
follicular phase of menstrual cycle 148
foot ulcers, diabetic 185
Forbes–Cori disease 376
forensic diagnosis, DNA technology 386
Frederickson classification of hyperlipidaemia 201, 206

Friedewald equation 201
fructosamine 186
fructose
  urinary 196
    intolerance, hereditary 196, 362
fumarylacetoacetase abnormality 373
furosemide test 69

galactorrhoea 340
galactose 375–6
  blood, raised (galactosaemia) 196, 260, 375–6
  urinary 196
galactose-1-phosphate uridyl transferase deficiency (galactosaemia) 196, 260, 375–6
α-galactosidase A deficiency 375
β-galactosidase deficiency 375
gallbladder carcinoma 264
gallstones 255, 263–4
gamma-globulins, electrophoresis 281
  CSF 331
  in disease 282, 283
  see also agammaglobulinaemia; hypogammaglobulinaemia; immunoglobulin G
gamma-glutamyltransferase (GGT) 254, 265, 266, 277
gangliosidoses 375
gastrectomy, complications 234, 241
gastric physiology/problems see stomach
gastrin 234, 235
  tumours secreting 234, 248
gastritis, chronic 234
gastrointestinal tract 233–49
  bicarbonate formation 63–4
  bleeding in upper GI tract, porphyrinuria 320
  digestion 233–9
  disorders causing malabsorption 239–48
  neonatal 358
  water handling/output 8
  see also specific regions
Gaucher's disease 375
gel electrophoresis
  DNA for Southern blots 383–4
  RNA 384
gender (sex) differences in test results 3
gene(s) 380, 383
  abnormalities see alleles; genetic causes and factors; genetic disorders; genetic tests
  inheritance patterns 380–1
gene therapy 371
general anaesthetics and malignant hyperpyrexia 379
general practice, point of care testing 395
genetic causes and factors
  diabetes 182, 183

hyperbilirubinaemia 261–2
   neonatal presentation 360
hyperthyroxinaemia 171
hyperuricaemia 303–4, 306
hypoalbuminaemia 283
hypoglycaemia 362
hypogonadism 150
iron overload 314–15, 317
lipid abnormalities
   hyperlipidaemias see hyperlipidaemias
   low HDL-cholesterol 210
metabolic disease see inborn errors of metabolism
porphyrias 318, 319, 320, 322, 379
see also familial studies; pharmacogenetics
genetic disorders, categories 380
genetic tests/diagnosis/screening 382–6
   examples 384–6
   prenatal 157
      cystic fibrosis 242, 369
   technology behind 383–4
genetics 380–3
   inheritance patterns 380–1
   molecular 382–3
genitalia, ambiguous/abnormal 138, 139, 153
gentamicin monitoring 345, 350
germ cell development
   females 147
   males 152
gestational diabetes mellitus see pregnancy
gigantism 119–20
Gilbert's syndrome 261–2
Gitelman's syndrome 86, 87
Glasgow criteria (pancreatitis) 239
glitazones 185
globulins, electrophoresis 281
   in disease 281, 282, 283
glomerulus 36
   dysfunction/disease
      in diabetes mellitus 184
      hyperuricaemia in 304
      metabolic acidosis in 66
      proteinuria in 295
   filtration 27
   filtration rate (GFR), normal
      neonatal 255
      reduced tubular function and 43
   filtration rate (GFR), reduced 43
      acute oliguria and 44–5
      normal tubular function and 42–3
      related to stage of renal failure 49
   function 36, 37
      tests 50–2
   see also filtration (subheading above)
   potassium in 82
glucagon 176, 177, 178
   stimulation test 123, 126
   tumours secreting 278

glucocerobrosidase deficiency 375
glucocorticoids (sometimes referred to as 'steroids') 128–9
   aldosteronism responsive to small doses of (GRA) 140, 141
   deficiency 135
   suppression test in hypercalcaemia 103
   tumour secreting 131
   use/therapy 137–8
      in hypercalcaemia 104
      side-effects 86, 137
      withdrawal/stopping, risks associated with 137–8
glucokinase 178
gluconeogenesis 178, 180
glucose 174–97
   administration
      in hyperkalaemia 92
      in parenteral nutrition 217
      see also dextrose saline
   administration in hypoglycaemia 195
      in diabetic coma 189–90, 190
   blood/plasma
      abnormal levels see hyperglycaemia; hypoglycaemia
      control 175
   blood/plasma, measurement/monitoring
      in diabetes 185
      in hyperlipidaemia 212
      in hypoglycaemia 196
      point of care 394, 395
   CSF 330–1
   distribution across cell membrane 14
   extracellular
      functions 174–5
      regulation 175–8
   impaired fasting 183
   impaired tolerance (and tolerance testing) 183
      in cortisol excess (Cushing's syndrome) 119
      in diabetes mellitus 191
      in growth hormone excess/acromegaly 119, 120, 191
   intake, systemic effects 178
   metabolism 174–8
      anaerobic 58, 180
      growth hormone effects 119, 177
      neonatal 361–2
      see also gluconeogenesis; glycolysis
   pleural fluid 333
   suppression test 120
   tolerance testing, see subheading above
   in urine see glycosuria
glucose-6-phosphatase deficiency see von Gierke's disease
glucose-6-phosphate 178
glucose-6-phosphate dehydrogenase deficiency 360, 379

α-1,4-glucosidase (maltase) deficiency 244, 376
β-glucosidase deficiency 375
glucuronates
   steroid conjugation with 129, 251
   urinary 196
glutamate 63
glutamine 63
γ-glutamyltransferase (GGT) 254, 265, 266, 277
gluten-sensitive enteropathy 240, 241
glycated haemoglobin 185–6
glycogen 174, 214
   breakdown (glycogenolysis) 178, 180
      in starvation 214
   storage
      disorders (glycogenoses) 362, 376–7
      in muscle 178, 180
   synthesis (glycogenesis) 178
glycogen phosphorylase deficiency see phosphorylase deficiency
glycolysis 174
   anaerobic 58, 180
glycopeptide antibiotic monitoring 350
glycosuria 175
   measurement/monitoring 196
      in diabetes 185
   in pregnancy 157–9
GM1/GM2 gangliosidoses 375
goitre 166
   euthyroid 171
gonad(s) see hypogonadism; hypothalamic–pituitary–gonadal axis; ovaries; sex hormones; testes
gonadotroph(s) 116
gonadotrophin(s), human chorionic see human chorionic gonadotrophin
gonadotrophin(s), pituitary 116, 144
   administration in ovulatory failure 161
   analogues 144
   deficiency 123–4, 124
      hypogonadism due to see hypogonadism
      treatment 126
   excess, hypogonadism due to (hypergonadotrophic hypogonadism), causes 150
   see also follicle-stimulating hormone; luteinizing hormone
gonadotrophin-releasing hormone (GnRH) 144
   test 153–4, 160
   use in infertility 161
Gordon's syndrome 135–6, 328
gout 302, 303, 303–4
   treatment 305
granulomatous thyroiditis 169, 170
granulosa cell tumours 343
Graves' disease 169

growth, children's
    arrested bone growth 276
    retardation 122–3, 124
growth hormone (GH; somatotrophin) 118–23
    actions 119
        carbohydrate metabolism 119, 174
    deficiency 118, 120–3
    excess 118, 119–20, 124
        diagnosis 119–20
        treatment 120
    secretion (normal) 116
growth hormone-releasing hormone (GHRH) 118, 119, 120
    measurement 120
gut see gastrointestinal tract
gynaecomastia 144, 340

haem
    metabolism 308–10
        disorders 317–22
    precursors, excretion 309
haematological disorders, lactate dehydrogenase raised activity 271, 279
haemochromatosis 260, 266, 314–15
    case study 315
    family studies 315, 317
    genetic tests 386
    primary/hereditary 314–15, 316–17
    secondary 315
haemoconcentration
    in isosmolar fluid loss 18
    laboratory evidence of 10
haemodialysis 53
haemodilution
    laboratory evidence of 10
    in pregnancy 157
haemofiltration 53
haemoglobin 309–10
    glycated 185–6
    inherited disorders affecting 386
    oxygen affinity (for haem) 77
    oxygen saturation, measurement by pulse oximetry 79
    related compounds/abnormal Hbs 79, 309–10
    in samples interfering with chemical tests 390
    synthesis 308–9
haemolysis 265
    anaemia in 312
    jaundice in 261, 265
        neonatal 360
    in samples of blood 390
haemorrhage/bleeding
    B-cell malignancy 293
    upper GI, porphyrinuria 320

haemosiderin 310
    accumulation in tissues (haemosiderosis) 314
hair, excess growth in females 150–1
haptoglobulin 281, 285
Hartmann's solution 11
Hartnup disease 226, 374–5
Hashimoto's thyroiditis 166–7
heart
    arrhythmias see arrhythmias
    failure 326
    HDL-cholesterol protective effect 205–6
    in hypokalaemia 87
    see also cardiovascular disease; coronary heart disease
heart failure, aldosteronism in 22
heavy chain (H) of Ig 287, 288
heavy chain disease 294
heavy metal poisoning 232
Helicobacter pylori infection 247
Henderson–Hasselbach equation 59
    blood bicarbonate calculated from 80
Henle's loops see loop of Henle
heparinized blood 390
hepatitis 256–7
    acute 256–7
        drug-induced acute hepatitis-like reaction 258
    alcoholic 257, 261, 266
    chronic 258, 266
        drug-induced 258
    liver enzymes in 265
    neonatal 360
    steatotic, non-alcoholic (= fatty liver) 261, 266
    viral see viral hepatitis
hepatocytes (liver cells) 250
    carcinoma 260, 266
    damage
        assessment 253, 254, 268–9, 277
        failure following 259–60
    proliferation assessment 268–9
    synthetic functions 251
hepatorenal syndrome 261
hereditary see entries under genetic
hermaphrodism, true 153
Hers' disease 377
hexokinase 178
hexosaminidase deficiency 375
HFE 314, 315, 386
high-density lipoprotein (HDL) 201, 204–6
    in metabolic syndrome X 184
high-density lipoprotein-cholesterol 205–6
    low, causes 210
hirsutism 150–1
histamine 234
histamine H2 receptor antagonists 234
histidinaemia 373

HMG-CoA reductase see 3-hydroxymethyl-3-methylglutaryl coA reductase
homocysteine 228, 327
homocystinuria 373
homogentisic acid, urinary 196, 373
homogentisic acid oxidase deficiency 373
hormones 115
    in glucose regulation 119, 175–7
    gut 234, 235
    neonatal deficiencies causing hypoglycaemia 361
    tests for excessive or deficient secretion 115
    tumours secreting see tumours
    see also endocrine function; endocrine system and specific hormones
human chorionic gonadotrophin 155–6
    assays in pregnancy 156
    in pregnancy 155
    stimulation test 154, 160
    tumours producing 342
        feminization due to 161
        gynaecomastia due to 340
Hunter's syndrome 375
Hurler's syndrome 375
hyaline membrane disease (neonatal respiratory distress syndrome) 157, 358
hybridization (nucleic acid) 383
    DNA on Southern blots 383–4
    RNA on Northern blots 384
hydatidiform mole 159
hydration status, monitoring 10, 300
hydrochloric acid, gastric secretion see stomach
hydrocortisone see cortisol
hydrogen breath test 244
hydrogen ion
    buffering see buffering
    concentration see pH
    disturbances see acid–base balance disturbances
    gastric secretion 64
    loss
        mechanisms 59
        metabolic alkalosis due to 73
    potassium and, relationship between 83, 83–4
    renal handling 38, 42, 61
        reabsorption/reduced secretion 42, 61
    sources (in metabolism) 58
hydroxybutyrate dehydrogenase 323
β-hydroxybutyrate 195
1-α-hydroxycholecalciferol, administration 109
25-hydroxycholecalciferol 97–8
hydroxycobalamin 228
5-hydroxyindole acetic acid (5-HIAA) 337
    elevated urinary 338
1-α-hydroxylase 97
    deficiency 106, 364

11-β-hydroxylase (CYP11B1) 138
    deficiency 128, 138, 153
        diagnosis 139–40
17-α-hydroxylase (CYP17) 138
    deficiency 139
21-α-hydroxylase (CYP21) 138
    deficiency 128, 138–9, 153
        diagnosis 139
4-hydroxy-3-methoxymandelic acid
        (HMMA; VMA) 335
    phaeochromocytoma 336, 337
3-hydroxymethyl-3-methylglutaryl coA
        (HMG-CoA) reductase 195, 204
    inhibitors (statins) 211, 212
5-hydroxytryptamine (serotonin)
    in carcinoid syndrome 338
    normal metabolism 337
5-hydroxytryptophan (5-HTP) 337
    in carcinoid syndrome 337
25-hydroxyvitamin D (25-
        hydroxycholecalciferol) 97–8
hyperaldosteronism see aldosterone
hyperalphalipoproteinaemia 209
hyperammonaemia, neonatal 365
hyperandrogenism see androgens
hyperbilirubinaemia 251, 252–3, 261–2
    conjugated 253, 262
        neonatal 360, 361
    inherited see genetic causes and factors
    jaundice in see jaundice
    unconjugated 252, 261–2, 264–5
        neonatal 359–60, 361
    see also kernicterus
hypercalcaemia 98–104
    causes 99–102
        hyperthyroidism 102, 168
        malignancy 99, 101, 293, 340
        parathyroid hormone-related protein
            99–100, 101, 103, 340
    clinical effects 98–9
        renal stones 55, 98, 100
    investigations 102–3
    neonatal 364
    treatment 103–4
hypercalciuria 109
    renal stones and 55
hypercapnic respiratory failure 78–9
hyperchloraemia 67, 80
hypercholesterolaemia
    cholesterol gallstones and 263
    familial 206–7, 213
        genetic tests 386
    polygenic 209
    predominant, in secondary
        hyperlipidaemia 210
hyperchylomicronaemia syndrome
        (chylomicron syndrome) 206, 213
hyperglycaemia
    in Cushing's syndrome 130

    in diabetes mellitus 184, 186–7
    transcellular water distribution in 14
hypergonadotrophic hypogonadism and its
        causes 150, 151, 160
hyperinsulinaemia, neonatal 361, 362
hyperinsulinaemic hypoglycaemia 193–4
hyperkalaemia 83, 90–3
    alkalosis and 24
    causes 90–2
        diabetic ketoacidosis 187, 190
    clinical features 92
    investigation 92
    neonatal 357
    treatment 92–3
hyperlipidaemias (dyslipidaemias) 206–13
    classification 201, 206
    in diabetes 184
    familial combined 207–8
    hyperuricaemia in 305
    investigation 211–12
    plasma osmolarity and osmolality in 12,
        13
    primary (familial/inherited forms) 206–9,
        213
        genetic tests 386
    secondary 209, 210
    treatment 210–11, 212, 227
hyperlipidaemias see dyslipidaemias
hyperlipoproteinaemia
    familial type IIa 207
    familial type III 208–9
hypermagnesaemia 112–13
hypermetabolic phase in trauma and sepsis
        215
hypernatraemia 29–30
    case study 31
    causes 17, 21, 29, 30
    euvolaemic 30
    hypervolaemic 30
    hypovolaemic 30
    investigation 29–30
    neonatal 357
hyperosmolality, plasma
    in hyperglycaemia 187
    hyperosmolal non-ketotic coma (HONK)
        188, 189, 190
hyperosmolar saline, emetic use, dangers 24
hyperoxaluria 55
hyperparathyroidism (PTH excess) 98, 102
    hypercalcaemia in 99–101, 103, 104
    hypocalcaemia in 104–6
    neonatal 364
    primary 100, 104, 106
    secondary 104–6
    tertiary 10–11
hyperphosphataemia 111
    in chronic renal failure 48
    in diabetic ketoacidosis 188
    hypercalcaemia and 102

    hypocalcaemia and 104, 106–7, 107
        treatment 109
    transient 276
hyperprolactinaemia (excess prolactin) 118,
        124, 125, 146–7, 160
    males 153
hyperproteinaemia, plasma osmolarity and
        osmolality in 12, 13
hyperpyrexia, malignant 379
hypertension 327–8
    management 328
    portal 259
    secondary causes 327–8
        Cushing's syndrome 131, 328
        in hypercalcaemia 99
        phaeochromocytoma 336
    in pregnancy 159
hyperthermia (hyperpyrexia), malignant 379
hyperthyroidism (thyrotoxicosis) 166,
        168–71
    causes 169–70
        secondary (TSH excess) 118, 340
    elderly 366
    hypercalcaemia 102, 168
    pathophysiology 170
    plasma thyroxine levels 164
    subclinical 170
    treatment 170
hyperthyroxinaemia, euthyroid 171–2
hypertonic ('more than normal') saline 11
    in polyuria, infusion test 34–5
hypertriglyceridaemia 204–5
    familial 208
    predominant, in secondary
        hyperlipidaemia 210
    severe, investigations and management
        212
hyperuricaemia 56, 303–6
    causes 303
    consequences 303
    investigation 305–6
    primary 303–4
    treatment 305
hyperventilation, respiratory alkalosis due to
        75, 76
hypervitaminosis A 224
hypervitaminosis D see vitamin D
hypervolaemic hypernatraemia 30
hypervolaemic hyponatraemia 26
hypoadrenalism see adrenal cortex
hypoadrenocorticism see Addison's disease
hypoalbuminaemia 253, 283–4
    causes 283
    consequences 284
        pharmacological 346
hypoaldosteronism (aldosterone deficiency)
        17, 19
    hyperkalaemia in 91, 92
    hyporeninism and 68, 71, 91, 135

hypoalphalipoproteinaemia 210
hypoandrogenism *see* androgens
hypocalcaemia 104–9
  causes 104–7
    chronic renal failure 48, 106
    postoperative 109
  clinical effects 104
  investigations 107
  neonatal 363–4
  treatment 107–9
hypocalciuric hypercalcaemia, familial 102
hypochloraemia 73, 80
hypodipsic hypernatraemia 21
hypogammaglobulinaemia 283, 290, 300
hypoglycaemia 192–7
  causes 193
    tumours *see* tumours
  CSF in 330
  definition 192
  in diabetes 186, 192–7
    coma 186, 189–90
    ketotic 180, 195
    symptoms 192
  investigation 192, 194–5, 196
  management 186, 190, 195–6
  neonatal 361–2
  reactive/functional 193, 194, 195
hypoglycaemic agents, oral 185
  overdose 186
hypogonadism (gonadal dysfunction)
  biochemical investigation 153–4
  females 149–52, 160
    hypergonadotrophic, and causes 150, 151, 161
    hypogonadotrophic (secondary) 118, 124, 126
      causes 150
      infertility treatment in 161
  males 152–3
hypogonadotrophic hypogonadism *see* hypogonadism
hypoinsulinaemic hypoglycaemia 193, 194
hypokalaemia 74, 83, 85–90
  alkalosis and 24, 74
  causes 85–7
    aldosteronism 23, 24, 85
    diabetic ketoacidosis 187–8
    ectopic ACTH secretion 86, 339
    potassium-losing diuretics 388
  clinical features 87
  hypercalcaemia and 98
  hyperchloraemic acidosis and 67
  investigation 74, 87–9
  neonatal 357
  treatment 89–90
hypomagnesaemia 113–14
  hypokalaemia and 88, 90
  neonatal 364

hyponatraemia 25–9
  appropriate 26
  artefactual 26
  causes 17, 18–19, 25–6
    diabetic ketoacidosis 188
    syndrome of inappropriate ADH secretion 25, 339, 356
  dilutional 18–19, 28
  euvolaemic 26, 28
  hypervolaemic 26
  hypovolaemic 26, 28
  investigation 26–8
  neonatal 356–7
  spurious (pseudohyponatraemia) 26, 292
  treatment 28–9
hypo-osmolality with incorrect i.v. fluid administration 18–19
hypoparathyroidism (PTH deficiency) 98, 102, 106–7
  hypocalcaemia in 105, 106–7, 107
  neonatal 364
  primary 106–7
hypophosphataemia 103, 111–12, 276
  clinical features 112
  familial, rickets in (= X-linked) 110, 111
  hypercalcaemia and 102
  hypocalcaemia and 104, 104–6
  treatment 112
hypophosphatasia 276
hypopituitarism 123–6
  causes 123–4
  consequences 124
  investigation 125–6
  treatment 126
hyporeninism–hypoaldosteronism 68, 71, 91, 135
hypotension
  in liver failure 259
  postural, in isosmolar fluid loss 18
hypothalamic–pituitary–adrenal axis 129
hypothalamic–pituitary axis, glucagon stimulation test 128
hypothalamic–pituitary–gonadal axis 144–6
  drugs affecting 161
hypothalamus
  adipsic hypernatraemia and the 21
  dysfunction, vs pituitary dysfunction 117–18
  reproductive function and the 144
hypothyroidism 118, 166, 166–8
  causes 166–7, 168
    secondary (TSH excess) 118, 124, 166
  compensated 167
  elderly 366
  laboratory investigations 168
  neonatal 167, 365–6
  pathophysiology 167

plasma thyroxine levels 164
  treatment 167
hypotonic ('less than normal') saline 11
hypouricaemia 307
hypovolaemia
  in isosmolar fluid loss 18
  in liver failure 259
hypovolaemic hypernatraemia 30
hypovolaemic hyponatraemia 26, 28
hypoxaemia
  neonatal 357–8
  respiratory failure in 78
hypoxanthine–guanine phosphoribosyl transferase (HGPRT) 302
  deficiency 304
hypoxia
  lactic acidosis in 67, 180
  tissue 180, 181

Ictostix 254
identification in test requesting
  clinician 388
  patient 388
IGF-1 *see* insulin-like growth factor-1
ileus, gallstone 264
imaging
  chronic pancreatitis 241
  gastrinomas 248
  phaeochromocytomas 337
iminoglycinuria 375
immune paresis 300
  B-cell malignancy 293
  plasma cell myeloma 294
immune system (and immune response) 280, 284–5, 286–9
  cellular response 286–7
  defects 290–1
    see also immune paresis
immunoassay, cortisol 129–30
immunoglobulin *see* antibodies *and specific Igs (below)*
immunoglobulin A 288, 289
  deficiency 240, 290
  increase (predominating over other classes) 289
immunoglobulin D 288
immunoglobulin E 288, 289
  in allergy and allergic disease 289
immunoglobulin G 288
  in CSF 331–2
  deficiency 290
  increase (predominating over other classes) 289
  neonatal 365
immunoglobulin M 288–9
  deficiency 290
  increase (predominating over other classes) 289
  neonatal 365

immunosuppressant monitoring 350
inborn errors of metabolism 368–79
    consequences/clinical effects/clinical
            importance 368–9
        acidosis 67
        hypoglycaemia in neonates/children
            361
        liver 260–1
    screening of neonates 369
    treatment principles 371
    when to suspect 369–70
indinavir stones 56
individuals (patients)
    variation between 2–3
    variation within 3
    see also patient
infants
    hypercalcaemia 102
    hypoglycaemia 362
    newborn see neonates
    premature see premature infants
infections
    C-reactive protein in 285, 332
    CSF biochemistry 330, 332
    in diabetes
        in aetiology 183
        as complication 184
    genetic tests 386
    H. pylori 247
    immune response see immune system
    intrauterine, neonatal jaundice due to
        360
    urinary tract, chronic, renal calculi
        associated with 55
infertility 159–61
    females 151, 159–60
        drug treatment 161
    males 152–3, 160–1
inflammation (inflammatory response)
        280–1, 284, 285
    cerebral tissue, non-purulent 331
    chronic, plasma protein electrophoresis
        282
    deficient components 290–2
inflammatory bowel disease 247, 275
    C-reactive protein in 285–6
inheritance see entries under genetic
inhibin 145
    ovarian and testicular tumours 343
injury (trauma), metabolic response 215
insulin
    actions 178
        genetic defects 182
    autoantibodies 182, 194
    C-peptide see C-peptide
    deficiency 182, 184
        absolute 182
    neonatal excess production
        (hyperinsulinaemia) 361, 362

in polycystic ovary syndrome 152
resistance syndrome see metabolic
        syndrome X
stimulation test
    combined with GnRH stimulation test
        154
    growth hormone response 123
therapy 190
    overdose 186
tolerance/stimulation/provocation test
        125–6, 195
    in Cushing's syndrome 134
    in hypopituitarism 125–6
tumours producing
    ectopic 340
    islet-cell see insulinoma
insulin-dependent diabetes mellitus (type I
        diabetes) 182
insulin-like growth factor-1 (IGF-1;
        somatomedin C) 119
    acromegaly screening 120
    hypoglycaemia due to ectopic production
        340
insulin-like growth factor-2 (IGF-2),
        tumours secreting 193
insulinoma 193–4, 195
    removal 195
intensive care, point of care testing 395
interactions, drug 347
intermediate-density lipoprotein 200, 201
intersex and ambiguous genitalia 138, 139,
        153
interstitial fluid 11
    electrolyte distribution between cells and
        11
    electrolyte distribution between plasma
        and 11
    excess see oedema
    see also extracellular fluid
intestine (bowel)
    absorption see absorption
    bicarbonate formation 63–4
    carcinoid tumours 338
    chloride reabsorption 64
    lymphomatous lesion 294
    potassium transport 82
        excessive loss from extracellular fluid
            into 87
    water handling/output 8
    see also colorectal carcinoma;
            contaminated bowel syndrome;
            inflammatory bowel disease; small
            intestine
intoxicants see toxins and drugs poisoning
intracellular fluid compartments 11
intrauterine infections, neonatal jaundice
        due to 360
intravenous fluid infusions,
        regimens/available forms 11

intrinsic factor 228, 233
    deficiency 243
inulin clearance 50–1
iodide
    sources 162
    in thyroid hormone synthesis 162
iodination, tyrosine 162
iodine 162
    intake
        deficiency 166
        excess 169, 170
    radioactive 170, 171
ions
    intra-/extracellular distribution 11
    renal tubular transport/exchange 37–8
    see also anion gap; cations and specific ions
iron 310–17
    absorption 238, 310
        increased 314
    deficiency 310, 312, 313
        anaemia of 315–16
        ferritin levels in 313
        porphyrinuria of 320
    distribution in body 310
    excretion 310–11
    in haem 208, 309
    metabolism 310–12
        investigating disorders of 315–16
    overdose 353
    overload 310, 311, 314–17
        causes 314, 353
        consequences (incl. deposition) 260, 314
        demonstration of increased stores 317
        ferritin levels in 313
        investigation 316–17
        syndromes 314–15
    plasma
        factors affecting concentration 311–12
        measurement 316
        transport in 311
    therapeutic administration 313–14
        parenteral, causing iron overload 314
iron-binding capacity 312
islet cells, pancreatic
    β-cell see beta-cell
    hormones synthesised by 175, 176
    neonatal overgrowth 362
    tumours producing 193–4, 195, 339
isoenzymes (and their determination) 269
    acid phosphatase 276
    alkaline phosphatase 275–6
    amylase 274
    creatine kinase 271–2, 323, 323–4, 325
    lactate dehydrogenase 271
isoniazid acetylation 350
isosmolal sodium-containing fluids, infusion
        26
isosmolar volume depletion and fluid loss
        16, 17–18

isosmotic transport in renal tubules 37
    water reabsorption 38
isotonic ('normal') saline 11, 19
    in hyperaldosteronism, infusion test 141

J chain of Ig 288
jaundice 252–3, 264–5
    haemolytic see haemolysis
    neonatal 261, 359–61
        in first 24 hours of life 360
        investigation 360–1
        physiological 359
    obstructive 264, 266
    as presenting feature 264–5
    various causes 262
Jod–Basedow syndrome 170

kaluria 84
kappa L chain 287
Kelley–Seegmiller syndrome 304
kernicterus (bilirubin encephalopathy) 252
    neonatal, risk factors 359
ketoacidosis, diabetic 180, 186–8
    hyperkalaemia 91
    management 186–8, 190
ketone production (ketosis) 178, 178–80, 214–15
    hypoglycaemia and 180, 195
    starvation and 214–15
ketonuria 196
Ketostix 196
kidney 36–54
    biochemistry of disorders 42–9
        pathophysiology 42
    calculi see calculi
    clinical features of disease 43–4
    diabetic disease (nephropathy) 184, 186
    disease/disorders/damage (in general)
        aminoaciduria due to 374
        biochemistry of see subheading above
        causing nephrotic syndrome 297
        in hypercalcaemia 98
        neonatal hyponatraemia due to acute disease 357
        rickets due to 96, 364
    function 36–42
        acid–base regulation 59, 60, 61–2
        elderly 366
        failure see kidney failure
        neonatal 355–7
        in pregnancy 157, 157–8
        vitamin D metabolism 37, 97
    function, tests 50–2
        in hyperuricaemia 305
    glucose metabolism 178
    impaired renal tubular response to ADH
        see nephrogenic diabetes insipidus

magnesium excretion/loss
    impaired 113
    increased 113
phosphate handling see phosphate
potassium handling see potassium
urate excretion 303
    reduced 304
water handling/output 8
see also nephropathy; renal vessels
kidney failure/dysfunction 44–9
    acute 44–5
        causes 46
        hyperkalaemia in 90–1
        investigation 46
        treatment 53
    chronic 47–9
        abnormal findings 47–9, 106
        causes 47
        hyperkalaemia in 90–1
        treatment 53–4
    cirrhosis and 261
    diagnosis 50–2
    hypoglycaemia in 193
    metabolic acidosis in 66
    proteinuria in 43, 395–6
    stages 49
Krebs' cycle 174, 175
Kupffer cells 250
kwashiorkor 216

labelling, specimen 392
laboratories
    methodological differences between 3–4
    sending specimen to 392
laboratory tests
    diagnostic value of abnormalities 4
    frequency/timing 1
    interpreting results 2–4
    requesting 1, 388
    samples for see samples
    significant changes 2, 4–5
    urgency criteria 2
labour induction 35
lactase deficiency 243–4
lactate
    CSF, in infection 332
    production 180
lactate dehydrogenase (LDH) 271
    malignancy 279, 342
    myocardial infarction 271, 323, 324, 325
    pleural fluid 33
lactation 155
lactic acidosis 58, 67, 180–2
lactogen, placental 155, 156
lactose 376
    intolerance 243
    urinary 196
lactotrophs 116
lambda L chain 287

Laron dwarfs 122
laxative abuse 247
lead poisoning, porphyrinuria 320
lecithin–cholesterol acyltransferase (LCAT) 204
    deficiency 210
Leiner's disease 291
leptin 220
Lesch–Nyhan syndrome 304
leucine sensitivity 362
leucodystrophy, metachromic 375
leukaemia, chronic lymphatic, in heavy chain disease 294
Leventhal–Stein syndrome 151–2
Leydig cells in hCG stimulation test 154, 160
Liddle's syndrome 328
    hypokalaemia 86
light chain (L) of Ig 287, 288
likelihood ratios 5–6
lipase 236, 274
    hepatic 204
    lipoprotein see lipoprotein lipase
    pancreatic 236, 238
        reduced activity 241, 242
lipid (fat) 198–213, 236–7
    absorption 236–7
        impaired see steatorrhoea
    faecal, estimation 237, 246
    measurements of plasma lipids 211–12
    metabolism 178–80, 202–6
        abnormalities see hyperlipidaemias
        growth hormone effects 119
        in liver 178, 179, 203–4, 250, 251
        nutrition and 214
    in parenteral nutrition 217
    solubility, absorption dependent on
        drugs 346
        nutrients 235
    storage disorders 375
    structure of plasma lipids 198
lipid-lowering drugs 210–11, 212, 227
    gallstones with 263
    see also specific types of drugs
lipoprotein 200–6
    electrophoretic mobility 200
        in hyperlipidaemia classification 200
    hepatic synthesis 251
    high-density see high-density lipoprotein
    intermediate-density 200, 201
    low-density see low-density lipoprotein
    metabolism 202–6
    very-low-density see very-low-density lipoprotein
    see also hyperlipoproteinaemia
lipoprotein (a) 201
lipoprotein lipase 203
    deficiency 206
β-lipotrophin 116

liquorice 86, 87
lithium monitoring 345, 349
liver 250–67
　biopsy *see* biopsy
　cirrhosis *see* cirrhosis
　disorders/diseases (in general) 250–67, 253–62
　　alcohol-related 257, 261, 266, 277
　　biochemical tests and investigations 253–5, 264–6, 275
　　cell damage in *see* hepatocytes
　　cell proliferation assessment 268–9
　　cholestatic *see* cholestasis
　　hypoglycaemia in 193
　　iron concentration in acute liver disease 312
　　neonatal 359–61
　　porphyrinuria 320
　function 250–3
　　failure 259–60
　function tests 253–5
　　new tests 255
　　in parenteral feeding 219
　metabolism 250–1
　　carbohydrate 177–8, 178–80
　　fat/lipid 178, 179, 203–4, 250, 251
　　ketosis 178–80
　　neonatal 359–60
　phosphorylase deficiency 377
　transplantation 260
liver cell *see* hepatocytes
loop of Henle 36, 39
　diuretics acting in 84
low-density lipoprotein (LDL) 201, 201–2
　Friedewald equation in calculation of 201
　metabolism/transport 204
　receptors 204, 205
　　mutations 206
lumbar puncture 329
lung
　cancer 333
　CO_2 control 59–60
　disorders/diseases (in general)
　　in alpha$_1$-antitrypsin deficiency 292
　　blood gas results affected by 77–8
　　fetal, immaturity 157
　　neonatal dysfunction 357–8
　　see also respiratory system
luteal phase of menstrual cycle 149
luteinizing hormone (LH) 116, 144
　excess/deficiency 118
　females
　　in menopause 149
　　in menstrual cycle 148, 149
　males
　　low 152
　secretion and function 145, 146
　measurement 154

lymphadenopathy, generalized, in heavy chain disease 294
lymphatic leukaemia, chronic, in heavy chain disease 294
lymphocytes *see* B-cells; T-cells
lymphocytic thyroiditis 169, 170
lymphoma, intestinal 294
lysosomal disorders 375, 376

McArdle's disease 376
macroamylaseaemia 274
macroglobulinaemia, Waldenström's 292, 294
magnesium 113–14
　abnormalities *see* hypermagnesaemia; hypomagnesaemia
　absorption 238
　loading test 113–14
　neonatal 364
　oral and i.v. replacement 114
　regulation 112
magnesium ammonium phosphate 55–6
malabsorption 239–48
　differential diagnosis 242–3
　hypoalbuminaemia 283
　investigation strategy 245–6
　luminal phase abnormalities causing 247
　mechanisms 240–1
　metabolic consequences *see* metabolic disorders
　mucosal phase abnormalities causing 247
　post-absorptive phase abnormalities causing 247
　of specific substances 243–4
　see also vitamin deficiency (*subheading below*)
　vitamin deficiency due to 222, 227, 237–8, 243, 244
males (men)
　androgen excess 138, 139
　daily basal metabolic rate 216
　fertility
　　elderly 367
　　problems 152–3, 160–1
　GFR measurement 51
　hypergonadotrophic hypogonadism 150, 151
　sexual development *see* sexual development
　testicular hormones 145–6
malignancy (cancer)
　adrenal 131
　B-cell 292–3
　bone *see* bone
　colorectal *see* colorectal carcinoma
　gallbladder 264
　hepatic (incl. infiltration) 260, 266
　hypercalcaemia in 99, 101, 293, 340
　hyperuricaemia in 304

　immune deficiency in 290
　lung 333
　meningeal 331
　pancreatic 239
　pleural effusions in 333
　prostatic 279, 340–1
　stomach 234
　thyroid 339, 343
　trophoblastic/molar 159, 170
malignant hyperpyrexia 379
malnutrition 216–21
　hypoalbuminaemia 283
　re-feeding syndrome 219–20
maltase deficiency 244, 376
manganese 231
　plasma enzymes in 279
mannitol 14
mannose-binding lectin 286
maple syrup urine disease 373
marasmus 216
masculinization *see* virilization
maturity-onset diabetes of the young 182
Mediterranean lymphoma 294
medium chain acyl-CoA dehydrogenase deficiency 378
medullary thyroid carcinoma 339
α-melanocyte-stimulating hormone 220
membrane
　capillary *see* capillary membrane
　cell
　　potassium and 83
　　water distribution across 13–14
men *see* males
MENIN mutation 339
meninges
　infection (meningitis) 330
　malignant infiltration 331
meningococcus 330
menopause 149, 367
menstrual cycle 148–9
　iron levels and 311
　ovulation in *see* ovulation
　sex hormones and 3, 148–9
menstrual period, absence (amenorrhoea) 149–50, 159
mercury toxicity 232
metabolic acidosis *see* acidosis, metabolic
metabolic alkalosis *see* alkalosis
metabolic disease
　inherited *see* inborn errors of metabolism
　liver 260–1
metabolic disorders
　acidosis in 67
　in diabetes 184
　　management 186
　inherited *see* inborn errors of metabolism
　jaundice due to 360
　in malabsorption 244–5
　　investigation 246–7

metabolic rate, basal *see* basal metabolic rate
metabolic syndrome X (insulin resistance/Reaven's syndrome) 183–4
   hyperuricaemia association 306
metabolism
   drug 346–7
   hepatic *see* liver
   hormones involved 176
   inborn errors *see* inborn errors of metabolism
   in starvation 214–15
   in trauma and sepsis 215
   tumour effects on 335–43
   see also specific substrates e.g. carbohydrate
metabolites of drugs, active/inactive 346–7
metachromic leucodystrophy 375
metals
   poisoning 232
   trace *see* trace elements
metastases, bone, hypercalcaemia 101
metformin 185
methaemalbumin 310
methaemoglobin 79, 309–10
   CSF 330
methanol poisoning 353
methionine 351
methodological differences between laboratories 3–4
methotrexate monitoring 350
methylenetetrahydrofolate reductase 228
   mutation 327
methylmalonic acidaemia 378
micelles 237
microalbuminuria 186, 296
   case study 296
micro-arrays 384
micronutrients *see* trace elements; vitamins
microvascular disease in diabetes mellitus 184
milk-alkali syndrome 101
mineral(s)
   neonatal balance/imbalance 363–4
   parenteral 217
   see also trace elements
mineralocorticoid(s) 129
   see also aldosterone
mineralocorticoid activity of a glucocorticoid (cortisol) 129
mitochondrial disorders 378
mivacurium sensitivity 277–8
molar pregnancy 159
molecular genetics 382–3
molybdenum 231–2
monoclonal B-cell proliferation 292
monoclonal gammopathy of undetermined significance 295
monoclonal proteinaemia *see* paraproteinaemia

monogenic disorders 380
mononuclear phagocytes (monocytes) in infection 286
monosaccharides 174
   digestion/absorption 235
   see also sugars
monounsaturated fatty acids 199
Morquio syndrome 375
motilin 235
mucopolysaccharidoses 375
mucosa, intestinal, absorption by 234–5, 235
   defective, causes 247
mucus secretion in vitamin A deficiency 223
multifactorial disorders 380
multiple alleles 382
multiple endocrine neoplasia (MEN; pluriglandular syndrome) 338–9
   MEN-1 339
   MEN-2 339
   phaeochromocytoma vs 336
multiple myeloma (myelomatosis) 101, 283, 292, 293–4, 300
multiple sclerosis 331
muscle (skeletal/striated)
   carbohydrate metabolism 178, 180, 181
   damage, troponin T and creatine kinase with, case study 324
   diseases 278–9
   protein 215
   rhabdomyolysis 272, 273
muscle phosphorylase deficiency 376
muscular dystrophy 278–9
   genetic tests 385
myelomatosis/multiple myeloma 101, 283, 292, 293–4, 300
myocardial infarction (MI) 269, 278, 323–5
   case studies of possible MI 4, 324, 326
   lactate dehydrogenase 271, 323, 324, 325
   point of care testing 394
myoglobin 309
   plasma 273, 309
      in myocardial infarction 325
   urinary 273
myophosphorylase deficiency 376

'Nago' isoenzyme 276, 279
nasal leakage of CSF (rhinorrhoea) 332
natriuretic peptides 326
   atrial 10
near-infrared spectroscopy 393
necrosis, hepatic, drug-induced 258
negative result
   false 5
   likelihood ratio 6
   predictive value 5
   true 5
Nelson's syndrome 129, 134
neonates (newborns) 355–67
   acid–base homeostasis 358

   blood gas estimations, specimen collection 79
   gastrointestinal tract 358
   glucose metabolism and disturbances 361–2
   hypothyroidism 167, 365–6
   Ig deficiency 290
   jaundice *see* jaundice
   liver function and disorders 359–61
   mineral balance/imbalance 363–4
   plasma proteins 364–5
   pulmonary function/dysfunction 357–8
   renal function 355–7
   respiratory distress syndrome 157, 358
   screening for inborn errors of metabolism 369
   thyroid function 365–6
   vitamin K deficiency 224
neonates
   point of care testing in special care baby units 395
   premature *see* premature infants
neoplasms *see* malignancy; tumours
nephrogenic diabetes insipidus 21
   causes 30
   investigations and management 30, 33, 34, 35
   polyuria in 30
nephron 36
   renal dysfunction and the 42
nephropathy
   diabetic 184, 186
   familial juvenile gouty 304
nephrotic syndrome 49, 297–8
   case study 297
   causes 297
   Ig deficiency 290
   plasma protein electrophoresis 283
nesidioblastosis 362
neural control of pituitary hormones secretion 117
neural tube defects 156
neuroblastomas 337
neuroleptic drugs 117
neurological complications
   liver disease *see* encephalopathy
   vitamin B_1 deficiency 225
neuronal-specific enolase 343
neuropathy
   diabetic 184–5
   vitamin B_6 excess 227
neuropeptide Y 220
neurotransmitters, drugs stimulating or blocking actions 117
neutrophils (polymorphonuclear neutrophil leucocytes) in infection 286
newborn infants *see* neonates
niacin 226–7, 229
nicotinamide 226–7, 229

nicotinic acid 211, 227
Niemann–Pick disease 375
night blindness 223
nitrogen in parenteral feeding
　　supplementation 217
　　urinary output measurement 219
nodules (thyroid), toxic 170
non-insulin-dependent diabetes mellitus
　　(type 2 diabetes) 182, 183
non-steroidal anti-inflammatory drugs
　　(NSAIDs), hyperuricaemia 305
noradrenaline (norepinephrine) metabolism
　　and actions 335–6
Northern blots 384
nucleic acids
　　hybridization see hybridization
　　synthesis 382, 383
　　　purines in 301, 302
　　see also DNA; RNA
nutrition/diet 214–32
　　assessment 215–16, 300
　　daily adult requirements 216, 217
　　in diabetes
　　　in oral glucose tolerance test 192
　　　as risk factor 183
　　in hyperlipidaemia management 210–11
　　in hyperuricaemia management 305
　　iron overload due to 315
　　in obesity management 220
　　support 216–20
　　　parenteral see parenteral feeding
　　see also absorption; digestion;
　　　malabsorption; malnutrition
nyctalopia 223

obesity 220–1
　　abdominal, in metabolic syndrome X 183
　　in Cushing's syndrome 130
　　vs Cushing's syndrome 133
　　treatment strategies 220–1
obstetrics see pregnancy
octreotide
　　ACTH-secreting carcinoid tumours 338
　　pituitary growth hormone-producing
　　　tumours 120
ocular problems, vitamin A deficiency 223
oedema 21–2
　　hereditary angioneurotic 291
　　investigation 300
　　pulmonary, blood gas results in 77
oestradiol 145
oestrogens 144, 145
　　menopause 149
　　menstrual cycle 148, 149
　　in pregnancy and lactation 155
　　puberty 147–8
older people see elderly
oligoclonal bands, CSF 331, 332
oligonucleotide probes, allele-specific 383

oliguria
　　acute 44–6, 53
　　chronic 48
omega-3 fatty acids 211
oocyte development 147
ophthalmological problems, vitamin A
　　deficiency 223
opiate overdose 353
opsonins 286
oral contraceptives 161
　　plasma iron and 311
oral medication, assays affecting by 388–9
organic acidurias 377–8
organophosphate exposure 278, 353
ornithine transcarbamylase deficiency 371,
　　372
orthostatic problems/effects, see entries under
　　postural
osmolality 12
　　faecal water, calculation 247
　　plasma 12, 52–3
　　　abnormalities, see also hyperosmolality;
　　　　hypo-osmolality
　　　hyponatraemia and 25
　　　measurement 12, 34
　　　solutes contributing to 7
　　　in water deprivation test 34
　　urine 53
　　　estimation 53
　　　in water deprivation and DDAVP tests
　　　　34
osmolar gap 12
osmolarity, plasma, calculated 12–13, 14
osmotic activity 7
osmotic diarrhoea 247
osmotic diuresis 9, 30, 33, 41–2
osmotic pressure 11–13
　　colloid see colloid osmotic pressure
　　units of measurement 12–13
osmotic pressure gradient
　　across cell membrane 13–14
　　colloid, decrease 22
osteitis fibrosa cystica 100
osteomalacia 105, 106
　　renal tubular causes 110
osteopenia, premature infants 364
osteoporosis 109–10
　　elderly 367
out-patient clinics and wards, point of care
　　testing 395
ovaries 148–52
　　function 148–9
　　　disorders 149–52
　　　elderly, decline 367
　　　granulosa cell tumours 343
　　hormones see sex hormones
overdose see toxins and drugs
overflow amino aciduria 374
overflow proteinuria 296

ovulation 149
　　failure (anovulation) 159
　　　drugs causing and treating 161
oxalate, urinary, high 55
oxidation, fatty acid 199
oximetry, pulse 79
oxoacid decarboxylation, deficient 373
oxygen, arterial blood 77
　　factors affecting results 77–8
　　saturation, measurement by pulse
　　　oximetry 79
　　see also hypoxaemia; hypoxia
oxygen therapy, respiratory acidosis 72
oxyhaemoglobin 309, 310
　　dissociation curve 77
oxytocin (Syntocinon) 35
　　neonatal hyponatraemia and 356

PABA test 239, 246
Paget's disease of bone 110
pain
　　abdominal 248–9
　　biliary (colic) 264
　　bone, in primary hyperparathyroidism
　　　100
palmar striae/xanthomata 209
pancreas 238–9
　　digestive enzymes/secretions 233–4, 236,
　　　238–9
　　　impaired activity 241–2
　　disorders (other than diabetes) 239,
　　　241–2
　　　differential diagnosis 242
　　exocrine function 238–9
　　hormones involved in glucose regulation
　　　175–6
　　islet cells see islet cells
　　malabsorption 239
　　　differential diagnosis 242–3
　　sodium bicarbonate secretion 64
pancreatic polypeptide 235
pancreatitis
　　acute 239
　　　case study 240
　　chronic 241
pancreolauryl test 239, 246
panhypopituitarism 123, 124
pantothenate 227, 229
paracetamol poisoning 351–3
paralysis, periodic see periodic paralysis
paraproteinaemia 283, 292–3, 342
　　causes 292, 294
　　'benign' 295
　　consequences 292–3
parathyroid hormone (PTH) 96, 97, 98,
　　99–100
　　abnormalities see hyperparathyroidism;
　　　hypoparathyroidism
　　in pseudohypoparathyroidism 107

parathyroid hormone-related protein 96, 98, 340
  hypercalcaemia induced by 99–100, 101, 103, 340
parenteral feeding 217–19
  iron overload due to 314
  monitoring and long-term complications 218–19, 256
paternity testing 386
patient
  self-testing 395
  in test requesting
    identification and location 388
      specimens see samples/specimens
  see also individuals
pellagra 226
penicillamine
  cystinuria 374
  Wilson's disease 231
pentolinium suppression test 337
pentoses, urinary 196
peptic ulcers 234
peptides
  as gut hormones 235, 238
  malabsorption 244
periodic paralysis
  hyperkalaemic 91
  hypokalaemic 87
peritoneal dialysis, ambulatory 53–4
peritoneal fluid accumulation 259
pernicious anaemia 228
peroxisome disorders 378
peroxisome proliferator-activated receptors 199
pH 58–9
  blood
    and haem affinity for oxygen 77
    measurement 80
  gastrointestinal 233
  urinary, and renal stone formation 54
  see also acid–base balance; acidosis; alkalosis
phaeochromocytomas 336–7
phagocytic cells in infection 286
pharmacogenetics 350–1
  inborn errors of metabolism and 378–9
pharmacokinetics 344
phenobarbital monitoring 345
phenylketonuria 372, 386
phenytoin monitoring 348
phosphate 110–12
  abnormal levels see hyperphosphataemia; hypophosphataemia
  buffering capacity
    blood 61
    urine 62, 63
  functions 111
  measurements in hypocalcaemia 107
  neonatal depletion 364

renal handling 38, 96, 110–11
renal handling abnormalities 112
  rickets due to 110
  restriction in chronic renal failure 53
  supplementation, neonatal 364
phosphofructokinase deficiency 377
phospholipids 200
  structure 198
phosphoribose diphosphate (phosphoribosyl pyrophosphate) 301
phosphoribosylamine 301, 304
phosphorylase (glycogen) deficiency
  hepatic 377
  muscle 376
pigment stones 263
pituitary gland 116–26
  elderly 366
  function
    evaluation 117
    vs hypothalamic dysfunction 117–18
  tumours see tumours
  see also hypothalamic–pituitary–adrenal axis; hypothalamic–pituitary axis; hypothalamic–pituitary–gonadal axis
pituitary hormones 116–26
  anterior 116–17, 144–5
    control 117
    reproductive function and 144–5
  anterior, disorders 123–6
    Cushing's syndrome associated with 118, 124, 131, 133, 134
  posterior 118–23
    control 116
    disorders 123
placenta, functional monitoring 155–6
placental alkaline phosphatase (Regan isoenzyme) 275–6, 276, 279, 343
placental lactogen 155, 156
plasma
  anion gap see anion gap
  drug levels in see drugs
  electrolyte distribution between interstitial fluid and 11
  fluorescence, porphyrias 320, 321
  hyperosmolality in hyperglycaemia 187
  osmolality and osmolarity see osmolality; osmolarity
  in renal disorders
    in reduced GFR (and normal tubular function) 43
    in reduced tubular function (and normal GFR) 43, 52
  see also specific components
plasma cell(s), in CSF, Ig synthesis 331
plasma cell myeloma (myelomatosis/multiple myeloma) 101, 283, 292, 293–4, 300
plasmids 383

pleural fluid 333
pluriglandular syndrome see multiple endocrine neoplasia
point of care testing 393–5
  advantages 393–4
  disadvantages 394
poisoning see toxins and drugs
polyclonal B cell response 292
polycystic ovary syndrome 151–2
polycythaemia due to erythropoietin secretion 340
polygenic disorders 380
polyglandular autoimmune syndrome 134
polymerase chain reaction (PCR) 384
  in genetic testing 385, 386
polymorphisms, DNA 383
polymorphonuclear neutrophil leucocytes in infection 286
polysaccharides 174
  digestion/absorption 235
    impaired 243
polyunsaturated fatty acids 199
polyuria 30–5
  causes 30
    chronic renal failure 47–8
    hypercalcaemia 98
    excess water loss due to 20
    hypernatraemia and 29
Pompe's disease (maltase deficiency) 244, 376
porphobilinogen (PBG) 309
  excessive production/excretion 318, 319
porphobilinogen (PBG) deaminase
  decrease/deficiency 318, 319, 321
  measurement 321, 322
porphobilinogen (PBG) synthase 309
  deficiency 318
porphyrias 317–22
  acute 317, 318–19, 321
    case study 318
    latent phase 318–19
  cutaneous 317, 318, 319–20, 321–2
  inherited 318, 319, 320, 322, 379
  investigations 320–1
porphyrin precursors, excretion 309
porphyrin screen 320
portal hypertension 259
positive result
  false 5
  likelihood ratio 6
  predictive value 5
  true 5
post-gastrectomy syndrome 234, 241
postoperative hypocalcaemia 109
postpartum thyroiditis 170
post-renal renal failure 45–6, 46
  treatment 53
postural (orthostatic) effects on blood tests 389

postural (orthostatic) hypotension in isosmolar fluid loss 18
postural (orthostatic) proteinuria 296
potassium 82–93
　abnormalities in plasma levels *see* hyperkalaemia; hypokalaemia
　administration (in hypokalaemia) 89–90
　　excess 91
　　intravenous 11, 89–90
　homeostasis 82–5
　　factors affecting 82–3
　　neonatal 357
　intake reduction 87
　intracellular 11
　measurement of plasma and urinary levels 84–5
　　in diabetes mellitus 190
　renal handling 38, 82–3, 83–4, 84–5
　　hyperkalaemia due to alterations in 90–1
　　hypokalaemia due to alterations in 85–6
　　reduced secretion in distal tubule 42
potassium-losing diuretics 84, 87
　hypokalaemia with 388
potassium-sparing diuretics 84
precision of method 5
predictive value 5
pre-eclampsia 159
pregnancy 155–9
　cholestasis in 255
　diabetes mellitus complicating 183
　　fetal/neonatal effects 362
　hyperparathyroidism 364
　iron levels in plasma 311
　thyroiditis following 170
　vitamin D deficiency 364
　see also fetus; prenatal tests
pregnenolone 127
premature infants
　drug metabolism 347
　Ig deficiency 290
　lactase deficiency of 243–4
　retinopathy 358
　rickets 364
prenatal tests and screening 156–7
　cystic fibrosis 242, 369
　inborn errors of metabolism 369
pre-renal renal failure 44–5, 46
　treatment 53
pressure, units of 397
primary care (general practice), point of care testing 395
primidone monitoring 345
probability (statistical) 2
procalcitonin 286
progesterone 145
　in infertility investigation 159
　in menstrual cycle 149
　in pregnancy and lactation 155

Prognostic Nutritional Index 216
prolactin 144
　deficiency 118, 124
　excess *see* hyperprolactinaemia
　in pregnancy and lactation 155
　secretion 116
　　ectopic 340
proliferative (follicular) phase of menstrual cycle 148
pro-opiomelanocortin 116, 220
propylthiouracil 170
prostate
　benign hyperplasia 341
　cancer 279, 340–1
prostate-specific antigen 340–1
prostatic acid phosphatase 279
protein(s)
　absorption 236
　　defective 244
　catabolism 280
　　in Cushing's disease 131
　CSF 331–2
　　individual protein measurement 331
　　synthesis abnormalities 331–2
　　total protein measurement 331
　dietary deficiency 216
　functions 280
　　buffering capacity 61
　metabolism 280
　　catabolism *see subheading above*
　　growth hormone effects on synthesis 119
　　hormones affecting 176
　plasma 280–95
　　blood samples for estimations 299–300
　　calcium binding to 94, 95
　　drug binding to 346
　　electrophoresis *see* electrophoresis
　　hepatic synthesis 251
　　indications for estimations 300
　　neonatal 364–5
　　thyroid hormone binding to 163
　　total *see* total protein measurement
　plasma, methods of assessment 281–3
　　electrophoresis 266
　　qualitative 281–3
　　quantitative 281
　skeletal muscle, assessment 215
　synthesis 280
　units of measurement 397
　urinary *see* proteinuria
　see also hyperproteinaemia; peptides
protein-losing enteropathy 244
　Ig deficiency 290
proteinuria 295–9
　apparent 297
　causes 43, 295–8
　in diabetes mellitus 186
　electrophoresis 281–3

investigations 298–9
rapid screening tests 298
transient 295–6
Proteus 56
prothrombin, low levels 251
prothrombin time 254, 266
proton pump inhibitors 234
protoporphyrin 309
　enhanced excretion (protophorphyria) 320, 321–2
provocation/stimulation tests (for deficient hormone secretion) 115
proximal tubules, function 36–7, 38, 42
　hypokalaemia associated with changes in 85, 86
　tests 52
pseudocholinesterase 277
pseudo-Cushing's syndrome 125–6, 134
pseudogout 306
pseudohermaphroditism
　female 138, 153
　male 153
pseudohyperkalaemia 90
pseudohypoadrenalism (pseudohypoaldosteronism) 91, 135–6
pseudohypoaldosteronism (pseudohypoadrenalism) 91, 135–6
pseudohypoglycaemia 196
pseudohypokalaemia 85
pseudohyponatraemia 26, 292
pseudohypoparathyroidism 107
pseudo-pseudohypoparathyroidism 107
psoriasis, hyperuricaemia in 304
puberty
　female 147–8
　male 152–3
　precocious 153
pulmonary medicine/disorders *see* lung; respiratory system
pulse oximetry 79
purgative abuse 247
purine
　dietary restriction 305
　metabolism 301–3
pus, CSF 331
pyloric stenosis 75, 80
　hypochloraemia 73, 80
　metabolic alkalosis 73, 75
pyridoxine *see* vitamin B_6

racial factors *see* ethnic/racial factors
radioactive iodine 170, 171
radiochromium-labelled EDTA, GFR calculation 51
radiology *see* imaging
random changes 3, 5
Ranson criteria (pancreatitis) 239

Raynaud's phenomenon, B-cell malignancy 293
Reaven's syndrome *see* metabolic syndrome X
recessive inheritance
    autosomal 381–2
    X-linked 382
rectal carcinoma *see* colorectal carcinoma
recumbency, hypoalbuminaemia 283
red cells *see* erythrocytes
re-feeding syndrome 219
reference ranges 2
refrigeration, blood samples 391
'Regan' isoenzyme (placental alkaline phosphatase) 275–6, 276, 279
rehydration, hypercalcaemia 104
renal vessels
    blood flow in
        reduced, and low glomerular filtration rate, responses 42
        and sodium balance 9–10
    damage causing aldosteronism 22–3
renin
    low (hyporeninism), and hypoaldosteronism 68, 71, 91, 135
    raised 140–1
renin–angiotensin system 9
reproducibility of results 5
reproductive system 144–54
Resonium-A 93
respiratory acidosis 64, 71–2
    compensatory changes in 76
    management 71–2
    mixed metabolic acidosis and 76, 77
    neonatal 358
respiratory alkalosis 74–6
    compensatory changes in 76
    neonatal 358
respiratory distress syndrome, neonatal 157, 358
respiratory failure 78–9
    acute 71
    chronic 71
    hypercapnic 78–9
    hypoxaemic 78
respiratory system
    disease, and blood gases 77–8
    neonatal dysfunction 357–8
    in pregnancy 157
    see also lung
restriction enzymes/endonucleases 383
restriction fragment length polymorphisms 383
reticuloendothelial iron overload 314, 317
retinol *see* vitamin A
retinopathy
    diabetic 184
    of prematurity 358
Reye's syndrome 261

rhabdomyolysis 272, 273
rheumatoid arthritis 333
rhinorrhoea 332
rhodopsin 223
riboflavine 226, 229
rickets 105, 106
    of prematurity 364
    vitamin D-dependent 106, 107
    vitamin D-resistant/hypophosphataemic 110, 111
Ringer's solution 11
mRNA (messenger RNA)
    Northern blots 384
    synthesis 383
Rotor syndrome 262, 361

salbutamol in hyperkalaemia 93
salicylate overdose 353
saline 11
    hyperosmolar, emetic use, dangers 24
    metabolic alkalosis responsive/non-responsive to 73, 74
    types and components 11
saline infusion test in hyperaldosteronism 141
salivary gland disorders and amylase 274
salt-loading test in hyperaldosteronism 141
samples/specimens 387–92
    collection
        blood *see* blood samples
        CSF 329
        errors in, causes and consequences 387
        faeces 392
        urine 391–2
    labelling 392
    requesting 1, 388
    sending to laboratory 392
Sanfilippo syndrome 375
sarcoidosis, hypercalcaemia 101–2
saturated fatty acids 199
Schilling test 228, 243
scoline apnoea 277–8, 279
scurvy 229–30
secretin 235, 238
    test 248
secretory diarrhoea 247
secretory phase of menstrual cycle 149
selenium 231
self-testing, patient 395
sensitivity, test 5, 6
sepsis, metabolic response 215
sequestrene *see* EDTA
serology, viral hepatitis 256–7
serotonin *see* 5-hydroxytryptamine
Sertoli cells 145, 152, 153
    tumours 343
severe combined immunodeficiency (SCID) 291

sex (gender)
    determination 147
        abnormalities 138, 139, 153
    differences in test results 3
        plasma enzymes 270
        plasma iron 311
sex chromosomes, normal and abnormal numbers 147
sex hormone(s) (gonadal hormones)
    androgens 129
    female (ovarian hormones) 145
        abnormalities 149–51
        in infertility investigations 159, 160
        menstrual cycle and 3, 148–9
        in pregnancy 155, 157
    male (testicular hormones) 145–6
        in infertility investigations 160, 161
    synthesis 145
    see also specific hormones
sex-hormone binding globulin 146
    conditions associated with abnormal levels 150, 151, 171
sex-linked inheritance 382
sexual development 147–53
    biochemical investigation of disorders 153–4
    females 147–52
        disorders 138, 139, 149–52, 153
    males 152
        disorders 138, 139, 152–3, 153
shock 215
shock-wave lithotripsy 264
short-gut syndrome 240–1
short stature 121, 122
SI units 397–8
sick euthyroid syndrome 171
    elderly 366
sickle-cell anaemia 386
sideroblastic anaemia, porphyrinuria 320
Siggard–Andersen acid–base chart for arterial blood 77
significance, statistical 2, 4–5
Sipple's syndrome 339
skeletal muscle *see* muscle
skin fold thickness, triceps 215
skin lesions
    porphyrias with 317, 318, 319–20, 321–2
    in vitamin A deficiency 223
    see also eczema
small airways obstruction 78
small intestine
    absorption *see* absorption
    surgical shortening 240–1
    transit time, increased rate 241
small vessel (microvascular) disease in diabetes mellitus 184
sodium 7–35, 356–7
    balance/homeostasis 7–35
        control 9–10

disturbances 16–35
    failure of mechanisms involved 19
    neonatal 356–7
    renal handling 38, 42
    total 7–8
    water homeostasis and, relation between 14–15
deficiency 16–21
distribution in body 10–15
    transmembrane 13
excess 21–5
    hypokalaemia associated with excess Na⁺ available for exchange 85, 86
fractional excretion (FEN) 16, 46
intake 7
    increased 24
    in intravenous fluids 11
    infusion (in hyponatraemia) 28–9
output 8
plasma, estimation 15
urinary, estimation 16, 18, 52–3
see also hypernatraemia; hyponatraemia
sodium bicarbonate
    administration
        in hyperkalaemia 92–3
        in metabolic acidosis 70, 190
        metabolic alkalosis due to 73
    secretion in pancreas/biliary tract 64
    see also bicarbonate
sodium/potassium exchange (and the Na⁺/K⁺ ATPase) 83
    hyperkalaemia related to 90
    hypokalaemia related to 85, 85–6, 86
soft tissue plasmacytoma 294
solubility
    in lipid see lipid
    in water, nutrient absorption depending on 235
solutes
    plasma osmolality and contribution of 7
    renal handling
        distal tubule/collecting duct 42
        proximal tubule 38
somatomedin C see insulin-like growth factor-1
somatostatin 176
somatostatin analogues
    ACTH-secreting carcinoid tumours 338
    pituitary growth hormone-producing tumours 120
somatotroph 116
somatotrophin see growth hormone
Somoygyi phenomenon 184
Southern blots 383–4
special care baby units, point of care testing 395
specificity, test 5, 6
specimens see samples/specimens
spermatogenesis 152

sphingomyelinase deficiency 375
spina bifida 156
spinal canal, blockage affecting CSF flow 331
spinal tap (lumbar puncture) 329
sprue, tropical 240
squamous cell carcinoma antigen 343
SRY (sex-determining region on Y chromosome) 153
starch 174
starvation 214–15
    hyperuricaemia in 304
    see also fasting
statins 211, 213
statistical significance 2, 4–5
stature, short 121, 122
steatorrhoea 105, 106, 240
    detection 237
    fat-soluble vitamin deficiency 223, 224
    investigations 242, 246
steatotic hepatitis, non-alcoholic (= fatty liver) 261, 266
stercobilinogen 253
steroids (steroid hormones)
    adrenocortical
        chemistry and synthesis 127–8
        physiology 128–9
    metabolism and inactivation in liver 251
    see also androgens; glucocorticoids; mineralocorticoids
stimulation tests (for deficient hormone secretion) 115
stomach
    disorders 234
    function 234
    H. pylori infection 247
    juices (incl. acid) secretion 64
    hyper- and hyposecretion 234
    post-gastrectomy syndrome 234, 241
stones see calculi
stools see faeces
stress
    hormones in 129
    mimicking Cushing's syndrome 133
striated muscle see muscle
struvite 55–6
Subjective Global Assessment 216
substance overdose see toxins and drugs
succinylcholine sensitivity 277–8, 379
sucrase–isomaltase deficiency 244
sugars
    inborn errors of metabolism 375–6
    reducing and non-reducing 174
    urinary 196
    see also disaccharides; monosaccharides
sulphaemoglobin 310
sulphate, steroid conjugation with 129, 251
sulphonylureas 185

suppression tests (for excess hormone secretion) 115
surfactant, pulmonary, and its deficiency 157
surgery
    adrenal tumours/adenomas 134, 141
    hypocalcaemia following 109
    pancreatic tumour (insulinoma) 195
    pituitary tumours/adenomas 134
    small bowel-shortening 240–1
suxamethonium sensitivity 277–8, 279
sweat, water loss 8
Syncathen see tetracosactrin stimulation test
syndrome X see metabolic syndrome X
Syntocinon see oxytocin
Système International d'Unités 397–8
systemic lupus erythematosus, C-reactive protein in 285–6

T-cells/lymphocytes 284
    deficiency 290–1
    infection 286
tacrolimus monitoring 345, 350
Tangier's disease 210
tartrate-labile acid phosphatase activity 276
Tarui's disease 377
tau protein 332
Tay–Sachs disease 375
teicoplanin monitoring 350
tendon xanthomata, familial hypercholesterolaemia 207
testes 152–3
    development 152
    dysfunction 152–3
    elderly, decline in function 367
    hormones see sex hormones
    Sertoli cell tumours 343
testosterone 145–6
    females 150, 151
        raised 151
    infertility investigations (males) 160
tetracosactrin (Syncathen) stimulation test 136, 137
    depot/prolonged 137
    short 137
    in 21-α-hydroxylase deficiency 139
tetrahydrofolate 227
thalassaemia, genetic tests 386
theophylline monitoring 345, 349
thiamine see vitamin B_1
thiazide diuretics 84
    hyperuricaemia with 304
thiopurine methyltransferase 350–1
thoracentesis 333
thrombolytic therapy 394
thrombosis, deep vein 326
thyroglobulin 162
    thyroid cancer 343
thyroid carcinoma 339, 343

thyroid function 162–73
   amiodarone effects 172, 348
   disorders 124, 166–72
     elderly 366
     hypercalcaemia 102
     neonatal 365–6
   tests 164–6
     factors interfering with 165–6
     neonatal 365–6
     strategies for and interpretation of 172–3
thyroid hormones 162–4
   abnormalities *see* thyroid function, disorders
   measurements 164, 164–5
     factors interfering with 165–6
     in hyperthyroidism 171
     in hypothyroidism 168
     interpretation of 172–3
   peripheral conversion 163
   protein binding in plasma 163
   resistance 167
   synthesis 162–3
   TSH secretion and effects of 164
thyroid-stimulating hormone *see* thyrotrophin
thyroidectomy, hypoparathyroidism and hypocalcaemia following 106
thyroiditis
   Hashimoto's/autoimmune 166–7
   subacute 169–70
thyrotoxicosis *see* hyperthyroidism
thyrotroph(s) 116
thyrotrophin (TSH; thyroid-stimulating hormone)
   deficiency (secondary hypothyroidism) 118, 124, 166
   excess (secondary hyperthyroidism) 118, 340
   neonatal 365
   pituitary tumours secreting 171
   plasma, measurement 164, 172
     in hyperthyroidism 170, 171
     in hypothyroidism 168
   secretion and its regulation 116, 163–4
thyrotrophin-releasing hormone (TRH) 144–5, 163–4
   measurements 165
   stimulation test 154, 171
thyroxine (T_4) 162
   euthyroid hyperthyroxinaemia 171–2
   measurements (plasma total and free) 164
     factors interfering with 165–6
     in hyperthyroidism 171
     in hypothyroidism 168
     interpretation of 172–3
   peripheral conversion 163
   plasma protein binding 163
   synthesis 162–3
   TSH secretion and effects of 164

thyroxine-binding globulin (TBG) 163
   measurements 164, 172
tissue hypoxia 180, 181
tobacco chewing 86
α-tocopherol *see* vitamin E
tolerance, drug 347
total iron-binding capacity (TIBC) 312
total protein measurement
   CSF 331
   plasma 281
     indications for estimation 300
toxic nodules 170
toxins and drugs handling in liver 251
toxins and drugs poisoning and overdose 351–3
   heavy metals 232
   hyperosmolar saline as emetic in, dangers 24
   hypocalcaemia due to 105
   liver damage (hepatotoxicity) 257, 258
   metabolic acidosis due to 65
   treatment 70
   vitamin excess *see* vitamins *and specific vitamins*
trace elements/metals 222
   in parenteral feeding 217
   plasma measurements 219
transaminases (aminotransferases) 253, 265–6, 270–1, 279
transcortin 128–9
transcription (DNA) 383
transcutaneous biosensors 393
transferrin 281, 310, 312, 312–13
   abnormal plasma concentrations 312–13, 316–17
   measurement 316–17
     in nutritional assessment 216
   receptor 313
     abnormal levels 313
transketolase activity, erythrocyte 226
transmembrane water distribution 13–14
transplantation, liver 260
transport function
   plasma protein 280
   renal tubular 37–8
transthyretin 295
transtubular potassium gradient (TTKG) 84–5, 92
transudates, pleural 333
trauma, metabolic response 215
tricarboxylic acid cycle 174, 175
triceps skin fold thickness 215
triglycerides
   hepatic metabolism 178, 179
   pleural fluid 333
   structure 198
   transport and metabolism 199, 236, 237
   see also hypertriglyceridaemia

tri-iodothyronine (T_3) 162
   measurements (plasma total and free) 164
     factors interfering with 165–6
     in hyperthyroidism 171
     in hypothyroidism 168
     interpretation of 172–3
   peripheral conversion 163
   plasma protein binding 163
   synthesis 162–3
   TSH secretion and effects of 164
triolein breath test 237, 243
trisomy 21, 156–7
trophoblastic tumours/molar invasion 159, 170
tropical sprue 240
troponins 325
   troponin T, case studies 4, 324, 326
true-positive or negative result 5
trypsin 238–9
   low levels 241
tryptase 278
tryptophan
   5-HT synthesis from 337
   Hartnup disease and 226, 374–5
tuberculosis, pleural fluid 333
tubules, renal
   acidosis 49, 68–9
     hyperchloraemic acidosis due to 67
   distal *see* distal tubules
   diuretic actions 84
   dysfunction
     acidosis due to 68
     aminoaciduria due to 374
     and normal GFR 43
     proteinuria 43, 295
     syndromes reflecting 49
   function 36, 36–7, 37–8
     acid–base regulation 61–2
     normal, and reduced glomerular filtration rate 42–3
     tests 34, 52
   impaired response to ADH *see* nephrogenic diabetes insipidus
   obstruction 45
   phosphate handling 38, 96
     rickets due to defect in 96, 364
   potassium handling 82–3, 84–5
   proximal *see* proximal tubules
tumour(s)
   adrenal 131, 140
     removal 134
   ectopic hormone production 86, 131, 134, 338, 339–40
   feminization caused by 161
   gastrointestinal 248–9
     hormone-secreting 87, 234, 248
     5-HT/serotonin-secreting 338

hypoglycaemia caused by 340
   islet cell *see* insulinoma
   non-islet cell 193, 195
hypokalaemia associated with 87
metabolic effects (in general) 335–43
pituitary 123, 124–5
   ACTH-producing 131
   growth hormone-producing 119, 120
   prolactin-producing 125, 146–7
   removal 134
   TSH-producing 171
trophoblastic/gestational 159, 170
   see also malignancy
tumour markers 340–3
   pleural fluid 333
turbidity, CSF 330
tyrosinaemia 373
tyrosinase deficiency 373
tyrosine iodination 162

UDP glucuronyltransferase (UGT) deficiency 261, 262

ulcer(s)
   diabetic 185
   peptic (gastroduodenal) 234
ulcerative colitis 245, 286
units of measurement 397–8
unsaturated fatty acids 199
uraemia
   definition 42
   mild 49
urate
   abnormal levels, hyperuricaemia; hypouricaemia
   excretion 303
   purine oxidation to 302
urea
   plasma, measurement 50
      in neonates 355–6
      in polyuria 33
   transmembrane distribution 13–14
   urinary excretion (24 hr), in nutritional assessment 216
   in parenteral nutrition 219
urea breath test 247
urea cycle disorders 371–2
   neonatal 365
uric acid
   drugs increasing excretion (uricosurics) 305
   stones 56, 303
uridine diphosphate glucuronyltransferase (UGT) deficiency 261, 262
urinary tract
   infection, chronic, renal calculi associated with 55
   obstruction, acute oliguria due to 45–6
urine
   albumin estimation 186

amino acids 372–3, 374
anion gap 66, 68–9
Bence-Jones proteins 296, 342
bilirubin 253, 254, 265
buffering 62–3
calcium loss in 94
in carcinoid syndrome, tests 338
chloride estimation 80
collection 391–2
concentration, disorder affecting mechanism of 49
cortisol estimation 132–3
glucose in *see* glycosuria
in hepatic disease, tests 254
ketones 196
myoglobin 273
neonatal/infant output 356
osmolality *see* osmolality
pH, and renal stone formation 54
in porphyrias, tests 318, 319, 321
potassium estimation *see* potassium
proteins *see* proteinuria
   in renal disorders
      reduced GFR (and normal tubular function) 43
      reduced tubular function (and normal GFR) 43, 52
sodium estimation 16, 18, 52–3
urobilinogen 254, 265
water excretion into, control 40–1
see also anuria; oliguria; polyuria
urobilinogen 253
   urinary 254, 265
Urobilistix 254
uroporphyrinogen 309
   accumulation 319
uroporphyrinogen decarboxylase deficiency 319
uroporphyrinogen III synthase deficiency 320
ursodeoxycholic acid 264
uterine infections, neonatal jaundice due to 360

vagus nerve 234
   gastrin 234
valproate monitoring 345, 349
Van den Bergh reactions 252
vancomycin monitoring 350
vanillyl mandelic acid *see* 4-hydroxy-3-methoxymandelic acid
variation, coefficient of 5
variegate porphyria 318–19, 319, 321, 322
vascular disease *see* cardiovascular disease
vasoactive intestinal polypeptide (VIP) 235
   tumours secreting 278
vasopressin *see* antidiuretic hormone
venepuncture (for blood sampling)
   effect on results of procedures before 388–9
   effect on results of technique of 389

venous stasis 389
venous thrombosis, deep 326
very-low-density lipoprotein (VLDL) 200
   in diabetes mellitus 184
   metabolism/transport 178, 179, 203–4
   nicotinic acid lowering levels of 211, 227
villi, intestinal 235
   atrophy 240
VIP *see* vasoactive intestinal polypeptide
viral hepatitis 256
   chronic 258
   hepatitis A (HAV) 256, 257
   hepatitis B (HBV) 256, 257
      case study 257
   hepatitis C (HCV) 256, 257
viral meningitis 330
virilization and masculinization 134, 138, 150, 151
   childhood 138
vitamin(s) 220–30
   absorption 237, 237–8
   classification 222–30
   deficiency 225–6
      causes 222, 225, 227, 237–8, 243, 244
   excess, causes 222
   fat-soluble *see* fat-soluble vitamins
   in parenteral feeding 217
      plasma measurements 219
   sources and function 225
   water-soluble *see* water-soluble vitamins
vitamin A (retinol) 223–4
   deficiency 223–4, 244
   excess 224
   sources and function 223
vitamin B complex 225–8
vitamin B_1 (thiamine) 225–6, 229
   deficiency 225–6, 229
   in nutritional support 219–20
vitamin B_2 226, 229
vitamin B_6 (pyridoxine) 227, 229
   administration lowering homocysteine levels 228, 327
   deficiency 227, 229, 327
vitamin B_{12} (cobalamins) 227–9, 233
   absorption 237
      impaired 227, 243
      administration lowering homocysteine levels 228, 327
      cobalt and 232
      deficiency 227, 228
vitamin C (ascorbate) 229–30
   deficiency 229–30, 315
   iron overload in 315
vitamin D (calciferol) 97–8, 224
   deficiency (impaired intake/absorption; inactivation) 105, 106, 224, 244
      case study 245
   maternal/neonatal 364

vitamin D (calciferol) (contd)
  excess (hypervitaminosis D) 224
    hypercalcaemia 99, 101
  metabolism 37, 97
    impaired 105, 106
  supplementation, neonatal 364
vitamin D-dependent rickets 106, 107
vitamin D-resistant (hypophosphataemic) rickets 110, 111
vitamin E (α-tocopherol) 224
  deficiency 224, 244
vitamin K 224, 251
volume of distribution 346
vomiting/emesis
  hyperosmolar saline to induce, dangers 24
  prolonged/chronic
    hypochloraemia due to 73, 80
    metabolic alkalosis due to 73, 75, 80
von Gierke's disease 305, 362, 376
  case study 376

Waldenström's macroglobulinaemia 292, 294
water 7–35
  balance/homeostasis 7–35
    control 8–9
    disturbances 16–35
  neonatal 356
  sodium homeostasis and, relation between 14–15
  total 7–8
  deficiency 16–21
  distribution in body 10–15
    transmembrane distributions 13–14
  excess 21–5
    features 25
  excretion, control 40–1
  faecal, osmolality calculation 247
  infusion in excess of sodium, babies 357
  intake 7
    high (water load) 41
  nutrient absorption depending on solubility in 235
  output 8
  reabsorption in kidney 38–9
  restriction/deprivation 40–1
    test employing 33–4, 52
  see also fluid
water-soluble vitamins 225–30
  absorption 237–8
weight
  gain in pregnancy 157
  loss in starvation 215
Williams' syndrome 102, 364
Wilson's disease 230–1, 260, 266
wolframin gene mutation 21
women see females

X-linked inheritance 382
xanthine 302
  increased excretion (xanthinuria) 307
xanthine oxidase 302
  deficiency 307
  inhibitors 302, 305
xanthine stones 56
xanthochromia, CSF 330, 332
xanthomata
  familial hypercholesterolaemia 207
  type III hyperlipoproteinaemia 209
xylose
  absorption test 235–6, 246
  urinary 196

Y chromosome, sex-determining region 153

zinc 230
Zollinger–Ellison syndrome 87, 234, 242, 248
zona fasciculata 127
zona glomerulosa 127
zona reticularis 127